Developments in Animal and Veterinary Sciences, 28

Biology of the Pancreas in Growing Animals

OTHER TITLES IN THIS SERIES

Developments in Animal and Veterinary Sciences, 28

Biology of the Pancreas in Growing Animals

Edited by

S.G. Pierzynowski
Department of Animal Physiology
Lund University
Lund, Sweden

and

R. Zabielski
Department of Animal Physiology
Warsaw Agricultural University
Warsaw, Poland

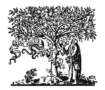

1999

ELSEVIER

Amsterdam–Lausanne–New York–Oxford–Shannon–Singapore–Tokyo

QL866
B55

ELSEVIER SCIENCE B.V.
Sara Burgerhartstraat 25
P.O. Box 211, 1000 AE Amsterdam, The Netherlands

First edition 1999

Library of Congress Cataloging in Publication Data
A catalog record from the Library of Congress has been applied for.

ISBN: 0-444-50217-3

♾ The paper used in this publication meets the requirements of ANSI/NISO Z39.48-1992 (Permanence of Paper).

Printed in the Netherlands

Preface

This book contains a compilation of papers presented during a satellite symposium to the 50th annual meeting of the European Association for Animal Production (EAAP), held in Zurich (Switzerland) in August 1999. The scientific programme was organised in association with the EAAP Commission on Animal Physiology.

The papers included in this book present the latest advances in the field of pancreas development, of its secretions and of the role of these secretions in digestion and nutrient metabolism, with a particular emphasis on domestic species used for animal production.

One of the main goals of the EAAP Commission on Animal Physiology is to offer a link between the scientists devoted to the biology of the main functions operating in animals and humans, and those who are more involved in the development of improved techniques for animal production. In other words, the aim of the Commission is to facilitate the use of recent advances in basic biological mechanisms for improving the efficiency and sustainability of animal production and the welfare of domestic animals.

The content of this book is well in line with the general policy of the Commission. Indeed, it includes a variety of approaches to the biology of the pancreas, from the cellular aspects of pancreatic development and the mechanisms controlling its endocrine and exocrine secretions, including knowledge obtained in rodents, to the effect of pancreatic secretion on growth and performance in domestic species used for meat production.

On behalf of the Commission on Animal Physiology, I wish to express my thanks to Prof. Pierzynowski and his colleagues, who in addition to organising the satellite symposium and editing this book were instrumental in the definition and animation of two of the sessions of the main programme of the Commission, within the 50th annual meeting of the EAAP.

Michel Bonneau
President
Commission on Animal Physiology

Preface

"Biology of the Pancreas in Growing Animals" presents the latest knowledge in the field of experimental pancreatology in growing animals. Most of the information originates from *in vivo* and *in vitro* studies, including recent developments in gastrointestinal endocrinology, molecular biology and immunocytochemistry.

Although the name *pancreas* has been used since the days of Aristotle in the fourth century BC, major progress in pancreatology started with the discovery about 100 years ago by I.P. Pavlov of the crucial role of vagal nerves, by W. von Boldyreff of the cyclic pattern of pancreatic secretion and by Bayliss and Starling of the hormonal control of the pancreas by secretin. The most significant discoveries of recent years described in this book include cloning of cholecystokinin (CCK) receptors and their localization in the vagal afferent fibres, and the description of several proteinase-sensitive CCK-releasing factors, including monitor peptide (MP) released by acinar cells, luminal CCK-releasing factor (LCRF) and diazepam-binding inhibitor (DBI), secreted intraduodenally by enterocytes. These factors appear to stimulate the release of CCK from the I-cells, as described in the article by T. Fushiki et al. entitled "Feedback regulation of pancreatic secretion".The activity of vagal fibres originates from the dorsal vagal complex in the brain stem, which appears to be the central site of the co-ordination of pancreatic secretory function.
Furthermore, intrapancreatic neurons expressing nitric oxide (NO) synthase and neuropeptides such as calcitonin-gene related peptide (CGRP) that play a major role in the control of pancreatic blood flow and integrity are mentioned by Dembinski, to emphasize the complex nature of the control of pancreatic secretion.

As most of the above-mentioned discoveries in pancreatology were made possible by various *in vivo* and *in vitro* preparations in different animals species, it was important to describe these experimental models and the article of Kato *et al.* elegantly provides this important information. Other important articles review the mechanisms of neural and hormonal intracellular signal transduction in acinar and ductular pancreatic cells in the process of water, electrolyte and enzyme secretion.

The dependency of exocrine pancreatic secretory function on the age of the animals and the composition of the diet, with different components inducing increases in specific activity and mRNA levels for various enzymes, is described, and it is suggested that posttranslational modulation of gene expression is responsible for the adaptation of enzyme secretion to the diet.

It has been proposed that the pancreas provides specific signals to affect feeding behaviour, such as neuropeptide Y (NPY), galanin, opioids, CCK, somatostatin, glucagon-like peptide and leptin, as described in an interesting article by C. Erlanson-Albertsson entitled "Appetite regulation and the pancreas".

In general, the 26 review articles of this book, authored by outstanding basic scientists and recognized pancreatologists, should serve as an excellent, comprehensive source of the most current information concerning the growth, development and function of the pancreas in growing animals. This book may also be of help for clinical pancreatologists in understanding the physiological and biochemical basis of disordered pancreatic function in man.

SJ Konturek

From the Editors

The idea of the book "Biology of the Pancreas in Growing Animals" was born a number of years ago, but the possibility to publish it arose just recently. Since our intention was to have the book ready for the corresponding Satellite Symposium to the 50th European Association of Animal Production Symposium, held in Switzerland in August 1999, the time for preparation was short. Therefore, first of all we would like to address our sincere thanks to the Authors, Reviewers, Technical Editors, and the ELSEVIER staff who have devoted their minds and hearts to completing this book on time. We would also like to give our heartfelt thanks to our sponsors for their support, and in particular The Swedish Institute, (Visbyprogrammet); Gramineer Int. AB, Sweden; The State Committee for Scientific Research (KBN), Poland and Solvay Pharmaceuticals, Germany.

Our intention was to describe the function of the pancreas in young animals. We intended to draw the attention of research workers and show them how different pancreatic secretion is in young animals in comparison with adult animals. We would like to highlight the fact that farm animals are generally used in production as young, growing animals. Thus their digestive specificity is different from that of adults and it is risky to make an interpolation of the results from the adult to the young or newborn.

While working on the book we did not pretend to compete with current fundamental handbooks in gastroenterology, in particular pancreatology. Our intention was rather to touch on some "white spots" in knowledge, or to point out certain aspects in a different, often controversial, way. The chapters of this book are either state-of-the-art articles or original scientific articles reflecting the originality of the Authors' thinking; thus the Reader will find, besides novel information, a lot of criticism and new ways of interpretation of classic processes, for instance those concerned with pancreatic feedback and appetite regulation.

We really hope the information contained and the controversies will prevent the book from being "neutral", and will serve to encourage an interdisciplinary discussion on the role of the pancreas in growth/developmental processes in young and newborn mammals, including young and newborn children. A better understanding of the challenging demands on the pancreas during animal development can help to bring a closer adjustment of production systems to the physiological needs of production animals.

SG Pierzynowski and R Zabielski

Institutions providing financial support

- The Swedish Institute, (Visbyprogrammet, 7391/1998(380/67), Sweden
- Gramineer Int. AB, Sweden
- The State Committee for Scientific Research (KBN), Poland
- Solvay Pharmaceuticals, Germany
- Department of Animal Physiology, Lund University, Sweden
- The Kielanowski Institute of Animal Physiology and Nutrition, Polish Academy of Science, Poland

Acknowledgements

The editors wish to thank Bengt Johansson for language revision and Ewa Sałek for professional help with the technical editing of the book.

Contributors

1. **Ahrén B** - Department of Medicine, University Hospital of Malmö, Lund University, SE-214 01 Malmö, Sweden.
2. **Barej W** - Department of Animal Physiology, Veterinary Faculty, Warsaw Agricultural University, Nowoursynowska 166, 02-787 Warsaw, Poland.
3. **Bilski J** - Chair of Physiology, Collegium Medicum, Jagiellonian University, Grzegórzecka 16, 31-531 Kraków, Poland.
4. **Blum J** - Division of Nutrition Pathology, Institute of Animal Breeding, University of Berne, Bremgartenstrasse 109a, 3012 Berne, Switzerland.
5. **Botermans J** - Department of Agricultural Biosystems and Technology, Swedish Univerity of Agricultural Sciences, P.O. Box 59, S-230 53 Alnarp, Sweden.
6. **Buddington R** - Mississipi State University, Department of of Biological Sciences, 39762 Missisipi State, USA.
7. **Dembiński A** - Chair of Physiology, Collegium Medicum, Jagiellonian University, Grzegórzecka 16, 31-531 Kraków, Poland.
8. **Donkin SS** - Nutrition and Metabolism, Department of Animal Sciences, Lilly Hall, Purdue University, West Lafayette, IN 47907, USA.
9. **Erlawanger KH** – Department of Preclinical Veterinary, University of Zimbabwe, P.O. Box MP187, Mount Pleasant, Harare, Zimbabwe.
10. **Erlanson-Albertsson Ch** - Department of Cell and Molecular Biology, Medical Faculty, University of Lund, P. O. Box 94, SE-221 00 Lund, Sweden.
11. **Fushiki T** - Laboratory of Nutrition Chemistry, Division of Applied Life Sciences, Graduate School of Agriculture, Kyoto University, Kyoto 606-8502, Japan.
12. **Gabert V** - Department of Animal Sciences, University of Illinois, Urbana, Illinois, 61801, USA.
13. **Gregory PC** - Department of Pharmacology Research, Solvay Pharmaceuticals GMBH, Hans-Bockler-Allee 20, D-30173 Hannover, Germany.
14. **Guilloteau P** - Laboratoire du Jeune Ruminant, Institut National de la Recherche Agronomique, 65 rue du St Brieuc, 35042 Rennes cedex, France.
15. **Hammon H** - Division of Nutrition Pathology, Institute of Animal Breeding, University of Berne, Bremgartenstrasse 109a, 3012 Berne, Switzerland.
16. **Harada E** - Department of Veterinary Physiology, Faculty of Agriculture,Tottori University, Tottori 680-0945, Japan.
17. **Hedemann MS** - Danish Institute of Agricultural Sciences, Department of of Animal Nutrition and Physiology, Research Centre Foulum, PO Box 50, 8830, Tjele, Denmark.
18. **Jakob S** - Institute of Animal Nutrition (450), Hohenheim University, Emil Wolf Strasse 10, D-70599 Stuttgart, Germany.
19. **Kamphues J** - Department of Animal Nutrition, Hannover School of Veterinary Medicine, Hannover, Germany.

20. **Kato S** - Department of Veterinary Physiology, School of Veterinary Medicine, Rakuno Gakuen University, Ebetsu, Hokkaido 069-8501, Japan.
21. **Karlsson S** - Department of Medicine, University Hospital of Malmö, Lund University, SE-214 01 Malmö, Sweden.
22. **Karlsson BW** - Department of Animal Physiology, Lund University, Helgonavägen 3B, S-223 62 Lund, Sweden.
23. **Konturek SJ** - Chair of Physiology, Collegium Medicum, Jagiellonian University, Grzegórzecka 16, 31-531 Kraków, Poland.
24. **Krogdahl Å** - Department of Biochemistry, Physiology and Nutrition, The Norwegian School of Veterinary Science, P. O. Box 8146, N-0033 Oslo, Norway.
25. **Le Huërou-Luron I** - Laboratoire du Jeune Ruminant, INRA, 65 Rue de Saint-Brieuc, 35042-Rennes Cedex, France.
26. **Lepine AJ** - Research and Development, The Iams Company, Lewisburg, OH, 45338
27. **Leśniewska V** - Department of Animal Physiology, Faculty of Veterinary Medicine, Warsaw Agricultural University, Nowoursynowska 166, 02-787 Warsaw, Poland.
28. **Mosenthin R** - Institute of Animal Nutrition (450), Hohenheim University, D-70593 Stuttgart, Germany.
29. **Naruse S** - Department of of Internal Medicine II, School of Medicine, Nagoya University, 65 Tsurumai-cho, Showa-ku, Nagoya, 466-8550, Japan.
30. **Olsen O** - Surgical Department C, Rigshospitalet, University of Copenhagen, DK -2100 Copenhagen, Denmark.
30. **Onaga T** - Department of Veterinary Physiology, School of Veterinary Medicine, Rakuno Gakuen University, Ebetsu, Hokkaido 069-8501, Japan.
31. **Płoszaj T** - Department of Animal Physiology, Faculty of Veterinary Medicine, Warsaw Agricultural University, Nowoursynowska 166, 02-787 Warsaw, Poland.
32. **Pierzynowski SG** – Department of Animal Physiology, Lund University, Helgonavägen 3B, 223 62 Lund, Sweden and Research and Development, Gramineer Int. AB, Ideon beta, S- 22370 Lund, Sweden.
33. **Podgurniak M** - and Department of Animal Physiology, Faculty of Veterinary Medicine, Warsaw Agricultural University, Nowoursynowska 166, 02-787 Warsaw, Poland.
34. **Pusztai A (**Prof. emeritus**)** - 6 Ashley Park North, Aberdeen, AB10 6SF, Scotland, UK.
35. **Rehfeld JF** - Department of Clinical Biochemistry, Rigshospitalet, University of Copenhagen, DK- 2100 Copenhagen, Denmark.
36. **Sundby A** - Department of Biochemistry, Physiology and Nutrition, The Norwegian School of Veterinary Science, P. O. Box 8146, N-0033 Oslo, Norway.
37. **Sangild PT** - Division of Animal Nutrition, Royal Veterinary and Agricultural University, 3 Grønnegaardsvej, DK-1870 Frederiksberg C, Denmark.
38. **Sauer WC** - Department of Agricultural, Food and Nutritional Science, University of Alberta, Edmonton, Alberta, Canada T6G 2P5.
39. **Studziński T** - Department of Animal Physiology, Faculty of Veterinary Medicine, Agricultural University of Lublin, Akademicka 12, 20-033 Lublin, Poland.
40. **Svendsen J** - Department of Agricultural Biosystems and Technology, P.O. Box 59, S-230 53 Alnarp, Sweden.
41. **Svendsen L** –Department of Agricultural Biosystems and Technology, P.O. Box 59, S-230 53 Alnarp, Sweden.

42. **Tsuzuki S -** Laboratory of Nutrition Chemistry, Division of Applied Life Sciences, Graduate School of Agriculture, Kyoto University, Kyoto 606-8502, Japan.
43. **Tabeling R -** Department of Animal Nutrition, Hannover School of Veterinary Medicine, Hannover, Germany.
44. **Takeuchi T -** Department of Veterinary Physiology, Faculty of Agriculture,Tottori University, Tottori 680-0945, Japan.
45. **Valverde Piedra JL –** Department of Animal Physiology, Faculty of Veterinary Medicine, Agricultural University of Lublin, Akademicka 12, 20-033 Lublin, Poland.
46. **Wang T -** College of Animal Science and Technology, Nanjing Agricultural University, Nanjing, China.
47. **Weström BR -** Department of Animal Physiology, Lund University, Helgonavägen 3B, SE-223 62 Lund, Sweden.
48. **Xu RJ -** Department of Zoology, The University of Hong Kong, Pokfulam Road, Hong Kong.
49. **Zabielski R -** The Kielanowski Institute of Animal Physiology and Nutrition, Instytucka 3, 05-110 Jabłonna n/Warsaw, Poland and Department of Animal Physiology, Faculty of Veterinary Medicine, Warsaw Agricultural University, Nowoursynowska 166, 02-787 Warsaw, Poland.
50. **Zhang SH -** Department of Human Physiology, Flinders University of South Australia, Adelaide, Australia.
51. **Żebrowska T -** The Kielanowski Institute of Animal Physiology and Nutrition, Instytucka 3, 05-110 Jabłonna n/Warsaw, Poland.

Contents

Biology of the Pancreas in Growing Animals
S.G. Pierzynowski and R. Zabielski (Editors)
© 1999 Elsevier Science B.V. All rights reserved.

Biology of the pancreas before birth

P.T. Sangild

Division of Animal Nutrition, Royal Veterinary and Agricultural University,
3 Grønnegaardsvej, DK-1870 Frederiksberg C, Denmark

The pancreas is an endocrine and exocrine organ that is essential for life *ex utero*. Hormones secreted into the circulation play a central role in maintaining homeostasis of energy and protein metabolism. Enzymes secreted into the gastrointestinal lumen are required for the hydrolysis of food macromolecules to allow nutrient absorption. In the fetus, nutrients are transferred across the placenta and not via the fetal gastrointestinal tract, and nutrient flow is relatively constant. Does this mean that the pancreas has little to do *in utero*? This review describes the main features of pancreatic development before birth in some large domestic species (pig, sheep, cow). A series of experimental studies on fetuses suggest that function of the endocrine pancreas is required for fetal nutrition and growth. However, both the endocrine and exocrine entities of the pancreas are relatively immature in structure and function, even in late gestation, and mature function is not present until several weeks after birth. Pancreatic development seems to be particularly rapid around the time of birth, and factors such as the fetal glucocorticoid levels, the events leading to birth, and the first intake of enteral milk stimulate these maturational changes.

1. TRANSITIONS IN THE ROLE OF THE PANCREAS AT BIRTH

The endocrine pancreas plays a key role in energy and protein metabolism via the effects of the insulin-glucagon system on the metabolic pathways of glucose and amino acids. This well-characterized function of the endocrine pancreas is particularly important in maintaining nutrient homeostasis during pre- and post-feeding cycles. The fetus does not experience such dramatic metabolic cycles and the variations that occur in the level of nutrients in the fetal circulation are smaller than those experienced by the mother. It seems that the endocrine pancreas may play a different role in fetal metabolism than it does in the metabolism of neonatal and adult animals.

The exocrine pancreas is essential for the hydrolysis of food constituents via its secretion of digestive enzymes into the intestinal lumen. It appears that the function of the exocrine pancreas can only be essential when the animal obtains a major part of its nutrient supply in the form of an enteral diet containing complex food carbohydrates, proteins and lipids. The fetus is essentially a parenterally nourished organism, with transfer of simple nutrients from the maternal circulation (e.g. monosaccharides, amino acids) across the fetal-placental barrier. Although the fetus swallows large amounts of amniotic fluid, which has a protein content of about 1%, this intake of luminal nutrients *in utero* remains rather small compared with that transferred across the placenta. In addition, there are indications that the breakdown of the relatively simple proteins and carbohydrates present in amniotic fluid occurs more by intracellular digestion than by enzymatic hydrolysis in the intestinal lumen [1]. The oral intake of amniotic fluid by the fetus is therefore unlikely to place any great demand on the ability of the pancreas to produce digestive enzymes before birth. Thus, the role of the exocrine pancreas must be quite different in the fetus compared with the neonate. The basic concepts of total parenteral nutrition before birth and of total enteral nutrition after birth are illustrated in Figure 1.

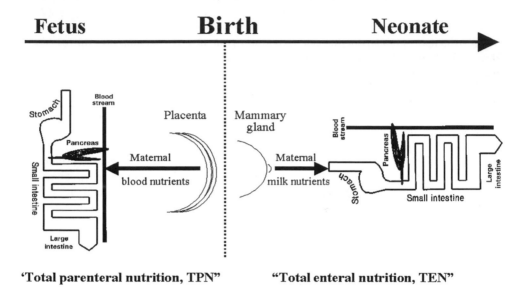

Figure 1. Schematic illustration of the nutritional transition around the time of birth. In the fetus, the supply of both oxygen and nutrients is transferred systemically and in a relatively constant manner to the fetus via the placenta ("total parenteral nutrition"). This results in a relatively quiescent gastrointestinal tract and pancreas. In the neonate, nutrients are transferred luminally and in a "meal-fashion" to the neonatal tissues via the lactating mammary gland and the neonatal gastrointestinal tract. The nutritional transition at birth leads to profound changes in the role of the endocrine and exocrine pancreas in sustaining growth and metabolism.

2. PANCREATIC MATURATION AT BIRTH IN DIFFERENT SPECIES

In growing animals, the development of the pancreas follows an inherited biological program. This genetic program can be modulated by regulatory signals (hormones) that act directly or in concert with nutritional changes. Overall, the characteristics of pancreatic development follow the same general pattern in all mammals. However, the time at which a certain structure or function appears in relation to birth varies widely among species and depends on the mode of organ development in each mammal, i.e. whether it is precocial (early-developing) or altricial (late-developing). In precocial rodents such as the guinea pig and spiny mouse, development of the endocrine and exocrine pancreas occurs relatively early, predominantly in fetal life, although the newborn pancreas may still exhibit some degree of immaturity [2,3]. Conversely, examples of species in which the pancreas develops late, predominantly in postnatal life, are mice, rats and mink [2-5]. Pancreatic development in the large domestic species (sheep, cow, pig, horse) and maybe also in humans [6] falls in between these two developmental extremes. In humans, some structural and functional characteristics of both the endocrine and exocrine pancreas develop before birth, while others develop after.

The developmental trajectory of pancreatic structure and function may or may not reflect essential biological needs during development. Generally, biological functions are "in the right place at the right time", but this is not true for a developing organ. The co-ordination of maturational processes in a whole series of interrelated organ structures may require that some cells and tissue structures develop "ahead of time" while others only appear just before they are required for normal body function. During development, the cells may be partly dysfunctional or refractory to stimulation since the developmental process could be disrupted if the normal pathways for stimulation and inhibition of cell function were fully functional during ontogeny. Thus, the biology of the pancreas before birth comprises a combination of two sets of structural and functional characteristics. One set plays an active role in the developing animal and is necessary for normal life to proceed (e.g. some of the hormonal functions of the endocrine pancreas). The other set of characteristics is present well ahead of the time when it is essential for normal body function (e.g. some of the digestive functions of the exocrine pancreas).

In this chapter, we shall briefly review the fetal development of the pancreas in the large domestic species. Emphasis will be put on the prenatal period, or the last trimester of gestation, because this period leads up to the time of birth when the demands on the pancreas increase enormously due to the transition to life *ex utero* and to enteral feeding. We will try to provide answers to two basic questions: 1) How does the endocrine and exocrine pancreas develop before birth? 2) Which factors modulate the prenatal development of the pancreas?

3. THE PRENATAL GROWTH OF THE PANCREAS

When an organ grows more rapidly than the body as a whole this often indicates a certain role in maintaining body homeostasis at this particular time, but during development, it may also suggest that this organ will be particularly important in the immediate future. Thus, the relative wet weight of the intestinal mucosa (relative to body weight) increases more than 2.5-fold during the final 3 weeks of gestation in preparation for enteral nutrition after birth [Sangild, Elnif and Buddington, unpublished results]. Somewhat unexpectedly, the corresponding relative wet weight of the fetal pancreas does not increase significantly during this period, either in pigs [Sangild, Elnif and Buddington, unpublished results, 7], or in calves [8, 9]. Does this mean that the final prenatal maturation of the pancreas is less important for life and nutrition in the immediate neonatal period than the small intestine? Not necessarily, but in the pancreas, rapid growth is clearly less well co-ordinated with the normal time of birth than in the small intestine.

The massive growth of the pancreas in newborn pigs (+80%) in response to the first 24 h of feeding on colostrum [10] suggests that the pancreas is more dependent on enteral stimulation for its growth and development than on the endocrine signals (or other signals) that lead up to birth. Relative pancreatic weight does not increase to a similar extent in response to the first 1-2 days of colostrum feeding in the calf (+ 20%) [8] or lamb (+20%) [11], so the pig may be somewhat extreme on this point. However, the fact that relative pancreatic weight is reduced in response to experimental ligation of the fetal oesophagus in lambs [12] indicates that luminal stimuli via fetal swallowing of amniotic fluid are important in modulating pancreatic growth in the fetus. This effect is only seen if amniotic fluid is absent from the gastrointestinal lumen for an extended part of gestation (e.g. the last trimester) and not after fetal oesophageal ligation for only 2-4 weeks in late gestation [Trahair and Sangild, unpublished results; Sangild, Elnif and Buddington, unpublished results]. The effect of luminal nutrition (and associated growth factors) on pancreatic growth therefore seems to be much more pronounced in the neonate than in the fetus. Prenatal infusion of colostrum whey, milk whey, amniotic fluid, saline or gastrin releasing peptide for 7 days into the gastrointestinal lumen also had very limited effects on pancreatic weight in a recent study on lamb fetuses [Trahair and Sangild, unpublished results]. This lack of response to luminal stimuli in the fetus is demonstrated in Figure 2.

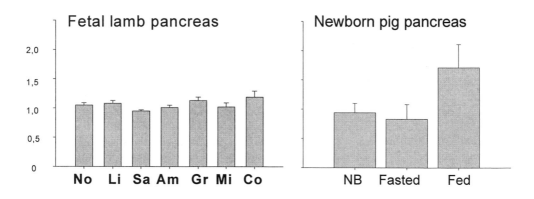

Figure 2. Relative wet weight of the pancreas (g/kg body weight, means ± SE, n = 5-7) in fetal lambs (left diagram) and neonatal pigs (right diagram). A) Lamb fetuses were infused for 7 days with either saline (*Sa*), amniotic fluid (*Am*), gastrin releasing peptide (*Gr*), milk whey (*Mi*) or colostrum whey (*Co*) at 85% gestation (term = 145 days). The 5 groups of infused lambs had very similar pancreatic weights to lambs swallowing normal amounts of amniotic fluid (*No*) and lambs receiving no luminal fluid at all after surgical oesophageal ligation (*Li*) [Trahair and Sangild, unpublished results]. B) The relative weight of the pancreas in pigs fed colostrum for 1-2 days (*Fed*) was increased by 60-80% in comparison with newborn pigs (*NB*) or pigs fasted for 1-2 days (*Fasted*).

The figure shows the relative weight of the pancreas in lamb fetuses infused with various fluids *in utero* [Trahair and Sangild, unpublished results] and in newborn piglets fed on colostrum for 1-2 days [7, 10].

Despite the marked differences between the pancreas and the small intestine in growth rate and response to luminal factors before term, the prenatal growth of both organs can be significantly affected by systemic factors such as the placental supply of nutrients and endocrine stimuli. Regarding the role of fetal nutrition, the results are somewhat conflicting. Fetal growth retardation in pigs [13] had a particularly detrimental effect on the growth of the pancreas (with no effect on the small intestine), resulting in fewer and smaller cells as well as retarded cell maturation. In fetal lambs, malnutrition of the pregnant ewe leads to lambs born with an elevated relative pancreas weight compared with lambs born from normally nourished ewes [14]. When restricted fetal nutrition was induced by carunclectomy, significant growth retardation was observed for the small intestine, with limited effects on the growth of the fetal pancreas [15].

IGF-I is known to play an important role in the growth of many tissues in adults, while in the fetus, IGF-II is more important than IGF-I in modulating growth. IGF-I and IGF-II act through the same receptor on the cell surface. In accordance with this, Peng *et al.* [16] showed that the concentrations of IGF-II mRNA in the fetal pig pancreas were much higher in the prenatal period than postnatally. Luminal infusion of IGF-I (up to 10 days) into the fetal sheep GIT raises plasma IGF-I [17], but has no effect on pancreatic weight and reduces intestinal weight. In another study, systemic infusion of IGF-I (for 10 days) increased pancreatic growth and had no effect on intestinal growth [Trahair and Owens, unpublished

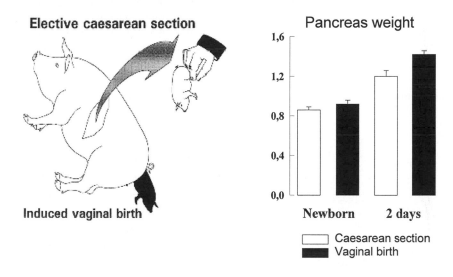

Figure 3. Relative wet weights of the pancreas (g/kg body weight, means ± SE, n = 15-20) in response to different modes of birth, elective caesarean section (open bars) or induced vaginal birth (filled bars) for pigs born at 105-115 days' gestation. There was no effect of gestational age at delivery and delivery mode on pancreas weight in newborn pigs. During the first 2 days after birth, the relative wet weight of the pancreas increased significantly more in pigs born vaginally (+54%) compared with corresponding pigs born by caesarean section (+30%).

results]. However, when IGF-I or IGF-II were administered to newborn pigs, there was a marked effect on the growth of the pancreas, without any effects on intestinal weight [18]. It seems that the responsiveness of the pancreas to growth stimulation by IGF peptides changes around the time of birth. In support of this hypothesis, two other peptides that have been shown to be trophic for the pancreas in adult animals, GRP and CCK [19, 20], were without effect in the fetal lamb [Trahair and Sangild, unpublished results] and the fetal guinea pig [21].

Based on the above results for fetal pancreatic growth in response to altered systemic or luminal nutrients and growth factors it can be hypothesized that birth itself plays an important role in making the pancreas more responsive to external stimuli. We have found support for this hypothesis by investigating postnatal pancreatic growth and enzyme content in pigs born after different modes of delivery. In this model we found that at 2 days after birth, the relative weight of the pancreas was significantly greater in those that had experienced the process of parturition (and the endocrine stimuli associated with it) compared with those born after elective caesarean section (Figure 3).

The observation that pancreatic growth during the first 2 days is not affected by the time of delivery (preterm or term) suggests that it is predominantly birth itself (transition to life *ex utero*) rather than fetal age, that makes the pancreas sensitive to growth stimulation by enteral factors. Our recent finding that the pancreas grows by 83% over the first 6 days after premature birth on enteral feeding but only 35% on total systemic (parenteral) nutrition [Sangild, Burrin, Elnif, Schmidt and Pedersen, unpublished results] supports this contention (Figure 4). In this experiment, the small intestine was even more sensitive to the lack of enteral nutrients than the pancreas, since the intestine gained 54% in relative weight for pigs fed enterally, while there was no intestinal gain for pigs fed entirely on systemic nutrients (Figure 4).

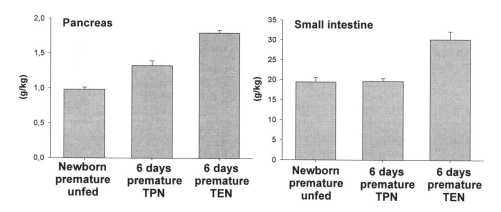

Figure 4. The effect of total enteral nutrition (TEN, sow's colostrum + sow's milk) and total parenteral nutrition (TPN, systemic nutrient infusion) on the relative wet weight of the pancreas and small intestine in prematurely delivered pigs (caesarean section at 106-108 days gestation) (g/kg body weight, means ± SE, n = 6-8). In contrast to the small intestine, the pancreas gains weight on TPN, albeit at a slower rate than on TEN.

4. PRENATAL DEVELOPMENT OF THE ENDOCRINE PANCREAS

The cells which produce the main endocrine hormones of the pancreas, insulin, glucagon, somatostatin and pancreatic polypeptide (PP), can be detected by immunohistochemistry from very early in gestation. In the pig pancreas, lightly stained cells can be found dispersed in the pancreatic parenchyma from 3-4 weeks of gestation [22,23]. More intense immuno-staining of the insulin and glucagon cells is not seen until 13 weeks' gestation (term = 16-17 weeks), and the cells do not start to cluster together in small islets until 10-13 days after birth [22]. At 3-4 weeks of gestation the somatostatin cells are fewer in number than the insulin and glucagon cells but they seem to reach adult number and intensity even before birth [22, 23]. The PP-immunoreactive cells differ from the cells containing the other three main hormones in that they are found at an earlier gestational age and are more numerous in the duodenal part of the pancreas than in the splenic part. Further, the porcine PP cells are also different in that they decrease in number during the first weeks after birth [23]. This pattern of development differs somewhat from that seen in the sheep pancreas where insulin and glucagon cells are the most numerous from early gestation while somatostatin and PP cellsare not present in any significant numbers until late gestation [24]. Interestingly, a

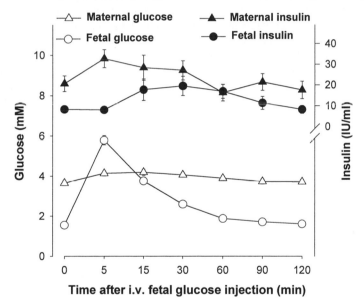

Figure 5. Blood glucose and plasma insulin levels (means ± SE, n = 8) in catheterized cows (*Maternal*) and their fetuses (*Fetal*) after injection of glucose (0.5 g/kg body weight) into the fetal circulation. The rise in fetal glucose levels results in a significant rise in fetal insulin levels. Glucose is transported over the placenta, but not insulin. Thus, some of the infused glucose will pass into the maternal circulation and result in a small increase in maternal insulin levels. The basal levels of both glucose and insulin are significantly lower in the fetal circulation than in the maternal circulation.

common feature of the fetal endocrine pancreas in both humans and pigs is that the 4 main hormones can be co-localised, not only to the same cells, but also to the same secretory granules [25]. With increasing age and maturation of the endocrine cells, structural differentiation of the secretory granules is associated with a gradual disappearance of the poly-hormonal granules. The first genuine mono-hormonal cell to appear in the porcine fetus is the PP cell (at 70 days' gestation) followed by the somatostatin-producing endocrine cell. Mature insulin- and glucagon-producing cells are only present after birth. In the adult, pancreatic endocrine cells produce only one of the four classic hormones.

Despite the obvious histological immaturity of the endocrine cell population, it seems beyond any doubt that the pancreatic hormones play a role in fetal growth and metabolism - at least in ruminants. Thus insulin secretion can be stimulated by both glucose and amino acids in the fetal lamb and calf during the last third of gestation [26,27].

Figure 5 shows how the fetal calf at 90% gestation responds to an intravenous glucose infusion with increased fetal insulin levels [Sangild, Schmidt, Jakobsen and Greve, unpublished results]. As indicated, part of the glucose infused into the fetus is readily transported across the placental circulation and results in a slight, but significant, elevation of not only maternal glucose levels, but also maternal insulin levels. Interestingly, peak insulin levels in the cow in response to this small elevation of maternal blood glucose occurred earlier (5 min after infusion) than the fetal insulin response to the large increase in fetal blood glucose (30 min after infusion). This may indicate that the beta cells in the fetal pancreas are less sensitive to stimulation than those in the maternal pancreas.

Fetal glucose uptake is relatively closely related to maternal glucose levels and this explains a large part of the mechanism whereby the nutritional level of the mother affects fetal metabolism and growth. High maternal glucose levels do not necessarily reflect a high feeding level but can actually be the result of inadequate feed intake and cold exposure. Thus, cold exposure in pregnant sheep leads to an increased birth weight in the lambs, probably because of the elevated glucose levels in the mother and the associated elevation of both glucose and insulin levels in the fetus [28]. However, after sustained high levels of maternal glucose the insulin-secreting capacity of the fetal pancreas decreases markedly [29]. Elevated fetal glucose levels therefore both stimulate (in the short term) and inhibit (in the longer term) insulin release [30]. In this manner the fetus protects itself from the effects of chronic high maternal glucose levels that may be induced by particular feeding habits or a diabetic state of the mother. The pronounced effects of pancreatectomy (surgical removal of the pancreas) also demonstrate that the fetal glucose-insulin system is essential in maintaining metabolic homeostasis and normal growth in fetal lambs. The body weight of such lambs is severely reduced at term and there is a significant inverse relationship between plasma insulin level and the levels of glucose and amino acids in both intact and pancreatectomised fetuses [31,32].

In the pig, it is more doubtful whether fetal insulin plays a major role in nutrient metabolism and growth. There is a relationship between lipogenesis and fetal insulin levels [27], but generally it appears that substrate availability from the sow, and not the fetal insulin level, is the rate limiting factor in fetal pig tissue growth. There is a poor insulin response to intravenous glucose infusion in the anaesthetised fetal pig [33] and a significant response is only seen in conscious fetuses [34]. This may be explained by the effect of an enhanced adrenaline secretion during anaesthesia, which is known to inhibit insulin release in fetal lambs [35].

In contrast to insulin, secretion of glucagon is stimulated by fetal stress in the prenatal pig (anaesthesia, hypoxia, acidaemia). Amino acid infusion stimulates glucagon release in both fetal pigs [36] and lambs [37]. Much less is known about the possible physiological role of fetal glucagon secretion and fetal somatostatin and PP secretion, but of course it cannot be ruled out that these hormones influence metabolism even in fetal life. Studies on fetal calves and pigs have shown that the plasma levels of glucagon, PP and somatostatin increase abruptly shortly before or at term [36,38], probably in preparation for life and nutrition *ex utero*. The increase in circulating somatostatin at this time may arise from both pancreatic sources of the hormone and from a number of extra-pancreatic tissues. The large increases in circulating levels of gut peptides such as gastrin and CCK (secreted from extra-pancreatic tissues) in the immediate prenatal period [38] are also candidates for a role in the prenatal adaptation of the pancreas, probably as a stimulators of pancreatic growth and secretion. However, the fact that the levels of the CCK_B/gastrin receptor in the pancreas increase 600-fold during the first 4 weeks of life in calves [39] suggests that the main effects of these hormones on pancreatic function must be related to postnatal life.

Hormones like epidermal growth factor (EGF) and gastrin are also produced by the fetal pancreas [40,41], but since the production of these hormones is low or disappears after birth, it is questionable whether they play a local physiological role in the development of the pancreas close to term, i.e. trophic effects. The presence of non-pancreatic hormones like EGF and gastrin in the fetal pancreas may just reflect a situation where the pancreas has not quite "found its own feet" and has not come to the point where it concentrates on producing key substances such as insulin, glucagon, PP and somatostatin. The fact remains that the fetal and newborn endocrine pancreas is immature in many respects and that it is unlikely to exhibit the same crucial role in the maintenance of steady-state nutrient metabolism in the prenatal period as it does in adult life.

5. PRENATAL DEVELOPMENT OF THE EXOCRINE PANCREAS

Quantitatively, the production of the hydrolases amylase, carboxyl ester hydrolase, anodal trypsinogen, chymotrypsinogen A and B, proelastase II, carboxypeptidase A and protease E is low in fetal pigs, but increases during the second half of fetal life [42,43]. Chymotrypsin is the most abundant protease during the prenatal period in pigs, and the enzyme is contained in secretory granules that are quite different from those in adult animals [44]. After birth, new proteinases appear after the first week, including chymotrypsin C, cathodal trypsin, and protease E, whereas elastase I is not found until 5 weeks after birth. Concomitantly with the above hydrolases, some as yet uncharacterised "fetal proteinases" with caseinolytic activity are present in fetal life and decrease in production postnatally [42,43].

During fetal development the entire gastrointestinal tract and pancreas produce a number of different protease inhibitors [45]. These inhibitors are generally identical to those found in the circulation, the majority of which may be produced by the liver [46]. The level of protease inhibitors in both the pancreas and other organs is highest in the fetal period [45], and this may reflect a particular need for the pancreas to protect itself from proteolytic degradation during early development when cell and tissue structures are still immature.

Like the pig, the fetal lamb shows significant increases in the pancreatic contents of amylase and chymotrypsin before term, while no trypsin can be detected [47]. In the fetal calf pancreas, the levels of trypsinogen, chymotrypsinogen, amylase and lipase remain very low before birth, and contrary to the other species, these enzymes do not increase in concentration during the final 3 weeks of fetal life [8; Sangild, Schmidt, Jakobsen and Greve, unpublished results].

Immediately after birth, the enzyme contents of the pancreas decrease in most species investigated, and this may reflect a birth-associated emptying of secretory granules [7,8,11,42]. In the following days the enzyme concentrations generally increase and this increase is in part stimulated by enteral feeding. Previously in this chapter, it was indicated that pancreatic growth is more sensitive to enteral stimuli after birth than before birth. This may be true for the maturation of pancreatic enzyme contents also. Thus, pancreatic levels of amylase in lamb fetuses at 85% gestation showed no significant change in response to 7 days of luminal infusion of amniotic fluid, gastrin releasing peptide, milk whey or colostrum whey in a study by Sangild and Trahair [unpublished results]. When a similar study was performed

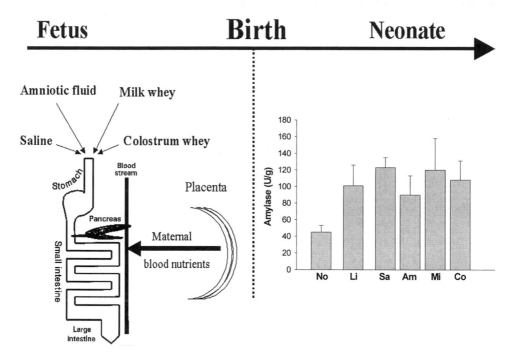

Figure 6. Concentration of amylase in fetal pig pancreas after luminal infusion of saline (*Sa*), amniotic fluid (*Am*), milk whey (*Mi*) or colostrum whey (*Co*) into the fetal gastrointestinal tract for 6 days at 90% gestation. All infused fetuses showed significantly higher enzyme contents than the unoperated normal fetuses (*No*), but were not different from fetuses which received no luminal fluid at all because of surgical eosophageal ligation (*Li*). The results indicate that factors other than enteral factors are important in controlling pancreatic amylase synthesis in the prenatal period of pigs.

in pig fetuses at 90% gestation [Sangild, Weström, Fowden and Silver, unpublished results] it was shown that pancreatic amylase concentrations were significantly higher in fetuses infused with saline, amniotic fluid, milk whey or colostrum whey than in unoperated fetuses (Figure 6). However, amylase concentrations were also elevated in fetuses which were prevented from receiving any luminal fluid at all by surgical oesophageal ligation. It appears that a factor associated with the fetal preparation (fetal cortisol levels) influenced amylase levels to a higher degree than the presence or absence of various enteral fluids.

Studies on pigs and lambs suggest that endogenous cortisol production in response to fetal surgery close to term may influence the maturation of the fetal exocrine pancreas. Thus, pancreatic amylase levels showed a significant correlation with fetal plasma cortisol levels in the study shown in Figure 6. Adrenal cortisol production normally increases dramatically in the weeks before term in all the large domestic species, and this prenatal rise in cortisol plays an important role in the enzymatic maturation of a number of tissues, including lungs, liver, kidneys and small intestine [1,7,48]. The fact that we did not find any effect of fetal surgery and luminal fluid infusion on amylase production in lamb fetuses (see earlier) can be due to the timing of this study. This experiment was carried out earlier in gestation (at 85% gestation) than the studies on pig fetuses (Figure 6), and at this time the adrenal cortex of the fetal lamb is still relatively unresponsive to the stress of surgery.

More specific studies on the fetal pig and lamb have now demonstrated that fetal glucocorticoid levels are important in stimulating the development of the exocrine pancreas. Newborn lambs in which the adrenal gland is removed during the last 4 weeks of gestation (fetal adrenalectomy) show a significant decrease (to less than 50%) in the amylase and chymotrypsin contents of the pancreas compared with normal newborn lambs [47]. Likewise, the contents of amylase and trypsin in the fetal pig pancreas show significant positive correlation with fetal plasma cortisol levels, and the enzyme contents are increased by fetal cortisol infusion and reduced by neonatal treatment with cortisol inhibitors [43]. It should be noted, however, that pancreatic enzymes other than amylase and trypsin remain unaltered after glucocorticoid manipulation. The effects of glucocorticoids are therefore highly specific for individual enzymes, and may depend on the presence of specific steroid response elements in the translational and post-translational processes involved in the synthesis of each hydrolase.

If the prenatal cortisol surge is important in the final maturation of the pancreas before term then we would expect to see that pigs delivered vaginally (high birth cortisol levels) have higher amylase and trypsin contents than pigs delivered by caesarean section (low birth cortisol levels). We have observed that at 2 days after birth, the levels of trypsinogen are significantly higher in pigs delivered vaginally at full term. Pancreatic amylase was also significantly elevated in 2-day-old vaginally-delivered pigs but only if delivery occurred prematurely (at 93% gestation). The hypothesis that each pancreatic enzyme is sensitive to cortisol induction only during a narrow "developmental window" is consistent with a number of publications on the effects of glucocorticoids on pancreatic enzymes in postnatal rats [49, 50]. These "developmental windows" are found mainly in the postnatal period in late-developing mammals, such as the rat, while they are found shortly before or just around the time of birth in domestic animals such as the pig and sheep.

6. CONCLUSION

The perinatal development of the pancreas is guided predominantly by an intrinsic genetic program, but this program is influenced by a number of external factors, including dietary changes and endocrine stimuli. Among the most prominent examples of external influences in farm animals are the effects of glucocorticoids in the fetus, of vaginal birth, and of colostrum feeding in the neonate on the exocrine pancreas in the pig. These factors act in concert with genetic signals to ensure that the relatively "quiescent" fetal pancreas will be well prepared for life and nutrition *ex utero*.

REFERENCES

1. J.F. Trahair and P.T. Sangild, Eq. Vet. J., Suppl., 24 (1997) 40.
2. W.H. Lamers, P.G. Mooren and R. Charles, Biol. Neonate, 47 (1985) 153.
3. W.H. Lamers, P.G. Mooren, H. Griep, E. Endert, H.J. Degenhart and R. Charles, Amer. J. Physiol., 251 (1986) E78.
4. J. Elnif, N. Enggaard Hansen, K. Mortensen and H. Sørensen, In: Biology, Pathology and Genetics of Fur Bearing Animals (eds. B.D. Murphy and B. Hunter). Hudson´s Bay Auction house, Rexdale, Canada, 1988.
5. J. Elnif and P.T. Sangild, Comp. Biochem. Physiol., 115A (1995) 37.
6. R.J. Grand, J.B. Watkins and F.M. Torti, Gastroenterology, 70 (1976) 790.
7. P.T. Sangild, Glucocorticoids and Development of Gastrointestinal Function. DSc thesis. The Royal Veterinary and Agricultural and University, Copenhagen, Denmark.
8. P. Guilloteau, T. Corring, R. Toullec and J. Robelin, Reprod. Nutr. Dev., 24 (1984) 315.
9. M. Schmidt, P.T. Sangild, H. Jacobsen, B. Avery and T. Greve, 14th Eur. Embryo Transf. Ass. (1998) 244.
10. E.M. Widdowson and D.E. Crabb, Biol. Neonate, 28 (1976) 261.
11. P.Guilloteau, T. Corring, P. Garnot, P. Martin, R. Toullec and G. Durand, J. Dairy Sci., 66 (1983) 2373.
12. C.G. Avila and R. Harding, J. Pediat. Gastroenterol. Nutr., 12 (1991) 96.
13. R.J. Xu, D.J. Mellor, M.J. Birtles, G.W. Reynolds and H.V. Simpson, J. Pediat. Gastroenterol. Nutr., 18 (1994) 231.
14. L. Clarke, D.P. Yakubu and M.E. Symonds, Reprod. Fert. Dev., 9 (1997) 509.
15. J.F. Trahair, T.M. DeBarro, J.S. Robinson and J.A. Owens, J. Nutr., 127 (1997) 637.
16. M. Peng, T. Abribat, E. Calvo, D. LeBel, M.F. Palin, G. Bernatchez, J. Morisset and G. Pelletier, J. Anim. Sci., 76 (1998) 1178.
17. J.F. Trahair, S.J. Wing, K.J. Quinn and P.C. Owens, Endocrinology, 152 (1997) 29.
18. R.J. Xu, D.J. Mellor, M.J. Birtles, B.H. Breier and P.D. Gluckman, Biol. Neonate, 66 (1994) 280.
19. A. Dembiński, P.K. Konturek and S.J. Konturek, Regul. Pept., 27 (1990) 343.
20. G. Varga, K. Kisfalvi, I. Pelosini, M. D'Amato and C. Scarpignato, J. Pharmacol., 124 (1998) 435.
21. M.K. Herrington, C.S. Joekel, J.A. Vanderhoof and T.E. Adrian, Pancreas, 11 (1995) 38.
22. J. Alumets, R. Håkanson and F. Sundler, Gastroenterology, 85 (1983) 1359.

23. M. Zabel, J. Surdyk-Zasada, I. Lesisz, E. Jagoda, T. Wysocka, J. Seidel, J. Zabel-Olejnik and J. Grzeszkowiak, Folia Morphol. (Warsaw), 54 (1995), 69.
24. S. Reddy, N.J. Bibby and R.B. Elliott, Q. J. Exp. Physiol., 73 (1988) 225.
25. A. Lukinius, J.L. Ericsson, L. Grimelius and O. Korsgren, Dev. Biol., 153 (1992) 376.
26. J.M. Bassett, Ann. Rech. Vet., 8 (1977) 362.
27. T.R. Kasser, G.J. Hausman, D.R. Campion and R.J. Martin, J. Anim. Sci., 56 (1983) 579.
28. G.E. Thompson, J.M. Bassett, D.E. Samson and J. Slee, Brit. J. Nutr., 48 (1982) 59.
29. J.P. Lips, H.W. Jongsma, J. Crevels and T.K. Eskes, Amer. J. Obstet. Gynecol., 159 (1988) 247.
30. T.D. Carver, S.M. Anderson, P.A. Aldoretta, A.L. Esler and W.W. Hay Jr, Ped. Res., 38 (1995) 754.
31. A.L. Fowden, X.Z. Mao and R.S. Comline, J. Endocrinol., 110 (1986) 225.
32. A.L. Fowden and W.W. Hay Jr, Q. J. Exp. Physiol., 73 (1988) 973.
33. C. Kuhl, P.J. Hornnes, S.L. Jensen and K.B. Lauritsen, Endocrinology, 107 (1980) 1446.
34. A.L. Fowden, R.S. Comline and M. Silver, Q. J. Exp. Physiol., 67 (1982) 225.
35. A.L. Fowden, J. Endocrinol., 87 (1980) 113.
36. M. Silver, A.L. Fowden, R.S. Comline and S.R. Bloom, J. Endocrinol., 108 (1986) 137.
37. J.M. Bassett, D. Madill, A.H. Burks and R.A. Pinches, J. Dev. Physiol., 4 (1982) 379.
38. P. Guilloteau, I. Le Huerou-Luron, G. Le Drean, M. Gestin, V. Philouze-Rome, A. Artiaga, C. Bernard and J.A. Chayvialle, Biol. Neonate, 74 (1998) 430.
39. M. Dufresne, C. Escrieut, P. Clerc, I. Le Huerou-Luron, H. Prats, V. Bertrand, V. Le Meuth, P. Guilloteau, N. Vaysse and D. Fourmy, Eur. J. Pharmacol., 297 (1996) 165.
40. M. Kapuścinski and A. Shulkes, J. Endocrinol., 145 (1995) 137.
41. M. Peng, M.F. Palin, S. Veronneau, D. LeBel and G. Pelletier, Dom. Anim. Endocrinol., 14 (1997) 286.
42. B.R. Weström, B. Ohlsson and B.W. Karlsson, Pancreas, 2 (1987) 589.
43. P.T. Sangild, B.R. Weström, A.L. Fowden and M. Silver, J. Pediat. Gastroenterol. Nutr., 19 (1994) 204.
44. J. Laine, G. Pelletier, G. Grondin, M. Peng and D. LeBel, J. Histochem. Cytochem., 44 (1996) 481.
45. B.G. Ohlsson, B.R. Weström and B.W. Karlsson, Biol. Neonate, 49 (1986) 292.
46. B.R. Weström, B.W. Karlsson and J. Svendsen, Biol. Neonate, 41 (1982) 22.
47. P.T. Sangild, B.R. Weström, M. Silver and A.L. Fowden, Reprod. Fert. Devel., 7 (1995) 655.
48. G.C. Liggins, Amer. J. Obstet. Gynecol., 126 (1976) 931.
49. P.C. Lee and E. Lebenthal, J. Nutr., 113 (1983) 1381.
50. E. Lebenthal and Y. Leung, J. Pediat. Gastroenterol. Nutr., 8 (1989) 1.

Biology of the Pancreas in Growing Animals
S.G. Pierzynowski and R. Zabielski (Editors)
© 1999 Elsevier Science B.V. All rights reserved.

Functional structure and growth of the pancreas in postnatal growing animals

R.J. Xu[a], T. Wang[b] and S.H. Zhang[c]

[a] Department of Zoology, The University of Hong Kong, Hong Kong, China

[b] College of Animal Science and Technology, Nanjing Agricultural University, Nanjing, China

[c] Department of Human Physiology, Flinders University of South Australia, Adelaide, Australia

The pancreas consists of two histologically distinct and functionally independent components, i.e., endocrine islets and exocrine acini. Cells in the endocrine islets produce hormones and regulate body metabolism via the blood circulation, while cells in the exocrine acini secrete digestive enzymes through the duct system into the duodenal lumen. The structure of the pancreas and its postnatal developmental changes in humans and laboratory rodents have been intensively reviewed in recent publications [1-3]. A similar review is lacking for the domestic animal species. This chapter focuses on the morphological structure of the pancreas in pigs and its growth and structural changes during the postnatal period. Wherever possible, information derived directly from studies of pigs is used, otherwise the species origin of the data is defined. Comparisons with other domestic animal species are made when information is available.

1. GENERAL MORPHOLOGY

The anatomical location of the pancreas in domestic animal species has been described in detail by Getty [4] and Bone [5]. In pigs the pancreas consists of a duodenal (right) lobe corresponding to the head of the human pancreas, and a splenic (left) lobe corresponding to the tail of the human pancreas. The duodenal lobe is located in the first duodenal loop and the splenic lobe extends leftward to the spleen. The two lobes are joined by a flat body located in the small curvature of the stomach. The portal vein passes through the pancreatic body (Figure 1). In pigs, the bile duct enters the duodenum alone, 1 to 2 cm from the pylorus. The accessory pancreatic duct (the duct of Santorini) opens from the duodenal lobe into the duodenum 10 to 13 cm posterior to the opening of the bile duct [6] (see chapter by Kato *et al.*). It enters obliquely from anterior to posterior and it does not open through a papilla. In some individuals there may be an additional pancreatic duct (the duct of Wirsung) entering the duodenum separately.

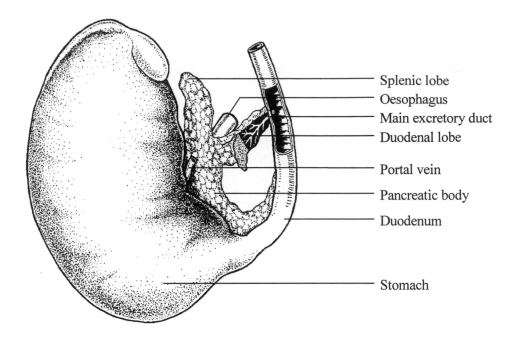

Splenic lobe
Oesophagus
Main excretory duct
Duodenal lobe

Portal vein

Pancreatic body

Duodenum

Stomach

Figure 1. A schematic diagram of the porcine stomach and pancreas. The pancreas consists of duodenal and splenic lobes joined by a flat body. The duodenal lobe is located in the first duodenal loop, where the pancreatic duct opens into the duodenal lumen. The splenic lobe of the pancreas extends leftward to the spleen. The pancreatic body is located in the small curvature of the stomach and the portal vein passes through it.

1.1. The exocrine pancreas

The exocrine component of the pancreas consists of tubuloacinar glands, organised in a fashion resembling a bunch of grapes, with the secretory acini corresponding to the grapes and the system of ducts corresponding to the stems. The gland is covered by fibroelastic connective tissue that passes into the gland and divides it into lobules. The (accessory) pancreatic duct extends almost the entire length of the pancreas and gives off branches to all lobules. These branches undergo further branching into long narrow intercalated ducts, which in turn branch before entering the terminal secretory acini.

The pancreatic acinus is a rounded structure composed of pyramidal epithelial cells (Figure 2). The acinar cells produce digestive enzymes and are notable for their large amounts of rough endoplasmic reticulum (rER) and extensive Golgi apparatus. The base of the acinar cell contains the nucleus and parallel cisternae of the rER, and thus the basal cytoplasm stains well with basic dyes such as haematoxylin. The apical portion stains with eosin due to the presence of numerous zymogen granules (Figure 2). The zymogen granules are most abundant in the resting gland and are reduced in number after feeding [7]. The intercalated duct begins within the acinus. The duct cell within the acinus is called the centroacinar cell and has a centrally placed nucleus and attenuated cytoplasm (Figure 3).

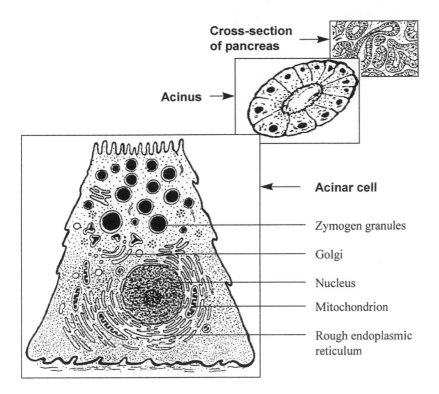

Figure 2. A schematic diagram of a pancreatic acinar cell. The cell is notable for its pyramidal shape, large amount of rough endoplasmic reticulum, extensive Golgi apparatus, and numerous zymogen granules in the apical region.

1.2. The endocrine pancreas

The endocrine pancreas consists of clusters of cells, called islets of Langerhans, scattered throughout the exocrine tissue. The islets have no duct system and their products are secreted directly into the blood stream. Immunohistochemical studies demonstrate that the islet contains four types of endocrine cells, i.e., A, B, D and PP cells, producing glucagon, insulin, somatostatin and pancreatic polypeptide, respectively [8]. The B cells are packed into the central region of the islet and the non-B cells are located in the peripheral region [9]. The islets are generally separated from the exocrine pancreas by a thin layer of connective tissue [10], but this connective tissue capsule is apparently absent in the pig [11].

The islets vary in size and shape, from clusters of a few cells to others that are macroscopically visible, and from spherical to ovoid [10]. The distribution of endocrine islets is not uniform in the pancreas of humans, laboratory rodents and pigs [9,10,12]. In pigs, the volume density of the endocrine islet is 1.0-1.2% in the duodenal lobe and 0.7-0.9% in the splenic lobe [13]. In the duodenal lobe the endocrine cells consist of 89-93% B cells, 7.0-13.7% A cells, 2.7-6.2% D cells and 3.9-5.4% PP cells, while in the splenic lobe the endocrine cells consist of 83-89% B cells, 11-23% A cells, 2.7-6.2% D cells and 1.0-3.1% PP cells [9].

Ultrastructural studies of the pancreatic islets in guinea pigs have shown that B cells contain irregularly shaped granules with a diameter of 350-550 nm, while A cells contain numerous spheroid granules with a diameter of 250-350 nm. D cells have elongated, axon-like processes that end at islet capillaries and contain small spheroid granules with a diameter of 150-250 nm. PP cells contain pale spheroid granules with a diameter of 100-200 nm [14].

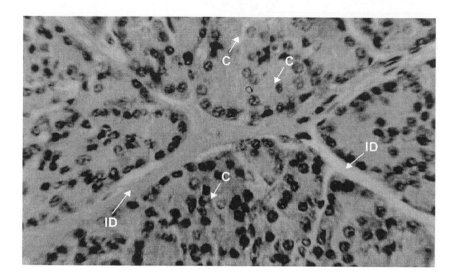

Figure 3. Light micrograph of a pancreatic section from a newborn pig (H/E stain; x 400). The intercalated duct (ID) leads from the pancreatic acinus and the cells forming the duct within the acinus are known as centroacinar cells (C).

2. ONTOGENY AND POSTNATAL DEVELOPMENT

The pancreas develops from the endodermal epithelium of the foregut that later becomes the duodenum. It appears initially as two epithelial-tissue buds at about 4 weeks post conception, the buds consisting of dense strands of epithelial cells [15]. Owing to differential growth of the duodenal wall, the ventral bud receives a more dorsal orientation soon after its formation and fuses with the dorsal bud, forming a single pancreatic primordium. The dorsal bud grows leftward to form the splenic lobe (tail), the ventral bud forms the main part of the duodenal lobe (head), and the part joining the two lobes forms the body.

Several vestiges of the two fetal pancreatic buds are still visible in adulthood. During later fetal development, the distal part of the duct draining the splenic lobe fuses with the one draining the duodenal lobe, forming a combined pancreatic duct. Such fusion may not occur, resulting in a main pancreatic duct and an accessory duct in some individuals. Another vestige of fetal development is the separate vascular supply of the duodenal lobe and the splenic lobe [16]. The non-uniform distribution of certain endocrine cells, such as PP cells and A cells, is probably also a result of the derivation of the pancreas from two separate buds.

2.1. Postnatal pancreatic tissue growth

Immediately after birth, the neonatal pancreas undergoes profound growth in various mammalian species, including pigs [17,18], cattle [19], goats [20] and rabbits [21]. In naturally suckled piglets, the absolute weight of the pancreas increases by 50-80% during the first postnatal day [17,22] and by 100-130% by the third postnatal day [18,23]. The growth rate of the pancreas during this early postnatal period is greater than that of the body as a whole, as indicated by a 30-70% increase in the ratio of pancreatic weight to body weight [18,24,25].

Further analysis of experimental data, including those from longer-term studies [26,27], shows that the postnatal pancreatic growth in pigs is biphasic (Figure 4). The first phase coincides with the immediate postnatal period, and the second with the postweaning period. An accelerated pancreatic tissue growth, as measured by relative pancreatic weight per unit body weight, occurs during both phases. It corresponds to the two important physiological challenges facing the digestive system in pigs during their postnatal life, i.e., switching from placental nutrition to oral nutrition at the time of birth and switching from a liquid milk diet to solid feed at the time of weaning. The accelerated pancreatic growth during these periods of time may well represent an adaptation process to meet these challenges.

During the first phase, pancreatic growth is mainly due to hyperplasia, while in the second phase both hyperplasia and hypertrophy contribute to the enlargement of the pancreas. In naturally suckled piglets, during the first three postnatal days pancreatic DNA content, an indicator of cellular population, increases significantly. Pancreatic cellular DNA synthesis, indicated by the incorporation of bromodeoxyuridine into cellular nuclei, is also active during this period [17,18]. In contrast, there is no significant increase in the ratio of either pancreatic weight to pancreatic DNA content or pancreatic protein content to DNA content, both being indicators of cellular volume. A longer-term study reveals that the pancreatic DNA content in pigs increases with age during the first 8 weeks of postnatal life, while the ratio of fresh pancreas weight to DNA content or pancreatic protein content to DNA content does not increase significantly until the 6th postnatal week [28].

The mechanism regulating postnatal pancreatic growth is not fully understood. During the early postnatal period pancreatic growth is apparently related to milk ingestion, as growth fails to occur if the newborn piglets are prevented from suckling and given water or 5% lactose solution only [17,22]. The trophic effect of milk ingestion may be mediated by the release of regulatory peptides. A postnatal surge in plasma concentrations of gastrin and cholecystokinin (CCK) occurs in suckling piglets [29] and milk-fed human infants [30]. Gastrin and CCK are known to stimulate pancreatic growth.

The trophic effect of oral ingestion of milk on pancreatic growth may also be mediated by milk-borne growth factors. A number of growth-promoting peptides and hormones, such as epidermal growth factor (EGF), insulin-like growth factors I and II (IGF-I and IGF-II) and insulin, have been found in mammary gland secretions in pigs [31,32]. The concentrations of these growth factors are generally high in colostrum, often several times higher than in the maternal blood circulation. There is evidence showing that these growth-promoting peptides are stable in the gastrointestinal lumen in suckling pigs [33,34] and can be absorbed into the blood circulation [35]. Specific receptors for these peptides have been found in rat pancreatic cells [36]. Oral administration of IGF-I or IGF-II stimulates pancreatic tissue growth in newborn pigs [37] and intraperitoneal injection of EGF stimulates pancreatic growth in rats [38]. In addition, the difference between the pig and the rat regarding postnatal pancreatic growth patterns apparently correlates with the growth factor concentration in the maternal milk [18].

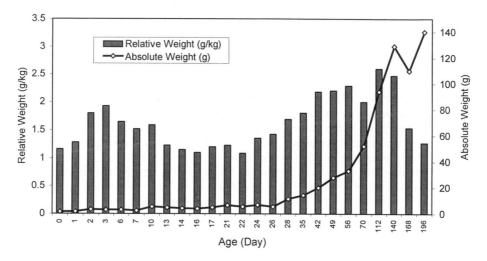

Figure 4. The pancreatic growth pattern in pigs during the first 28 weeks of postnatal life. Data, presented as the absolute organ weight (g) and the relative organ weight per unit body weight (g/kg), are derived from multiple studies [Ref: 17,18, 22, 24-27, 39-42].

2.2. Ontogeny and development of the exocrine pancreas

A systematic study of the ontogeny of the exocrine pancreas in domestic animals is not available. In humans at 7 weeks of gestation the fetal pancreas consists of tubules and masses of undifferentiated epithelial cells [1]. No zymogen granules are detectable at this stage of development. Subsequently the tubules grow out to form exocrine acini at 14 to 16 weeks of gestation. The acinar cells mature rapidly, with an increase in the number of zymogen granules and an accumulation of basophilic material. In pigs the pancreas appears at 4 weeks of gestation, but no ducts or acini are seen in the pancreatic primordia at this early stage of development [8]. By the time of birth, however, the exocrine pancreas is well developed in the pig, with a well-formed duct system and numerous zymogen granules accumulated in the acinar cells [43].

During the immediate postnatal period the exocrine pancreas undergoes a dramatic morphological change and functional maturation (Figure 5). During the first 3 days after birth in naturally suckled piglets the pancreatic acinar size increases by 29% and the number of cells per acinus increases by 27%, although the size of the acinar cells remains unchanged [17]. The acinar cell proliferation rate, as indicated by the cellular incorporation of bromodeoxyuridine, also increases significantly during this period. In association with the enlargement of the acinus and active acinar cell proliferation there is a rapid acinar cell maturation, as shown by an increased basophilic staining and granulation, an indication of increased synthesis and storage of enzymes [43].

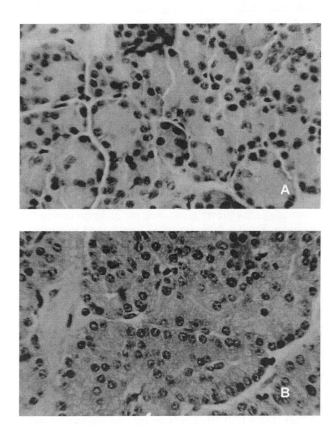

Figure 5. Light micrographs of a pancreatic section from a newborn pig (A) and a 3-day-old pig (B) with H/E stain (x 400). During the first 3 days after birth, there is a significant change in the morphological structure, with an enlargement of pancreatic acini and thickening of the pancreatic duct system. Increased basophilic staining and granulation of the acinar cells is seen, an indication of increased enzyme synthesis and accumulation.

Factors affecting the development of the exocrine pancreas are numerous, with intestinal luminal nutrients, intestinal regulatory peptides and glucocorticoids possibly playing a major role [44,45]. In addition, prenatal growth retardation appears to have an impact on fetal pancreatic development and functional maturation at birth. Compared with controls, prenatal growth retarded piglets have a disproportionately small pancreas at birth, due to a reduced number and size of acinar cells [46]. Both the total pancreatic enzyme content and the enzyme content per acinar cell are markedly reduced. Similar results are also seen in human infants and laboratory rodents with prenatal growth retardation [47,48].

2.3. Ontogeny and postnatal development of the endocrine pancreas

The ontogeny of pancreatic endocrine cells in the pig has been studied with immunohistochemical techniques by Alumets *et al.* [8]. A schematic illustration of the development of the endocrine pancreas in the fetal pig is shown in Figure 6. At 4 weeks of gestation A, B and D cells occur in the dorsal pancreatic primordium of the fetal pig, while PP cells occur in the ventral pancreatic primordium. At this early stage of fetal development the A, B and D cells are intermingled and densely packed, but they are subsequently dispersed in the pancreatic parenchyma during the following 2-4 weeks. At 10 weeks of gestation A, B and D cells appear in the duodenal portion of the pancreas, which is derived from the ventral bud. Small islet-like nests appear, but not until 2 weeks after birth does the islet show the adult pattern, i.e., with B cells occupying the central core and non-B cells distributed in the periphery. At this stage of development many B cells still remain scattered in the exocrine parenchyma, while in adult pigs very few B cells are found outside the islets.

At an early stage of fetal development the ventral pancreatic bud differs from the dorsal bud in that no A, B, or D cells occur [8]. The PP cells appear in the ventral bud at 4 weeks of gestation, and they are disseminated throughout the growing exocrine parenchyma during the subsequent 2-4 weeks of fetal development. From a fetal age of 13 weeks until parturition, the duodenal portion of the pancreas derived from the ventral bud is rich in PP cells, some of which are arranged in clusters, while others are scattered in the exocrine parenchyma. Two weeks after birth the PP cells occur as single cells in the exocrine parenchyma or in small clusters within or outside the islets. The PP cells do not appear in the dorsal pancreatic bud and the corresponding splenic portion of the pancreas until the 13th week of gestation. They remain few in number in this location throughout fetal development. A similar ontogenic pattern for the endocrine pancreas is seen in buffaloes [49].

The pancreatic dorsal bud seems to be wholly made up of densely packed endocrine cells at an early fetal development stage (4 weeks of gestation), and no duct or acinus is visible. During subsequent stages, the endocrine cells are separated from each other, probably as a result of invasive growth of the exocrine parenchyma [8]. In newborn pigs the endocrine cells constitute 1.2% of the total pancreatic cell population in pigs, of which A and B cells each contribute 48.5% and D cells contribute 3.0% [37]. In newborn rats the endocrine cells constitute 2.5% of the total pancreatic volume and the endocrine islets consist of 27, 67 and 6% A, B and D cells, respectively [50]. In 1-week-old hamsters the endocrine islets constitute 2.7% of the pancreatic volume and the endocrine islets consist of 12, 82 and 6% A, B and D cells respectively [10].

Prenatal development of the endocrine pancreas is affected by maternal nutrition during pregnancy. Newborn rat pups from mothers fed with an isocaloric low protein diet (8% vs.

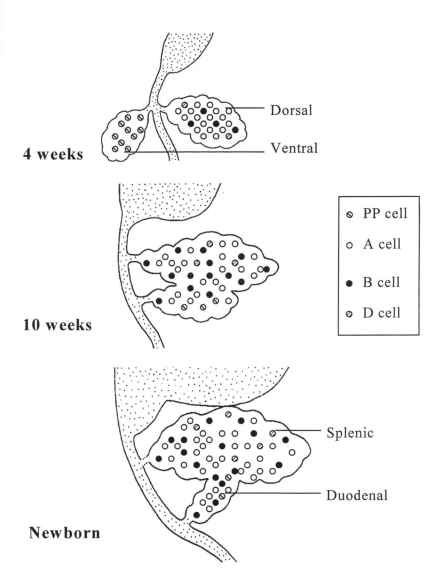

Figure 6. A schematic diagram illustrating pancreatic development in fetal pigs. The pancreas develops from the endodermal epithelium of the foregut initially as two separate epithelial tissue buds. The two buds subsequently fuse and form a single gland. Glucagon (A), insulin (B), and somatostatin (D) cells originate from the dorsal bud and pancreatic peptide (PP) cells originate from the ventral bud. The endocrine cells are dispersed in the pancreatic parenchyma during the fetal stage and the endocrine islets are formed shortly after birth.

20%) or a 50% restriction in feed intake during pregnancy show a reduction in pancreatic endocrine cell proliferation, islet size, islet vascularisation and insulin secretion capacity of islet cells when compared with control pups [51-53]. The damage to the endocrine pancreas during fetal life is apparently permanent because a normal diet from birth to adulthood restores the body weight and the weight of the pancreas but fails to restore a normal insulin response to an oral glucose challenge.

The postnatal development of the endocrine pancreas in pigs has not been systematically examined. In hamsters the total volume of endocrine islets increases progressively during the postnatal period until adulthood; however, the volume density of the endocrine islets and the number of islets per unit area of pancreatic tissue sections are several times greater in 1-week-old hamsters than in 8-week-old and adult animals [10]. The size of the islet also increases with age during the postnatal period but the size of the islet cells remains unchanged, suggesting an increase in cell number per islet during this period [10]. The proportion of endocrine cells represented by each cell type does not change during the postnatal period.

Studies of laboratory rats have shown that the pancreatic weight and the proportion of the pancreas occupied by islet tissue are greater in the male than in the female [54]. However, the maximal glucose-stimulated insulin secretion is similar in both sex groups, suggesting that insulin secretion capacity per unit islet cell mass is greater in females than in males. A fall in insulin secretion capacity per unit islet cell mass occurs with age and this age-related change seems to be independent of sex. No difference in the structure of pancreatic islets is seen in adult pigs of different breeds but the density of islets in the pancreas varies with breed.

3. CONCLUSION

During the postnatal period the animals face two important physiological challenges, i.e., switching from placental nutrition to oral nutrition at the time of birth and switching from a liquid milk diet to solid feed at the time of weaning. To adapt to these challenges the pancreas undergoes rapid tissue growth and morphological and functional changes. Prenatal nutritional status and postnatal milk ingestion appear to have a significant impact on pancreatic development. Prenatal growth retardation is associated with a disproportionate reduction in pancreatic tissue mass and endocrine cell population. The long-term impact of prenatal growth retardation on the pancreas remains to be investigated.

REFERENCES

1. E. Lebenthal (ed), Textbook of Gastroenterology and Nutrition in Infancy, Raven Press, New York, 1981.
2. E. Lebenthal (ed.), Human Gastrointestinal Development, Raven Press, New York, 1989.
3. L. R. Johnson (ed.), Physiology of the Gastrointestinal Tract (3rd ed.), Raven Press, New York, 1994.
4. R. Getty (ed), The Anatomy of the Domestic Animals (5th ed.), Saunders, Philadelphia, 1975.

5. J. F. Bone, Animal Anatomy and Physiology (3rd ed), Prentice Hall, New Jersey, 1988.
6. M.W. Sloss, Am. J. Vet. Res., 15 (1954) 578.
7. F. Sachelarie, T. Trandaburu, A. Petrescu and G.P. Negulescu, Analele Institutului de Biologie si Nutritie Animala Balotesti, 16 (1993) 179.
8. J. Alumets, R. Hakanson and F. Sundler, Gastroenterology, 85 (1983) 1359.
9. H. Miyamoto, M. Mikasa and Y. Miyamoto, Jpn. J. Zootechnical Sci., 60 (1989) 1016.
10. L. Massa, H. Del Zotto, C.L.A. Gomez Dumm and J. J. Gagliardino, Pancreas, 14 (1997) 58.
11. A. Falorni, G. Basta, F. Santeusanio, P. Brunetti and R. Calafiore, Pancreas, 12 (1996) 221.
12. S.A. Bencosme and E. Liepa, Endocrinology, 57 (1955) 588.
13. H. Miyamoto, M. Mikasa and T. Ishibashi, Jpn. J. Zootechnical Sci., 60 (1989) 255.
14. D. Baskin, K.C. Gorray and W.Y. Fujimoto, Anat. Rec., 208 (1984) 567.
15. S. Falkmer, R. Hakanson and F. Sundler, Evolution and Tumor Pathology of the Neuroendocrine System, Elsevier, Amsterdam, 1984.
16. L. Orci, Diabetes, 31 (1982) 538.
17. J.N. Mubiru and R.J. Xu, Biol. Neonate, 71 (1997) 317.
18. J.N. Mubiru and R.J. Xu, Com, Biochem. Physiol. A, 120 (1998) 699.
19. P. Guilloteau, H.L. I. Le, J.A. Chayvialle, A. Mouats, C, Bernard, J.C. Cuber, J. Burton, A. Puigserver and R. Toullec, Reprod. Nutr. Dev., 3 (1992) 285.
20. V. Lopez, E. Martinez-Victoria, M.D. Yago, M.J. Lupian and M. Manas, Arch. Physiol. Biochem., 2 (1997) 210.
21. E.M. Karkashan, W.K. MacNaughton and D.G. Gall, Biol. Neonate, 6 (1992) 395.
22. E.M. Widdowson and D.E. Crabb, Biol. Neonate, 28 (1976) 261.
23. I. Tarvid, P.D. Cranwell, L. Ma and R. Vavala, Proc. VIth Int. Sym. Digest. Physiol. Pig (1994) 199.
24. R.P. Chapple, J.A. Cuaron and R.A. Easter, J. Anim. Sci., 67 (1989) 2956.
25. R.P. Chapple, J.A. Cuaron and R.A. Easter, J. Anim. Sci., 67 (1989) 2985.
26. R.G. Shields, K.E. Ekstrom and D.C. Mahan, J. Anim. Sci., 2 (1980) 257.
27. C.P. McMeekan, J. Agri. Sci., 30 (1940) 276.
28. T. Corring, A. Aumaitre and G. Durand, Nutr. Metab., 22 (1978) 231.
29. R.J. Xu and P.D. Cranwell, Comp. Biochem. Physiol. B, 98 (1991) 615.
30. A. Aynsley-Green, Amer. J. Clin. Nutr., 41 (1985) 399.
31. R.J. Xu, Reprod. Fertil. Dev., 8 (1996) 35.
32. R.J. Xu, Food Rev. Int., 14 (1998) 1.
33. W.H. Shen and R.J. Xu, Life Sci., 59 (1996) 197.
34. W.H. Shen and R. J. Xu, Life Sci., 63 (1998) 809.
35. R.J. Xu and T. Wang, J. Pediat. Gastroenterol. Nutr., 23 (1996) 430.
36. J. Mossner, C.D. Logsdon, I. D. Goldfine and J.A. Williams, Gut, 28 (1987) 51.
37. R.J. Xu, D.J. Mellor, M.J. Birtles, B.H. Breier and P.D. Gluckman, Biol. Neonate, 66 (1994) 280.
38. A. Dembiński, H. Gregory, S. J. Konturek and M. Polański, J. Physiol., 325 (1982) 325.
39. K.R. Cera, D.C. Mahan and G.A. Reinhart, J. Anim. Sci., 68 (1990) 384.
40. R.C. Efird, W.D. Armatrong and D.L. Herman, J. Anim. Sci., 6 (1982) 1380.
41. R.C. Efird, W.D. Armatrong and D.L. Herman, J. Anim. Sci., 6 (1982) 1370.
42. M. Gestin, I.L. Huerou-Luron, J. Peiniau, G.L. Drean, V. Rome, A. Aumaitre and P. Guilloteau, J. Nutr., 127 (1997) 2205.

26

43. J.N. Mubiru, PhD Thesis, The University of Hong Kong, Hong Kong, 1997.
44. S.G. Pierzynowski, B.R. Weström, J. Svendsen, L. Svendsen and B.W. Karlsson, Int. J. Pancreatol., 18 (1995) 81.
45. P.T. Sangild, B.R. Weström, A. L. Fowden and M. Silver, J. Pediat. Gastroenterol. Nutr., 19 (1994) 204.
46. R.J. Xu, D.J. Mellor, M.J. Birles, G.W. Reynolds and H.V. Simpson, J. Pediat. Gastroenterol. Nutr., 18 (1994) 231.
47. E. Lebenthal, M. Nitzan, B.L. Chrzanowski and B. Krantz, Pediat. Res. 14 (1980) 1356.
48. G. Boehm, U. Bierbach, H. Senger, I. Jakobsson, I. Minoli, G. Moro and N. C. R. Raiha, J. Pediat. Gastroenterol. Nutr. 12 (1991) 324.
49. C. Lucini, L. Castaldo, O. Lai and G. de Vico, J. Anat., 192 (1988) 417.
50. R.C. McEvoy and K. L. Madson, Biol. Neonate, 38 (1980) 248.
51. S. Dahri, A. Snoeck, B.B. Reusens, C. Remacle and J.J. Hoet, Diabetes Suppl., 40 (1991) 115.
52. J. J. Hoet, S. Dahri, A. Snoeck, B. B. Reusens and C. Remacle, Bull. Mem. Aced. R. Med. Belg., 147 (1992) 174.
53. A. Garofano, P. Czernichow and B. Breant, Diabetologia, 40 (1997) 1231.
54. E.P. Reaven, D.L. Curry and G.M. Reaven, Diabetes, 36 (1987) 1397.

Biology of the Pancreas in Growing Animals
S.G. Pierzynowski and R. Zabielski (Editors)

Pancreatic hormones (insulin and glucagon) in calves: ontogenetic changes and nutritional effects*

J. W. Blum and H. Hammon

Division of Nutrition Pathology, Institute of Animal Breeding,
University of Berne, Bremgartenstrasse 109a, 3012 Berne, Switzerland

The review summarizes general aspects (synthesis, regulation of secretion, metabolism, effects) of pancreatic hormones (insulin, glucagon, somatostatin, pancreatic polypeptide, pancreastatin, amylin) in calves. Furthermore, it concentrates on ontogenetic changes of insulin and pancreatic glucagon (during the fetal stage and neonatal stage, in veal calves, in suckling calves, and during weaning). In addition, factors regulating the secretion of insulin and glucagon and the influence of nutrition (energy, carbohydrates, proteins and amino acids, fats, minerals and trace elements) on the insulin and glucagon status in calves are reviewed. Moreover, the review deals with changes of the insulin status in metabolic disorders (diabetes mellitus, insulin resistance) of calves, in genetic dwarfs, and in calves with reduced growth performance due to subacute and chronic infections.

ABBREVIATIONS

AA, amino acids; EHGC, euglycaemic-hyperinsulinaemic glucose clamps; FA, fatty acids; GH, growth hormone; GI, gastrointestinal; HGC, hyperglycaemic glucose clamps; IGF-I, insulin-like growth factor-I; MCR, metabolic clearance rate; mRNA, messenger RNA; MR, milk replacer; NEFA, non-esterified fatty acids; PP, pancreatic polypeptide; SS, somatostatin; TG, triglycerides; T_3, 3.5.3'-triiodothyronine; T_4, thyroxine.

1. INTRODUCTION

Besides its exocrine functions, the pancreas has essential endocrine functions. The endocrine part is organized as discrete islets (of Langerhans) which contain at least four types of cells [1-6]. A morphological study by Bonner-Weir and Like [1] of the bovine pancreas from fetus to adult documented the presence of two distinct types of pancreatic islets: large islets (100 to 1600 μm in diameter), in interlobular connective tissue, and small islets (25 to 200 μm in diameter), enmeshed in the exocrine tissue. Large islets (consisting primarily of

*The studies were supported by the Swiss National Science Foundation (Grants No. 32.30188.90, 32.36140.92, 32.051012.97), Berne, Switzerland; the Schaumann Foundation, Hamburg, Germany; F. Hoffmann-La Roche, Basle, Switzerland; Novartis (formerly Ciba Geigy AG), Basle, Switzerland; Gräub AG, Berne, Switzerland; and the Swiss Federal Veterinary Administration, Liebefeld-Berne, Switzerland.

well-granulated B cells) decrease in relative volume with increasing age and in mature cattleare seldom seen. The overall relative volume of endocrine tissue is age-dependent and ranges from 30% in the 6th month of the fetus to 10% in the neonate and 5% in mature cattle. Small islets contain B cells whose cytoplasmic granularity increases with increasing fetal age, significantly decreases just prior to birth, and subsequently increases again a few weeks after birth. The B cells of the small islets are uniquely characterized by junctional complexes in close association with large numbers of desmosomes. The junctional complexes have been shown to consist of macula occludens (focal tight junctions) enclosing nexuses (gap junctions). The two types of islets differ in distribution, times of growth and times of B cell granularity and may be indicative of functional differences.

The four main cell types of the pancreas produce different peptide hormones [2]. The most numerous of the islet cells are the B cells, which synthesize insulin. A cells synthesize glucagon, D-cells synthesize somatostatin (SS) and F cells synthesize pancreatic polypeptide (PP). Immunohistochemical analyses of the pancreas obtained from calves at different ages have shown specific localization of insulin, glucagon, SS, and PP within the islets of Langerhans [7-9] (Hammon and Blum, unpublished observations) and the islets of Langerhans are especially concentrated to the left lobe [5,7].

Besides insulin, glucagon, SS, and PP there are other hormones and hormone-like substances (especially gastrointestinal hormones and neuropeptides) localized in A, B, D or F cells, albeit normally only in small amounts [4]. Insulin-like growth factor-I (IGF-I) appears to be present in the pancreas of calves, according to immunohistochemistry studies, and appears to have a localization similar to that of insulin (Hammon, Breier and Blum, unpublished observations). Whether IGF-I is produced in the calf pancreas is not yet clear, because we could not detect IGF-I mRNA in 8-day-old calves [10], but IGF-I mRNA has been demonstrated in the porcine pancreas during fetal and neonatal stages [11]. Noradrenaline-, acetylcholine-, and β-endorphin-releasing neurons are also present [4,12]. It is notable that the bovine pancreas is densely innervated with parasympathetic and sympathetic nerves, which are involved in the physiological control of insulin, glucagon, SS, and PP secretion in calves [13-19]. There is also evidence that single cells are basically able to produce more than one hormone [4]. Thus in the bovine pancreas serotonin co-localizes with glucagon and PP in A and F cells, besides being present alone in EC cells [20].

Pancreatic peptide hormones, which are influenced by gastrointestinal (GI) hormones and related peptides [2,21-22] are important metabolic regulators. The importance of insulin and glucagon for the homeostatic control of energy, carbohydrate, protein, and lipid metabolism and of circulating glucose, fatty acid (FA), and amino acid (AA) concentrations in mature ruminants has been reviewed [3,23]. Their main primary assignment is to provide the organism with substrates (especially glucose, FA, and AA) for energy metabolism and for synthetic purposes, including growth.

Whereas there is considerable information on the physiology of insulin, knowledge about glucagon, SS, and PP, and especially other pancreatic hormones in young calves, is scarce or nonexistent. This review summarizes elementary knowledge of the physiological aspects of pancreatic hormones. It concentrates especially on the physiology of insulin and to some extent of glucagon in young calves.

2. PANCREATIC HORMONES: GENERAL ASPECTS

2.1. Insulin

Insulin is a peptide hormone consisting of two chains (A,B), with 21 and 30 AA, respectively, which are connected by two disulfide bridges [2]. Although the monomer form is considered to be the biologically active form, insulin also exists in di-, tetra-, and hexamer forms, which are connected by zinc. There are differences in the AA composition among species, but the differences are small, e.g., bovine, sheep, equine, and canine insulin differ only in positions 8, 9, and 10 of the A chain [6]. Therefore the biological differences are not very species-specific.

After synthesis of preproinsulin, proinsulin is formed and transferred to the Golgi apparatus, where it is packaged into granules which contain insulin and the connecting (C-) peptide (33 AA). Whereas insulin and C-peptide are secreted postprandially, fasting causes a rapid fall in insulin and C-peptide secretion [2]. The most important factor stimulating the secretion of insulin is a rise of plasma glucose concentration, as early shown in milk-fed calves, too [24,25] and starch-rich rations enhance insulin secretion more than lipid-rich rations [26]. In calves, the insulin response during intravenous glucose tolerance tests has been shown to depend on age, but is modified by various other factors [27]. Factors which inhibit glucose transport into and utilisation by B cells also inhibit insulin release. Most of the other factors stimulate insulin secretion only in the presence of sufficient glucose. Upon stimulation, especially by glucose, insulin is biphasically secreted, i.e., in the first min stored insulin is released and in the second phase the insulin newly synthesized during prolonged stimulation is released [2].

Whole meals provoke a greater insulin response than the oral administration of glucose, indicating that other nutritional factors (such as AA and FA) stimulate insulin secretion [2], as also shown in veal calves [28-30]. Insulin secretion is enhanced by oral arginine administration in veal calves (Hüsler and Blum, unpublished observations), but glycine, serine, and leucine may have an even greater effect [31]. However, the effect of AA on insulin secretion is smaller than of glucose [32,33]. Volatile FA (such as propionate) stimulate insulin secretion in preruminants and mature ruminants, including preruminant calves [34,35]. Various secretagogues other than glucose, such as β-adrenergic agonists, typically only stimulate the acute release [2]. In addition, pancreatic glucagon directly stimulates insulin release [2].

Because the oral administration of glucose provokes a larger insulin response than its parenteral administration, GI factors (especially hormones, including gastrin, cholecystokinin, secretin, and glucose-dependent insulinotropic polypeptide) are important [2,36]. However, glucose-dependent insulinotropic polypeptide, which is the most potent factor in humans [36], does not seem to be a secretagogue in ruminants [21]. On the other hand, SS markedly inhibits insulin secretion, as also shown in calves [19].

It is well known that insulin secretion is enhanced in situations of insulin resistance, such as if excessive growth hormone (GH) and cortisol are produced, to compensate for reduced effects on target tissues [2]. This is also the case if β-adrenergic agonists are administered, as also shown in calves [37].

The pancreas is innervated by the autonomous nervous system and increased cholinergic activity after food intake, associated with enhanced release of acetylcholine, increases insulin secretion, i.e., the parasympathetic innervation to the pancreas plays an important part in the control of insulin release in response to hyperglycaemia [5]. Insulin concentrations steadily increase in calves after the administration of non-metabolizable 2-deoxy-D-glucose (which mimics hypoglycaemia by blocking the supply of glucose to the brain), an effect which is parasympathetically mediated [38]. Propionate-stimulated insulin secretion in calves is in part, too, mediated by parasympathetic nervous system activation through muscarinic receptors, because it can be blocked by atropine, but not by phentolamine, propranolol or hexamethonium [39].

There is also sympathetic innervation of the calf pancreas [40]. Noradrenaline, adrenaline and synthetic α-adrenergic agonists inhibit insulin release through interaction with α-adrenergic receptors on B cell membranes, whereas synthetic β-adrenergic agonists stimulate insulin secretion through interaction with β-adrenergic receptors on B cell membranes [2], as also shown in calves [37,41-43]. In cattle there is also evidence for inhibition of insulin secretion by dopaminergic agonists, such as aminotetraline analogues [44]. Adrenaline, after release from the adrenal medulla, reaches B cells through the blood circulation, noradrenaline in addition after release from sympathetic nerves in the pancreas. Dopamine may be released from mast cells, which in cattle contain abundant amounts of this amine in most tissues. In addition, in calves the effect of insulin can directly (i.e., independently of changes in the activity of the sympathetic and parasympathetic nervous systems) be enhanced by neurotensin [45]. Importantly, normal plasma ionised calcium is needed for stimulus-secretion coupling, as shown in cows [46], but hypocalcaemia is not an important problem in calves.

The insulin that has not interacted with receptors and been taken up by target cells is degraded to AA primarily in the liver and kidneys. Insulin has a half-life of about 10 min in the circulation [6]. In preterm calves, compared with calves born at term, the metabolic clearance rate (MCR) of insulin is reduced [47].

Whereas proinsulin has a direct biological effect which is about one-tenth that of insulin, the C-peptide is not biologically active [48]. The main metabolic functions of insulin are anabolic, because it stimulates the (oxidative and non-oxidative) conversion of glucose, FA, and AA to their storage form, i.e., glycogen, triglycerides (TG), and protein, respectively. Through modification of the activity of various enzymes, insulin facilitates glucose oxidation and glycogen synthesis (in liver and muscle), inhibits glycolysis and gluconeogenesis, stimulates FA uptake (by stimulation of the endothelial lipoprotein lipase) and lipogenesis and inhibits lipolysis. It stimulates AA uptake (in most tissues, except the liver) and protein synthesis, and inhibits protein degradation (and thus urea formation).

Although gluconeogenesis is inhibited, it is not fully suppressed by insulin in ruminants [3], not even in pre-ruminant (veal) calves [28,49-51]. Furthermore, ketogenesis is reduced and therefore acetoacetate and β-hydroxybutyrate concentrations decrease in response to insulin administration. Net effects are a decrease in blood glucose, FA, TG, β-hydroxybutyrate, AA, and urea concentrations, as also shown in calves [52]. Concentrations of galactose and fructose, too, decrease in response to insulin administration [4].

The effects of insulin are associated with reduced plasma concentrations of potassium and inorganic phosphate, because these minerals are taken up especially by the skeletal muscles [4]. Except in brain, liver, (bovine) mammary gland, red and white cells, the uptake of glucose by cells of other tissues is not possible without insulin, which facilitates the transfer of glucose from the plasma into cells by stimulation of the insulin-dependent glucose transporter-4 [53]. Effects on the liver are especially important because the pancreatic venous effluent first passes directly to the liver. It is well-known that insulin counteracts the effects of glucagon, enhances postprandial depression of GH secretion, as shown in calves [54] and stimulates hepatic IGF-I production. The stimulatory effects of insulin on growth may be direct, on selected tissues, or indirect, such as by regulation of the production of IGF-I [55].

2.2. Glucagon

Pancreatic glucagon consists of a single chain of 29 AA. There is considerable homology in AA composition among species. Besides the pancreas, there are other organs that produce glucagon: thus, gut glucagon with the same AA sequence as pancreatic glucagon is produced in the stomach and the small intestine produces an immunologically similar glucagon, called glicentin or enteroglucagon [6], as also shown in calves [8]. Like other hormones, glucagon is first produced as a precursor peptide and then packaged in the Golgi apparatus in the form of secretory granules.

The main factor stimulating pancreatic glucagon synthesis and secretion is a fall in the plasma glucose concentration, such as occurs after prolonged periods without food [6]. Pancreatic glucagon has therefore also been termed the "hunger hormone". Pancreatic glucagon secretion, at least in humans, increases some time after food intake and when the blood glucose concentration starts to decrease. A sluggish rise in plasma glucagon concentrations was observed in calves, too, if food was withheld for 48 h, confirming that calves react to energy deficiency in the same way as other species [38]. In cortisol-treated, thyroidectomized (diabetic) calves the administration of 2-deoxy-D-glucose (which reduces cellular glucose uptake) caused a marked rise in plasma pancreatic glucagon concentrations [38].

The A cells require insulin for glucose entry. This explains why in states of insulin deficiency, because of decreased entry of glucose into the A cells, glucagon secretion is paradoxically elevated. Nevertheless, hyperglycaemia typically inhibits pancreatic glucagon release, as also shown in calves [45], although effects are small (Kaufhold and Blum, unpublished observations). Pancreatic glucagon is furthermore inhibited by increased plasma non-esterified fatty acid (NEFA) and TG concentrations, i.e., if glucagon stimulates lipolysis, it is secondarily inhibited by feed-back from the NEFA [4].

On the other hand, pancreatic glucagon (similar as insulin) secretion is increased after protein ingestion and thus by increased plasma AA levels [6]. Glucagon secretion in calves is stimulated by propionate and responses to propionate were greater in calves fed milk and grain than in those fed only milk [35]. Pancreatic glucagon secretion is in addition stimulated by several GI hormones besides secretin, and is inhibited by SS. Furthermore, both the sympathetic and parasympathetic nervous systems stimulate pancreatic glucagon secretion, as shown in calves [14,41]. The positive effects of adrenaline and noradrenaline on secretion are mediated by α-adrenergic receptors on A cell membranes. The propionate-induced rise in pancreatic glucagon secretion in preruminant calves is mediated by α-adrenergic receptors, because it can be blocked by phentolamine, but not by propranolol, atropine or hexamethonium [39].

In calves, glucagon secretion is also slightly increased by neurotensin and this effect is probably direct, i.e., independent of changes in the activity of the sympathetic and parasympathetic nervous systems [45]. In contrast to pancreatic glucagon, studies in man and dogs indicate that the secretion of enteroglucagon is stimulated postprandially, even after glucose loads, and insulin-induced hypoglycaemia does not enhance its secretion [6].

If not taken up by target cells, glucagon is degraded in the liver and kidneys and disappears from the circulation with a half-life of about 5 min [6].

The most important effects of glucagon are to ensure sufficient glucose availability for the organism [6]. These effects are exerted primarily in the liver and involve a decrease in hepatic glycogen synthesis and an increase in glycogenolysis and hepatic gluconeogenesis. Whereas the stimulation by pancreatic glucagon of propionate used for gluconeogenesis was similar in preruminant and ruminant calves, the stimulation by glucagon of lactate metabolisation for gluconeogenesis was decreased as the ruminant stage approached [49,50].

Glucagon stimulates proteolysis in skeletal muscle, whereby AA, after deamination (resulting in enhanced urea synthesis), are provided as substrates for hepatic gluconeogenesis, as also shown in ruminants [3]. As a consequence, pancreatic glucagon (whose secretion is enhanced after protein ingestion and increased plasma AA levels) through stimulation of gluconeogenesis with AA as the main substrate, neutralises the postprandial hypoglycaemia-inducing effect of insulin. Furthermore, pancreatic glucagon stimulates glycogenolysis in skeletal muscle, which is followed by increased lactate formation. Furthermore, pancreatic glucagon in high amounts inhibits glucose or acetate use for lipogenesis and stimulates lipolysis, but effects in ruminants are equivocal [3]. In noncompensated insulin deficiency, this may be followed by marked ketogenesis and ketoacidosis [2]. Thus, effects of pancreatic glucagon on glucose, lipid and protein metabolism are opposite to those of insulin.

2.3. Somatostatin

Somatostatin is a peptide composed of 14 AA and, besides occurring in the pancreas, is present in the GI tract and the brain [6]. The presence of immunoreactive SS in the pancreas and GI tract of calves has been documented [5,7,56-58]. Ontogenetic changes in SS concentrations in plasma of calves have been described by Guilloteau *et al.* [2122,57]. The secretion, at least in humans, is enhanced after ingestion of nutrients (especially glucose and AA), by GI hormones, by insulin and glucagon, and by adrenaline, noradrenaline and acetylcholine [6]. Based on studies in humans and dogs, the secretion is relatively sluggish. After release, SS is very rapidly (with a half-life of <5 min) cleared from the circulation.

The main effects of SS are the rapid inhibition of the secretion of insulin, glucagon, PP, and of its own secretion, besides inhibition of the secretion of other hormones, such as GH, adrenocorticotropic hormone, and thyroid stimulating hormone [4, 6]. Inhibition by SS of the secretion of insulin, glucagon, and PP was also demonstrated in calves [19]. Effects of SS on glucagon secretion are greater than on insulin secretion. Furthermore, SS inhibits digestive and absorptive processes in the GI tract by inhibition of GI motility and of the secretion of digestive enzymes [6]. Thus, in calves SS inhibits the effects of secretin on the flow of exocrine pancreatic juice and amylase activity and also inhibits cholecystokinin-pancreocymin effects, pancreatic excretion of water and proteins and amylase activity in milk-fed calves [59]. As a consequence of a high SS status, the intermediary provision of nutrients and glucose homeostasis are expected to be impaired. Recent advances in knowledge on SS in calves during fetal, perinatal, preruminant stages and at weaning have recently been reviewed [21,22].

2.4. Pancreatic polypeptide

Pancreatic polypeptide consists of 36 AA and is only produced in the pancreas [6]. Ontogenetic changes in PP concentrations in the plasma and pancreas of calves and regulation of the secretion have been described by Bloom *et al.* [38] and Guilloteau *et al.* [21,22,57]. The secretion is stimulated by hypoglycaemia and inhibited by hyperglycaemia and thus often behaves similarly to pancreatic glucagon. On the other hand, its secretion is stimulated after meals by the combined action of GI hormones (cholecystokinin, secretin, and gastrin) as well as by acetylcholine, released by parasympathetic neurons. Proteins have a marked effect, whereas fats and carbohydrates have only small effects on PP secretion. The secretion is inhibited by SS.

Effects of PP are mainly exerted on the GI tract, i.e., PP inhibits the secretion of pancreatic enzymes and the contraction of the gall bladder and modifies GI motility and gastric emptying. Recent advances in knowledge about PP in calves during the fetal, perinatal, preruminant stages and at weaning have been reviewed [21,22].

2.5. Pancreastatin

This peptide of about 50 AA obviously derives from chromogranin A, a secretory protein present in various endocrine and neuroendocrine cells [4,6]. It exerts paracrine effects on the endo- and exocrine pancreas and directly inhibits glucose-stimulated insulin secretion and pancreocymin-stimulated secretion of pancreatic enzymes, but may stimulate pancreatic glucagon secretion. Studies in calves have to our knowledge not yet been performed.

2.6. Amylin

This peptide is produced in B cells and in cells of the GI tract and consists of 37 AA [4,6]. There are marked species differences with respect to AA composition. In B cells the amyloid peptide is stored together with insulin in secretory granules and co-secreted with insulin, but the amounts are much smaller (about 1%) than of insulin. The secretion is inhibited by SS. This hormone modifies insulin secretion (inhibition as well as stimulation) and in rats modifies appetite. Studies in calves have to our knowledge not yet been performed.

3. INSULIN AND GLUCAGON IN CALVES

3.1. Insulin and glucagon during the fetal stage

Insulin is integral to satisfactory fetal growth, hypoinsulinaemia and hyperinsulinaemia causing reduced and enhanced fetal growth, respectively [60]. Insulin production in the bovine fetal pancreas changes during development. Thus, insulin mRNA levels/g tissue decreased from the first to third trimester in association with a concomitant increase in exocrine pancreatic tissue growth, but in cell-free synthesis experiments the concentration of the translation products of immunoreactive insulin was not different [61]. There was a 2- to 3-fold rise of preproinsulin mRNA between the first and second trimester, falling again in the third trimester to levels similar to those in mature cattle [62]. The amount of immunoreactive insulin in pancreatic tissue in the first trimester bovine fetus was similar to that in mature cattle (8 and 6 U/g wet tissue). Concentrations increased up to the third trimester and reached levels (39 U/g wet tissue) which were 7-fold higher than in mature cattle. In relation to protein, concentrations decreased between the mid-second and the third trimester, which was interpreted to be the consequence of a relative decrease in the endocrine portion of the pancreas compared to the rapidly growing exocrine pancreas.

Immunoreactive insulin could be detected in all trimesters in fetal blood serum, but in contrast to the pancreas, concentrations remained stable at about 20 mU/l. On the basis of these studies it may be concluded that the endocrine pancreas synthesizes insulin during all stages of fetal development, pancreatic (U/g pancreas), but not serum, concentrations of immunoreactive insulin increase progressively during fetal development, and the ontogeny of preproinsulin mRNA is paralleled by that of pancreatic immunoreactive insulin (U/g pancreas). Insulin stimulates transplacental transport of glucose and AA by enhancing their uptake by fetal tissues [60]. Effects of insulin may in part be indirect through stimulation of growth factors, such as IGF-I.

Pancreatic glucagon and an immature form are detected early during development of the bovine fetus [7, 63-65]. The presence of both insulin and glucagon (together with PP and SS) in the pancreas and circulation early in bovine fetal life suggests that these hormones are important in intra- and extra-pancreatic metabolism.

3.2. Insulin and glucagon during the neonatal period

After birth, a shift from glucose to a carbohydrate-fat mixture as the major energy source necessitates major metabolic rearrangements, affecting glucose, lipid and protein metabolism. Thus, newborn calves are characterised by hypoglycaemia, and high plasma NEFA acid, but low TG, phospholipid, and cholesterol levels [66,67]. Furthermore, gluconeogenesis in neonates is essential for glucose homeostasis because lactose intake is insufficient [68] and glucose is also important in neonatal calves for thermoregulation [69]. However, glucose is spared because the contribution of glucose oxidation to the total energy expenditure in neonates (at least in humans) is small [70]. Insulin and glucagon are known to play a major role in the metabolic adaptations of the neonate in general, including calves.

Various studies on metabolic and endocrine traits that are dependent on feeding have recently been performed in neonatal calves, including studies on insulin and glucagon [71-84], as recently reviewed [85]. Colostrum contains high amounts of various growth factors and hormones, including insulin and glucagon [71,73,78,86-89]. We have found insulin receptor mRNA in the small intestine of 8-day-old calves (Cordano, Hammon and Blum, unpublished observations) and the insulin receptor number (based on ligand binding) in the small intestine and colon of 8-day-old calves was higher in those fed colostrum than those given milk replacer (MR), besides being associated with a greater absorptive capacity for xylose [79,80]. However, colostral insulin seems not to be intestinally absorbed and bovine insulin is not absorbed, even if administered in pharmacological amounts with milk or buffer [73], in contrast to findings reported earlier [90]. Effects of colostral insulin, for example on gut closure [91], may thus be mediated by intestinal receptors. Nevertheless, plasma insulin concentrations increase after ingestion of the first meal [92] and on d 1 of life, hyperinsulinaemia was more marked in MR-fed than colostrum-fed calves because of greater hyperglycaemia, due to a greater lactose intake, if MR was given [73,78].

Neurally mediated insulin release (secondarily caused by the administration of 2-deoxy-D-glucose) was greatly reduced or absent in 1-d-old calves and much lower than in older calves, whereas the capacity to release pancreatic glucagon (and PP) was fully developed at this age. Glucagon responses were even greater than in older calves, and the release of pancreatic glucagon (and of PP) was suppressed by intravenous glucose infusions [14].

The enhanced capacity to release glucagon in response to glycaemic stimuli, in association with a sluggish insulin release, both of which are glucose-dependent, may have considerable biological significance for glucose homeostasis and especially for protection against hypoglycaemia, which is seen also in neonatal calves [67]. During the first week of life plasma insulin concentrations postprandially increased more when colostrum was fed than only MR or water, demonstrating prolonged effects of colostrum feeding [78,93]. On the other hand, insulin concentrations decreased immediately if food was withheld from 1 or 8 day old calves for 24 h [93-95]. The data demonstrate that insulin in neonatal calves responds to nutritional changes in basically the same way as in mature monogastrics of other species, but the glucose-insulin relationship is less developed than in older calves. On the other hand, newborn calves (day 1 of life) in comparison with older (7-day-old) calves are relatively resistant to insulin, which may be explained by high levels of plasma adrenaline, released at birth [96], but may also be the consequence of elevated cortisol concentrations. However, the decrease in plasma glucose in response to intravenous insulin injections in preterm calves was greater than in calves born at term, which was explained by higher plasma insulin levels (as a consequence of reduced MCR) and a reduced or even missing response of adrenaline, adrenocorticotropic hormone, and cortisol to correct the hypoglycaemia [47].

There are only limited data available on pancreatic glucagon levels in neonatal calves [72, 97]. In our studies plasma glucagon concentrations transiently increased in response to the first meal, increased more in calves fed colostrum rather than MR, and concentrations were higher during the first 3 days of life in calves fed high amounts of colostrum from the first milking instead of colostrum obtained from milkings 1 to 6 of lactation [67,78,81] (Rauprich, Hammon and Blum, unpublished observations). This indicates that the glucagon status depends on colostrum feeding intensity and on colostrum components. On the other hand, plasma glucagon concentrations on the ensuing days of life increased more in calves fed MR than in those fed colostrum.

3.3. Insulin and glucagon in suckling calves

We have studied metabolic, enzymatic and endocrine traits in suckling Simmentaler calves during the first 3 months of life in a cow-calf operation [67]. Plasma glucose concentrations increased transiently on d 1 of life and then remained stable. There were transient elevations in plasma glucagon concentrations from d 1 to d 14 of life, then concentrations returned to those measured at birth. Insulin concentrations increased on d 1 of life and then remained at this level up to d 84 of life. Mean plasma insulin concentrations were lower than normally found in veal calves. On the other hand, concentrations of insulin during the 3rd month were higher than could normally be measured in calves raised for potential breeding. The pattern of insulin and glucagon concentrations in female and (castrated and intact) male Angus calves in two other cow-calf herds was very similar to that in Simmentaler calves (Egli and Blum, unpublished observations). The data obtained in this study indicated considerable differences in the ontogenic pattern of glucose and insulin concentrations when veal calves were compared with calves raised for potential breeding. There may be specific effects of suckling, as indicated by differences in metabolic and endocrine traits in suckling and bucket-fed veal calves [98].

3.4. Insulin resistance, hyperglycaemia, glucosuria, and galactosuria in veal calves

Veal calves are pseudomonogastrics and thus rapidly absorb glucose, FA, and AA in the small intestine. The utilisation of these substrates requires subtle homeostatic metabolic control. However, in veal calves glucose-insulin relationships are often grossly abnormal, and postprandially a transient type-II-like diabetes may develop [30,51,98,100-107]. Thus, plasma glucose concentrations often increase markedly during fattening in bucket-fed calves fed twice daily. Plasma glucose concentrations were much lower in calves fed at least 6 times/24 hours than in calves fed the same amounts of MR only 2 times/24 hours, demonstrating that feeding frequency is important. In addition, insulin/glucose ratios during 8-hour postprandial periods increased markedly in bucket-fed calves, but remained stable in suckling calves, and were much lower in the latter, indicating an absence of insulin resistance in these, but not in bucket-fed calves. Thus, marked and sudden postprandial glucose loads could obviously not be handled by older veal calves. Glucosuria and galactosuria occurred, especially towards the end of fattening, if plasma glucose increased to above 1.5 g/l (kidney threshold), indicating energy loss and reduced energy utilisation. Glucose clearance was markedly reduced, especially postprandially. Glucose tracer kinetics during euglycaemic-hyperinsulinaemic clamps (EHGC) demonstrated reduced insulin-dependent glucose oxidation and enhanced storage of glucose as glycogen. Insulin concentrations increased excessively after feed intake, especially towards later phases of fattening in calves fed twice daily. Mean insulin concentrations were lower in calves fed 6 times than 2 times/24 h with the same amount of food. However, in hyperglycaemic clamps (HGC), glucose-stimulated insulin responses were not age-dependently enhanced. Hyperinsulinaemia was primarily due to enhanced secretion, because in EHGC the MCR was not reduced and the $t_{1/2}$ of insulin (after intravenous injection) was normal, with no difference pre- and postprandially. Towards the end of fattening, the plasma glucose concentration remained elevated even in the presence of extremely high circulating amounts of insulin, indicating development of insulin resistance with increasing age. The hypoglycaemia-inducing effects of insulin at 3 h after MR intake were smaller than before feeding, i.e., insulin resistance was primarily a postprandial problem. In accordance, insulin-dependent glucose utilisation, measured by EHGC (and thus about 15 h after the last meal) did not change in an age-dependent manner - in contrast to the postprandial situation.

The aetiology of insulin resistance in veal calves is most likely multifactorial. There may be a constitutionally based and an age-dependent reduction in the ability of veal calves to handle high amounts of absorbed nutrient components, especially glucose; i.e., a high feeding intensity may be the overall cause of insulin resistance. It may be speculated that insulin resistance protects the calf from excess metabolic loads of absorbed nutrients.

Hyperinsulinaemia after MR intake was greater than after oral administration of lactose or oral and parenteral administration of glucose, although plasma glucose concentrations were lower, indicating that factors other than lactose or glucose contribute to insulin resistance. Although a high lactose intake was not the only factor causing hyperinsulinaemia, feeding during the fattening period caused a reduction in the insulin receptor number (not affinity) in skeletal muscle.

It is well known that a high fat intake in man and rats is an important cause of insulin resistance, but this has been questioned for calves [100,101]. However, high protein intake may be a cause as well [108].

Cr(III) deficiency seems not to be involved, because supplementation of a synthetic Cr(III) preparation [containing Cr(III), nicotinic acid, glycine, glutamic acid and cysteine] did not reduce postprandial hyperglycaemia and hyperinsulinaemia (Blum and Bruckmaier, unpublished observations). Iron excess as an aetiological factor for insulin resistance could be excluded because insulin resistance developed in calves fed only 20 mg iron/kg MR.

High amounts of circulating insulin in themselves are likely to be important, since insulin down-regulates its own receptors. Glucose-dependent insulinotropic polypeptide (GIP) could also be excluded, because its postprandial rise was similar in calves fed normal or high amounts of lactose, its postprandial rise at the start and end of fattening was comparable and GIP is not insulinogenic in ruminants. Furthermore, GH and cortisol excesses (which are known to cause insulin resistance) could be excluded as aetiological factors of insulin resistance. However, markedly higher amounts of noradrenaline and dopamine excreted during 24 h/kg$^{0.75}$ in the urine at the end than at the start of fattening indicated enhanced sympathetic activity with increasing age, which may contribute to the age-dependent increase in insulin resistance.

Because a normal insulin status (concentration, effect) is required for the stimulation of anabolic processes, it is somehow surprising that high growth rates are possible under conditions of marked insulin resistance. IGF-I, whose concentrations increase continuously during fattening in veal calves [103], may mediate some of the effects of insulin under high-intensive feeding conditions. However, glucagon, IGF-I, GH and prolactin concentrations were lower in calves fed MR twice/day compared with calves fed the same amount of MR at least 6 times/day, i.e., IGF-I concentrations behaved differently to insulin [98,106] (Kaufhold and Blum, unpublished observations). Interestingly, glucagon, GH and prolactin concentrations were lower in calves fed MR twice/day compared with calves fed the same amount of MR at least 6 times/day, indicating that suckling per se may have specific effects.

3.5. Diabetes mellitus in calves

Diabetes mellitus (type I) is a rare clinical disease in cattle, including calves, and mainly occurs in association with pancreatic injuries and infections, such bovine virus diarrhoea and mucosal disease or after recovery from foot and mouth disease [4,108]. There may be rare cases of congenital diabetes mellitus in calves. Thus, glucosuria, hyperglycaemia and unmeasurably low insulin concentrations were found in 2-day-old twin Simmentaler calves (Blum, unpublished observations).

Glucocorticoids directly inhibit insulin secretion, induce insulin resistance [109], as also shown in calves, and in several species induce overt type I diabetes mellitus after prolonged administration, but this is hardly the case in calves [110]. However, the diabetes mellitus can be induced in calves by combined thyroidectomy and glucocorticoid (cortisol) administration [38,110,111]. In this situation plasma concentrations of insulin decreased, whereas those of glucagon and PP increased [38]. However, the changes were reversed if T_4 was substituted. If 2-deoxy-D-glucose was administered, plasma insulin concentrations did not rise, whereas plasma glucagon and PP concentrations increased. The increased plasma glucagon levels probably made a secondary contribution to the hyperglycaemia in thyroidectomized and cortisol-treated calves. This study also indicated that A and F cells become insensitive to glucose in the absence of insulin.

3.6. Insulin in iron-deficient veal calves

A low iron intake with milk or MR diets in veal calves is necessary to produce white meat. The consequences of a marked iron deficiency are reduced O_2 transport (by haemoglobin), O_2 storage (by myoglobin) and O_2 utilisation (by enzymes of the respiratory chain). In iron-deficient calves the deficiency was characterised by anaemia, reduced O_2 consumption, reduced growth and physical performance, increased lactate formation, reduced cell-mediated

38

immune reactions, and increased infection rates [85]. Interestingly, an increased insulin-dependent glucose utilisation was found [28]. Furthermore, insulin concentrations in iron-deficient calves were often reduced [112]. Together with enhanced metabolic clearance rates of GH, a reduced rise in IGF-I in response to exogenous bovine GH, and low basal plasma concentrations of insulin, IGF-I, and often of 3.5.3'-triiodothyronine (T_3) were seen, besides metabolic changes (especially of glucose). These endocrine changes may contribute to low average daily gains and reduced feed utilisation in markedly iron-deficient calves. The enhanced insulin-dependent glucose utilisation in iron-deficient calves is in line with the well-known decrease in insulin-dependent glucose utilisation seen in states of iron overload, such as haemochromatosis in man.

3.7. Calves raised for potential breeding

The change from milk to roughage-concentrate diets results in reduced feeding intensity and energy intake and causes metabolic and endocrine changes [21,22,113-116]. After weaning, volatile FA (especially acetate) are increasingly utilised for energy and fat synthesis. Furthermore, use of lactate for gluconeogenesis [49,117], effects of insulin on glucose utilisation and utilisation of glucose for fat synthesis and for energy are reduced when calves become true ruminants. Compared with veal calves, calves raised for potential breeding were characterised by lower blood plasma concentrations and reduced or lacking postprandial increments of glucose, lower insulin, IGF-I and to some extent T_4 and T_3 concentrations and higher concentrations of NEFA, β-hydroxybutyrate, globulin, haemoglobin, iron, and GH [104]. Increased concentrations of NEFA, and decreased concentrations of insulin, IGF-I, T_4 and T_3 in part probably reflected a lower energy intake of calves raised for potential breeding than of veal calves.

3.8. Insulin in dwarf and sick calves

To what extent a reduced insulin production and effects on target tissues contribute to genetically reduced growth (dwarfs) is equivocal. Reduced insulin concentrations have in fact been measured and there is also evidence for insulin resistance in some of these cases, but other factors contribute to the phenomenon [118,119].

There is a transient increase in insulin concentrations immediately after endotoxin administration in calves [95,120], but as in other species, concentrations are most often decreased in subacute and chronic infectious diseases due to ingestion of less feed, energy and protein. This has been demonstrated in calves with diarrhoea [121], pneumonia [66] and Sarcocystosis [58] and (in combination with other metabolic and endocrine changes) this most likely contributes to low growth performance.

REFERENCES

1. S. Bonner-Weir and A.A. Like, Cell Tissue Res., 206 (1980) 157.
2. D. Porte and J.B. Halter, The endocrine pancreas and diabetes mellitus, In: Textbook of Endocrinology , R.H. Williams (ed.), W.B. Saunders Co., Philadelphia, 1981.
3. R.P. Brockman, Pancreatic and adrenal hormonal regulation of metabolism, In: Control of Digestion and Metabolism in Ruminants, L.P. Milligan, W.L. Grovum and A. Dobson (eds.), Prentice Hall, Englewood Cliffs, 1986.

4. U. Fischer, Pankreas, In: Veterinaermedizinische Endokrinologie, Döcke F. (ed.), G. Fischer Verlag, Jena, 1994.
5. T. Hiratsuka, M. Abe, K. Takehana, K. Iwasa and A. Kobayashi, Okjimas Folia Anatom., 72 (1986) 285.
6. D. Greco and G.H. Stabenfeldt, The endocrine system, In: Textbook of Veterinary Physiology, J.G. Cunningham (ed), W.B. Saunders Co., Philadelphia, 1997.
7. S.N. Reddy and R.B. Elliott, Australian J. Biol. Sci., 38 (1985) 237.
8. N.W. Bunnett and F.A. Harrison, Q. J. Exp. Physiol., 71 (1986) 433.
9. C. Domenghini and S. Arrighi, Acta Histochem., 96 (1994) 287.
10. P. Cordano, H. Hammon and J.W. Blum, Tissue distribution of insulin-like growth factor mRNA in 8-day old calves, In: Growth in Ruminants: Basic Aspects, Theory and Practice for the Future, J.W. Blum, T. Elsasser and P. Guilloteau (eds.), University of Berne, Berne, 1998.
11. M. Peng, T. Abribat, E. Calvo, D. LeBel, M-F. Palin, G. Bernatchez, J. Morisset and G. Pelletier, J. Anim. Sci., 76 (1998) 1178.
12. A.K. Tung and E. Cockburn, Diabetes, 33 (1984) 235.
13. T.E. Adrian, S.R. Bloom and A.V. Edwards, J. Physiol., 344 (1983) 25.
14. S.R. Bloom and A.V. Edwards, J. Physiol., 314 (1981) 23.
15. S.R. Bloom and A.V. Edwards, J. Physiol., 314 (1981) 37.
16. S.R. Bloom, A.V. Edwards and N.J.A. Vaughan, J. Physiol., 236 (1974) 611.
17. S.R. Bloom, A.V. Edwards and R.N. Hardy, J. Physiol., 280 (1978) 9.
18. S.R. Bloom, A.V. Edwards and R.N. Hardy, J. Physiol., 280 (1978) 37.
19. S.R. Bloom, A.V. Edwards and J. Järhult, J. Physiol., 308 (1980) 29.
20. S. Nakajima, N. Kitamura, J. Yamada, T. Yamashita and T. Watanabe, Acta Anatom., 131 (1988) 235.
21. P. Guilloteau, I. Le Huërou-Luron, R. Toullec, J.A. Chayvialle and J.W. Blum, Regulatory peptides in young ruminants, In: Ruminant Physiology: Digestion, Metabolism, Growth and Reproduction, v. W. Engelhardt, S. Leonhard-Marek, G. Breves and D. Giesecke (eds.), F. Enke Verlag, Stuttgart, 1995.
22. P. Guilloteau, I. Le Huërou-Luron, R. Toullec, J.A. Chayvialle, R. Zabielski and J.W. Blum, J. Vet. Med. A, 44 (1997) 1.
23. T.E.C. Weekes, Hormonal control of glucose metabolism, In: Physiological Aspects of Digestion and Metbaolism in Ruminants, T. Tsuda, Y. Sasaki and R. Kawashima (eds.), Academic Press, Inc., San Diego, 1991.
24. J.W. Young, E.O. Otchere, A. Trenkle and N.L. Jacobsen, J. Nutr., 100 (1970) 1267.
25. T.N. Kumalu and A.H. Trenkle, Nutr. Rep. Int., 18 (1978) 243.
26. J. Grizard, P. Patureau-Mirand and R. Pion, Ann. Biol. Anim. Bioch. Biophys., 16 (1976) 593.
27. U. Reinicke, Der intravenöse und modifizierte Glukosetoleranztest beim Milchrind - Einflussfaktoren und Beziehungen zur Milchleistung, Thesis in Veterinary Medicine, Freie Universtät Berlin, 1993.
28. R. Hostettler-Allen, L. Tappy and J. W. Blum, J. Nutr., 123 (1994) 1656.
29. A. Oshibe, K. Hodate, A. Yamada, S. Ando and S. Oshio, J. Anim. Physiol. a Anim. Nutr., 76 (1996) 1511.
30. D. Hugi, R.M. Bruckmaier and J.W. Blum, J. Anim. Sci., 75 (1997) 469.
31. T. Kuhara, S. Ikeda, A. Ohneda, T. Tsuda and Y. Sasaki, Asian J. Anim. Sci., 2 (1989) 231.

32. J. Grizard, R. Toullec, P. Guilloteau and P. Patureau-Mirand, Reprod. Nutr. Develop., 22 (1982) 475.
33. R. Guilhermet and R. Toullec, Reprod. Nutr. Developm., 23 (1983) 341.
34. D.D. Johnson, G.E. Jr. Mitchell, R.E. Tucker and R.W. Hemken, J. Anim. Sci., 55 (1982) 1224.
35. Owens, J.L. Sartin, R.J. Kemppainen, K.A. Cummins, F.F. Bartol and M.A. Bowman, Amer. J. Vet. Res., 47 (1986) 263.
36. L.M. Morgan, P.R. Flatt and V. Marks, Nutr. Res. Rev. 1 (1988) 79.
37. U.V. Zimmerli and J.W. Blum, J. Anim. Physiol. a Anim. Nutr., 63 (1990) 157.
38. S.R. Bloom, A.V. Edwards and A.S. Fielding, J. Physiol., 318 (1981) 395.
39. H. Sano, N. Hattori, Y. Todome, J. Tsuruoka, H. Takahashi and Y. Terashima, J. Anim. Sci., 71 (1993) 3414.
40. S.R. Bloom, A.V. Edwards and R.N. Hardy, J. Physiol., 269 (1977) 131.
41. S.R. Bloom and A.V. Edwards, J. Physiol., 362 (1985) 311.
42. J.W. Blum and N. Flückiger, Eur. J. Pharmacol., 151 (1988) 177.
43. G. Scholtysik, F. Regli, R.M. Bruckmaier and J.W. Blum, J. Vet. Pharmacol. a Therapeut., 21 (1998) 477.
44. J.W. Blum, Eur. J. Pharmacol., 105 (1984) 239.
45. A.N. Blackburn, S.R. Bloom and A.V. Edwards, J. Physiol., 314 (1981) 11.
46. J.W. Blum, R.B. Wilson and D.S. Kronfeld, J. Dairy Sci., 56 (1973) 459.
47. E. Richet, M-J. Davicco, M. Dalle and J-P. Barlet, Reprod. Nutr. Develop., 25 (1985) 427.
48. A.E. Kitabchi, Metabolism, 26 (1977) 547.
49. S.S. Donkin and L.E. Armentano, J. Anim. Sci., 73 (1995) 546.
50. S.S. Donkin and L.E. Armentano, J. Anim. Sci., 75 (1997) 3082.
51. D. Hugi, L. Tappy, H. Sauerwein, R.M. Bruckmaier and J.W. Blum, J. Nutr., 128 (1998) 1023.
52. Y. Chilliard, D. Durand, C. Audigier, S. Auboiron and D. Bauchart, Ann. Zootech., 42 (1993) 208.
53. J-F. Hocquette, M. Balage and P. Ferré, Proc. Nutr. Soc., 55 (1996) 221.
54. A. Oshibe, K. Hodate, S. Ando and S. Ashio, J. Anim. Physiol. a Anim. Nutr., 73 (1995) 243.
55. D.J. Hill and R.D.G. Milner, Pediatr. Res., 19 (1985) 879.
56. P. Guilloteau, J.A. Chayvialle, D. Durand, C. Bernard, R. Toullec, A. Mouats and D. Bauchart, Reprod. Nutr. Developm., 28 Suppl. 1 (1988) 163.
57. P. Guilloteau, I. Le Huërou-Luron, J.A. Chayvialle, A. Mouats, C. Bernard, J.C. Cuber, J. Burton, A. Puigserver and R. Toullec, Reprod. Nutr. Developm., 32 (1992) 285.
58. T.H. Elsasser, R. Fayer, T.S. Rumsey and A.C. Hammond, Domest. Anim. Endocrinol., 7 (1990) 537.
59. M-J. Davicco, J. Lefaivre and J-P. Barlet, Ann. Rech. Vet., 11 (1980) 123.
60. B.H. Breier and B.W. Gallaher, Endocrine control of fetal growth, In: Growth in Ruminants: Basic Aspects, Theory and Practice for the Future, J.W. Blum, T. Elsasser and Guilloteau P. (eds.), University of Berne, Berne, 1998.
61. M.L. Frazier, R.A. Montagna and G.F. Saunders, Biochemistry, 20 (1981) 367.
62. J. D'Agostino, J.B. Field and M.L. Frazier, Endocrinology, 116 (1985) 1108.
63. A.K. Tung, J.L. Ruse and E. Cockburn, Can. J. Biochem., 58 (1980) 707.

64. L.C. Lopez, M.L. Frazier, C.J. Su, A. Kumar and G.F. Saunders, Proc. Natl. Acad. Sci., 80 (1983) 5485.
65. A.K. Tung and K.P. Siu, Biochem. Biophys. Res. Commun., 125 (1984) 524.
66. J.W. Blum, R.M. Bruckmaier and M. Moser, Deutsche Tierärztliche Woschenschrift 103 (1997) 115.
67. C. Egli and J.W. Blum, J. Vet. Med. A, 45 (1998) 99.
68. J. Girard, Biol. Neonate, 50 (1986) 237.
69. R.L. Stanko, M.J. Guthrie, C.C.Jr. Chase and R.D. Randel, J. Anim. Sci., 70 (1992) 3007.
70. J.B. Goudever, E.J. Sulkers, T.E. Chapman, V.P. Carnielli, T. Efstatopoulos, H.J. Degenhart and J.J. Sauer, Pediatr. Res., 33 (1993) 583.
71. H. Ronge and J.W. Blum, J. Anim. Physiol. a Anim. Nutr., 60 (1988) 168.
72. S. Oda, H. Satoh, T. Sugawara, N. Matsunaga, T. Kuhara, K. Katoh, Y. Shoji, A. Nihei, M. Ohta and Y. Sasaki, Comp. Biochem. Physiol., 94 (1989) 805.
73. R. Grütter and J.W. Blum, Reprod. Nutr. Develop., 31 (1991) 389.
74. C.R. Baumrucker and J.W. Blum, J. Endocrinol., 140 (1994) 15.
75. C.R. Baumrucker, M.H. Green and J.W. Blum, Domest. Anim. Endocrinol., 11 (1994) 393.
76. H. Hammon and J.W. Blum, Amer. J. Physiol., 273 (1997) E130.
77. H. Hammon and J.W. Blum, Biol. Neonate, 73 (1998) 121.
78. H. Hammon and J.W. Blum, J. Nutr., 128 (1998) 624.
79. H. Hammon and J.W. Blum, Intestinal IGF type 1 and type 2 and insulin receptors in neonatal calves: effects of feeding colostrum for different duration or only milk replacer. In: The somatotrophic axis (Proceedings of the 3rd International Conference on Farm Animal Endocrinology), Brussels, 1998.
80. H. Hammon, C. Bühler, G. Rossi and J.W. Blum, Effects of different colostrum supply on xylose absorption, small intestinal histomorphometry, and IGF-I and insulin receptors in neonatal calves, In: Growth in Ruminants: Basic Aspects, Theory and Practice for the Future (J.W. Blum, T. Elsasser and P. Guilloteau (eds.), University of Berne, Berne, 1998.
81. H. Kühne, H.M. Hammon, R.M. Bruckmaier, C. Morel, Y. Zbinden and J.W. Blum, Intestinal absorptive capacity, metabolic and endocrine traits, and growth performance in neonatal calves fed low or high amounts of colostrum or only milk replacer, In: Growth in Ruminants: Basic Aspects, Theory and Practice for the Future, J.W. Blum, T. Elsasser and P. Guilloteau (eds.), University of Berne, Berne, 1998.
82. A. Rauprich, H. Hammon and J.W. Blum, Metabolic and endocrine effects of low and high colostrum feeding intensity in neonatal calves, In: Growth in Ruminants: Basic Aspects, Theory and Practice for the Future, J.W. Blum, T. Elsasser and P. Guilloteau (eds.), University of Berne, Berne, 1998.
83. A. Rauprich, H. Hammon and J.W. Blum, Metabolic and endocrine effects of feeding a milked-based formula compared with colostrum in neonatal calves, In: Growth in Ruminants: Basic Aspects, Theory and Practice for the Future, J.W. Blum, T. Elsasser and P. Guilloteau (eds.), University of Berne, Berne, 1998.
84. I. Zanker, H. Hammon and J.W. Blum, Effects of time-point of first colostrum intake on plasma insulin-like growth factor-I (IGF-I), IGF-binding proteins (IGFBPs) and insulin in neonatal calves, In: Growth in Ruminants: Basic Aspects, Theory and Practice for the Future J.W. Blum, Elsasser T. and P. Guilloteau (eds.), University of Berne, Berne, 1998.
85. J.W. Blum and H. Hammon, Domest. Anim. Endocrinol. (in press).

42

86. P.V. Malven, H.H. Head, R.J. Collier and F. Buonomo, J. Dairy Sci., 70 (1987) 2254.
87. W.M. Campana and C.R. Baumrucker, Hormones and growth factors in bovine milk, In: Handbook of Milk Composition, R.G. Jensen (ed.), Academic Press, New York, 1995.
88. M. Ollivier-Bousquet, INRA Prod. Anim., 6 (1993) 253.
89. P-Y. Vacher and J.W. Blum, Milk Sci. Int., 48 (1993) 423.
90. A.E. Pierce, P.C. Risdall and B. Shaw, J. Physiol., 171 (1964) 203.
91. H. Tyler and H. Ramsey, J. Dairy Sci., 76 (1993) 2736.
92. H. Hartmann, J. Hubald, H. Meyer and H. Little, Arch. Exp. Vet., 34 (1980) 777.
93. U. Hadorn, H. Hammon, R.M. Bruckmaier and J.W. Blum, J. Nutr., 127 (1997) 2011.
94. M. Kinsbergen, H.P. Sallmann and J.W. Blum, J. Vet. Med. A, 41 (1994) 268.
95. M. Kinsbergen, R.M. Bruckmaier and J.W. Blum, J. Vet. Med. A, 41 (1994) 530.
96. R.S. Comline and A.V. Edwards, J. Physiol., 198 (1968) 383.
97. X.Z. Mao, S.Z. Li, Z.K. Zhu and W.L. Qin, J. Vet. Med. A, 41 (1994) 405.
98. J.N. Kaufhold and J.W. Blum, Metabolic and endocrine changes in veal calves fed by automate or by bucket, In: Growth in Ruminants: Basic Aspects, Theory and Practice for the Future (J.W. Blum, T. Elsasser and P. Guilloteau (eds.), University of Berne, Berne, 1998.
99. M.S. Wijayashinghe, N.E. Smith and R.L. Baldwin, J. Dairy Sci., 67 (1984) 2949.
100. J. Doppenberg and D.L. Palmquist, Livest. Prod. Sci., 29 (1991) 151.
101. D.L. Palmquist, J. Doppenberg, K.L. Roehrig and D.J. Kinsey, Domest. Anim. Endocrinol., 9 (1992) 233.
102. H. Ronge and J.W. Blum, Acta Endocrinol., 121 (1989) 153.
103. R. Hostettler-Allen, L. Tappy and J.W. Blum, J. Anim. Sci., 72 (1994) 160.
104. D. Hugi and J.W. Blum, J. Vet. Med. A, 44 (1997) 99.
105. D. Hugi, V.D. Bracher, L. Tappy and J.W. Blum, J. Anim. Physiol. a Anim. Nutr., 78 (1997) 42.
106. D. Hugi, S.H. Gut and J.W. Blum, J. Vet. Med. A, 44 (1997) 407.
107. J.N. Kaufhold and J.W. Blum, Fructo-oligosaccharide supplementation in veal calves: effects on metabolic and endocrine traits, In: Growth in Ruminants: Basic Aspects, Theory and Practice for the Future, J.W. Blum, T.Elsasser and P. Guilloteau (eds.), University of Berne, Berne, 1998.
108. W.J.J. Gerrits and J.W. Blum, The role of protein intake in the development of insulin resistance in preruminant calves, In: Growth in Ruminants: Basic Aspects, Theory and Practice for the Future (J.W. Blum, T. Elsasser and P. Guilloteau (eds.), University of Berne, Berne, 1998.
109. J.E. Madigan and N.O. Dybdal, Endocrine and metabolic diseases, In: Large Animal Internal Medicine, Bradford P.S. (ed.), The CV Mosby Company, St. Louis, 1990.
110. K. Sternbauer, J. Luthman and S.O. Jacobsson, J. Vet. Med., 45 (1998) 441.
111. R.S. Comline, A.V. Edwards and P.W. Nathanielsz, J. Physiol., 208 (1970) 33.
112. A.V. Edwards, P.W. Nathanielsz and N.J.A Vaughan, J. Endocrinol., 51 (1971) 511.
113. A. Ceppi and J.W. Blum, J. Vet. Med. A, 41 (1994) 443.
114. D.W. Webb, H.H. Head and C.J. Wilcox, J. Dairy Sci., 52 (1969) 2007.
115. I.C. Hart, S.V. Morant and J.H.B. Roy, Anim. Prod., 32 (1981) 215.
116. B.H. Breier, P.D. Gluckman and J.J. Bass, J. Endocrinol., 119 (1988) 43.

117. J.W. Blum, Nutritional, metabolic, endocrine and hematological aspects in suckling calves, veal and weaned calves, In: Growth in Ruminants: Basic Aspects, Theory and Practice for the Future, J.W. Blum, T. Elsasser and P. Guilloteau (eds.), University of Berne, Berne, 1998.
118. S.S. Donkin, D.S. Black, R.B. Greenfield and C. Agca, J. Anim. Sci., 76 Suppl. 1, J. Dairy Sci., 81 Suppl. 1 (1998) 137.
119. J.W. Blum, B. Kovacs, P. Nett, M. Schenk and G. Stranzinger, Metabolic and endocrine changes in a dwarf calf, In: Growth in Ruminants: Basic Aspects, Theory and Practice for the Future, J.W. Blum, T. Elsasser and P. Guilloteau (eds.), University of Berne, Berne, 1998.
120. A.C. Hammond, T.H. Elsasser, M.C. Lucy, C.C.Jr. Chase and T.A Olson, Growth in Ruminants: Basic Aspects, Theory and Practice for the Future, J.W. Blum, T. Elsasser and P. Guilloteau (eds.), University of Berne, Berne, 1998.
121. D.C. Kenison, T.H. Elsasser and R. Fayer, Amer. J. Vet. Res., 52 (1991) 1320.
122. A. Gutzwiller and J.W. Blum, Amer. J. Vet. Res., 57 (1996) 560.

Biology of the Pancreas in Growing Animals
S.G. Pierzynowski and R. Zabielski (Editors)
© 1999 Elsevier Science B.V. All rights reserved.

45

The role of apoptosis in pancreatic development

J.L. Valverde Piedra and T. Studziński

Department of Animal Physiology, Faculty of Veterinary Medicine,
Agricultural University of Lublin, Akademicka 12, 20-033 Lublin, Poland

The molecular mechanisms involved in pancreatic apoptosis remain largely unknown. The exact role of apoptosis in the structural and functional formation and modelling of the pancreas in the neonatal period is unknown as well, although it has been shown recently that apoptotic processes participate in the development of the pancreas in the neonatal rat. Clusterin is a multifunctional glycoprotein which participates in the differentiation and morphogenesis of the pancreas, but its precise function during the period of fetal development, neo- and postnatal life has not been established. The increased expression of clusterin synthesis during the first 11 days of neonatal life in the rat is very interesting. It may be related to the rather protracted fetal pattern of clusterin synthesis in this species. One would like to know what pattern of clusterin synthesis might be present in other species, such as domestic animals and humans. Although no data are available, one could speculate that it might be shorter in new-born pigs, calves, horses *et cetera*, because they are at a more advanced stage of general development at the time of birth. This is an intriguing subject for further study.

1. APOPTOSIS

Apoptosis is a specific type of cell death, different from necrosis in that it does not involve primary cell membrane disintegration and tissue inflammatory reactions. The term apoptosis was introduced in analogy with the loss of leaves from deciduous trees and in Greek means "leaves falling from trees" [1]. Cell apoptosis is sometimes called a suicidal (or physiological) and active (or programmed) cell death. It is a process that appears to involve a sequence of energy-consuming events, resulting in DNA degradation and cell death with little or no associated inflammatory response [1].

Apoptosis is morphologically and biochemically distinct from necrosis, which is an accidental event caused by, for example, exposure to mechanical injury or toxic chemicals. Necrosis evokes an inflammatory process in the vicinity of the cell, induced by substances such as cytokines and other components released from the cell. Cell death by apoptosis is a highly specific process for removing redundant, senescent, changed and deleterious cells from the organism. Apoptosis (along with mitosis) maintains and determines the amount of epithelial cells and tissue homeostasis [2]. Tissue hyperplasia and atrophy can result from inhibition or potentiation of apoptosis, respectively. Ineffective apoptotic elimination of genetically altered cells appears to contribute to malignant transformation [3,4].

Morphological changes may be observed in the nucleus and cytoplasm of the apoptotic cell. The cell shrinks, becomes denser, and in the cell nucleus the chromatin becomes pyknotic and packed into homogenous masses located close to the nuclear envelope. The cell nucleus often breaks into fragments while microvilli disappear and protrusions containing organelles are formed on the cell surface [5,6]. These protrusions often contain nuclear fragments and tend to break off, becoming apoptotic bodies. These morphological changes are followed by secondary necrosis *in vitro* and enable the identification of apoptosis. The discrimination between live, early apoptotic, late apoptotic and necrotic cells is possible by combined cell staining with certain fluorochromes such as propidium iodide and Hoechst 33342. The accessibility of nuclear DNA to these fluorochromes depends on the cell membrane's integrity and permeability. The nuclei of live and early apoptotic cells are labelled with differing intensity by Hoechst 33342 fluorochrome, which evokes blue fluorescence, whereas the nuclei of late apoptotic and necrotic cells are labelled mainly by propidium iodide, which induces red fluorescence. Thus discrimination between stages of apoptosis and between necrosis and apoptotic changes is possible [5].

Apoptotic bodies undergo phagocytosis under physiological conditions without any symptoms in neighbouring epithelial cells, while *in vitro*, in tissue cell culture, these morphological changes are followed by secondary necrosis. These apoptotic changes occur rapidly, and because they last only 2-4 hours, are difficult to detect. Release of cellular constituents from apoptotic bodies and apoptotic cells to the surrounding space is very rare or absent, and is not accompanied by inflammatory reactions.

2. THE PHYSIOLOGY OF APOPTOSIS IN THE PANCREAS

The molecular mechanisms involved in pancreatic apoptosis remain largely unknown. The exact role of apoptosis in the structural and functional modelling of the pancreas in the neonatal period is unknown as well, although it has been shown recently that apoptotic processes participate in the development of the pancreas in the neonatal rat [7,8].

Clusterin is a multifunctional glycoprotein which participates in the differentiation and morphogenesis of the pancreas [8,9]. However, its precise function during the period of fetal development, neo- and postnatal life has not been established.

Results of recent work show that clusterin is synthesised and released by the exocrine pancreas [8]. Its strong overexpression during pancreatic development might be involved in the selection of cells destined to survive [9]. A fine balance between cell replication and cell death determines pancreatic structure and functional readiness at the moment of birth. The increased expression of clusterin mRNA at this time suggests that the glycoprotein is responsible for the control of this balance.

After birth, the rate of duct, islet, and acinar cell proliferation remains fairly constant during the first few weeks and then declines after weaning [10]. As the results recently obtained in the rat show, the levels of clusterin mRNA are high during pancreatic cell proliferation and differentiation, suggesting that in the pancreas this protein functions as a crucial antiapoptotic agent in these processes. Thus it may influence cell differentiation and proliferation as well as cell death and survival [9].

Clusterin mRNA expression is strong in late fetal life and remains high for the first two weeks of postnatal life in the rat [8]. Its antiapoptotic function during the development of the pancreas and in pancreatitis is well documented. Reddy *et al.* [11] demonstrated a modified form of clusterin with nuclear localisation, which suggests the possibility of direct involvement in gene regulation.

Clusterin mRNA expression has not been detected in the healthy pancreas, but after 6 h duration of pancreatitis strong stimulation, reaching a maximum at 24-28 h, has been observed, followed by a progressive decrease to undetectable levels. Clusterin has been detected in pancreatic juice and pancreatic homogenates from rats with acute pancreatitis, but not in healthy rats [8].

There is a lack of information regarding the physiological mediators of pancreatic cell apoptosis in either health or disease. The proapoptotic Bax gene is clearly expressed in the normal healthy pancreas [12]. The antiapoptotic genes Bcl-2 and Mcl-1 are not observable in normal physiologically functional acinar cells when analysed by immunocytochemical methods [12]. Pancreatic cell apoptosis could be triggered by Bax genes as in many other cells of different tissues, but these genes would be controlled and repressed by the antiapoptotic genes.

Most of what is known about apoptosis in the pancreas is derived from research on pathophysiological models of pancreatitis. Pancreatitis results from acinar cell injury and is accompanied by morphological alterations typical of apoptosis and necrosis. Acute pancreatitis is associated with release to the extracellular space of digestive enzymes, leading to propagation and intensification of the acinar cell injury, followed by an inflammatory process and necrosis. By studying various animal models of acute pancreatitis, induced by different methods such as pancreatic duct obstruction, stimulation with supra-maximal doses of caerulein, or a choline-deficient, ethionine-supplemented diet, it has been possible to gain new information about the apoptosis and necrosis of acinar cells and discern a basic relationship between these two processes in experimental acute pancreatitis [13].

The studies of Kaiser *et al.* [13] suggest that apoptosis in the pancreas, unlike in other organs, can be associated with mild evidence of inflammation and low infiltration by inflammatory cells. This is connected with the possibility that acinar cells, in contrast to other types of cells, maintain a balance between the mild symptoms of inflammation, characteristic of acute pancreatitis, and those of the necrosis that follows. Acinar cells may be able to release some chemotactic factors in precisely regulated amounts, which evoke only mild inflammation or even counteract inflammation. At the same time they are able to control the process leading to apoptosis, which may minimise the level of inflammation and the severity of the pancreatitis. In this way, acinar cells may be provided with a sophisticated defence mechanism based on the substitution of inflammation by apoptosis, which is safer for the pancreas due to more advanced conservation of integrity of the acinar cells and a lower rate of cell death. Apoptotic mechanisms counteract severe inflammatory development accompanied by necrotic disintegration of the acinar cells, which is always connected with the release of a whole spectrum of digestive enzymes. This is fatal not only for the pancreas and for other organs, but for the whole organism [13].

Deregulated apoptosis has been implicated in several diseases of the pancreas such as pancreatitis and pancreatic cancer [2]. Acute or chronic pancreatitis is accompanied by typical changes, with cells showing signs of apoptosis and necrosis.

Ligation of the common bile pancreatic duct in the opossum (*Didelphis virginiana*) results in severe, frequently lethal pancreatitis, while the same procedure in the rat produces a relatively mild form of pancreatitis. In the experiments of Kaiser *et al.* [13] morphological examination of the pancreas after common bile-pancreatic duct ligation indicated only mild injury, including the presence of moderate oedema and infiltration, mostly with macrophage-like cells. There was little evidence of necrosis, however, and neither fat necrosis nor haemorrhage. Common bile-pancreatic duct ligation in the opossum results in both macroscopic and microscopic changes characteristic of acute pancreatitis, such as oedema, inflammatory cell infiltration, haemorrhage, fat necrosis, acinar cell injury and necrotic disintegration.

Common bile-pancreatic duct ligation in the rat induced relatively little necrosis, affecting at most 14.6% of the acinar cells on the third day after ligation. In contrast, common bile-pancreatic duct ligation in the opossum resulted in extensive necrotic injury, encompassing at most 49.8% of the acinar cells on the seventh day after ligation. Widespread disintegration of acinar cell membranes was observed with focal confluence of membranes among neighbouring cells, and symptoms of syncytial transformation and dilatation of intracellular organelles. These changes are typical of necrosis.

Gel electrophoresis of genomic DNA from necrotic cells resulted in no ladder-like pattern characteristic of apoptosis but rather a general degradation of genomic DNA into small-sized fragments, typical of necrosis. Using the Tunel technique based on *in situ* DNA nick and labelling and nuclear morphology, it was noted that in the rat, apoptosis is biphasic. The maximal value reached represented a 231-fold increase in the value noted in control rats. Using electron microscopy, DNA gel electrophoresis and two other quantitative techniques (nuclear morphology; DNA nick and labelling), it was possible to distinguish between apoptosis and necrosis of the acinar cells. In the opossum, widespread disintegration of acinar cell membranes was noted, with other symptoms more typical of necrosis than apoptosis.

Clusterin has been described as a secretory protein present in semen, plasma, cerebrospinal fluid, milk and urine, and in pancreatic juice during acute pancreatitis. This protein has also been identified in pancreatic homogenates from rats after 24 h of pancreatitis, but not in healthy rats [8]. Although little is known about the function of stimulated synthesis of clusterin in the pancreas during pancreatitis it is reasonable to believe that it may be involved in a defence mechanism aimed at protecting the pancreas against apoptosis and necrotic degradation of acinar cells. Such an antiapoptotic function has been demonstrated in some tissues and cells under the influence of apoptotic factors [9].

A strong of expression clusterin has been induced by various apoptotic factors such as ceramide, staurosporine, cycloheximide and oxidative stress [8]. These results support the hypothesis that clusterin protects against apoptotic cell death and is not dependent on the pathway by which apoptosis is evoked.

During ontogeny and development of multicellular organisms, organogenesis requires the atrophy and elimination of cells in order to provide the structural remodelling necessary for the selection of those cells destined to survive. Strong expression of clusterin synthesis at the stage of advanced fetal development in rats and during the first 11 days of neonatal life is evidence of its developmental role as an antiapoptotic factor, determining through stimulation of cell replication the architecture of the pancreas.

The increased clusterin synthesis seen during the first 11 days of neonatal life in the rat is very interesting [8], considering the rather protracted fetal pattern of clusterin synthesis in this species. One would like to know more about the pattern of clusterin expression in other species, such as domestic animals and humans. Although no data are available, one may speculate that this pattern may be shorter in new-born pigs, calves, horses *et cetera* because they are at a more advanced stage of general development at the time of birth. It is worth mentioning that the maturation and development of the digestive tract in the new-born rat also are more protracted in the neonatal period. For example, the time until closing of the jejunal pores to macromolecular transport, which is 19-21 days in neonatal rats, lasts only hours in calves and piglets.

One could also speculate about clusterin secretion in colostrum and milk, a possible role in its resorption from the digestive tract and its relationship with the time of closure of the jejunal pores to macromolecular transepithelial transport. Perhaps two sources of clusterin exist, one connected with acinar cells and the other with the mammary gland and colostrum or milk feeding. Further research is necessary for these questions to be answered.

REFERENCES

1. J.F. Kerr, A.H. Wyllie and A.R. Currie, Brit. J. Cancer, 26 (1972) 239.
2. J.A. Blake and G.J. Gores, Amer. J. Physiol., 273 (Gastrointest. Liver Physiol. 36) (1997) G1174.
3. L.E. French, A. Chonn, D. Ducrest, B. Baumann, D. Belin, A. Wohlwend, J.Z. Kiss, A.P. Sappino, J. Tschopp and J.A. Schifferli, J. Cell Biol., 122 (1993) 1119.
4. D.E. Jenne and J. Tschopp, Trends Biochem. Sci., 17 (1992) 154.
5. T. Motyl, Post. Biol. Kom., 25 (1998) 315.
6. J. Kawiak, G. Hoser and T. Skórski, Folia Histochemica et Cytobiologica, 36 (1998) 99.
7. L. Scaglia, C.J. Cahill, D.T. Finegood and S. Bonner-Weir, Endocrinology, 138 (1997) 1736.
8. E.L. Calvo, G.V. Mallo, F. Fiedler, D. Malka, M.I. Vaccaro, V. Keim, J. Morisset, J.C. Dagorn and J.L. Iovanna, Eur. J. Biochem., 254 (1998) 282.
9. L.E. French, A. Wohlwend, A.P. Sappino, J. Tschopp and J.A. Schifferli, J. Clin. Invest., 93 (1994) 877.
10. P.S. Oates and R.G. Morgan, J. Anat., 167 (1989) 235.
11. K.B. Reddy, G. Jin, M.C. Karode, J.A. Harmony, P.H. Howe, Biochemistry, 35 (1996) 6157.
12. S. Krajewski, M. Krajewska, A. Shabaik, T. Miyashita and H.G. Wang, J.C. Reed, Amer. J. Pathol., 145 (1994) 1323.
13. A.M. Kaiser, A.K. Saluja, A. Sengupta, M. Saluja and M.L. Steer, Amer. J. Physiol., 269 (Cell Physiol. 38) (1995) C1295.

Biology of the Pancreas in Growing Animals
S.G. Pierzynowski and R. Zabielski (Editors)

Pancreatic regeneration after tissue damage

A. Dembiński and S.J. Konturek

Chair of Physiology, Collegium Medicum Jagiellonian University,
Grzegórzecka 16, 31-531 Kraków, Poland

Clinical studies of early stages of acute pancreatitis are almost impossible in practice. Most information we do have is based on experimental models. For this reason several animal models were developed to study acute pancreatitis, which at least in part, mimic the etiological factors and morphological changes observed during acute pancreatitis in humans. These models include: caerulein-induced pancreatitis, injection of ethionine, ligation of the main pancreatic duct, retrograde injection of sodium taurocholic acid into the pancreatic duct, ischaemia-reperfusion of the pancreas, intravenous L-arginine infusion and others.

It is generally assumed that an attack of acute pancreatitis with injury and loss of acinar cells is followed by full recovery of the structure and function of the exocrine pancreas. Spontaneous regeneration is observed after single and repeated episodes of pancreatitis. Endogenous and exogenous cholecystokinin (CCK) in several models of pancreatitis was shown to accelerate pancreatic regeneration after injury. The effect of epidermal growth factor (EGF) is similar to that observed after CCK administration. Overexpression of transforming growth factor-β (TGF-β) is biphasic during the course of pancreatic regeneration after damage, with early and late peaks. Pancreatic damage in the early phase of pancreatitis is due in part to the inhibition of cell proliferation, possibly mediated by TGF-β, and in the later phase due to TGF-β-stimulated EGF formation. Prolonged excitation of sensory nerves as well as the presence of their main mediator, calcitonin gene related peptide (CGRP), disturbs pancreatic regeneration after acute pancreatitis and leads to pancreatic functional insufficiency typical of chronic pancreatitis. Platelet activating factor (PAF) plays an important role in the pathogenesis of acute pancreatitis, probably by reducing the blood flow and increasing vascular permeability in the pancreas, thus delaying the regeneration of the pancreas. Hepatocyte growth factor (HGF) overexpression is observed in the course of pancreatic regeneration but its role in this process remains obscure. Secretin, the hormone involved physiologically in pancreatic bicarbonate secretion is a weak stimulant of pancreatic regeneration. Acinar cell proliferation during the late regeneration after pancreatitis is mediated, at least in part, by paracrine release of insulin-like growth factor (IGF-1) from fibroblasts. Polyamines synthesized in the pancreas during its recovery after acute pancreatitis and unspecific pancreatic injury show the ability of the tissue to regenerate with an increase in phospholipase D. However, this last effect does not seem to be directly related to polyamine metabolism in the pancreas. The mechanism whereby somatostatin has beneficial effects in pancreatitis is still not clear. The beneficial effect of somatostatin on pancreatic acinar cells after acute pancreatitis has been observed, despite the fact that it causes a decrease in the pancreatic blood flow. Nitric oxide (NO) can confer protection against the development of acute pancreatitis, probably through improvement of the pancreatic microcirculation, while lipopolysaccharide (LPS) pretreatment, as well as oxidative stress may aggravate experimental acute pancreatitis. Repeated episodes of acute pancreatitis may lead to chronic insufficiency of this organ. The process of regeneration of the endocrine pancreas varies depending on the circumstances.

Our knowledge abut regeneration of the pancreas after it is damaged is still fragmentary and further investigation is needed in this field.

1. HISTOPATHOLOGY OF THE PANCREAS AFTER DAMAGE

Most cases of pancreatic tissue damage are related to acute, and to some extent chronic pancreatitis. According to the Atlanta classification of 1992 [1] acute pancreatitis is an acute inflammatory process of the pancreas, with variable involvement of other regional tissues or remote organ systems. We have little information on lesions of the human pancreas in early mild acute pancreatitis, and in the early stages it is hard to distinguish between mild interstitial pancreatitis and severe necrotizing pancreatitis because of the progression observed in both grades of acute pancreatitis. Pancreatic necrosis can be diffuse or local and is typically associated with fat necrosis. In the mild form fat necrosis is minimal and scattered in the oedematously enlarged gland. Necrosis involves the interlobular fatty tissue. Necrosis in small veins leads to oedema, swelling and granulocytic infiltration of the wall with subsequent thrombosis and haemorrhage [2]. Acute fluid collection occurring early in the course of acute pancreatitis is located in or near the pancreas. In infectious pancreatitis, a scattered acinar cell necrosis without fat necrosis may be seen [3]. In acute necrotizing pancreatitis necrosis is seen predominantly in peripancreatic tissue, while the parenchyma of the gland is less affected. In some cases there is a discrepancy between the high degree of extraperitoneal necrosis and the comparative normality of residual portions of the pancreas. It has been suggested that the duct system is disrupted and the secretion of the surviving pancreas causes enzymatic destruction of extrapancreatic tissues, which contributes to the high mortality in the disease [4]. Necrotic areas within the pancreas usually resolve slowly and may induce interlobular fibrosis. This process has been named as the necrosis fibrosis sequence [5] and if it takes place repeatedly may evolve into chronic pancreatitis.

According to the classification of Marseille [6] chronic pancreatitis is characterized morphologically by irregular sclerosis, with destruction and permanent loss of exocrine parenchyma, which may be focal, segmental or diffuse. It can be combined with varying degrees of dilatation of the duct system. All types of inflammatory cells may be present in varying degrees, as well as, intraductal protein plugs and calculi (calcification), oedema and focal necrosis. They may be sterile or infected. It is interesting that the islets of Langerhans are relatively well preserved when compared to the degree of acinar destruction.

2. REGENERATIVE POTENTIAL OF THE PANCREAS

The phenomenon of regeneration is common in biology. In contrast to physiological regeneration involved in the normal cell turnover of various tissues, regeneration under pathophysiological conditions is always preceded by tissue damage. Cell replication to compensate for the loss of cells patterns formation in such a way as to renew the tissue architecture, and inflammation to remove the tissue debris is necessary to restore normal organ structure and function. The integration of these processes in a complex network in time and space, leading to normal tissue structure and function, is called regeneration. The resolution and outcome of fat necrosis depend on its localization and size. In mammals, only a few tissues have the ability to regenerate fully after damage. The proliferative capacity of the pancreas is low, but under the appropriate conditions, pancreatic parenchymal cells can enter the cell cycle and this can lead even to hyperplastic growth [7]. After pancreatic damage leading to loss of more than 50% of the tissue mass, replication occurs in different pancreatic cell types as a part of the regeneration process.

Small peripancreatic fat necroses resolve entirely. In larger areas that do not spontaneously dissolve, the macrophages are replaced by a thin layer of granulation tissue within 10-20 days of the onset of the disease. Subsequently the granulation tissue produces a fibrotic capsule that gradually increases in thickness and forms a visible wall. Pancreatic pseudocysts contain enzyme-rich pancreatic juice, which suggests that a connection persists to a pancreatic duct, ruptured during the acute phase of inflammation. Infections most often occur between day 4 and 20, early during the development of pseudocysts, when the liquefied areas are demarcated only by a rim of macrophages or a thin layer of granulation tissue. Some pancreatic pseudocysts, with or without a connection to the pancreatic duct, may persist without expanding or leading to symptoms.

Clinical and postmortem studies of early pancreatitis are difficult and very often impossible to perform. For this reason early damage and eventual subsequent repair is investigated mainly on experimental models which do not fully mimic changes observed in the human pancreas. It is generally accepted that in most cases the pancreas needs about one month to recover completely from acute experimental pancreatitis, which is consistent with observations in acute pancreatitis in humans. The changes in pancreatic tissue observed in experimental acute oedematous pancreatitis are shown in Figure 1. This caerulein-induced model of acute pancreatitis, initially described by Lambel and Kern [8], is typified by gross oedema, leukocyte infiltration and cell vacuolization (panel B). Twenty days later pronounced regeneration of the pancreas without signs of inflammation (panel C) is observed.

Using thin-section electron microscopy, shortly (30 minutes) after the onset of caerulein infusion, large vacuoles are observed in the Golgi area, and are later distributed throughout the cytoplasm. These vacuoles were found to be acid phosphatase-positive and to be labelled by antibodies directed against digestive zymogens [9]. These studies suggest that hyperstimulation of secretagogues with caerulein leads to the intracellular activation of digestive enzymes, and this may be an important step in the development of acute pancreatitis. In most cases these changes persist for 10 to 15 days, and the return of pancreatic enzymes to control levels in the plasma is an early sign of pancreatic tissue recovery.

3. MODELS USED TO STUDY PANCREATITIS

The list of etiological factors for acute pancreatitis is long. The most common aetiologies are biliary tract disease and alcoholism. Other aetiologies, such as, obstruction of the pancreatic duct, infections, toxins and vascular diseases are rare and in about 10%-30% of patients, the aetiology remains unknown. Several protocols have been established to induce acute experimental pancreatitis which at least in part mimic the etiological factors and morphological changes observed during acute human pancreatitis.

A   B

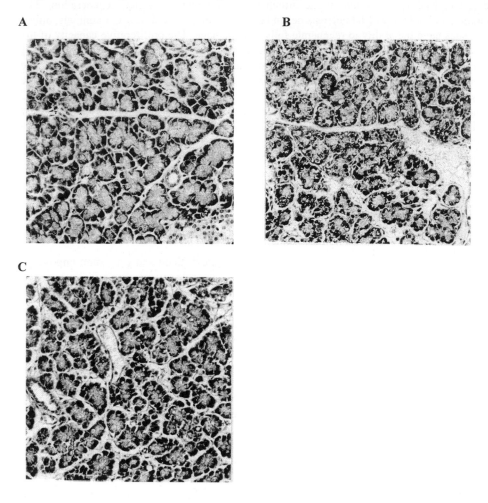

C

Figure 1. Pancreatic acinar cells of control rats (panel A), in rats infused for 6 h with caerulein (10 µg/kg/hour sc) (panel B) and in rats 20 days after pancreatitis induction (panel C).

The first model that demonstrated the regenerative ability of the pancreas was the partial pancreatectomy model [10]. In this method there is full agreement with observations on human pancreata, revealing an increased mitotic index in association with pathological alterations such as acute and chronic pancreatitis. After pancreatectomy the total mass of the organ is not restored, even after long periods of time [11], suggesting only limited regeneration of this organ. Proliferation of acinar cells is most pronounced after 90% resection but lasts only for 2 to 5 days following resection. In contrast to other models used in pancreatic regeneration studies, surgical resection is usually accompanied by a slight inflammation of the organ, particularly at the resection boundaries where regeneration in terms of cell replication is most predominant. This suggests that pancreatic tissue regeneration is correlated with inflammation and it is assumed that cytokines and growth factors secreted by inflammatory cells play an important role in the regulation of pancreatic repair.

The next model of experimental pancreatitis is caerulein-induced acute pancreatitis, described by Lambel and Kern [8] and later modified by Wood *et al.* [12]. Infusion or injection of the cholecystokinin (CCK) analogue, caerulein (an amphibian skin decapetide structurally and functionally related to CCK) over a period of 6 h leads to around 50% loss of pancreatic tissue, followed by a restoration of the organ after two weeks [13]. In this and subsequent models used in pancreatic regeneration studies inflammatory infiltration of the tissue is observed. It is of interest that pancreatic damage in the rats is completely repaired, even after repeated treatment with caerulein [13,14]. This strongly suggests that the regenerative capacity of the pancreas is high. After caerulein infusion, interlobular and intralobular oedema are observed in the tissue, accompanied by perivascular leukocyte infiltration and vacuolization, due to uncontrolled fusion of zymogen granules and the formation of autophagic vacuoles in over half of the acinar cells [13]. Pancreatic oedema and vacuolization reach a maximum immediately after caerulein infusion, whereas leukocyte infiltration reaches a peak 24 h after the end of caerulein infusion, tending to regress through the remainder of the experiment, and showing only small changes after two weeks when compared to control. Autoradiographic quantification of labelling indices demonstrates predominant incorporation of the label during the first 2 days in intralobular duct cells and periacinar fibroblasts. Labelling indices in acinar cells are not significantly elevated during the initial regenerative period, but starting on the second day they are 100-fold elevated over a period of 4 days. Pancreatic blood flow in this type of pancreatitis is strongly reduced immediately after the development of pancreatitis, followed by a significant increase.

The first model that gave basic information about experimental pancreatitis was the injection of ethionine combined with feeding a protein-free diet [15]. The disadvantage of this model was the 10-day period of induction, in which the occurrence of parenchymal cell damage, inflammation and regeneration was difficult to analyze. Regeneration is seen in this model on the second day of feeding with a standard diet, with a peak on the fifth day. The increased labelling indices in fibroblasts and inflammatory cells reaches a peak earlier than in acinar cells (on the third day). This pattern of response may be explain as an indirect effect of an inflammatory reaction of the degenerating pancreas affecting the duct and interstitial cells first, before the proper regeneration of acinar cells starts, resulting in repair of the destroyed organ [16].

Another approach to inducing pancreatic tissue damage, used by Banting and Best [17], is by ligation of the main pancreatic duct, which results in atrophy of the acinar tissue with preservation of the islets of Langerhans. An innovation of this method is partial ligation, which induces atrophy only in the occluded segment and can be used to study tissue regeneration in both the atrophic and nonatrophic portions of the pancreas [18].

Many cases of human acute pancreatitis do well with conventional therapy. However, some necrohaemorrhagic forms have a fatal outcome, and in these cases no treatment has been shown to be of value. Among the different models of pancreatitis the one based on an old Heinckel technique [19] of retrograde injection of sodium taurocholic acid into the pancreatic duct of the rat fits well with this description, because it produces a necrohaemorrhagic pancreatitis, with death of all animals within 36 h. After infusion of taurocholic acid, pancreatic necrosis was progressive and quantified. It appeared as dispersed foci of coagulative necrosis with only slight acute inflammatory infiltrate or none at all. Necrotic foci were localized in the centrilobular areas, and when confluent, only a rim of viable peripheral acini was seen. In some animals there was fat necrosis with saponification [20]. This model of pancreatitis is sometimes classified as the lethal form [21], and for this reason is useless in determination of pancreatic regeneration after damage.

The role of ischaemia in the pathogenesis of acute pancreatitis remains unclear. Microvacular perfusion failure is a hallmark of experimental and clinical pancreatitis. Ischaemia alone may not initiate pancreatic inflammation but the pancreatitis is associated with changes in pancreatic blood flow. Some studies have demonstrated that it can cause pancreatic cellular necrosis and a drop in intestinal pH [22]. There is evidence that ischaemia-reperfusion injury can produce acute pancreatitis in animal models incorporating complete pancreatic ischaemia for varying lengths of time followed by reperfusion [23]. This model of pancreatitis induces leukocyte adherence to the walls of interlobular veins, forming plaques constituting 39% of the observed venular cross-section. Leukotriene antagonists prevent leukocyte adherence. Radical scavengers also prevent the arterial constriction and leukocyte adherence to the venular endothelium observed in this model [23]. Tissue damage during ischaemia-reperfusion injury is due not only to oxygen radical production and activation of polymorphonuclear leukocytes; disturbances in calcium homeostasis are also a possible mechanism for cellular injury, as well as the release of proteolytic enzymes. As usual, the final common pathophysiological pathway is cell injury through lipid peroxidation and membrane disruption, with breakdown of the microcirculation leading to organ dysfunction. Ischaemia of 2 hours followed by reperfusion of the pancreas for 5 days led to the development of histologically verified haemorrhagic-necrotizing pancreatitis in all animals, with a mortality of 50% [24]. There is a lack of information about regeneration processes taking place in this model of pancreatitis, which is closely correlated with changes observed in the clinic.

Other models are usually a modification of those described above. In pancreatitis induced by L-arginine infusion, for example [25], which inflammation and damage are observed three days after infusion, and continuous tissue atrophy becomes visible at the site of previous pancreatic necrosis, with simultaneous regeneration of the pancreas, mainly around the Langerhans islets.

A common lesion found under a variety of pathophysiological conditions in the pancreas is the so-called tubular complex [26]. It is accepted that these structures are remnants of acinar cells, and it has been proposed that these are undifferentiated acinar cells, with the capability of proliferation and subsequent differentiation into normal acinar cells. This assumption is based on the finding that the epithelial cells of tubular complexes are partly labelled with tritiated thymidine, a finding which could not be demonstrated in another study, however [26].

4. PANCREATIC REGENERATION AFTER INJURY

4.1 Spontaneous regeneration after single and repeated episodes of acute pancreatitis

A single infusion of a supramaximal dose of caerulein decreases DNA synthesis, an index of cell proliferation, by nearly 50%. This is followed by a significant increase in DNA

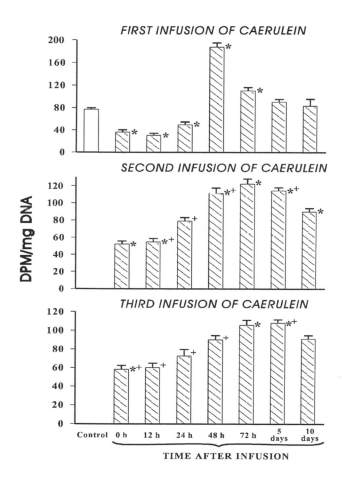

Figure 2. DNA synthesis in the rat pancreas after 1st, 2nd, and 3rd induction of pancreatitis. *p<0.05 compared to control $^{+}$p<0.05 compared to value observed after 1st infusion of caerulein.

58

synthesis 48 h later, returning to control on the fifth day (Figure 2). This increase in DNA synthesis is consistent with the observation of Wellmer *et al.* [27] who studied mitotic activity by the labelling index of [³H] thymidine and found that in acinar cells this index increased between the second and fifth day after caerulein administration. In addition they observed an enhanced activity of fibroblasts 24 h after the induction of pancreatitis. Immediately after cessation of the caerulein infusion, plasma amylase activity is significantly increased and pancreatic amylase activity is reduced by 57%. Both, plasma amylase (Figure 3) and pancreatic amylase content in this type of experimental pancreatitis are back to control after 10 days, indicating almost complete regeneration of the pancreas.

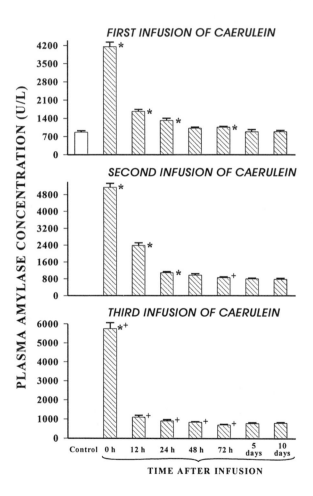

Figure 3. Plasma amylase activity in the rat pancreas after single and repeated caerulein-induced pancreatitis. *p<0.05 compared to control ⁺p<0.05 compared to value observed after 1st infusion of caerulein at the same time of observation.

At the termination of 5 h caerulein infusion, pancreatic blood flow is reduced by about 61% when compare to control rats, and this is followed by a significant increase, reaching a peak on the 5th day after pancreatitis induction (Figure 4). In these rats, a significant decrease is observed in RNA and DNA contents two days after pancreatitis development, returning to control two weeks later. Histologically, in rats infused with caerulein, the interlobular and intralobular oedema was accompanied by perivascular leukocyte infiltration and vacuolization. Pancreatic oedema and vacuolization reached a maximum immediately after infusion, whereas leukocyte infiltration reached a peak 24 h after the end of caerulein infusion, followed by regress, with only small changes on the tenth day of the experiment. Histological signs of regeneration appeared 12 h after the development of pancreatitis, reaching a peak on the third day. These results are in keeping with the morphological changes observed by others [28,29] who demonstrated that the regenerative process starts 48 h after a single caerulein infusion and is almost complete 10 days later.

Pancreatitis induced a second and third time at 10 days intervals resulted in less pronounced signs of inflammation [13]. It must be pointed out that in the presented data, one of the most accepted markers of pancreatic tissue damage, an elevation in plasma amylase activity, (Figure 3) was unexpectedly increased, with a peak at immediately after subsequent caerulein infusion. This inconsistency between pancreatic condition and plasma amylase concentration can be explained by a smaller drop in pancreatic blood flow after each consecutive induction of pancreatitis (Figure 4) and followed by an earlier increase in this parameter. The improvement in pancreatic blood flow facilitated the removal of active digestive enzymes from the pancreatic tissue and protected the pancreas against damage from these enzymes. For the same reason the initial peak of plasma amylase was followed by significantly earlier reduction in this parameter after repeated episodes of pancreatitis. Histological signs of pancreatic damage such as oedema, leukocyte infiltration and vacuolization were less pronounced when compared to the first or second administration of caerulein, but a delay was observed in the start of regeneration processes in the pancreas after each consecutive pancreatitis induction [30]. Regeneration processes were significantly less extensive, reaching their highest value 10 days after the last caerulein infusion. This may be because the damage was less pronounced after the second and third caerulein infusion, as histologically determined. It is possible that when there is less tissue damage the involvement of growth promoting factors in tissue repair is reduced, and consequently regeneration delayed. This means that repeated induction of pancreatitis leads to the development of adaptation processes, as manifested by both biochemical and histological changes; there was constant progress in these changes after each consecutive peptide infusion.

The results presented confirm findings from various laboratories [27,31], indicating that in this model of experimental pancreatitis there is reversible self-destruction of the gland followed by spontaneous regression of the inflammation and a subsequent regeneration process. The most interesting point in the data presented above is that the pancreas is able to adapt to repeated insults of acute inflammation and exhibits spontaneous regeneration.

60

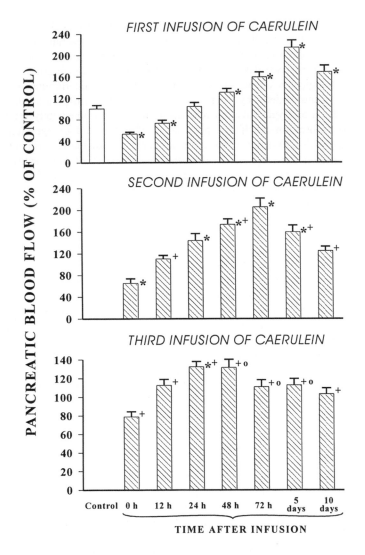

Figure 4. Pancreatic blood flow in the rat pancreas after single and repeated caerulein-induced pancreatitis. *p<0.05 compared to control $^+$p<0.05 compared to value observed after 1st infusion of caerulein at the same time of observation.

4.2 Involvement of cholecystokinin in pancreatic regeneration after acute experimental pancreatitis

Acinar cells of the adult exocrine pancreas have a relatively low resting mitotic activity [32] but under certain circumstances they can divide rapidly. These circumstances include, among the others, postnatal development [33] and responses to the administration of several hormones and peptides [34,35]. The regenerative response of the damaged pancreas is probably triggered by complex mechanisms involving gastrointestinal hormonal peptides, among which CCK seems to be the most important. During caerulein-induced pancreatitis (Figure 5) plasma amylase activity, as expected, is significantly elevated, exhibiting a

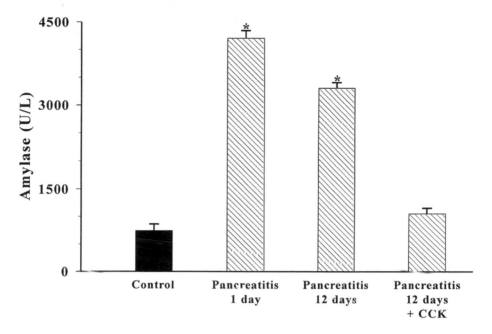

Figure 5. Amylase activity in control animals and 12 days after caerulein-induced pancreatitis in rats injected with saline or caerulein (600 ng/kg every 8 hr sc). *p<0.05 compared to control.

significant drop after 12 days but remaining above the control value. In rats injected with caerulein in therapeutic doses, 600 ng/kg every 8 hr sc, in the course of regeneration, almost full reduction of amylase to control values is observed. The described results are similar to the observations of Morisset et al. [28] who demonstrated a faster return of total pancreatic amylase content to control after caerulein-induced pancreatitis in rats injected with caerulein (1µg/kg every 8 hours); and also to the observations of Majumdar et al. [34] in ethionine-induced pancreatitis. In another model of pancreatitis induced by L- arginine [25] Hegyi et al. described how administration of low doses of cholecystokinin-octapeptide (CCK-8) increased the inflammatory signs in the early phase of pancreatitis, but subsequently diminished the level of atrophy and accelerated the processes of regeneration in this model of pancreatitis. In the results of Majumdar et al. [34], regeneration was observed 7 days after cessation of ethionine and their data relating to thymidine kinase activity are consistent with our data relating to total RNA and DNA contents after caerulein injection, exhibiting almost full restoration of the said parameters to control 12 days after caerulein-induced pancreatitis

(Figures 6 and 7). The study of Morisset *et al.*[28] presented for the first time complex data on pancreatic tissue recovery during the period lasting up to 23 days after caerulein-induced pancreatitis, and demonstrated acceleration of regeneration by endogenous release of CCK. Endogenous CCK release was achieved by feeding the animals a soya bean trypsin inhibitor. This suggests a physiological importance of endogenous CCK in regeneration processes. Furthermore, increased plasma CCK levels have been reported in chronic pancreatitis in humans [36]. In the model presented in the studies of Morisset *et al.* [28], DNA synthesis was increased by 247%, and by 306% 3 days later, and, which is very interesting, thymidine incorporation into DNA was still greater than control 40 days after the development of pancreatitis. It must also be noted that chymotrypsin seems to be an exception to this rule of tissue priority, because its content is restored to control after 3 days of rest. This rapid induction of chymotrypsin is probably the result of the induction of its gene expression [37]. Data obtained using the specific CCK receptor antagonists L364,718 and CR 1409 [38], provide strong support for the physiological role of endogenous CCK in regeneration processes. Low doses of L364,718 did not prevent regeneration but higher doses strongly inhibited spontaneous regeneration by blocking the receptors for endogenous CCK. Moreover, recently Nakano *et al.* [39] showed that exogenous caerulein administration after CCK receptor blockade by loxiglumide accelerates pancreatic tissue recovery in caerulein-induced pancreatitis. Loxiglumide, in these experiments, significantly suppressed the recovery of pancreatic weight and DNA content. When loxiglumide treatment was followed by 3 days

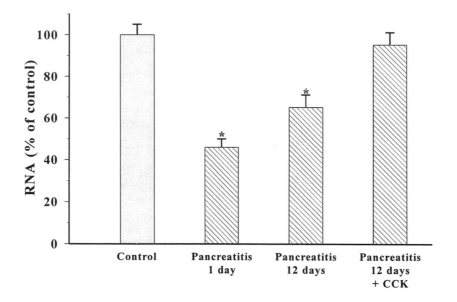

Figure 6. Total RNA level in control animals and 12 days after initiation of caerulein-induced pancreatitis in rats injected with saline or caerulein (600 ng/kg every 8 hr sc). *p<0.05 compared to control.

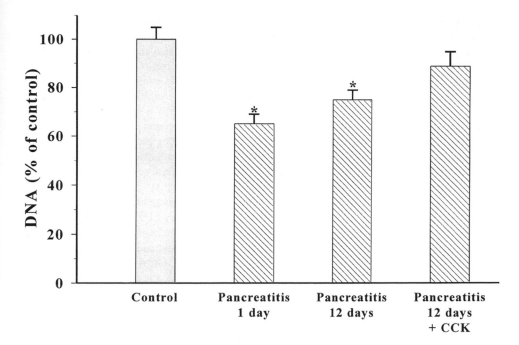

Figure 7. Total DNA level in control animals and 12 days after initiation of caerulein-induced pancreatitis in rats injected with saline or caerulein (600 ng/kg every 8 hr sc). *p<0.05 compared to control.

of CCK-8 injections, pancreatic protein and DNA content recovered to levels comparable to control. On the other hand in these experiments CCK-8 treatment had no significant influence on pancreatic enzyme contents. In 1998 Myasaka at al. [40] observed that after pancreatic duct occlusion in rats lacking CCK-A receptor gene expression, regeneration of the pancreatic tissue is retarded and there is no modification of the initial phase of acute pancreatitis.

Finally, as discussed above, data suggest that endogenous and exogenous CCK may represent efficient treatment to accelerate pancreatic regeneration in some cases of mild acute pancreatitis.

4.3 The role of epidermal growth factor (EGF) in pancreatic regeneration after acute pancreatitis

EGF a 53-amino acid single-chain polypeptide originally isolated from the submandibular glands of male mice [41], has also been found in duodenal Brunner's glands, kidneys and in several biological fluids, including saliva, milk, urine, gastric juice and duodenal juice [42,43]. Significant quantities of EGF have been noted in the human [44] and animal [45] pancreas, and in pancreatic juice. This peptide is a powerful mitogen and an inhibitor of gastric acid secretion [46]. EGF also modulates exocrine pancreatic secretion [47] as well as stimulating pancreatic growth [48], acting directly on the pancreatic acinar cells. EGF and

EGF receptor immunoreactivity have been detected in the apical surface of ductal cells and in the acinar cells of the normal pancreas and an increased expression of the EGF receptor was found in patients with acute and chronic pancreatitis [49,50]. Also in rats with caerulein-induced pancreatitis an enhanced expression of EGF and mRNA for EGF was demonstrated by immunochemistry, and RT-PCR in pancreatic tissue [51]. The stimulation of pancreatic growth by EGF is evidenced by an increase in pancreatic DNA synthesis, and nucleic acid content.

In a previous study [52], we found that EGF given before and during induction of pancreatitis protects against caerulein-evoked pancreatic damage, as evidenced by improvement of biochemical and histological parameters. Salivectomy, which is known to eliminate the major source of endogenous EGF in rats, increased the severity of pancreatitis caused by caerulein overstimulation, suggesting that a deficiency of endogenous EGF aggravates the course of pancreatitis. In caerulein-induced pancreatitis pancreatic DNA synthesis was reduced, and this was partly reversed by exogenous EGF administration. Our observation are supported by the study of Liu *et al.* [53] who demonstrated that treatment with EGF may prevent septic complication in acute necrotizing pancreatitis.

The activation of leukocytes plays a crucial role in various forms of tissue injury. In pancreatitis the activation of leukocytes was shown to be associated with a rapid production of cytokines such as Il-1, Il-6 and TNF-α, within the pancreas and systemically [54]. Il-1 is a

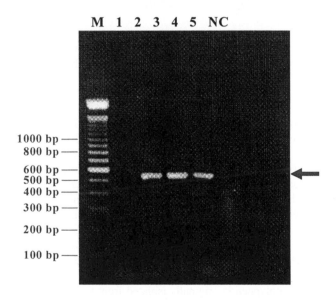

Figure 8. Expression of IL-1β in the rat pancreas during caerulein-induced pancreatitis. M.=marker: Gibco 100 bp ladder, lane 1: control rat, lane 2: 0 h, lane3: 48 h, lane 4: 5 days, lane 5: 10 days.). Similar data were obtained in other vehicle- and caerulein-infused rats.

well-known component of acute inflammation and plays a role in the induction of the release of other members of the cytokine cascade [55]. IL-1β is expressed in the rat pancreas during hormone-induced pancreatitis until the fifth day of regeneration (Figure 8). Blockade of Il-1 by use of a naturally occurring receptor antagonist almost completely eliminates the rise in serum of Il-6 and TNF-α levels and decreases the severity of experimental acute pancreatitis. As presented in Figure 9, caerulein-induced pancreatitis resulted in an increase in plasma IL-1β concentration.

Administration of EGF during pancreatitis development reduced the leukocytic infiltration in pancreatic tissue and also suppressed the cytokine cascade, as evidenced by a reduction in plasma IL-1β level. This effect is well correlated with the protective action of EGF in pancreatic tissue. This accurate correlation between serum cytokine levels and the severity of pancreatitis is in good agreement with observations in experimental and clinical studies [56]. Paradoxically salivectomy in caerulein-induced pancreatitis resulted in a decrease in plasma IL-1β concentration. This can easily be explained by significantly increased tissue damage, as evidenced by biochemical and histological findings and a substantial decrease in pancreatic blood flow, causing a very slow washout of interleukins from the damaged pancreas.

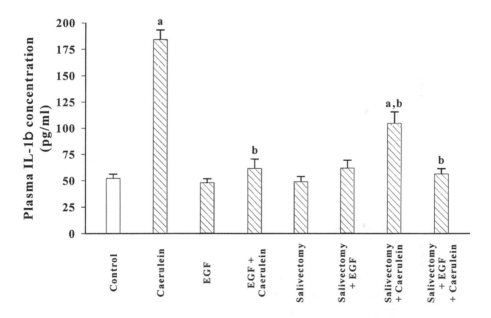

Figure 9. Effect of caerulein, salivectomy, and EGF alone or in combination on plasma IL-1β concentration in rats. [a]p<0.05 compared with control. [b]p<0.05 compared with caerulein given alone.

There is a lack of information in the literature as to whether EGF treatment after induction of pancreatitis can affect the pancreatic tissue regeneration. An answer to this question is essential before EGF can be used in the therapy for acute pancreatitis, and we are trying to answer this question in an on-going study. The mild oedematous pancreatitis induced by caerulein infusion was found to be accompanied by initial hyperaemia [57], followed by a severe reduction in pancreatic circulation [58]. As seen in Figure 10, salivectomy combined with caerulein-induced pancreatitis produced a greater and more prolonged decrease of

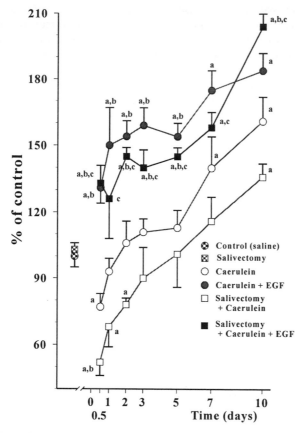

Figure 10. Pancreatic PBF in sham-operated or salivectomized rats treated during caerulein-induced pancreatitis (caerulein 10 µg/kg/h for 5 h) with placebo, or EGF (given three times daily at a dose of 10 µg/kg each). [a]P<0.05 compared with control, [b]P<0.05 compared with caerulein-induced pancrea-titis, [c]P<0.05 compared with caerulein-induced pancrea-titis combined with salivectomy.

pancreatic blood flow when compared with sham-operated rats. Exogenous EGF prevents the drop in pancreatic blood flow. A sufficient blood flow is crucial for the physiological function of the pancreas and its disturbance is involved in the pathophysiology of this organ, leading to the activation and release of lysosomal and exocrine enzymes, causing pancreatic autodigestion and the production of reactive species [59]. We conclude that in the presented data a regulatory effect of EGF on pancreatic blood flow can be observed. The major finding is that exogenous EGF reduces the damage to the pancreas after the induction of pancreatitis and accelerates the recovery of the pancreas from this damage. This is evidenced by an increase in DNA synthesis (Figure 11) induced by exogenous EGF, a decrease in DNA synthesis caused by salivectomy in rats with caerulein-induced pancreatitis, and by changes in total RNA, DNA and protein contents.

Plasma amylase activity (Figure 12) also increased following induction of pancreatitis in all groups of rats between 24 h and 3 days but later tended to return to control values. The reduction in plasma amylase activity was faster after addition of exogenous EGF, as evidenced by a significant difference in this activity after 7 and 10 days. Salivectomy tended to delay the reduction in plasma amylase activity but without reaching statistical significance

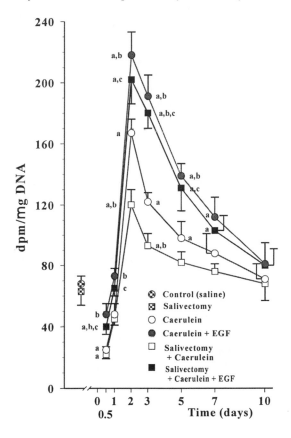

Figure 11. DNA synthesis in the same groups of rats as in Figure 10. [a]P<0.05 compared with control, [b]P<0.05 compared with caerulein-induced pancreatitis, [c]P<0.05 compared with caerulein-induced pancreatitis combined with salivectomy.

in any period tested. Histological findings are closely correlated with biochemical data showing a beneficial role of EGF in acute pancreatitis, but it should be mentioned [60] that longer (4 weeks) treatment with EGF in mature Goetingen minipigs leads to enlargement and increase in height in epithelial interlobular ductal cells of the pancreas, with accumulation of glycoconjugates in the columnal cells, which is similar to changes observed in chronic pancreatitis. Overexpression of the EGF receptor [61] in human pancreatic cancer is also associated with an increase in EGF and TGF-α levels. For these reasons the dose and duration of EGF treatment must be carefully considered. Very strong support for the importance of EGF in resolution of pancreatitis is provided by the demonstration of an EGF mRNA signal during the development of acute caerulein-induced pancreatitis (Figure 13). This seems to be a signal for the initiation of the early phase of pancreatic repair by this growth factor.

Serum IL-1β levels (Figure 14) were increased 12 h after caerulein infusion, both in sham-operated and salivectomized rats. These levels rose for three days and remained elevated above control until the 10th day after the induction of pancreatitis. The addition of EGF caused a significant reduction in the IL-1β when compare to sham-operated animals. This accurate correlation between serum cytokine level and the severity of the pancreatitis is in good agreement with observations in experimental and clinical studies made by others [56,62]. Thus the mode by which EGF action accelerates regeneration after acute pancreatitis depends, at least in part, on the suppression of the cytokine cascade, as evidenced by the reduced plasma IL-1β level.

In summary, EGF in the pancreas exhibits protective activity, similar to that observed in the stomach [63], and accelerates the regeneration of pancreatic cells.

4.4 The role of transforming growth factor-β (TGF-β) in pancreatic regeneration

TGF-βs form a family of structurally related peptides that include at least 3 distinct isoforms, termed TGF-β1, TGF-β2, TGF-β3. The growth factor TGF-β1, which is the predominant form of the TGF-β family, is considered a multifunctional cytokine, implicated in the regulation of many cellular processes including cell growth differentiation and the composition of the extracellular matrix [64]. TGF-β1 also plays an important role in tissue repair by promoting angiogenesis and stimulating the synthesis of different matrix components such as fibronectin, tensin, collagens and proteoglycans [65,66]. It simultaneously inhibits matrix degradation by decreasing the synthesis of proteases and increasing the levels of protease inhibitors. All these events may have a local effect on the tissue injury, leading to excessive scarring and fibrosis. Increased expression of TGF-β1 was reported in liver cirrhosis [67] but little is known about the role of TGF-β1 in acute pancreatitis. There are indications that TGF-β1 may play an important role at the site of tissue injury by chemotaxis of inflammatory cells. This property may have an aggravating effect on the course of acute pancreatitis. The ability to promote the deposition of cellular matrix seems to be important in subsequent events of acute pancreatitis, such as remodelling and regeneration of pancreatic tissue. Van Laethem *et al.* [68] reported that the course of acute caerulein-induced pancreatitis in mice was not influenced by TGF-β1 when this cytokine was administered systematically.

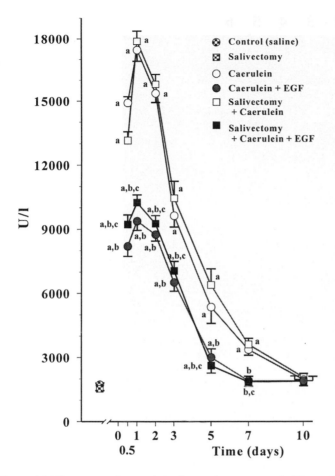

Figure 12. Plasma amylase activity in rats in groups as in Figure 10. Mean ± SEM of 8-10 observations. [a]P<0.05 compared with control, [b]P<0.05 compared with caerulein-induced pancreatitis, [c]P<0.05 compared with caerulein-induced pancreatitis combined with salivectomy.

On the other hand, Logsdon et al. [69] showed that TGF-β1 inhibits the growth of pancreatic acinar cells. Detection of TGF-β1 transcripts in early phases of pancreatitis (Figure 15), when acute oedema and neutrophil infiltration occur [51], suggests that this cytokine may be an important for the increase in vascular permeability and the accumulation of protein in oedematous pancreatic tissue as well as the observed decrease in DNA synthesis, pancreatic blood flow and the subsequent increase in plasma amylase activity [51]. It is possible that the

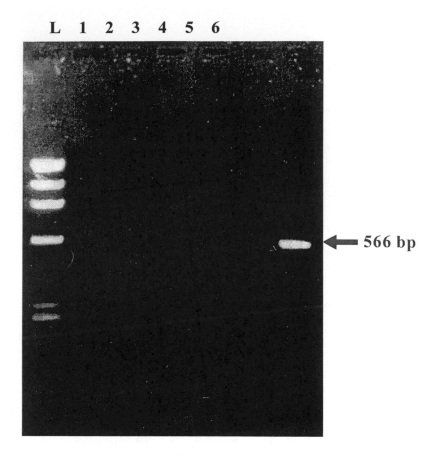

Figure 13. Typical record of RT-PCR analysis of EGF mRNA in the pancreatic tissue of intact control rats infused with saline (lane 1) and in the pancreatic tissue after 1, 2, 3, 4 and 5 h of caerulein infusion to evoke pancreatitis (lane 2-6). Similar data were obtained in other vehicle- and caerulein-infused rats.

initial expression of TGF-β1 leads to activation of the EGF gene and an increased formation in the pancreatic tissue, to stimulate the regeneration of the injured pancreas. It is interesting to note that enhanced expression of TGF-β1 was observed in humans during the course of acute pancreatitis [70], which suggests that this cytokine has a role in repair processes. This is supported by our experimental findings [71], showing that TGF-β1 in normal pancreatic tissue was present only in a few ductal cells, but immediately after the termination of caerulein infusion, during the development of pancreatitis, there was a 3-fold increase in the

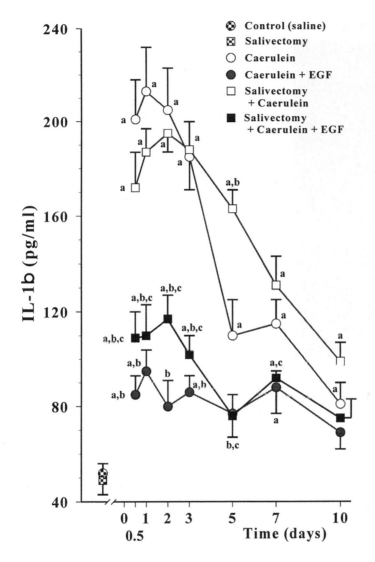

Figure 14. Plasma Il-1β concentration in rats as in Figure 10. P<0.05 compared with control,
bP<0.05 compared with caerulein-induced pancreatitis, cP<0.05 compared with caerulein-
induced pancreatitis combined with salivectomy.

number of TGF-β1 positive cells in pancreatic tissue. During the next 48 h, a further increase
in expression was observed. After 72 h there was a progressive decline in TGF-β1 expression,
followed by a marked increase on day 10 after the induction of pancreatitis. Muller Pilasch *et
al.* [72] and Menke *et al.* [73] also found that inhibition of TGF-β1 with neutralizing
antibodies only reduced the amount of stromelysin transcripts throughout the pancreatic
regeneration areas, which suggests that remodelling during pancreatic regeneration involves
the deposition of proteases that degrade the extracellular matrix, and in particular stromelysin.

L 1 2 3 4 5 6

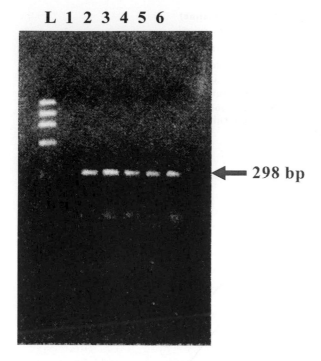

← 298 bp

Figure 15. Typical record of RT-PCR analysis of TGF-β1 mRNA in the pancreatic tissue of intact control rats infused with saline (lane 1) and in the pancreatic tissue after 1, 2, 3, 4 and 5 h of caerulein infusion to evoke pancreatitis. Similar data were obtained in other vehicle- and caerulein-infused rats.

In summary, the results presented indicate that; 1. acute pancreatitis is associated with the up-regulation of TGF-β1 transcription. 2. expression of TGF-β1 is biphasic, with an early peak and a second peak during pancreatic regeneration. 3. Pancreatic damage in the early phase of pancreatitis is probably due, in part, to an inhibition of cell proliferation mediated by TGF-β1. 4. In the later phase, an enhanced expression of TGF-β1 stimulates the synthesis of extracellular matrix components. In caerulein-induced pancreatitis, the repair of pancreatic acinar and duct cells occurs as a consequence of earlier expression of EGF.

4.5 Role of sensory nerves and calcitonin gene-related peptide (CGRP) in protection and regeneration of pancreatic tissue

The function of primary sensory neurons is to receive and transmit information from the external and internal environment and thereby contribute to maintenance of homeostasis. The excitation of thin, unmyelinated sensory nerves is followed not only by conduction of nerve activity to the central nervous system but also by the release of neuromediators from the activated peripheral endings themselves, and this process is the basis for a local "axon reflex"[74]. Thin, unmyelinated sensory fibres have a special sensitivity to capsaicin [75].

Low doses of capsaicin result in the stimulation of sensory nerves, accompanied by the release of CGRP and other neuromediators [75-77], whereas high doses of capsaicin lead to ablation of sensory nerves, with a decrease in plasma and tissue levels of CGRP [78-79]. The stimulation of sensory fibres as well as the administration of exogenous CGRP were found to exert a protective effect in different experimental models of gastric ulcer [80-82], whereas the ablation of sensory nerves aggravated gastric mucosal lesions induced by various ulcerogenic factors [83-84], and prolonged healing of gastric ulcers [85].

We found capsaicin and CGRP to have a similar effect in the pancreas. Activation of sensory nerves [86] or treatment with CGRP [87] before and during induction of acute pancreatitis by caerulein attenuated the pancreatic damage, whereas deactivation of sensory nerves aggravated the severity of the pancreatitis. Stimulation of sensory nerves reduced pancreatic oedema, which was seen as a limitation of the increase in pancreatic weight and protein content. That there was less damage to the pancreatic tissue was also evidenced by higher DNA synthesis and a reduction in plasma amylase activity. Vasodilatation and preservation of the pancreatic blood flow play an important role in the beneficial effect of sensory nerve stimulation on the pancreatic tissue. Our study showed that activation of sensory nerves increases pancreatic blood flow and reduces activation of neutrophils, as measured by rosette formation. Neutrophils play a crucial role in various forms of tissue damage [88]. After activation they adhere to the vascular endothelium and contribute to tissue injury by reducing blood flow via occlusion of microvessels, and by releasing noxious mediators. Pretreatment with CGRP before induction of acute pancreatitis results in an effect on pancreatic tissue similar to that of sensory nerve stimulation by low doses of capsaicin [87]. Morphological features and biochemical parameters showed improvement in the condition of the pancreas, whereas deactivation of sensory nerves contributed to an increased severity of the acute pancreatitis. Histological examination revealed interlobular oedema in all cases, and severe intralobular oedema in almost all animals. Leukocytic infiltration and vacuolization of acinar cells were also pronounced in animals with deactivated sensory nerves and induced pancreatitis [87]. The deleterious effect on the pancreatic tissue of ablation of sensory nerves during the development of caerulein-induced pancreatitis was completely reversed by pretreatment with exogenous CGRP, and the pancreatic condition was even better than after caerulein given separately [87].

In contrast to the protective effects on pancreatic tissue of CGRP administration before and during the induction of acute pancreatitis, treatment with CGRP after the induction of acute pancreatitis aggravated pancreatic damage [52]. Pancreatic cell proliferation was decreased, leading to a decrease in DNA synthesis (Figure 16); and the pancreatic blood flow was reduced (Figure 17), whereas the plasma interleukin-1β concentration (Figure 18) was maximally increased. The plasma amylase activity (Figure 19) was higher than in the group treated with caerulein alone, but a significant difference was found only between animals treated with CGRP before and after caerulein infusion. This dual effect of CGRP on the course of caerulein-induced pancreatitis seems to be mainly dependent on CGRP-evoked vascular dilatation and the severity of the microvascular damage. CGRP is known to be a potent vasodilator [89,90] and its administration, before and during infusion in our study prevented the decrease in pancreatic blood flow. The improvement in pancreatic circulation before vascular damage reduced pancreatic ischaemia and allowed the removal of active

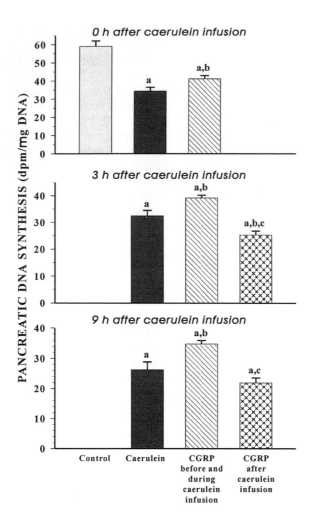

Figure 16. Effect on DNA synthesis in the pancreas of CGRP given before and during or after caerulein infusion. [a]P<0.05 compared with control, [b]P<0.05 compared with caerulein given alone at the same time of observation, [c]P<0.05 compared with animals treated with CGRP before and during caerulein infusion at the same time of observation.

digestive enzymes and mediators of inflammation from the pancreatic tissue, leading to a reduction in pancreatic damage. On the other hand, caerulein-induced pancreatitis led to tissue and vascular damage and for this reason administration of vasodilators such as CGRP increased plasma protein leakage from injured vessels to the pancreatic tissue, causing pancreatic oedema, a reduction in pancreatic blood flow and an increase in pancreatic ischaemia. These findings are in agreement with studies performed Cambridge *et al.* [91] and Newbold *et al.* [92] who found that treatment with CGRP enhances the effect of mediators increasing vascular permeability, leading to the production of oedema. Moreover there is a growing amount of evidence suggesting that CGRP released from unmyelinated afferent sensory nerves may cause neurogenic inflammation [93] and can contribute to a chronic inflammatory response [94].

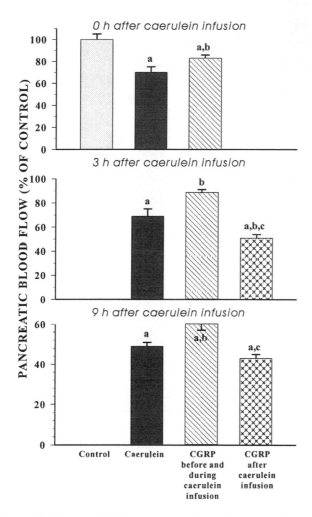

Figure 17. Effect of CGRP given before and during or after caerulein infusion on pancreatic blood flow. [a]P<0.05 compared with control, [b]P<0.05 compared with caerulein given alone at the same time of observation, [c]P<0.05 compared with animals treated with CGRP before and during caerulein infusion at the same time of observation.

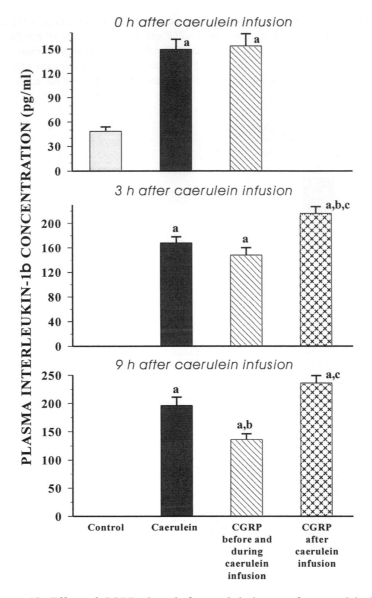

Figure 18. Effect of CGRP given before and during or after caerulein infusion on plasma interleukin-1β concentration. [a]P<0.05 compared with control, [b]P<0.05 compared with caerulein given alone at the same time of observation, [c]P<0.05 compared with animals treated with CGRP before and during caerulein infusion at the same time of observation.

Foci of chronic inflammatory cells are a common component in the pancreas in chronic pancreatitis. Some of them are closely associated with nerves, causing damage to the perineurium and removing the barrier that separates the inner compartment of the nerve from the surrounding tissue [95]. Moreover, in chronic pancreatitis, a remarkable increase in the density and staining intensity of CGRP, VIP and NPY immunoreactive fibres has been observed in clinical [96] as well as experimental [97] studies. These data prompted us to study whether administration of CGRP or stimulation of sensory nerves after repeated episodes of acute pancreatitis was able to affect pancreatic regeneration. Five episodes of acute caerulein-induced pancreatitis were induced with an interval of one week between each, and two weeks after the last induction a morphological and biochemical examination of the pancreata was performed. The pancreata of control animals receiving placebo showed almost full recovery and no significant difference was found between them and intact animals. In rats treated with stimulatory doses of capsaicin, regeneration of the pancreata was delayed. Pancreatic DNA synthesis was decreased, as was pancreatic amylase (Figure 20) and faecal chymotrypsin activity (Figure 21). A similar but less pronounced effect was observed after administration of CGRP. These results suggest that prolonged activity of sensory nerves, as well as the presence of their main mediator, CGRP, disturbs the pancreatic regeneration after acute pancreatitis and leads to the pancreatic functional insufficiency typical of chronic pancreatitis.

4.6 Other factors influencing pancreatic tissue injury and regeneration after acute pancreatitis

It has been reported [98] that pancreatic acinar cells, when stimulated by caerulein or cholecystokinin, release a substantial amount of platelet activating factor (PAF). PAF is a low-molecular-weight phospholipid exhibiting potent biological effects, including platelet and neutrophil aggregation, systemic hypotension and capillary leakage [99], leading to haemorrhagic damage in the gastrointestinal tract. Emanueli *et al.* [100] reported that an injection of PAF into the superior pancreaticoduodenal artery induced changes in the rabbit pancreas characteristic of acute pancreatitis. In our study [58] we observed that exogenous PAF injected intraperitoneally inhibited the pancreatic blood flow to the same extent as in caerulein-induced pancreatitis. Pretreatment with TCV-309, a specific PAF blocker [101], before caerulein infusion significantly reduced the drop in pancreatic blood flow (Figure 22). Plasma amylase activity was significantly increased after caerulein or PAF administration. Pretreatment with TCV-309 diminished this increase to some extent (Figure 23). TCV-309 pretreatment before administration of PAF almost completely prevented the alterations in pancreatic weight and protein content caused by PAF. The pancreas appeared normal, and histologically only slight oedema and cellular infiltration or acinar cell vacuolization were noticed. These results indicate that PAF plays an important role in the pathogenesis of acute pancreatitis, probably by reducing the blood flow and increasing vascular permeability in the pancreas. In the same way, this factor is able to delay regeneration of the pancreas after injury.

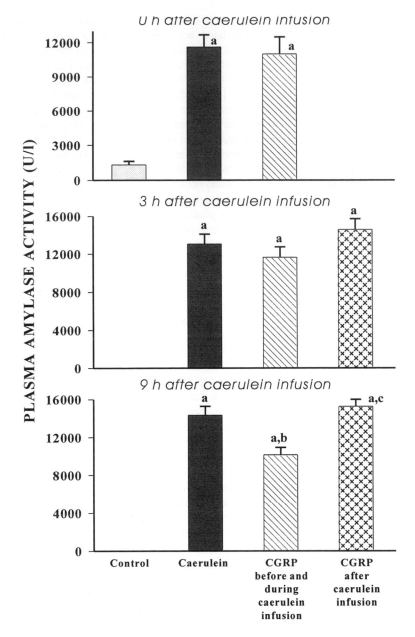

Figure 19. Effect of CGRP given before and during or after caerulein infusion on plasma amylase activity. [a]P<0.05 compared with control, [b]P<0.05 compared with caerulein given alone at the same time of observation, [c]P<0.05 compared with animals treated with CGRP before and during caerulein infusion at the same time of observation.

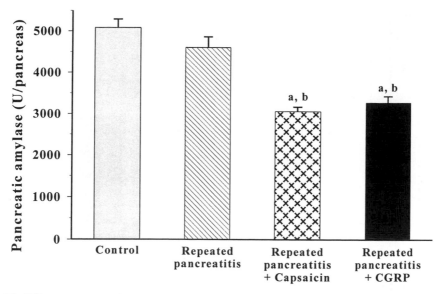

Figure 20. Effect on pancreatic amylase activity of sensory nerve stimulation by capsaicin and administration of CGRP during pancreatic regeneration after repeated induction of acute pancreatitis. [a]$P<0.05$ compared with control, [b]$P<0.05$ compared with repeated pancreatitis alone.

Hepatocyte growth factor (HGF) is a 97-kDa heterodimer originally identified in the serum of various species on the basis of its capacity to stimulate hepatocyte proliferation [102]. HGF stimulates the proliferation of keratinocytes, biliary duct epithelial cells, melanocytes, and endothelial cells, but it does not affect fibroblast proliferation [103,104]. HGF was shown to be a potent mitogen for normal human pancreatic cells *in vitro* [104] which suggested that this substance may play a physiological role in pancreatic growth. Overexpression of HGF was observed between the fifth and seventh day after caerulein-induced pancreatitis [105]. In contrast, fibroblast growth factor-2 expression was increased between the first and third day after pancreatitis development and in these experiments TGF-α exhibited the most prolonged overexpression. These results indicate that the highly coordinated process of regeneration after pancreatitis may be influenced by a sequential induction and expression of peptide growth factors and their receptors. Ueda *et al.* determined serum levels of HGF, C-reactive protein (CRP) and IL-6 at the time of admission in humans with acute pancreatitis. HGF was as useful as CRP and more than IL-6 for detection of severe pancreatitis and for predicting hepatic dysfunction [106]. Actually HGF is under clinical evaluation in patients with gastrointestinal and pancreatic diseases [107] but its role in regeneration processes in the pancreas after pancreatitis remains obscure. It is interesting that CCK-receptor antagonists such as proglumide and benzotript had a strong effect on caerulein-induced necrotizing pancreatitis in mice [108]. Both antagonists had a protective effect, even when they were injected after caerulein. In comparison to CCK-receptor antagonists, secretin had a lesser

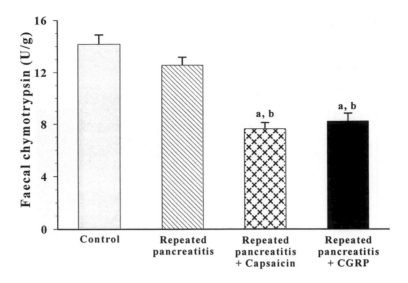

Figure 21. Effect on faecal chymotrypsin activity of sensory nerve stimulation by capsaicin and administration of CGRP during pancreatic regeneration after repeated induction of acute pancreatitis. [a]P<0.05 compared with control, [b]P<0.05 compared with repeated pancreatitis alone.

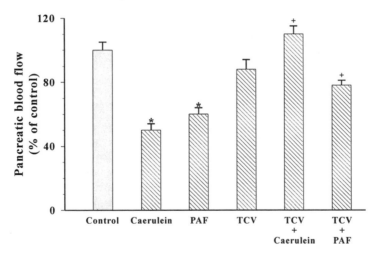

Figure 22. Pancreatic blood flow of rats infused for five hours with saline, caerulein (10 μg/kg/h sc), platelet activating factor (50 μg/kg/h ip), TCV-309 (50 μg/kg/h ip), or a combination of TCV-309 plus caerulein or platelet activating factor. Asterisk indicates effect on caerulein-induced pancreatitis regarding serum amylase concentration and pancreatic weight.significant decrease below the control value. Cross indicates significant increase above the value obtained with caerulein or platelet activating factor.

Similarly, the histological changes in pancreatitis after secretin injections were only slightly ameliorated. Taking electron microscopic studies [108] into consideration as well, it can be concluded that secretin, the hormone involved physiologically in pancreatic secretion, is a weak stimulant of pancreatic regeneration.

Pancreatic regeneration after caerulein-induced pancreatitis is characterized by transient fibroblast proliferation followed by replication of the acinar cells. The mechanism that coordinates regeneration is incompletely understood. Insulin-like growth factor 1 (IGF-1) mRNA levels increased over 50-fold during regeneration after acute pancreatitis [109], reaching a maximum on the second day. Immunohistochemically, IGF-1 was localized in

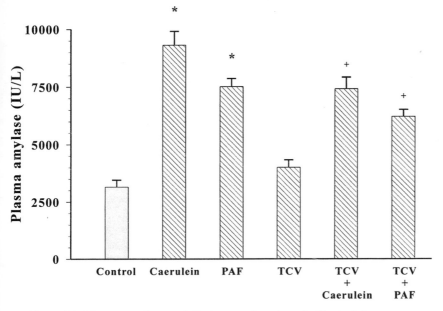

Figure 23. Plasma amylase activity in experiments as in Figure 16.

fibroblasts within the areas of interstitial tissue. Possible paracrine regulation was confirmed by stimulation of acinar cell proliferation with fibroblast-conditioned medium, which was partially inhibited by an IGF-1 antagonist. In addition, Menke *et al.* [105] found that IGF-1 mRNA is overexpressed during pancreatic regeneration but down-regulated in the normal adult pancreas. It can be concluded that acinar cell proliferation during the late regeneration after pancreatitis is mediated at least in part by paracrine release of IGF-1 from fibroblasts.

The importance of polyamines in pancreatic tissue growth and regeneration was shown by Jurkowska *et al.* [110]. Treatment with the inhibitor of polyamine synthesis alpha-difluoromethyl ornithine (DFMO) during induction of pancreatitis did not worsen the tissue damage. However, when this treatment was prolonged up to 14 days during the recovery period after pancreatic injury the spontaneous regeneration tested biochemically and histologically was reduced. In rats with acute pancreatitis treated with DFMO during 14 days, lower pancreatic weight and RNA content, which are signs of microscopic injury, correspond to an increased phospholipase D activity. These results indicate the involvement of polyamines in pancreatic recovery after acute pancreatitis and unspecified pancreatic injury with an increase in phospholipase D. However, this last effect does not seem to be directly related to polyamine metabolism in the pancreas, as there was a lack of effect of DFMO on phospholipase D activity in an *in vitro* study.

The mechanism whereby somatostatin has beneficial effects in pancreatitis is still not clear. The studies of Rodriguez *et al.* [111] give indirect evidence for the importance of this peptide in pancreatic regeneration. In a pancreaticobiliary duct ligation model of experimental pancreatitis they found a beneficial effect of somatostatin, but not due to a direct action of this peptide on pancreatic acinar cells. It must be noted that somatostatin decreases the pancreatic blood flow, which is one of the most important factors involved in augmentation of acute pancreatitis. Therefore the beneficial role of somatostatin is questionable.

Transgenic mice bearing the INF-γ gene expressed in the pancreatic islets exhibit a remarkable pattern of damage, proliferation, and differentiation in the pancreas [112]. INF-γ mice are characterized by inflammation-induced islet cell loss concomitant with hyperglycaemia and duplication of various stages of insulin-dependent diabetes mellitus [113]. Unlike most islet destruction accompanying pathological conditions, however, islet cells in INF-γ mice have a unique capacity to regenerate from proliferating ducts. The exocrine components adjacent to islets become filled with small ductules and often seem to arise from differentiated acini. The ductules exhibit hyperplasia and become surrounded by nests of fibroblasts. These changes resemble some of those observed in chronic pancreatitis [114]. Studies on the regenerating pancreas of γ-interferon transgenic mice [113] provided important evidence that supports the role of INF-γ and cytokines released by activated macrophage in the regulation of TGF-α and EGF-receptor-mediated pathways.

Nitric oxide (NO) has been shown to play a significant role in inflammation. To clarify the role of NO in acute pancreatitis the serum concentration of NO_x (NO_2^- plus NO_3^-) and TNF-α was investigated, and the grade of pancreatitis in caerulein-induced pancreatitis in mice pretreated with lipopolysaccharide (LPS) or not [115]. LPS pretreatment aggravated the pancreatitis in association with a transient increase in serum TNF-α, which was followed by a gradual increase in NO. This elevation in NO concentration was inhibited by NO synthase inhibitor (L-NNA). L-NNA increased serum amylase activity, a marker of pancreatitis severity. The effects of L-NNA were reversed by L-arginine, an NO donor. These results suggest the involvement of NO in the resolution of acute pancreatitis. This is supported by the study of Liu *et al.* [116], showing that NO could confer protection against the development of haemorrhagic pancreatitis, probably through improvement of the pancreatic microcirculation. It must be also noted that LPS causes the release of pancreatic phospholipase A_2 into blood plasma, the activation of phospholipase A_2 in pancreatic tissue and stimulates apoptosis of acinar cells [117].

Pancreatic oxidative stress with depletion of pancreatic glutathione is an early feature in all tested models of acute pancreatitis [118]. Therefore it was important to find evidence of oxidative stress in human acute pancreatitis by analyzing blood samples. Brangaza *et al.* [119] showed that oxidative stress pervades the vascular compartment in patients with acute pancreatitis, and in these patients a significant reduction in ascorbic acid, selenium, β-carotene and other antioxidants was shown.

Repeated episodes of acute pancreatitis may lead to chronic insufficiency of this organ. Chronic pancreatitis is morphologically characterized, among other things, by destruction and permanent loss of exocrine parenchyma. This permanent loss of cells excludes any significant ability of the pancreas to regenerate. Moreover, these changes may be associated with dilatation of segments of the duct system. Slater *et al.* [120] performed studies to determine whether pancreatic parenchymal epithelial cells in human chronic pancreatitis tissues retain a biologically significant capability to proliferate. Using an *in vitro* labelling method with bromodeoxyuridine and conventional immunohistochemistry it was shown that the loss of parenchymal epithelium occurring in chronic pancreatitis is not caused by a primary failure of pancreatic "stem cell" proliferation but is due to disproportional attrition of differentiated parenchymal epithelial cells by a mechanism, possibly stromal in origin, which remains unidentified.

All the changes described above in acute pancreatitis and subsequent regeneration processes were related to the exocrine pancreas. The proliferative capacity of adult pancreatic islet cells is limited [121], although the formation of new islets from cells associated with the ductal epithelium is achievable, even in the adult gland. Neogenesis-associated proteins were found to be expressed early in the neogenic process, before the ductal cell proliferation. It is interesting that beta-cell regeneration after 48-h glucose infusion in mildly diabetic rats is not correlated with functional improvement [122]. Using immunolabelling techniques Woolfe-Coote *et al.* [123] showed that PP and somatostatin occurred during development before glucagon, and a noticeable increase in duct cell proliferation and endocrine cell volume but no increased replication of endocrine cells was observed during regeneration processes. In contrast, in a mouse experimental model with destruction of pancreatic beta-cells [124] the ability of beta cell to regenerate was demonstrated, occurring mostly through the proliferation of pre-existing intra-islet beta-cells. In conclusion, the regeneration processes of the endocrine pancreas varied according to the circumstances.

These various avenues of investigation have greatly enhanced our knowledge about processes of damage and regeneration in pancreatitis, but our knowledge is still fragmentary and further investigation is needed in this field.

REFERENCES

1. E.L. Bradley III, Arch. Surg., 128 (1993) 586.
2. G. Klöppel and E.L. Bradley III. (eds.), Acute pancreatitis: Diagnosis and Therapy. Raven Press, New York, 1994.
3. A.B Jensin, H.S Rossenberg and A.L Notkins, Lancet, 2 (1980) 354.
4. N. Maclean, Brit. J. Surg., 64 (1977) 345.
5. G. Klöppel and B Maillet, Virchows Arch., 420 (1992) 1.
6. M.W. Singer, K. Gyr and H. Sarles, Gastroenterology, 89 (1985) 683.
7. A. Dembiñski and L.R. Johnson, Endocrinology, 105 (1979) 769.
8. M. Lambel and G.F. Kern, Virchows Arch., 373 (1977) 97.
9. O. Watanabe, F.M. Baccino, M. L. Steer and J. Meldolesi, Amer. J. Physiol., 246 (1984) G457.
10. E. Di Mattei, Giornale Reale Acad. Med. Torino Ser., 3 (1985) 476.

11. M. Lehy, P.J. Fitzgerald, Am. J. Pathol., 53 (1968) 513.
12. J. Wood, R. Garcia and T.E. Solomon, Gastroenterology 82 (1982) 1213.
13. A. Dembiñski, Z. Warzecha , P.Ch. Konturek, P. Ceranowicz and S.J. Konturek,
14. R. Tomaszewska and J. Stachura, J. Physiol. Pharmacol., 47 (1996) 455.
15. H.P. Elsasser, D. Puplat, G. Adler and H.F. Kern, Cell tissue Res., 262 (1990) 143.
16. P.J Fitzgerald, In: R.J. Gross (eds.) Regulation of organ and tissue growth, New York, Academic Press, 1972.
17. P.J Fitzgerald, K. Vinijchaikul, B. Carol and L. Rosenstock, Am. J. Pathol., 52 (1968) 1039.
18. P.G. Banting and C.H. Best, Amer. J. Physiol., 59 (1922) 479.
19. G.T Hultquist, V. Karlsson, A.C. Hallner, Exp. Pathol., 17 (1979) 44.
20. K. Heinkel, Klin. Wochenschr., 31 (1995) 815.
21. J.C. Rueda, L. Ortega, J.M. Arguello, A.J. Torres, I. Landa and J.L. Balibrea, Virchows Arch., 23 (1991) 117.
22. H.J. Aho, M. L. Konkensalo and T.L. Nevalainen, Scand. J. Gastroenterol.,15, (1980) 411.
23. M.T. Toyama, M.P.N. Levis, A.M. Kusske, A.M. Reber, S.W. Ashley and H.A. Reber, Scand. J. Gastroenterol., 219 (1996) 20.
24. K. Kusterer, T. Poschmann, A. Friedman, M. Enghofer, S. Zendler and K.H. Usadler, Amer. J. Physiol., 265 (1993) G165.
25. T.F. Hoffmann, R. Leiderer, A.G. Harris and K. Messmer, Microsc. Res. Tech., 37 (1997) 557.
26. P. Hegyi, T. Tajas, K. Jarmay, I. Nagy, L. Cako and J. Lonovics, Int. J. Pancreatol., 22 (1997) 193.
27. S. Willemer, H.P. Elsasser, H.F. Kern and G. Adler, Pancreas, 2 (1997) 669.
28. S. Willemer, H.P. Elsasser and G. Adler, Eur. Surg Res., 24 (1994) 29.
29. G. Jurkowska, G. Grondin, S. Masse and J. Morisset, Gastroenterology, 102 (1992)550.
30. C.W. Imre, Gastroenterology, 10 (1994) 496.
31. R. Tomaszewska, A. Dembiñski, Z. Warzecha, S.J. Konturek, P. Ceranowicz, P.K. Konturek and J. Stachura, Pol. J. Pathol., 48 (1997) 95.
32. G. Adler, T. Hupp and H.F. Kern, Virchows Arch., 382 (1979) 31.
33. C.P. Leblond and B.E Walker, Physiol. Rev., 36 (1956) 255.
34. T.E. Solomon and L.R. Johnson (eds.), Physiology of gastrointestinal tract, New York, Raven Press, 1981.
35. A.P.N. Majumdar, G.D. Vesenka and M.A. Dubick, Pancreas, 2 (1987) 199.
36. A.B. Dembiñski and L.R. Johnson, Endocrynology, 106 (1980) 323.
37. A. Schafmayer, H.D. Backer, M. Werner, U.R. Folsh and W. Creutzfeldt, Digestion, 32 (198) 36.
38. S. Rosiewicz, V.H. Levan and R.A. Liddle, Amer. J. Physiol., 251 (1986) G70.
39. G. Jurkowska, G. Grondin and J. Morisset, Pancreas, 7 (1992) 295.
40. S. Nakano, Y. Kihara and M. Otsuki, Pancreas, 16 (1998) 169
41. K. Miyasaka, M. Ohta, K. Tateishi, A. Jimi and A. Funakoshi, Pancreas, 16 (1998) 114.
42. S. Cohen, J. Biol. Chem., 237 (1962) 1555.
43. H.S. Gregory, C.R. Walsh and C.R. Hopkins, Gastroenterology, 77 (1979) 315.
44. A.G. Kaselberg, D.N. Orth, M.E. Gray and M.T. Stahlnan, Pancreas, 33 (1985) 315.

45. Y. Hirata and D.N. Orth, Clin. Endoc. Metabol., 48 (1979) 667.
46. J. Jaworek, S.J. Konturek, W. Bielański, J. Bilski and M. Hładij, Int. J. Pancreatol., 11 (1992) 9.
47. A. Dembiński, D. Drozdowicz, H. Gregory, S.J. Konturek and Z. Warzecha, J. Physiol., 278 (1986) 347.
48. S.J. Konturek, J. Jaworek, T. Brzozowski and H. Gregory, Amer. J. Physiol., 246 (1984) G580.
49. A. Dembiński, H. Gregory, S.J. Konturek and M. Polański, J. Physiol., 325 (1982) 35.
50. M. Korc, H. Friess, Y. Yamanaka, M.S. Kobrin, M. Büchler and H.G. Berger, Gut, 35, (1994) 1468.
51. M. Ebert, H. Freiss, M.W. Büchler and M. Korc, Dig. Dis. Sci., 40 (1995) 2134.
52. P.Ch. Konturek, A. Dembiński, Z. Warzecha, P. Ceranowicz, S.J. Konturek, J. Stachura and E.G. Hahn, J. Physiol. Pharmacol., 48 (1997) 59.
53. Z. Warzecha, A. Dembiński, P. Ch. Konturek, P. Ceranowicz, S.J. Konturek and J. Stachura, R. Tomaszewska, J. Physiol. Pharmacol., 50 (1999) 49.
54. Q. Liu, G. Djuricin, C. Nathan, P. Gatusso, R.A. Weinstein and R.A. Prinz, J. Surg. Res., 69 (1997) 171.
55. J. Norman, M. Franz, A. Riker, P.J. Fabri and W.R. Gower, Surg. Forum, 45 (1994) 148.
56. A. Kingsnorth, Gut, 40 (1997) 1.
57. D.L. Helath, D.H. Cruickshank, A. Jehanli, A. Shenkin, C.W. Imrie, Pancreas, 66 (1993) 41.
58. W. Trudo Knofel, N. Kollias, A.L. Warshaw, H. Waldner, N.S. Nishioka and D.W. Rattner, Surgery, 116 (1994) 904.
59. S.J. Konturek, A. Dembiński, P.J. Konturek, Z. Warzecha, J. Jaworek, P. Gustaw, R. Tomaszewska and J. Stachura, Gut, 33 (1992) 1268.
60. H. Waldner, Eur. Surg. Res., 24 (1992) 62.
61. L. Vinter-Jensen, C.O. Juhl, P.S. Teglbjærg, S.S. Poulsen, E.Z. Dajani and E. Nexo, Gastroenterology, 113 (1997) 1367.
62. M. Korc, B. Chandrasekar, Y. Yamanaka, H. Friess, M. Büchler and H.G. Berger, J. Clin. Invest., 90 (1992) 1352.
63. H.P. Greval, K. Malak, A.M. El Din, M. Ohman, A. Salem, L. Gabor and A.O. Gabor, Surgery, 115 (1994) 213.
64. P.Ch. Konturek, S.J. Konturek, T. Brzozowski and H. Ernst, Eur. J. Gastroenterol. Hepatol., 7 (1995) 933.
65. D.M. Kingsley, Gen. Dev., 8 (1994) 133.
66. J.A. Bernard, R.M. Lyons and H.L. Moses, Biophys. Acta, 1032 (1990) 79.
67. R.A. Ignotz, J. Massague, J. Biol. Chem., 263 (1986) 3039.
68. M.J. Czaja, F.R. Weiner and K.C. Flanders, J. Cel. Biol., 108 (1989) 2477.
69. J.L. Van Leathem, P. Robberecht and A. Resibois, J. Deviers, Gastroenterology, 110 (1996) 476.
70. C.D. Logsdon, L. Keyes and R.D. Beauchamp, Amer. J. Physiol., 262 (1992) G364.
71. H. Friess, Z. Lu, E. Riesle, W. Uhl, A.M. Bründler, L. Horvath, L.I. Gold, M. Korc and M.W. Büchler, Ann. Surg., 227 (1998) 95.
72. P.Ch. Konturek, A. Dembiński, Z. Warzecha, A. Ihlm, P. Ceranowicz, S. J. Konturek, J. Stachura and E.G. Hahn, Digestion, 59 (1998) 110.
73. F. Müller Pillasch, T.M. Gress, H. Yamaguchi, M. Geng and G. Adler, Pancreas, 15 (1997) 168.

74. A. Menke, H. Yamaguchi, T. M. Gress and G. Adler, Gastroenterology, 113 (1997) 295.
75. P. Holzer, Pharmacol. Rev., 43 (1991) 143.
76. J. Ren, R.L. Young, D.C. Lassiter and RF Harty, Gastroenterology, 104 (1993) 485.
77. P. Holzer, B.M. Peskar, B.A. Peskar and R. Amann, Neurosci. Lett., 108 (1990) 195.
78. J.R. Grider, Amer. J. Physiol., 266 (1994) G1139.
79. S.J. Wimalawansa, Peptides, 14 (1993) 247.
80. C. Sternini, J.R. Reeve jr and N. Brecha, Gastroenterology, 93 (1987) 852.
81. P. Holzer and I.T.Lippe, Neuroscience, 27 (1988) 981.
82. P. Holzer, M.A. Pabst and I.T. Lippe, Gastroenterology, 96 (1989) 1425.
83. G. Clementi, M. Amico-Roxas, A. Caruso, V.M. Cutuli and S. Maugeri, Prato A, Eur. J. Pharmacol., 238 (1993) 101.
84. T. Brzozowski, S.J. Konturek, J. Pytko-Poloñczyk and Z. Warzecha, Scand. J. Gastroenterol., 30 (1995) 6.
85. J. Szolcsányi and L. Barthó, In: Gastrointestinal Defense Mechanisms, G. Mózsik, O. Hänninen and T. Jávor (eds.), Pergamon Press and Akadémiai Kiadó, Oxford and Budapest, 1981.
86. K. Takeuchi, K. Ueshima, T. Ohuchi and S. Okabe, Gastroenterology, 106 (1994) 1524.
87. A. Dembiñski, Z. Warzecha, P.Ch. Konturek, P Ceranowicz and S.J. Konturek, Int. J. Pancreatol., 19 (1996) 179.
88. Z. Warzecha, A. Dembiñski, P. Ceranowicz, P.Ch. Konturek, J. Stachura, S.J. Konturek and J. Niemiec, J. Physiol. Pharmacol., 48 (1997) 775.
89. P.H. Guth and Yale J. Biol. Med., 65 (1992) 677.
90. S.D. Brain, T.J. Williams, J.R. Tippins, H.R. Morris and I. MacIntyre, Nature, 313 (1985) 54.
91. P. Holzer and P.H. Guth, Circ. Res., 68 (1991) 100.
92. H. Cambridge and S.D. Brain, Brit. J. Pharmacol., 106 (1992) 746.
93. P. Newbold and S.D. Brain, Brit. J. Pharmacol., 108 (1993) 705.
94. L.A. Chahl, Pharmacol. Ther., 37 (1988) 275.
95. E.A. Mayer, H. Raybould and C. Koelbel, Dig. Dis. Sci., 33 (1988) 71S.
96. D.E. Bockman, in Diagnostic procedures in pancreatic disease, P. Malfertheiner, J.E. Domínguez-Muñoz, H.-U. Schulz and H. Lippert, (eds.), Springer-Verlag, Berlin-Heidelberg, 1997.
97. M. Büchler, E. Weihe, H. Friess, P. Malfertheiner, E. Bockman, S. Müller, D. Nohr and H.G. Beger, Pancreas, 7 (1992) 183.
98. R. De Giorgio, C. Sternini, A. L. Widdison, C. Alvarez, N.C. Brecha, H.A. Reber and V.L. Go, Pancreas, 8 (1993) 700.
99. H.D. Soling, W. Fest, J. Biol and Chem., 30 (1986) 16.
100. N.L. Karnowski, A. Leaf, L.C. Bolis (eds.), Biological membranes; aberations in membrane structure and functions, New York, Liss, 1988.
101. G. Emanuelli, G. Montrucchio, E. Gaia, L. Dughera, G. Corvetti and L. Gubetta, Am. J. Pathol., 134 (1989) 315.
102. J. Casals-Strenzel and H. Hener, Prog. Biochem. Pharmacol., 22 (1988) 58.
103. T. Nakamura, K. Nawa and A. Ichihara, Biochem. Biophys. Res. Comm., 122 (1984) 1450.
104. R.A. Furlogn, Bioessays, 14 (1992)613.

105. M.R. Vila, T. Nakamura and F.X. Real, Lab. Invest., 73 (1995) 409.
106. A. Menke, H. Yamaguchi, T. M. Gress and G. Adler, Pancreas, 18 (1999) 28.
107. T. Ueda, Y. Takeyama, Y. Hori, J. Nishikawa, M. Yamamoto and Y. Satoh, J. Gastroenterol., 32 (1997) 63.
108. M. Matsuno, G. Shiota, K. Umeki, H. Kawasaki, H. Kojo and K. Miura, Res. Commun. Pathol. Pharmacol., 97 (1997) 25.
109. C. Niederau, L.D. Ferrell and J.H. Grendell, Gastroenterology, 88 (1985) 1192.
110. C.U. Ludwig, A. Menke, G. Adler and M.P. Lutz, Amer. J. Physiol., 276 (1999) G193.
111. G. Jurkowska, G. Rydzewska and A. Andrzejewska, J. Physiol. Pharmacol., 48 (1997) 789.
112. M.E. Rodriguez, A.I. Alvaro, G. Bodega and E. Arilla, Life Sci., 61 (1997) 225.
113. D. Gu and S. Sarvetnick, Development, 118 (1993) 33.
114. M. Arnush, D. Gu, Ch. Baugh, S.P. Sawyer, B. Mroczkowski, T. Krahl and N. Sarvetnick, Lab. Invest., 74 (1996) 985.
115. J.E. Oertel, G.C. Heffes and V.C. Oertel, In: S.S. Sternberg (eds.) Diagnostic surgical pathology, Raven Press, New York, 1989.
116. Y. Kikuchi, T. Shimosegawa, A. Satoh, R. Abe, T. Abe, M. Koizumi, T. Toyota, Pancreas, 12 (1996) 68.
117. X. Liu, I. Nakano, H. Yamaguchi, T. Ito, M. Goto, S. Koyangi, M. Kinjoh, H. Nawata and Dig. Dis. Sci., 40 (1995) 2162.
118. V.J.O. Laine, K.M. Nyman, H.J. Peuravuori, K. Henriksen, M. Parvinen, T.J. Nevalainen, Gut, 38 (1996) 747.
119. J.M. Braganza, Curr. Op. Gastroenterol., 6 (1990) 763.
120. J.M. Braganza, P. Scott, D. Bilton, D. Schofield, Ch. Chaloner, N. Shiel, L. Hunt and T. Bottiglieri, Int. J. Pancreatol., 17 (1995) 69.
121. S.D. Slater, R.C. Williamson and C.S. Foster, J. Pathol., 186 (1998) 104.
122. L. Rosenberg, Microsc. Res. Tech., 43 (1998) 337.
123. C. Bernard, C. Thibault, M.F. Berthault, C. Magnan, C. Saulnier, B. Portha, W.F. Penicauld and A. Ktorza, Diabetes, 47 (1998) 1058.
124. S. Wolfe-Coote, J. Louw, C. Woodroof and D.F. du Toit, Microsc. Res. Tech., 43 (1998) 322.
125. M. Wafuri, K. Yamamoto, J.I. Miagava, Y. Tochino, K. Yamamori, Y. Kajimioto, H. Nakajima, H. Watada, I. Yoshiuchi, N. Itoh, A. Namaba, M. Kuwajima, Y. Yamasaki, T. Hanafusa, Y. Matsuzawa and Diabetes, 48 (1997) 1281.

Biology of the Pancreas in Growing Animals
S.G. Pierzynowski and R. Zabielski (Editors)
© 1999 Elsevier Science B.V. All rights reserved.

Characteristics of *in vivo* and *in vitro* experimental models[*]

S. Kato[a], T. Onaga[a], R. Zabielski[b,c], V. Leśniewska[b] and P. Guilloteau[d]

[a]Department of Veterinary Physiology, School of Veterinary Medicine,
Rakuno Gakuen University, Bunkyodai-Midorimachi, Ebetsu,
Hokkaido 069-8501 Japan

[b]Department of Animal Physiology, Faculty of Veterinary Medicine,
Warsaw Agricultural University, Nowoursynowska 166, 02-787 Warsaw, Poland

[c]The Kielanowski Institute of Animal Physiology and Nutrition,
Polish Academy of Sciences, Instytucka 3, 05-110 Jabłonna, Poland

[d]Laboratoire du Jeune Ruminant, Institut National de la Recherche Agronomique,
65 rue du St Brieuc, 35042 Rennes cedex, France

In this chapter, *in vivo* and *in vitro* experimental models for the study of the exocrine pancreas in various animal species are reviewed. For the intact animal models, some anatomical details of the pancreatic duct system, which are important for the surgical preparation necessary for collection of pancreatic juice, are explained. Several techniques for collecting pancreatic juice are described, with their relevance to specific animal species. The advantages and disadvantages of various materials used for cannulas and catheters for collecting pancreatic juice are presented. For the vascular perfused models, some anatomical details of the vascular supply system are described, and the techniques used for preparation and perfusion, including the apparatus and composition of perfusates. As models for the study of cellular mechanisms, the characteristics of pancreatic segments, dispersed acinar cells and dispersed acini preparations are presented, as well as the techniques used.

Systematic research into the functions of the exocrine pancreas, i.e. the pancreatic acini (synthesis and release of pancreatic enzymes and secretion of chloride-rich fluid) and ducts (secretion of bicarbonate-rich fluid), only began in the last hundred years using whole animal preparations. These preparations were necessary to study the secretory response of pancreatic juice to changes in various conditions: diets, stages of life, environments, diseases etc. and the role of pancreatic juice in the nutrition. The factors found to regulate pancreatic secretions in intact animals were investigated to see whether they acted directly on the pancreas or not. To simplify the interpretation by excluding interference from other organs, isolated perfused preparations or pancreatic segment preparations were developed. However, isolated pancreas and pancreatic segments still contain the endocrine portion, which regulates exocrine functions, as later became known. To study direct effects on acinar cells, preparations of dispersed single acinar cells and acini were developed. The development of these

---

[*] The help of Mr. H. Inoue in drawing figures is gratefully acknowledged.

90

experimental models led to significant progress in animal and human pancreatology. The purpose of this chapter is to review and characterise experimental models for studying the functions of the exocrine pancreas.

1. *IN VIVO* EXPERIMENTAL MODELS

1.1. Anatomy of the pancreatic duct system in different animal species
The pancreas consists of lobules loosely united by the interlobular connective tissue. It is both an endocrine and an exocrine gland. The endocrine part (comprising only 2 % of the pancreas tissue) consists of numerous pancreatic islets (groups of epithelial cells) scattered throughout the exocrine pancreas. The exocrine pancreas is composed of pancreatic acini and a branched secretory duct system. Pancreatic acinar cells synthesise, store and release pancreatic enzymes and enzyme precursors into the ducts, and ductal cells support the juice with water and electrolytes. The pancreatic secretory duct system transports the juice into the duodenum. It is a tree-like system; the smallest ducts contact the pancreatic acini and combine into intralobular and then perilobular ducts that meet to form a pancreatic duct or ducts leading the juice out into the duodenum. There are considerable differences between species concerning the topography of the pancreatic duct system in experimental animals. The pancreas develops from the embryonic duodenum via two bud-like primordia, one dorsal and one ventral. Each primordium communicates individually with the duodenum. The duct of the ventral primordium is the pancreatic duct (formerly Wirsung's duct) and opens together with the bile duct through the major duodenal papilla. The duct of the dorsal primordium is the accessory pancreatic duct (formerly Santorini's duct) and opens through the minor duodenal papilla [1]. In the later stages of fetal development the two pancreatic primordia fuse into one organ, and the duct system evolves in a species-specific manner.

1.1.1. Dogs
In most dogs (84%), according to Nelson and Bishop [2], two separate pancreatic ducts remain [1], but in some only the accessory pancreatic duct is present. The pancreatic duct that meets the duodenum together with the bile duct through the major duodenal papilla is small, and secretes a very small amount of pancreatic juice. In most surgical techniques this duct is ligated: a fragment of the pancreatic duct and its orifice a few millimetres in size can be seen on the lesser curvature of the duodenum, sometimes even without preparation of the right pancreatic lobe. The accessory pancreatic duct is in fact considerably larger than the aforementioned pancreatic duct, and has its own opening into the duodenum through the minor duodenal papilla, located 2.3 to 8 cm distal to the major duodenal papilla. To access the duct for cannulation, a little separation of the pancreas from the duodenum is necessary.

1.1.2. Cats
In the cat, the pancreatic duct is always present. It is located in the right pancreatic lobe and enters the duodenum through the major duodenal papilla. The accessory pancreatic duct is present in only 20 % of the cats examined [1] (Figure 1).

1.1.3. Pigs
In the pig, only one functional accessory pancreatic duct is usually described (Figure 1). X-

ray examination techniques could not demonstrate the pancreatic duct in any of 15 pigs, including mixed breeds of both sexes [3]. However, in Swedish landrace x Duroc piglets, a functional pancreatic duct has been observed in ca. 15% of operated animals at autopsy [4, Pierzynowski, Zabielski - unpublished data]. The accessory pancreatic duct leaves the right lobe of the gland and ends at the minor duodenal papilla in the descending duodenum, 20-25 cm distal to the pylorus [1]. At first its localisation may cause some trouble, because the duct is situated deep in the pancreatic tissue and is neither visible nor palpable. The duct is exposed for catheterisation after gentle separation of the last part (1-1.5 cm) of the right pancreatic lobe from the lesser curvature of the duodenum.

1.1.4. Horses
The pancreas of the horse has two secretory ducts. The pancreatic duct, the larger of the two, enters through the major duodenal papilla. The accessory pancreatic duct enters through the minor duodenal papilla, almost opposite the major duodenal papilla [1] (Figure 1).

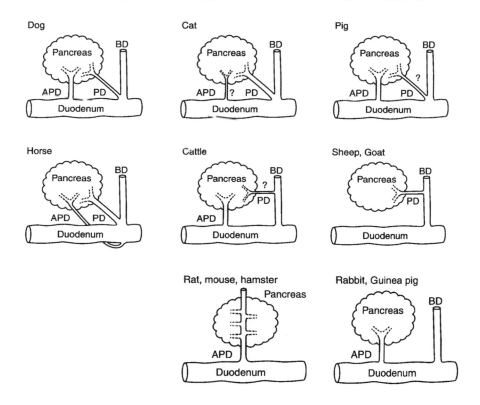

Figure 1. Schematic presentation of the pancreatic duct system in various animal species. PD: pancreatic duct, APD: accessory pancreatic duct, BD: bile duct ?: duct present only in certain animals.

1.1.5. Cattle

In the cow, both pancreatic duct systems may exist; however, the accessory pancreatic duct (Figure 1) drains the greater part of the pancreatic juice. This duct enters the duodenum separately through the minor duodenal papilla, which is located 30-40 cm distal to the major duodenal papilla, which enters the duodenum about 60 cm from the pylorus [3]. In most cannulated cows and calves (Friesian, Simmental and Jersey) the accessory pancreatic duct is hidden between pancreatic lobuli, but its duodenal orifice is palpable in the distal part of the right lobe. X-ray studies have revealed that a considerable percentage of cattle possess a pancreatic (Wirsung's) duct that opens into the bile duct [3]. This small connection is usually not ligated during surgery due to the difficult surgical approach and negligible volume of pancreatic juice secreted this way [5]. In our studies, we have observed the pancreatic duct in ca. 5% Friesian calves. Data of pancreatic juice secretion from these animals were excluded from analyses.

1.1.6. Sheep and goats

In sheep and goats, a short pancreatic duct joins the bile duct about 5 cm proximal to the major duodenal papilla, forming the common bile duct [6] (Figure 1). A thin-walled single pancreatic duct is placed deep within the lobuli. Cannulation of the pancreatic duct in these species is difficult or even impossible. On the other hand, the bile duct and the common bile duct are easy to locate and prepare. Therefore in these species, cannulation of the common bile duct instead of the pancreatic duct is performed. However, such a procedure necessitates ligation of the bile duct just above the pancreatic duct orifice and bypassing of the bile into the duodenum.

1.1.7. Rats, mice and hamsters

In the rat, mouse and hamster, a variable number of interlobular ducts open into the bile duct forming a common biliary-pancreatic duct [7] (Figure 1). Pure pancreatic juice can be collected by cannulation similar to that in small ruminants, except in mice, which are too small for cannulation.

1.1.8. Rabbits

In rabbits, the pancreatic duct enters the duodenum some 35 to 40 cm distal to the entrance of the biliary duct (Figure 1) [8]. Rabbits are anatomically classified as animals having an accessory pancreatic duct only. However, small pancreatic ducts communicating directly with the duodenum probably exist, because proteolytic enzymes continue to be found in the duodenal lumen 4 weeks after ligation of the pancreatic duct, in concentrations comparable to those found in non-ligated controls [9].

1.1.9. Guinea pigs

In guinea pigs, the pancreatic secretions drain into a series of ducts ultimately ending in the short and narrow (1 mm in diameter) pancreatic duct, which is formed by the convergence in the cranial lobe of the main duct from each lobe. The duct empties into the ascending portion of the duodenum about 7 cm distal to the duodenal papilla of the common bile duct. There is no other pancreatic duct in the guinea pig [10] (Figure 1).

The pancreas in animals is a relatively fixed organ (with a short mesentery) deeply situated between the duodenum and liver in the right upper part of the abdomen. The whole gland is between the duodenum and liver in the right upper part of the abdomen. The whole gland is delicate, richly innervated and vascularized; thus rough impatient manipulation during surgery may disturb local circulation and innervation, damage pancreatic tissue, and at worst cause pancreatitis. In all investigated species, longer incisions in the abdominal wall facilitated exposition of the pancreas for catheterisation (a dorsoparacostal incision in the right flank or an incision along the white line is most commonly used). Near the orifice of the pancreatic duct there is an abundance of blood vessels; thus any bleeding in this area may seriously complicate catheterisation of the duct. Moreover, gentle preparation of the duct avoiding damage to the lobuli markedly shortened postsurgical recovery in our studies.

1.2. Materials for implantation

The materials used for constructing catheters or cannulas mostly depend on the surgical method selected for catheterisation. For collection of pancreatic juice through a catheter inserted into the pancreatic duct via a duodenal cannula (Figure 1) a wide, stainless steel cannula is recommended [11]. Stainless steel is well tolerated by the tissues and resistant to digestive juices and biting. Such cannulas in dogs may function properly for several years. Some researchers have used Thomas type cannulas made of polyvinyl chloride (PVC) or polymethylmethacrylate (PMM) (Perspex, Plexiglas, and Metaplex) but these materials appeared to be less durable than steel, which is especially important in dogs. Magee and Naruse [12] successfully used Thomas type cannulas made of aluminium. According to Thomas [11], a short glass tube was inserted through the duodenal cannula into the pancreatic duct One end of the glass cannula was fitted with an olive-shape thickening to prevent the tube sliding from the duct. At present, polyethylene (PE) or PVC tubing is used instead of glass, e.g. Magee and Naruse [12] used the top (last 8-10 cm) of a cardiovascular catheter. Catheters made of PE and PVC are elastic, neutral to tissues and not fragile. Tubing (PE, PVC, and silicone) good for preparing catheters for chronic implantation is available in a wide range of sizes. Although Teflon tubing (polytetrafluoroethylene, PTFE) is well tolerated by the tissue, it is not recommended because of its lack of elasticity and propensity to bend easily. Silicone tubing which is very elastic, resistant and very well tolerated by tissues is most commonly used for chronic cannulation. Silicone is available as tubing, plates, powder and glue; and easy cutting and gluing make it possible to devise custom-made cannulas. However, thin-walled silicone tubing is easily bent (e.g. close to the rib or between the abdominal muscles) which may block juice flow; thus it is necessary to select the inner and outer diameter with care. Medical grade silicone materials, tubing and glue have been used by many researchers with good results. PE is available for acute studies but not suitable for chronic studies, though it is a little cheaper and easier to insert into the duct than silicone. Its stiffness is a disadvantage, as with Teflon, leading to injury to the duct and blockage of pancreatic duct flow just in front of where the tip is inserted into the duct. Tubing made of elastic PVC is not tolerated as well as silicone or PE, although the technology for producing PVC for medical purposes has improved markedly in recent years.

1.3. Methods for pancreatic juice collection and surgical techniques

In general, methods for pancreatic juice collection are based either on exposure of the duodenal papilla for temporary catheterisation or chronic modification of the pancreatic duct outlet. In the former method, the catheter is inserted into the pancreatic duct only for

Table 1

Comparison of the three methods most frequently used for collection of pancreatic juice in experimental animals (from Zabielski *et al.* [15] with modifications)

	Thomas' method	Duodenal pouch method	Direct catheter method
Method:			
- References	Thomas, 1941 [11]; Scott, 1940 [18] Hill and Taylor, 1957 [44] Lehmann and Klein, 1977 [35]	Dragstedt *et al.*, 1930 [13] Preshaw and Grossman, 1965 [20] Herrera *et al.*, 1968 [21] St-Jean *et al.*, 1992 [5] Hee *et al.*, 1985 [38]	Routley *et al.*, 1952 [14] Butler *et al.*, 1960 [39] Corring *et al.*, 1972 [34] Comline *et al.*, 1969 [47] Pierzynowski, 1983 [45] Green and Miyasaka, 1983 [48]
- Principle	Temporary intubation of pancreatic duct via a wide duodenal cannula	Preparation of duodenal pouch containing pancreatic duct orifice	Chronic implantation of a catheter in the pancreatic duct
- Reintroduction of juice	By natural way, after removing the collection tubing	By various duodenal cannulas	By duodenal cannula, needs support
Surgery:			
- Surgical procedure	Simple, continuity of the tissues minimally affected	Extensive preparation of tissues, interruption of duodenal continuity	Simple, precise preparation of pancreatic duct, continuity of tissues minimally affected
- Postsurgical recovery- Handling of operated animals	Smooth (No mortality) No special requirements	High mortality (25-85%) Frequent cleaning of cannulas	Smooth (mortality < 3%) Frequent control of juice flow
Animals:			
- Species	Dog, sheep, pig	Dog, pig, cattle	Rat, dog, cat, pig, cattle, sheep, horse

Table 1 (continued)
Comparison of the three methods most frequently used for collection of pancreatic juice in experimental animals (from Zabielski *et al.* [15] with modifications)

	Thomas' method	Duodenal pouch method	Direct catheter method
- Age	Adult; not recommended for Fast-growing and fat animals	Growing and adult	Any age, including newborns
Collection of pancreatic juice:			
- Start after surgery	4 weeks	Few days	Immediately after catheter implantation
- Preparation for collection	Catheterisation of the papilla	None	None
- Animal immobilisation	Severe (Pavlov stand)	Minimal or unnecessary	Minimal or none (animal's own cage)
- Juice purity	Pure and nonactivated	Contains duodenal juice (~10%), controversial for precise enzymological studies	Pure and nonactivated
- Functioning of animal	Many years	Several weeks	Several weeks
- Complications that may exclude animal from the study	Rare, damage to the papilla after impatient cannulation	Frequent (see text)	Blockage and rejection of the catheter
Applications for a particular aim of study:			
- Interdigestive secretion/ neurohormonal regulation	Recommended	Not recommended due to extensive tissue preparation during surgery	Recommended
- Feeding studies	Not recommended	Possible	Recommended
- Gastrointestinal perfusion	Not recommended	Possible	Recommended
- Long collections (e.g. 24 h)	Impossible	Possible	Possible

collection of juice, and between experiments the juice flows in its natural way into the duodenum (e.g. method proposed by Thomas [11]). In the latter method, the pancreatic juice is permanently drained by a surgically modified system of leading ducts (e.g. duodenal pouch method of Dragstedt *et al.* [13] and direct catheter method of Routley *et al.* [14]). A brief comparison of these methods is shown in Table 1 [15]. These methods were first developed using dogs. Because of its size, compliance and pancreatic anatomy, the dog is still the animal species of choice for studies of exocrine pancreatic secretion.

1.3.1. Dogs

1.3.1.1. Exposure of the duodenal papilla

Thomas [11, 16] developed the method of duodenal papilla exposure for collection of pancreatic juice in dogs. In this method, pancreatic juice is collected through a permanent duodenal fistula, leaving the pancreas and its ducts in their normal relations to the duodenum and to their nerve and blood supply. The surgical approach for this method in the dog consists of ligation of the pancreatic (Wirsung's) duct and implantation of a wide Thomas cannula on the greater curvature of the duodenum, just in front of the minor duodenal papilla (Figure 2).

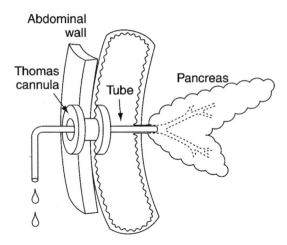

Figure 2. Schematic drawing of method for collection of pancreatic juice in the dog, as described by Thomas [11,16].

Fastening of the cannula and exteriorization through the abdominal wall must be very exact to place the minor duodenal papilla in the centre of the field of vision in the cannula; otherwise further catheterisation of the papilla will be difficult or even impossible. Collection of pancreatic juice can be made after a minimum recovery of 4 weeks. This period is necessary for the pancreas to adapt to the ligation of the pancreatic duct and for proper healing around the cannula. During recovery and between experiments the cannula is closed with a stopper, and the pancreatic juice flows into the duodenum.

Before the experiment, the dog is restrained in a Pavlov stand. The animal must be immobilised in a stand during collection of pancreatic juice, so previous training is necessary. Once trained, however, a dog may be used successfully for many years. The cannula is opened and flushed with a small amount of body-warm saline and the accessory pancreatic duct orifice on the papilla is localised. A glass tube is carefully inserted into the duct (Figure 2) and suspended by threads clipped to the external collar of the Thomas cannula. Originally, the top of the tube had a small olive-like thickening made over a gas burner to protect the tube from sliding off. In subsequent modifications a plastic tube was used instead of glass. The tube is connected to rubber, or later plastic, extension tubing to lead the pancreatic juice into collecting tubes. The Thomas cannula is left open during the entire collection; thus this method cannot be used for feeding experiments. Some authors closed the cannula with special stoppers for feeding experiments; however it was very difficult to keep the tube inside the duct due to increased duodenal motor activity and flow of digesta.

After the experiment, the tube is removed from the duct, the Thomas cannula is closed with a stopper, and the pancreatic juice enters the duodenum in the natural way. This smooth reintroduction of pancreatic juice is a great advantage of the Thomas method, since the main difficulty in other methods is often the reintroduction of pancreatic juice. Another advantage is that juice collected is pure and nonactivated; thus it can be used for enzymological studies. The implantation of a Thomas cannula is simple, and postsurgical complications are fairly rare. On the other hand, some experience of catheterisation of the pancreatic duct is needed. The structure of the duodenal papilla is very delicate, and any damage to it may seriously hinder subsequent catheterisation. If the catheter is inserted too deeply into the duct it may block the smaller branches of the accessory pancreatic duct; juice will then remain in the branches, which may cause oedema and at worst acute pancreatitis. When the cannula is implanted in animals that are too young, the papilla may move from the centre of the Thomas cannula a few months after surgery, making it impossible to catheterise the duct at all. This method proposed by Thomas is still often used for investigation of pancreatic juice secretion in dogs.

1.3.1.2. Pancreatic fistula

In 1898, Pavlov transplanted the duodenal papilla into the skin, forming a permanent pancreatic fistula by modification of the pancreatic duct orifice [17]. The surgery consisted of dissecting out an oval piece of the duodenal wall containing the orifice of the accessory pancreatic duct and transplanting it into the skin of the cranial portion of the abdominal wall. Collections were started soon after surgery. Pancreatic juice was collected into containers placed on the right flank, close to the transplanted fragment. This method had serious disadvantages: pancreatic juice was not reintroduced into the gastrointestinal tract, and thus the dogs lost water, electrolytes and enzymes and were dead within a few weeks; proteolytic enzymes were activated by contact with the duodenal mucosa and caused tryptic ulceration of skin around the transplanted fragment; and the dogs could lick the secretion and induce ascending duct infection. Pavlov's method is not used nowadays, but many investigators have subsequently modified it. Dragstedt *et al.* [13] and Routley *et al.* [14] proposed the most essential techniques. A fragment of the duodenum (duodenal pouch) containing the pancreatic duct orifice was isolated by the former and a thin elastic catheter was chronically implanted into the pancreatic duct by the latter.

1.3.1.3. Duodenal pouch

A duodenal pouch represents a separated segment of duodenum containing the pancreatic papilla, which is closed at both ends and into which the pancreatic fluid drains. This new type of pancreatic fistula in dogs was described by Dragstedt *et al.* [13] in 1930. A portion of the proximal part of the duodenum including the biliary and pancreatic papilla was isolated by separating it from the stomach and distal part of the duodenum.

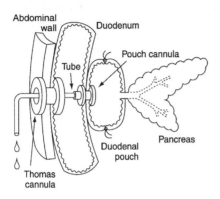

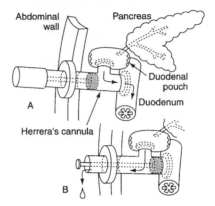

Figure 3. Schematic drawing of method for collection of pancreatic juice in the dog, as described by Preshaw and Grossman [20].

Figure 4. Schematic drawing of method for collection of pancreatic juice in the dog, as described by Herrera *et al.* [21] in the dog. When juice is not being collected, it is guided into the duodenum by a shorter plug (A). During experiments, a longer plug changes the direction of the flow to the outside, for collection (B).

The pyloric portion of the stomach was excised, and the distal part of the duodenum was anastomosed with the gastric stump. The common bile duct was implanted into either the stomach or the distal part of the duodenum. Secretion from the pouch was evacuated via a cannula. Scott [18] included only the accessory pancreatic duct in the isolated segment of duodenum, allowing part of the secretion to drain into the intestine by way of the pancreatic duct. Consequently digestion proceeded normally, and the severe systemic disturbances associated with the loss of pancreatic secretion were considerably diminished. However, it was impossible to collect the entire secretion. Wood and Forster [19] ligated the pancreatic duct and thereby made it possible to collect total secretion. This method was modified by Preshaw and Grossman [20]. The size of the pouch was reduced and pancreatic juice was permitted to flow into the duodenum between experiments. Furthermore, the pylorus, the proximal duodenum and the orifice of the bile duct were left untouched. This became a standard method for decades for studies in dogs and other species. In the dog, according to Pershaw and Grossman [20], the pancreatic (Wirsung's) duct was ligated, the duodenum was cut 2 cm proximal and 2 cm distal to the accessory (Santorini's) pancreatic duct orifice, and the two stumps of the duodenum were joined by end-to-end anastomosis. A small pouch (a few millilitres) was formed from an excised part of the duodenum. The duodenal pouch was connected to the duodenum by means of a small metal cannula that drained juice from the pouch into the duodenum. Another wide metal cannula was implanted into the duodenum vis-à-vis the outlet of the smaller cannula (Figure 3). After surgery the wide cannula was kept closed and was opened only for collection of pancreatic juice. Although the surgical procedure was more complex than that proposed by Thomas, the collection of juice was simple: after opening the wide cannula, one end of a special metal tubing was inserted into a cannula draining the pouch and the other end was connected to collecting bags.

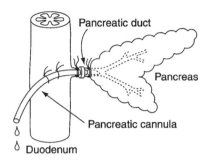

Figure 5. Schematic drawing of direct catheterization into the duct for collection of pancreatic juice. Described by Routley *et al.* [14] in the dog.

Herrera *et al.* [21] modified this method by replacing the two separate cannulas with a single T-shape metal cannula. One flanged end of the cannula was implanted in the duodenum, and the flanged end of the side arm was inserted into the duodenal pouch to drain the juice. Two plugs were used to fasten the cannula and control the direction of juice flow; a shorter plug allowing evacuation of juice from the pouch into the duodenum was used between experiments (Figure 4-A), and a longer one was used during collection (Figure 4-B).

These models described by Preshaw *et al.* [20] and Herrera *et al.* [21] are characterised by their usefulness in that the flow of pancreatic juice into the duodenum is maintained between experiments and the juice is collected without any difficulty during experiments, though an extensive surgical procedure is necessary. However, many complications arising from preparation of the duodenal pouch have been reported. Postoperative mortality as high as 25 to 85 % has been reported because of the extensive surgical procedure [22]. Functional fistulae between the pouch and duodenum, avascular necrosis of the duodenal pouch, ulceration through the walls of the pouch, leakage from the pouch and duodenum, and precipitation of calcium salts inside the cannula may develop after a time. These complications hinder the animals from use in experiments and from continuing good health [5,21,23]. One of the major disadvantages is that pure pancreatic juice can not be collected. Almost 10% of the entire secretion in collected juice can be duodenal juice, and trypsinogen is activated by enterokinase produced by the duodenal pouch. Another possible disadvantage is the disruption of continuity in the duodenum, that can affect duodenal motility and the duodeno-pancreatic neural reflexes. Despite these drawbacks these methods are often used, mostly for studies with feeding and intragastric and intraduodenal infusion, in many animal species.

1.3.1.4. Chronic catheterisation of the pancreatic duct

The technique proposed by Routley et al. [14] was based on chronic implantation of an elastic catheter into the pancreatic duct. As with Thomas' method, it was possible to collect pure and nonactivated pancreatic juice suitable for enzymatic analysis, including electrophoresis and chromatography. In the dog, according to the method of Routley et al. [14] (catheter method), the accessory pancreatic duct was cannulated with a polyvinyl resin plastic tubing, bypassing the duct sphincter after gentle separation of the duct from the adjacent tissues near its duodenal orifice, to a distance of 2 cm. The pancreatic duct was ligated. Two silk ligatures were put under the duct, the duct was incised and the catheter inserted into the duct (Figure 5). The top of the catheter was cut obliquely and supported with a narrow ring glued approximately 5 mm from the top, protecting the catheter from sliding out. The catheter was then inserted into the duct along with this ring and fixed by means of ligatures just proximal and distal to the ring. The free end of the catheter was exteriorised through the right flank just distal to the last rib. Another collar glued approximately 15 cm from the catheter's top was supported by two silk ligatures to immobilise the catheter between the abdominal muscles. In the second part of surgery, a similarly constructed catheter was implanted into the stomach and its free end was exteriorised. The two free ends of the catheters were joined by a shunt after surgery, for reintroduction of juice into the gastrointestinal tract through the gastric cannula. The loop was protected by a gauze and muslin coat made to fit the dog. For collection the loop was disconnected and the gastric catheter plugged with a wooden plug. By means of this technique it was possible to use animals for collections a few days after surgery. Restraint in Pavlov's cage for collections was unnecessary and the entire study could be made on a freely moving animal in its own box.

The advantages of the catheter method compared with the duodenal pouch method are reduced operative trauma and maintenance of intact gut tissues. Thereby intestinal innervation and motility are retained. As a result the animals can eat soon after recovery from anaesthesia, allowing the catheter method to be used in young animals, since neonates cannot tolerate the long postoperative starvation required by the pouch technique [24]. Moreover, this method permits the collection of pure nonactivated pancreatic juice. Recently, Gabert et al. [25] compared the parameters of swine pancreatic juice collected using the "pouch" and catheter methods. Juice volume, bicarbonate output and total activity of pancreatic enzymes (trypsin, chymotrypsin, carboxyl ester hydrolase and colipase) were markedly higher in the latter method. This suggests that enterotomy during pouch preparation severed essential neural pathways regulating the amount of pancreatic secretion, and that pancreatic trypsin activated by pouch enterokinase markedly depressed (2 to 3-fold) the activity of the other pancreatic enzymes.

Routley's catheters function for 2 to 3 months if the animal receives proper care, which is much shorter than with the Thomas cannula. The most frequent cause of catheter failure is reflux of duodenal content into the pancreatic catheter and pancreatic ducts, leading to blockage of juice flow, oedema of the pancreas and pancreatitis. This problem arises because of reintroduction of pancreatic juice without an intermediary sphincter. The installation of one-way valves in the catheter was ineffective. Better results were obtained with permanent collection of pancreatic juice in a retention container and continuous reintroduction of the juice by means of a peristaltic pump, in sheep [26] and rats [27]. In this method, the animal was kept in modified metabolic cage (the rat in a Bollman cage) and a peristaltic pump placed nearby pumped the juice into the duodenum at a low, constant rate. Although this method is satisfactory in mature ruminants in which secretory fluctuation is very small, even after meals, it is otherwise difficult to set the rate of the pump, since pancreatic secretion shows marked oscillations (periodic pancreatic secretion and food-stimulated secretion) during the day [12,27,28]. There have also been attempts to produce complicated servomechanisms for precise adjustment of the rate of infusion of pancreatic secretions. The infusion can be automated and permanently controlled by computer, but the animal has to be immobilised in a metabolic cage. Another solution to prevent the reflux of duodenal content was a silicone T-shape perforated duodenal cannula introduced by Pierzynowski *et al.* [4] (Figure 7). The long perforated arm of the cannula implanted in the duodenal lumen almost completely prevents a rapid increase in pressure in the arm connected to the pancreatic catheter. Only during maximal contractile activity of the duodenum during phase III of the migrating motor complex (MMC) may the duodenal contents flow into the side arm of the cannula for a moment [28]. Perforated duodenal T-cannulas were successfully used in piglets and calves of different ages [4,28,29,30], and also for reintroduction of bile in sheep. However, reintroduction of pancreatic juice by means of perforated T-cannulas in rats and sheep failed, probably due to low secretion and high viscosity of the juice (unpublished).

1.3.2. Cats
In cats the duodenal papilla of the accessory pancreatic duct is small and difficult to catheterise in the conscious animal according to the method of Thomas. According to Konturek *et al.* [31] the bile duct was ligated and a duodenal bypass for bile was made.

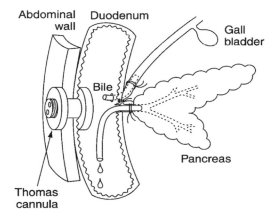

Figure 6. Schematic drawing of method for collection of pancreatic juice in the cat, described by Konturek *et al.* [31].

A Thomas type cannula was implanted and a catheter made of polyethylene tubing inserted into the pancreatic duct and fixed with sutures. A free end of tubing was kept in the duodenum and the cannula plugged (Figure 6).

Thus between experiments pancreatic juice flowed via the catheter into the duodenum. Before each experiment the Thomas cannula was opened, flushed with saline and the free end of the catheter gently removed with fine tweezers for collection of juice. The juice could be collected for one to three months, after which the polyethylene tubing dropped out of the duct.

1.3.3. Pigs

Early collections of pancreatic juice from conscious pigs were made through a plastic tubing cannula implanted into the accessory pancreatic duct by the method of Routley [32, 33,34]. Marcenac et al. [32] returned the collected juice intraduodenally using a U-tube, and collected for 18 days. Wass [33] collected all the pancreatic juice and did not return it to the duodenum. This resulted in the death of pigs within 5 to 8 days. Corring [34] reintroduced the juice into the duodenum by means of a pump and collected for 30 to 45 days. The Thomas cannula method was also applied to the pig [35]. Winnicki et al.[36] implanted accessory pancreatic duct catheters without incising the duct in pigs. After localisation of the orifice of

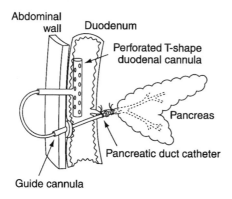

Figure 7. Schematic drawing of method for collection of pancreatic juice in the pig described by Pierzynowski et al. [4].

the accessory pancreatic duct, the duodenum was incised on the greater curvature. A polyethylene catheter was inserted from the lumen side of the duodenum into the pancreatic duct and secured with ligatures, similarly to the method of Konturek et al. [31] in the cat. The incision in the duodenum was closed and a free end of the catheter exteriorised and connected to a duodenal cannula for reintroduction of juice. The authors did not examine how long the catheter could function, since the animals were killed 14 days after surgery. Żebrowska et al. [37] and Hee et al. [38] made duodenal pouches to permit long-term collection of pancreatic secretions in growing pigs. In the former, a re-entrant cannula was formed on either side of a short pouch to allow flow of digesta, and a pouch cannula was connected to the re-entrant cannula. In the latter, a re-entrant cannula made of silicone tubing with a one-way valve was placed within 3 cm of the normal entry point of the pancreatic duct on the anastomosed intestine. Both pouch and re-entrant cannulas were exteriorised and connected with a U-shaped stainless steel tubing. During the 4-month study, pancreatic secretions were persistent and meal-induced secretion patterns were sustained, and the cannulas were still functional when the pigs reached live weights of greater than 100 kg. This method was used recently by Gabert *et al.* [25]. Pierzynowski *et al.* [4] reported a surgical model which enabled the long-term collection of pure pancreatic juice under natural conditions from the first week of life until several weeks after weaning. According to their method, the pancreatic duct was carefully separated from the adjacent tissue, and 2-5 mm from the orifice a silicone catheter (o.d. 0.64-1.19 mm. i.d. 0.3-0.64 mm) was inserted 5-10 mm into the duct. A duodenal perforated T-cannula made of Silastic tubing was implanted directly distal to the pancreatic duct. Both cannulas were exteriorised through the wound between the ribs, the T-shaped duodenal cannula directly and the ductal catheter through an abdominal guide cannula fixed between the peritoneal paries and the muscle layer in the dorsal part of the incision (Figure 7).

1.3.4. Cattle

The method of Routley *et al.* [14] was applied in calves with an improvement in the reintroduction of pancreatic juice. Butler *et al.* [39] reintroduced pancreatic juice into the duodenum to avoid degradation of pancreatic enzymes, instead of the stomach where Routley *et al.* returned the juice in dogs. Wass [40] collected bovine pancreatic juice for enzymologic study through the polyethylene catheter implanted into the accessory pancreatic duct, without returning the juice to the intestine. Although this method is not suitable for quantitative physiological studies, it allows collection of large volumes of pancreatic juice. McCormick and Stewart [41] inserted both outflow and inflow polyethylene cannulas into the duct. However, several calves had pancreatic ducts of such short length that only the outflow cannula could be inserted. In these calves the inflow cannula was introduced into the duodenum. The best cannula stayed in place only 6 weeks and some were lost within a few days. Ternouth *et al.* [42] collected pancreatic juice continuously from a pancreatico-duodenal pouch and returned it through a duodenal cannula. Thivend and Mathieu [43] developed a new cannula that permits only a small fraction of the pancreatic juice to be sampled, the rest passing normally into the intestinal lumen. With this cannula, they were able to obtain regular secretion for more than two months with no change in pancreatic juice composition. St-Jean *et al.* [5] fitted Holstein steers (300-400 kg body weight) with Herrera type cannulas. The pouch was made of an 8-cm segment of the duodenum containing the orifice of the accessory pancreatic duct. In some of the animals, the connections between the branches of the pancreatic duct and bile duct were occluded during surgery, although there were no differences in the pancreatic secretion of these steers in comparison with steers without occlusion. The formation of a functional fistula between the duodenal pouch and the duodenum was detected approximately 4 months after surgery. The fistula resulted in accumulation of ingesta in the duodenal pouch. Implantation of a polypropylene mesh between the pouch and the duodenum prevented the formation of a fistula.

For our studies [30], calves were fitted with accessory pancreatic duct catheters at ages ranging between 4 days and 3 months, according to the method of Pierzynowski for the pig (Figure 7). The orifice of the accessory pancreatic duct was located by palpation and the duct separated from surrounding tissues to a length of 10 mm. After incision of the duct the top of the catheter (20-25 mm) was inserted and secured with two silk ligatures. The pancreatic catheter (23 cm long) was constructed of Silastic tubing 3 x 2 mm in diameter and the inserted portion had 1.2-mm perforations. Two silicone cuffs were glued behind the last hole on the catheter to ensure proper fixation, and a ring (10 mm in diameter) was mounted in the middle of the catheter to stabilise the catheter between the abdominal muscles. The perforated T-cannula was implanted with a double purse-string suture made longitudinally in the duodenum, 7-8 centimetres distal to the accessory pancreatic duct orifice [30]. The pancreatic catheter and duodenal cannula were exteriorised through separate small incisions and the laparotomy site was closed. The exteriorised free ends were protected with silicone collars and the duodenal cannula plugged with a silicone stopper. The pancreatic catheter was connected to the duodenal cannula one day after surgery and between experiments to enable free flow of pancreatic juice. The catheter and cannula were disconnected every day for 1 to 2 hours and cleaned, and the juice flow through the catheter was checked without disconnecting it several times a day. Most catheters functioned successfully for at least two months and in some animals for more than 3 months. In adult cows the surgery was performed in local anaesthesia, after premedication, on the standing animal. The catheter was 30 cm in length and 0.4 x 0.6 mm in diameter, and the surgical procedure was similar to that in calves. Experiments were started 4-5 days after surgery, and during the experiments the animals were kept in their own boxes without restraint. The duodenal cannula was disconnected and a 4-ml plastic tube was attached to the free end of the pancreatic catheter for collection of juice. The plastic tube was changed at every sampling occasion. The duodenal cannula was connected to a peristaltic pump by means of thin silicone tubing for the reintroduction of juice. A 0.1 - 0.2-ml juice sample was taken for analysis and the remainder was infused at the rate of secretion.

1.3.5. Sheep and goats

In small ruminants (sheep, goat) the pancreatic juice reaches the duodenum along with bile, via the common bile duct. Hill and Taylor [44] collected pancreatic juice using the Thomas technique. The common duct was ligated between the junction of the cystic and hepatic ducts and the entrance to the pancreatic duct. Bile was drained from the apex of the gall bladder into the intestine through polythene tubing. Pierzynowski [45] modified the method of Routley for collection of pure pancreatic juice in sheep. After finding the orifice of the common bile duct in the duodenum and the orifice of the pancreatic duct in the common bile duct they were separated from the adjacent tissues. One pair of silk ligatures was put on the bile duct above the orifice of the pancreatic duct and the lumen of the duct closed, and the other pair was put on the common bile duct below the orifice of the pancreatic duct for fixation of the pancreatic catheter.

A pancreatic catheter made of silicone tubing (3.6 x 2.0 mm in diameter, 35 cm in length) was inserted into the common bile duct and secured with ligatures. Another catheter of identical size was implanted into the apex of the gall bladder for collection of bile. For reintroduction of pancreatic juice and bile, Plexiglas cannulas were implanted into the duodenum and jejunum, respectively (Figure 8).

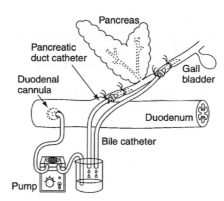

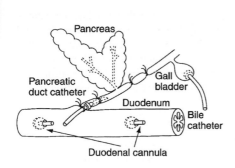

Figure 8. Schematic drawing of method for collection of pancreatic juice in the sheep as described by Pierzynowski [45].

Figure 9. Schematic drawing of method for collection of pancreatic juice in the sheep as described by Kato and Young [26].

During collection the catheters were disconnected from intestinal cannulas and the cannulas closed with stoppers. Kato and Young [26] inserted the bile catheter into the bile duct, instead of the gall bladder, and implanted a single duodenal cannula for reintroduction of both juice and bile. Their duodenal cannula was made of silicone tubing (2 x 4 mm in diameter). The juice and bile were permanently collected into a bottle attached to the animal's cage, and the collection was slowly infused into the duodenum by means of a peristaltic pump (Figure 9). A similar surgical technique was proposed by Naranjo *et al.* [46] in preruminant goats. Compared to the techniques described earlier, the major difference was in the location of the cannula for reintroducing juice and bile. In this case, Silastic tubing (1 x 2 in diameter) was inserted into the common bile duct towards the duodenum, allowing normal function of the sphincter of Oddi and preventing reflux from the duodenum (Figure 10). This method could be used for 4 weeks to collect juice in preruminant goats.

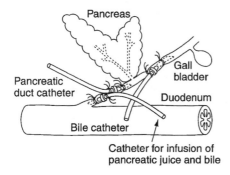

Figure 10. Schematic drawing of method for collection of pancreatic juice in the sheep as described by by Narajno *et al.* [46].

1.3.6. Horses

Comline *et al.* [47] studied exocrine pancreatic secretion in anaesthetised and conscious horses. Silicone tubing was inserted into the pancreatic duct by the method of Routley and the accessory duct was ligated in some preparations so that the total secretion was diverted through the catheters. The juice collected was returned to the duodenum through the silicone cannula implanted in the duodenum. It was reported that recovery from the operation was rapid and that secretion of juice continued for over three months without deterioration in the animal's health.

1.3.7. Rats

The anatomy of the biliary and pancreatic ducts in rats is comparable to that in sheep and goats. Methods for pancreatic juice collection in rat are based on Routley's technique [27,48] and taking into account the anatomy of the ducts, the methods are similar to those used in small ruminants. Onaga *et al.* (1993) implanted thin silicone tubing (0.5 x 1.0 mm in diameter), first in the common bile duct, close to its duodenal orifice, secondly in the bile duct between the liver and pancreas, and thirdly in the upper jejunum in Wistar rats. Pure pancreatic juice and bile were then first collected via two catheters into a small glass container and then reintroduced into the upper jejunum by means of a peristaltic pump. Permanent restraint of the rat in a modified Bollman's cage was necessary for several days before surgery and all the time after the operation. An interesting method for pancreatic juice collection in rats was described by Ormai *et al.* [49]. They proposed a cannula with an original construction that does not require the rat to be restrained in a Bollman's cage between experiments. Ormai's cannula was glued from a polyethylene tubing and it was composed of a main arm placed intraperitoneally and two side arms. The main arm connected the common pancreatic duct with the duodenum, and free ends of both side arms were exteriorised. For protection against biting the exteriorised ends of the cannula were protected with a metal thimble, sutured to the skin on the right flank. Bile was bypassed to the duodenum with polyethylene tubing, with one end implanted in the bile duct and the opposite end inserted through the stomach into the duodenum. Between experiments the free ends of the side arms were plugged and covered with thimbles, and the animals were kept in their own cage without restraint and provided with free access to food and water. During experiments, the rats were moved to the Bollman's cage, and the thimble removed. For collection of juice the arm of the pancreatic side was unplugged, and the plug in the arm of the duodenal side was replaced with a longer one, stopping the flow of juice through the main arm into the duodenum. According to Ormai *et al.* their catheters functioned successfully for about two weeks.

1.4. Secretion of pancreatic juice in animals prepared with different methods

Table 2 presents the amounts of pancreatic juice collected with different techniques in different animal species. This table shows that the amounts of juice obtained by temporary drainage of the ovine and canine pancreatic duct according to Thomas [12,50] are larger than those obtained by chronic catheterisation with a duodenal pouch [51] or pancreatic duct according to Routley *et al.* [52]. The secretion of pancreatic juice in calves catheterised according to Herrera *et al.* was similar to that in calves prepared according to Routley *et al.* It also should be pointed out that the mean secretion of pancreatic juice in rats using the methods of Ormai *et al.* [49] and Onaga *et al.* [27]) was similar, although Onaga *et al.* used a peristaltic pump for smooth reintroduction of the juice into the gastrointestinal tract. We are aware that comparison of parameters in pancreatic juice other than juice volume (e.g., protein, bicarbonate, and enzyme activities) may be substantially influenced by the differences in analytical methods used in different laboratories [53]. Therefore for illustration we recommend the comparative study (pouch versus catheter method) carried out in the same laboratory [54,55]. In this study, the pigs prepared with the pouch method secreted substantially less juice, with a lower pH and a much lower activity of trypsin, colipase and carboxyl ester hydrolase than the pigs prepared with the catheter method.

Table 2
Averaged outflow of pancreatic juice in different animal species according to technique used for cannulation of the pancreas.

Species	Age or size	Juice flow	Cannulation method	Reference
Dogs	(adult)	150-400 ml/24 h	Pa	Markowitz, (1954) [17]
"		0-2 ml/10 min*	Th	Magee, (1983) [12]
"		0.5-2.5 ml/15min*	He	Konturek, (1986) [51]
Calves	(1-4 w)	0.7-1.9 ml/5 min*	Ro	Zabielski, (1993) [28]
"	(7 d)	297 ml/12 h	He	Ternouth, (1973) [23]
"	(63 d)	602 ml/12 h	He	Ternouth, (1973) [23]
"		1000 ml/24 h	Ro	McCormick, (1967) [41]
Steers	(~ 360 kg)	100 ml/h	He	St-Jean, (1992) [5]
Cows	(~ 450 kg)	260-410 ml/h	Ro	Pierzynowski, (1988) [4]
Sheep	(~ 50 kg)	13-30 ml/h	Ro	Pierzynowski, (1983) [45]
"	(38-58 kg)	1.3 ml/10 min	Ro	Kato (1984), [52]
"	(adult)	3.1 ml/15 min	Th	Magee (1961), [50]
Piglets	(0-4 w)	0.5 ml/kg/h	Ro	Pierzynowski, (1990) [24]
	(9 w)	2.5 ml/kg/h	Ro	Pierzynowski, (1990) [24]
Pigs	(80-90 kg)	23-120 ml/h	Wi	Winnicki, (1994), [37]
Goats	(4 w)	1.5 ml/min	Ro	Naranjo, (1986), [46]
Rats	(300 g)	0.43 ml/h	Ro	Ormai, (1986), [49]
"	(250 g)	18-25 µl/3 min*	Ro	Onaga (1993), [27]

*takes into account periodic fluctuations in pancreatic juice secretion
d-days, w-weeks, mo-months, He-Herrera, Pa-Pavlov, Ro-Routley, Th-Thomas, Wi-Winnicki.

In contrast, the amylase and lipase activities and the total protein output were slightly greater in the juice collected through the pouch. A major difference between the methods was that trypsin and chymotrypsin were fully active in pancreatic juice obtained through the pouch, whereas virtually no trypsin or chymotrypsin activity was detected in pancreatic juice collected through the catheter. The presence or absence of hormonal feedback or alteration to the extrinsic innervation of the upper gastrointestinal tract may have influenced pancreatic secretion. The differences between the collection methods observed in this study may affect the response of the exocrine pancreas to a change in diet composition, feeding regimen or application of a particular secretagogue and should be taken into consideration in future studies with either method.

2. *IN VITRO* EXPERIMENTAL MODELS

2.1. Perfusion of the pancreas
The first *in vitro* preparation of the pancreas as tissue slices was used in the 1930s to study pancreatic metabolism. However, pancreatic fluid secretion clearly cannot be studied in slices because ductal integrity must be maintained in order to collect and measure the secretory product. Therefore perfused models of isolated pancreas have been used in various species. The greatest advantage of this model in comparison with the intact animal models is the possibility to study function without possible interference from other organs. The disadvantage may be the requirement of considerable surgical skill to isolate and perfuse the pancreas. The object is to obtain an organ as near to normal as possible and to sustain it under conditions approximating the normal. The preparation consists of an isolated pancreas cannulated into its vascular and ductal system, the perfusion apparatus and the perfusate.

2.1.1 Isolation and cannulation techniques
The pancreas receives its blood supply from a number of sources, which makes perfusion of the gland impossible without considerable surgical preparation. Although there are some

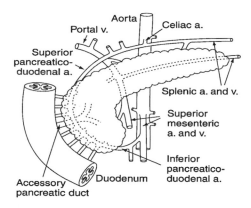

Figure 11. Schematic drawing of vascular supply of the canine pancreas.

differences between different species, blood is generally supplied to the pancreas from the celiac arterial system and the superior mesenteric arterial system. In the former system, a branch from the splenic artery supplies part of the body and left lobe, and the superior pancreaticoduodenal branch of the hepatic artery supplies part of the body and the right lobe of the pancreas. In the latter system, the inferior pancreaticoduodenal artery supplies the uncinate process and the rest of the right lobe of the gland (Figure 11). The details have been described by Babkin and Starling [56], Goldstein [57], Nardi *et al.* [58], Hermon-Taylor [59], Grenier *et al.* [60], Rao and Elmslie [61], Augier *et al.* [62] and Eloy *et al.* [63] for the dog; by Case *et al.* [64] for the cat; by Kanno [65] for the rat; by Jensen *et al.* [66] for the pig; by Saito [67] for the rabbit and by Matsumoto and Kanno [68] for the guinea pig.

2.1.1.1. Dogs

Babkin and Starling [56] perfused a canine pancreas by way of the superior pancreaticoduodenal artery using a heart lung preparation. Nardi *et al.* [58] perfused part of the canine pancreas through an isolated segment of aorta. The gland remained within the body of the animal. Hermon-Taylor [59] developed a model entirely separated from the animal, consisting of the isolated pancreas and a short attached portion of the duodenum. Splenic and superior mesenteric arteries were used for arterial inflow and the portal vein for venous drainage. The splenic artery was cannulated retrogradely distal to the left lobe of the pancreas and the superior mesenteric artery was cannulated retrogradely beyond the origin of the inferior pancreaticoduodenal vessel. In this model, pancreatic anoxia is prevented by transferring from blood supply through the aorta to artificial perfusion through the arterial cannula without any delay (Figure 12).

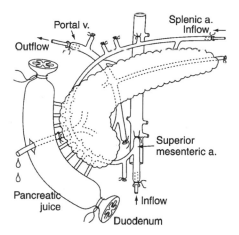

Figure 12. Schematic drawing of vascular and ductal cannulations for perfusing canine pancreas described by Hermon-Taylor [59].

The dog's own blood at its normal haematocrit (Ht) was infused at the rate of 20-25 ml/min (about 0.2ml/min/g pancreas) using a peristaltic pump. The venous flow was led from the portal vein to the oxygenator and recirculated to the pancreas. Rao and Elmslie [61] modified the method developed by Hermon-Taylor, the major change being excision of the duodenum, a minor one being aortic perfusion rather than through the splenic and mesenteric arteries. The splenic artery and the superior mesenteric artery were ligated and divided at the points where arterial cannulas were inserted in the method of Hermon-Taylor. After ligation and dissection of unnecessary blood vessels and attachments to other organs, the gland was completely isolated, leaving the blood supply intact. The aorta was cannulated distal to the superior mesenteric artery. The right branch of the portal vein was cannulated and the left one was ligated. After collection of blood for primary perfusion through the distal cannula, the proximal aorta was ligated and divided (Figure 13).

The interval between ligation of the aorta and the start of perfusion was usually between 3-5 minutes. The dog's own blood diluted with physiological salt solution to 10-20% Ht was infused at the rate of 30-50 ml/min (about 0.5-0.7 ml/min/g pancreas) in the recirculating system.

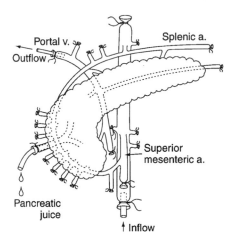

Figure 13. Schematic drawing of vascular and ductal cannulations for perfusing canine pancreas as described by Rao and Elmslie [61].

As the duodenum is a major site for the production of hormones that act on the exocrine pancreas, any response by a pancreas/duodenum preparation could be brought about indirectly through an effect on the release of duodenal hormones or through local reflexes. The advantage of the preparation containing only the pancreas is that any pancreatic response must be due to a direct effect on the gland. Eloy *et al.* [63] improved the perfusate and the method of perfusion using the preparation of pancreas only. A suspension of homologous canine erythrocytes in an artificial culture medium at 25% Ht was perfused without recirculation in "once-through" system. Bovine serum albumin (4%) and dextran (50%) were added in order to maintain the correct oncotic pressure in the perfusate. Whole blood contains metabolic and hormonal factors of unknown quantities that have been responsible for fluctuations in the haemodynamical perfusion conditions and in the results, as far as hormonal or metabolic studies were concerned. Perfusion without recirculation of the perfusate implies elimination of any contamination of the perfusate by hormonal or metabolic pancreatic secretion, and moreover, the composition of the perfusate remains constant throughout the experiment. Teranishi [69] perfused Krebs-Henseleit solution without adding erythrocytes. Augmentation of oxygenation by cooling of the perfusate was needed.

2.1.1.2. Cats

The possibility to change the ionic conditions of the pancreas in intact animals is limited. The isolated gland, however, can be exposed to a wide range of osmotic pressures and electrolyte concentrations. Case *et al.* [64] developed a perfused preparation of isolated cat pancreas to investigate the mechanism of ionic secretion. Although a short portion of duodenum remained attached to the pancreas in this preparation, the vascular branches to the duodenum from the vessels lying between the duodenum and the right lobe of the pancreas were ligated, in contrast to that described by Hermon-Taylor in dogs. The vascular system in cats is similar to that of dogs. Circulation through the isolated pancreas was maintained by pumping saline solution through the celiac and superior mesenteric arteries and collecting the effluent from a retrograde catheter in the superior mesenteric vein (Figure 14).

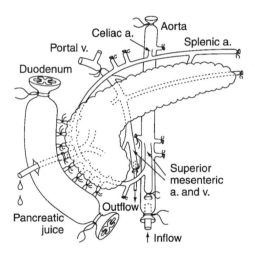

Figure 14. Schematic drawing of vascular and ductal cannulations for perfusing the cat pancreas described by Case *et al.* [64].

The route of inflow was similar to that described by Rao and Elmslie in dogs, but the route of outflow was different; the mesenteric vein was used instead of the portal vein. Perfusion was made with physiological saline without the addition of erythrocytes, at the rate of 4-6 ml/min and a pressure of 30 mmHg. Pancreatic secretion was stimulated by administration of secretin at a rate of 10 µg/min. In response to continuous secretin infusion, for up to 6 hrs the preparation secreted a juice which was similar to that obtained *in vivo*, with the exception that the bicarbonate concentration decreased and the chloride concentration increased over time, even when the rate of secretion remained constant. Dextran was added to the perfusate at a concentration of 6 % in an attempt to minimise the development of oedema, which could have affected the concentration of secretin reaching the pancreatic cells. Using this preparation, the relationship between the osmolality of the perfusate and the secretory response was shown. The osmolalities of perfusate and secretion were identical over a range of 450 mOsm/kg, but the electrolyte concentration of the secretion was always slightly higher than that of the perfusate. Variations in perfusate osmolality produced inverse changes in the secretion rate, between 600 mOsm/kg, at which secretion ceased, and 150 mOsm/kg, at which the rate of secretion was highest. At perfusate osmolalities below 150 mOsm/kg secretion declined rapidly.

2.1.1.3. Pigs

The isolated perfused preparation of porcine pancreas was first described by Jensen *et al.* [70]. The pancreas without duodenum was perfused through its entire arterial supply, i.e. the splenic, the gastroduodenal, and superior mesenteric arteries, and was drained through its complete portal venous system. The aorta was ligated proximal to the celiac artery and cannulated distal to the superior mesenteric artery. The common bile duct was ligated and divided close to duodenum. The accessory pancreatic duct was dissected and catheterised. The pancreatic gland was perfused in a "once-through" system with a Krebs-Ringer bicarbonate buffer supplemented with dextran, 5 %, human serum albumin, 0.1 %, and pyruvate, fumarate and glutamate at concentrations of 5 mmol/l each. Preparations with a functionally intact vagal nerve or both a vagal and splanchnic nerve supply have been also been developed to study the role of VIPergic nerves in the control of fluid and bicarbonate secretion [71], the effect of GRP on exocrine secretion and its release from the pancreas [72], and the effect of peptides on vagally-induced exocrine secretion [73].

2.1.1.4. Rats

Rats have frequently been used for studies of the pancreas because of their low cost and the ready availability of well-established strains. The perfused model was first described by Kanno [65], who recorded the transmembrane potential and amylase output of acinar cells. The inlet of the vascular perfusion was the superior mesenteric artery and outlet was the portal vein. Krebs-Henseleit solution was perfused at a constant pressure of about 120 mmHg, provided by a large reservoir. The inlet for perfusion of the common duct was the hepatic end of the duct and the outlet was the duodenal end. The common duct was flushed with the Krebs-Henseleit solution at a constant pressure of 5 cm H_2O. A cannula was inserted into the duodenal lumen at the intestinal end to drain off the duodenal contents (Figure 15). This flushing preparation was improved to allow simultaneous measurement of pancreatic protein output and juice flow [74]. This was done by ligating the hepatic end of the common duct and collecting the pancreatic juice from the duodenal end of the duct following cannulation with a stainless steel tube. The superior mesenteric artery and the celiac artery were used as inlets for the vascular perfusion in this preparation, and the outlet was the portal vein (Figure 16). At this time, both the superior mesenteric artery and the celiac artery were used for the inlets in the flushing preparation as well. The rate of vascular flow in both preparations was kept constant at 1 ml/min with the aid of a peristaltic pump. These preparations were further improved by isolating the duodenum [75, 76].

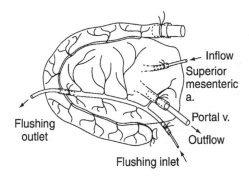

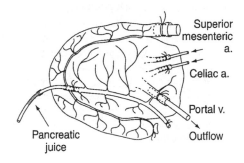

Figure 15. Schematic drawing of vascular and ductal cannulations for perfusing the rat pancreas as described by Kanno [65]. In this preparation the common duct was flushed with Krebs-Henseleit solution at a constant pressure.

Figure 16. Schematic drawing of vascular and ductal cannulations for draining the rat pancreas as described by Kanno [65]. In this preparation pure pancreatic juice was collected.

Tournut *et al.* [77] simplified the surgical procedure for the draining preparation. The pancreas was separated from the spleen, stomach, and intestine after ligation of the splenic coronary, superior mesenteric arteries and celiac trunk beyond their pancreatic division. The aorta was cannulated for arterial infusion below the origin of the superior mesenteric artery. This preparation was perfused in situ. An advantage of this technique is that the preparation can be set up faster and more easily than the ex-vivo-isolated perfused preparation.

2.1.1.5. Rabbits

In rabbits, a technique for perfusion of the isolated pancreas was first reported by Saito [67]. The stem arteries in the pancreas start from the superior mesenteric and the celiac arteries. From the superior mesenteric arterial system, the inferior pancreaticoduodenal branch supplies a larger part of gland, anastomosing with the branch of the celiac artery. The entire system of stem veins in the pancreas run into the portal vein. Thus perfusate was infused into the gland's arterial supply via a cannula in the superior mesenteric artery and drained through the portal vein. This preparation consists of pancreas, duodenum and attached rectum (Figure 17).

The perfusion was carried out with Krebs-Henseleit solution at a constant pressure of 25 mmHg in a "once-through" system. In this preparation, spontaneous secretion was obtained for up to 7 hr without external stimulation. Although the rate of juice flow increased and the amylase output decreased with time during the first 2 hrs, remaining relatively constant for the following 5 hr, these secretory rates were very similar to those obtained in anaesthetised animals. Fichaux *et al.* [78] also reported an *in vitro* method for studying endocrine and exocrine function in the perfused isolated rabbit pancreas. This preparation is the pancreas-duodenum-stomach-spleen complex. Considering the objective of the perfused organ preparation, an isolated pancreas with less other organs would be better to evaluate direct effects on the pancreas.

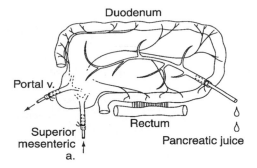

Figure 17. Schematic drawing of vascular and ductal cannulations for perfusing the rabbit pancreas described by Saito [67].

2.1.1.6. Guinea pigs

The pancreas of the guinea pig was also perfused by Matsumoto and Khan [68]. The inlet of the vascular perfusion was the celiac artery, and the outlet was the portal vein. The rate of vascular flow was kept constant at 2 ml/min using a peristaltic pump.

2.1.2. Perfusion apparatus

A simple apparatus consists of reservoir, oxygenator, heat exchanger, pump and thermostatic perfusion chamber. The perfusate in the reservoir is supplied with a gas mixture of 95% O_2 and 5% CO_2, cooled to augment oxygenation and mixed with stirrer. A peristaltic pump is convenient to produce and maintain the required flow rate through the experimental circuit. The perfusate is heated to about 37 °C with a heat exchanger that is placed in front of the pancreas, and there is an air trap just before the pancreas (Figure 18).

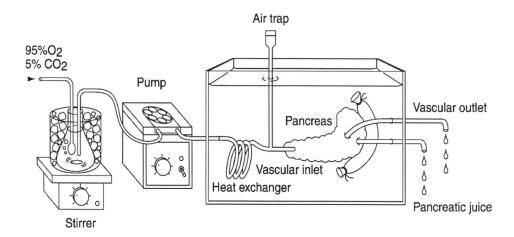

Figure 18. Schematic drawing of the apparatus used for perfusion of the pancreas.

2.1.3. Composition of the perfusate

The isolated blood-perfused gland is a most suitable preparation in which to investigate the relationship between blood flow and secretion, as all the variables may be rigorously controlled. It also allows the vasomotor response of the pancreatic vessels to be studied without interference from secondary effects caused by alterations in the blood pressure. In recent studies on exocrine pancreas, Krebs-Ringer solution containing 5% erythrocytes was used in dogs [79] and Krebs-Ringer bicarbonate solution containing 15% erythrocytes in pigs [73]. In the study of cellular mechanisms of pancreatic secretion, the presence of erythrocytes and protein in the perfusate presents certain difficulties in experimentation and in the interpretation of results. For example, manipulation of electrolyte concentrations in the perfusate is only possible when erythrocytes are absent. To overcome these problems a technique was devised using a perfusate consisting only of a balanced salt solution with added glucose. The necessary oxygen supply to the gland is obtained from that carried in physical solution during perfusion at high rates of flow. The low viscosity of the solution enables this to be achieved at modest hydrostatic pressure [80]. In recent studies on the exocrine pancreas, the following perfusates without erythrocytes were used; a Krebs-Ringer bicarbonate solution in cats [81] and rabbits [78] and a Krebs-Henseleit solution in rats [82] and guinea pigs [68]. Dextran-70 at 3 to 5% and/or albumin at 0.1% was added to the buffer.

2.2. Pancreatic segment preparation

Initially the secretory function of the pancreas *in vitro* was studied using slices or fragments of the gland. Fragment preparations are still used as an easy technique. Recently Ohbo *et al.* [83] used the preparation of pancreatic tissue segments isolated from sheep, rats, hamsters, field voles and mice to study the effects of saturated fatty acids on pancreatic amylase release. A middle part of the pancreas (about 2 g) from sheep or the whole pancreas from other animal species was removed and cut into small segments with fine scissors in oxygenated HEPES buffered saline solution (HBSS) at 37 °C. Tissue segments of 20 mg were preincubated for 20 min at 37 °C in a tissue basket, the bottom of which consisted of a piece of plastic mesh (mesh size: 150μm). After preincubation, the tissue baskets were transferred to a 10-ml plastic test tube containing 2 ml oxygenated HBSS and incubated for 10 min, after which the basket was transferred to the next tube. This procedure was repeated successively. In this preparation the dose-response relationship can be tested by increasing the concentration of secretagogues in successive tubes. This preparation can easily be made from any kind of animal and several sets of experiments can be carried out simultaneously. In spite of these advantages, the preparation can not be used for evaluation of fluid secretion because collection of pure pancreatic juice is impossible. Neither can direct effects of secretagogues on acinar cells be determined, because the preparation consists of heterogeneous tissues containing acinar cells, centroacinar cells, duct cells, endocrine cells, nerve terminals, ganglion cells and so on.

2.3. Preparations of dispersed pancreatic acinar cells and acini

An advance in the study of pancreatic function *in vitro* was the development of a technique for preparing dispersed pancreatic acinar cells [84]. This preparation consists of a homogenous suspension of dispersed single acinar cells which retain their responsiveness to pancreatic secretagogues for up to 5 hrs [85]. Dispersed pancreatic acinar cells have been prepared in various species, including rats, mice, guinea pigs, rabbits and sheep, with a minor modification of the technique developed by Amsterdam and Jamieson [84]. In the original method, a Krebs-Ringer bicarbonate (KRB) solution equilibrated with 95% O_2 and 5% CO_2 (to pH 7.4) and containing 14 mM glucose, a complete L-amino acid supplement, and 0.1 mg of soya bean trypsin inhibitor per ml was used. $MgCl_2$ and $CaCl_2$ concentrations were adjusted as required. Crude collagenase or bovine-plasma albumin were dissolved and dialysed at 4 °C against KRB solution containing the appropriate concentrations of bivalent cations, and centrifuged at 1000 x g for 15 min to remove particulate matter. Pure collagenase, hyaluronidase, and soya bean trypsin inhibitor were added as salt-free powders. Media used for incubation of cells after dissociation contained 100 U of potassium penicillin G per ml and 50 μg of streptomycin sulphate per ml. All glassware that the tissue and cells contacted was siliconized. Dissociation of the tissue involved two sequential digestions with collagenase-hyaluronidase, with an interposed chelation of bivalent cations by EDTA, and was completed by application of mild shearing forces produced by gentle pipetting. In the first digestion, the pancreas was trimmed free of fat and mesentery, and 4.8 ml of the enzyme mixture (0.75 mg of crude collagenase per ml and 1.5 mg of hyaluronidase per ml in KRB solution containing 0.1 mM Ca^{2+} and 1.2 mM Mg^{2+}) was inoculated at room temperature (23°C) into the interstitium of 0.8 g of tissue so as to distend the gland and rapidly expose the majority of its lobules to the enzymes. The distended gland and excess enzyme solution were transferred to a 25-ml Erlenmeyer flask, equilibrated with 95% O_2-5% CO_2, and incubated at 37°C for 15 min with agitation at 130 oscillations per min. During this time, the tissue structure did not collapse, although the gland softened, probably due to progressive hydrolysis of the intercellular matrix. For bivalent cation removal and replacement, the soft tissue was next incubated twice for 5 min at 37 °C in 8 ml of KRB buffer without Ca^{2+} and Mg^{2+} and containing 2 mM EDTA. Bivalent cations were subsequently replaced by briefly washing the tissue twice with 8 ml of KRB solution containing 0.1 mM Ca^{2+} and 1.2 mM Mg^{2+}. In the second digestion, fresh collagenase and hyaluronidase (4.8 ml with 0.1 mM Ca^{2+} and 1.2 mM Mg^{2+}) at concentrations of 1.25 mg/ml and 2.0 mg/ml, respectively, were added and incubation was continued for 45-55 min at 37 °C (enzyme concentrations were increased to compensate for fluid carried over from the previous step). At this time the tissue structure disintegrated and a fine suspension of lobules and many single cells resulted. The end point was indicated by the free movement of cells within the remaining tissue pieces. Single cells were readily liberated by sequential passage through pipettes with tip diameters of 1.3 mm and 0.9 mm (5 times in each). Duplicate aliquots of the cell suspension were then layered over two 8-ml columns of KRB solution containing 4% bovine-plasma albumin, 1 mM Ca^{2+}, and 1.2 mM Mg^{2+} in conical centrifuge tubes, and centrifuged at 50 x g for 5 min to form pellets of packed cells. This step rapidly and quantitatively separated the cells from the enzyme mix and cell debris and placed them in a protective environment. After two further washes of the pooled cells in 8 ml of the above solution, they were suspended in Krebs-Ringer bicarbonate buffer containing 1% bovine-plasma albumin, 2.5 mM Ca^{2+}, and 1.2 mM Mg^{2+}. All subsequent incubations were performed at 37 °C with agitation at 60 oscillations per min.

However, it was observed that single acinar cells lose their polarity and lack secretory responsiveness [86]. A method for preparing dispersed pancreatic acini, as a preparation highly responsive to secretagogues, was developed by a modification of the technique for preparing dispersed cells [87]. Dispersed acini represent clumps of pancreatic acinar cells containing 10-20 cells/clump [85]. The pancreas is removed, trimmed of adipose and connective tissue, and injected with 5 ml of a HEPES-buffered Ringer solution containing 70-80 U/ml of purified collagenase, 0.1 mg/ml of soya bean trypsin inhibitor (SBTI), and 1.0 mg/ml of BSA and enriched with Eagle's MEM amino acids and 2 mM glutamine. The pH of the medium is adjusted to 7.4 with NaOH. Injected glands are incubated in three successive 5-ml volumes of the injection medium for a total of 90 min at 37 °C, gassed at 15-min intervals with 100% O_2, and shaken continuously at 60 cycles/min. Final dissociation of the pancreas is effected by pipetting the tissue successively through a siliconized 10-ml glass pipette and a siliconized Pasteur pipette with a narrowed tip. The resulting suspension of acini is filtered through 100-μm nylon mesh to remove undissociated tissue and rinsed twice in 10 ml of HEPES-Ringer with BSA and SBTI to remove subcellular debris. These acini preparations consist mainly of acinar cells, although a small number of centro-acinar cells and terminal duct cells are also included, and preserves secretory responsiveness which is comparable to that of the intact organ preparation. Freshly prepared dispersed acini can be used for at least 5 hrs *in vitro* and have been very useful to investigate the mechanism of action of various secretagogues. Highly purified collagenase should be used. If crude collagenases contaminated with protease are used, single acinar cells and pseudo-acini consisting of only 3-4 acinar cells are produced. These cells lose their polarity and lack secretory responsiveness [86].

The dispersed acini preparation can be examined in two different experimental systems, namely incubation experiments and perifusion experiments. In the incubation experiments, the secretory response is assessed by measuring enzyme activity released into the media over a set stimulation period with various concentrations of secretagogues. In the perifusion experiments, an aliquot of acini suspension is loaded onto a millipore filter (5μm pore size) held in a plastic holder, and perifused with the medium solution at a set rate using a peristaltic pump. The perifusate is collected for enzyme analysis. This procedure has the advantage that a population of pancreatic acini can be subjected to a continuous flow of material *in vitro*, thereby both supplying fresh modifier and removing the products of the response, as is likely to happen *in vivo*. Moreover the outflow is collected continuously into fractions that are then analysed, permitting constant monitoring of the dynamics of the system.

2.4. Comparison of *in vitro* pancreatic exocrine preparations

A comparison of *in vitro* pancreatic exocrine preparations is shown in Table 3.

Although preparations of perfused pancreas require considerable surgical skill, they retain a responsiveness similar to that of intact animals, and make it possible to collect pure pancreatic juice. Therefore, this preparation is recommended for simultaneous measurements of juice flow and enzyme output, and for demonstration of secretory responses to secretagogues at a low, physiological concentration. This preparation is also suitable for studies of the influence of the endocrine pancreas on the neighbouring exocrine pancreas. Preparations of pancreatic segments can easily be made from any kind of animals and are recommended for comparative studies on the secretory responses of different kinds of animals and for studies on dose-response relationships, ranging from pharmacological to toxic doses of secretagogues. Dispersed pancreatic acini are obtained by milder digestion than acinar cell preparations and share most of the advantages of acinar cell preparations. One of the major differences lies in their responsiveness to secretagogues; dispersed pancreatic acini retain higher sensitivity than single cell preparations. Therefore, preparations of dispersed pancreatic acini are to be preferred for studies on dose-response relationships for pharmacological to toxic doses of secretagogues, studies on direct effects of secretagogues and of drugs on acinar cells, and studies on the receptor level.

Table 3
Comparison of *in vitro* pancreatic exocrine preparations

| | Preparations | | | |
	Perfused pancreas	Segments	Dispersed acini	Acinar cells
Complexity of preparation	Complex	Simplest	Simple	Simple
Limitation of animals	Limited	Not limited	Not limited	Not limited
Exclusion of endocrine Interference	Impossible	Impossible	Possible	Possible
Taking samples from one animal	Only one	Multiple	Multiple	Multiple
Leakage of digestive Enzymes	None	A little	Substantial	Substantial
Polarity	Retained	Retained	Retained	Lost
Responsiveness to Secretagogues	Same as intact animal	Close to intact organ	Close to intact organ	Very low
Regulation of cellular ionic Environment	Difficult	Possible	Easy, strictly	Easy, strictly
Hypoxia	None	Partial	None	None
Cell count	Impossible	Impossible	Impossible	Possible
Collection of pure juice	Possible	Impossible	Impossible	Impossible

CONCLUSIONS

Whole animal preparations have been necessary for various pancreatic studies on physiology, nutrition and pathophysiology. Three main methods for collection of pancreatic juice have been used: the Thomas method, duodenal pouch method and catheter method. In the Thomas method, pure and nonactivated juice can be collected and pancreatic juice enters the duodenum in the natural way when juice is not collected. However, this method can not be used for feeding experiments because it is very difficult to keep the collecting tube inside the duct, due to the increased duodenal motor activity and flow of digesta. In the pouch method, pancreatic juice enters the duodenal pouch through the duodenal papilla and the juice is collected without any difficulties. However, an extensive surgical procedure is necessary and pure pancreatic juice can not be collected. The catheter method does not require complex surgical skills and permits the collection of pure, nonactivated pancreatic juice. In this method, pancreatic juice is reintroduced into the duodenum without an intermediary duct sphincter. Therefore reflux of duodenal contents into the pancreatic catheter causes blockage of juice flow. If a valve that functions similarly to the duct sphincter is devised, the catheter method seems to be better than the others in any kind of animal or experiment for the collection of pure pancreatic juice.

The vascular perfused model of the isolated pancreas was developed to exclude possible interference from other organs. Although preparing this model requires complex surgical skills, it maintains the favourable morphological arrangement and the polarity of all cells that exist *in situ*. This preparation also retains responsiveness to physiologically low concentrations of secretagogues, and is therefore suitable for studies both on fluid and enzyme secretion and on the relationship between the endocrine and exocrine function of the pancreas.

Preparations of pancreatic segments, dispersed acinar cells and dispersed acini were developed for studies of the direct effects of secretagogues on acinar cells and of the cellular secretory mechanisms of acinar cells. These preparations can be made from any kind of animal and make it possible to carry out several sets of experiments simultaneously, because many preparations can be made from one animal. The pancreatic segments are easier to prepare than the other two preparations, but still contain endocrine tissue. In dispersed acinar cells, population of cells can be purified to homogeneity and studied in the absence of other cell types. However, dispersed acinar cells lose their cellular polarity and therefore are not suitable for measuring the functions that reflect their polarity. In contrast, dispersed acini retain their cellular polarity and a higher sensitivity to secretagogues than dispersed acinar cells. Therefore dispersed pancreatic acini are to be preferred for studies of acinar cell function at the cellular level.

Further contrivances of pancreatic experimental models, both *in vivo* and *in vitro,* will promote the progress of exocrine pancreatic research.

REFERENCES

1. R. Nickel, A. Schummer, E. Seiferle (eds.), The viscera of the domestic mammals, Verlag Paul Parey, Berlin Hamburg, Germany, 1979.
2. S.W. Nielsen and E. J. Bishop, Amer. J. Vet. Res., 15 (1954) 266.
3. W.M. Wass, Amer. J. Vet. Res., 26 (1965) 67.
4. S.G. Pierzynowski, B.R. Westrom, B.W. Karlsson, J. Svendsen and B. Nilsson, Can. J. Anim. Sci., 68 (1988) 953.
5. G. St-Jean, D.L. Harmon, J.P. Peters and N.K. Ames, Amer. J. Vet. Res., 53 (1992) 2377.
6. I.W. Caple and T.J. Heath (eds.), Biliary and pancreatic secretions in sheep: their regulation and roles, The University of New England Publishing Unit, Sydney, 1975.
7. R.M. Case and B.E. Argent, Methods Enzymol., 192 (1990) 256.
8. P.J. Manning, D.H. Ringle and C.E. Newcomer (eds.), The Biology of the laboratory rabbit, Academic Press, San Diego, 1994.
9. C. Arvanitakis and J. Folscroft, Experientia, 34 (1978) 77.
10. G. Cooper and A.L. Schiller (eds.), Anatomy of the guinea pig, Harvard University Press, Cambridge, Massachusetts, 1975.

11. J.E. Thomas, Proc. Soc. Exp. Biol. Med., 46 (1941) 260.
12. D.F. Magee and S. Naruse, J. Physiol., 344 (1983) 153.
13. L.R. Dragstedt and M.L. Montgomery, J.C. Ellis, Proc. Soc. Exper. Biol. and Med., 28 (1930) 109.
14. E.F. Routley, F.C. Mann, J.L. Bollman and J.H. Grindlay, Surg. Gynec. Obstet., 95 (1952) 529.
15. R. Zabielski, V. Leśniewska and P. Guilloteau, Reprod. Nutr. Dev., 37 (1997) 385.
16. J.E. Thomas and J.O. Crider, J. Pharmac. Exp. Ther., 87 (1946) 81.
17. J. Markowitz (eds.), Experimental Surgery., The Williams and Wilkins Company, Baltimore, 1954.
18. V.B. Scott, J. Lab. Clin. Med., 25 (1940) 1215.
19. L.P. Woods, J.H. Foster and J. Surg. Res., 3 (1963) 9.
20. R.M. Preshaw and M.I. Grossman, Gastroenterology, 48 (1965) 36.
21. F. Herrera, D.R. Kemp, M. Tsukamoto, E.R. Woodward and L.R. Dragstedt, J. Appl. Physiol., 25 (1968) 207.
22. R.E. Niebergall, S. Teyssen and M.V. Singer, Lab. Anim. Sci., 47 (1997) 606.
23. J.H. Ternouth, H.L. Buttle, Brit. J. Nutr., 29 (1973) 387.
24. S.G. Pierzynowski, B.R. Westrom, J. Svendsen and B.W. Karlsson, J. Pediatr. Gastroenterol. Nutr., 10 (1990) 206.
25. V.M. Gabert, M.S. Jensen, H. Jorgensen, R.M. Engberg and S.K. Jensen, J. Nutr., 126 (1996) 2076.
26. S. Kato and B.A. Young, Agriculture and Forestry Bulletin, Feeder's Day Rep., 62 (1983) 97.
27. T. Onaga, R. Zabielski, H. Mineo and S. Kato, The temporal coordination of interdigestive pancreatic exocrine secretion and intestinal migrating myoelectric complex in rats., XXXII Congress of the International Union of Physiological Sciences, Glasgow, Great Britain,, 1993), pp. 95.1/P, 83.
28. R. Zabielski, T. Onaga, H. Mineo and S. Kato, Exp. Physiol., 78 (1993) 675.
29. P. Podgurniak, S.G. Pierzynowski, Chin. Med. Sci. J., 8 (1993) 75.
30. R. Zabielski, et al., Exp. Physiol., 77 (1992) 807.
31. S.J. Konturek, J. Dubiel and B. Gabrys, Acta. Physiol. Pol., 21 (1970) 484.
32. L.N. Marcenac, A. Jondet and G. Leroy, Bull. Acad. Vet., 5 (1959) 281.
33. W.M. Wass, Amer. J. Vet. Res., 26 (1965) 1106.
34. T. Corring, A. Aumaitre and A. Rerat, Ann. Biol. Anim. Biochim. Biophys., 12 (1972) 109.
35. L. Lehmann and H.D. Klein, Res. Exp. Med., 171 (1977) 173.
36. T. Winnicki, Medycyna Wet., 50 (1994) 37.
37. T. Żebrowska, A.G. Low and H. Żebrowska, Brit. J. Nutr., 49 (1983) 401.
38. J.H. Hee, W.C. Sauer, R. Berzings and L. Ozimek, Can. J. Anim. Sci., 65 (1985) 451.
39. H.C. Butler, D.C. Brinkman and P.A. Klavano, Amer. J. Vet. Res., 21 (1960) 205.
40. W.M. Wass, Amer. J. Vet. Res., 26 (1965) 1103.
41. R.J. McCormick and W.E. Stewart, J. Dairy Sci., 50 (1967) 568.
42. J.H. Ternouth, R.C. Siddons and J. Toothill, Proc. Nutr. Soc., 30 (1971) 89A.
43. P. Thivend and C.M. Mathieu, Ann. Biol. Anim. Biochim. Biophys., 13 (1973) 187.
44. K.J. Hill and R.B. Taylor, J. Physiol., 139 (1957) 26.
45. S. Pierzynowski, Ann. Wars. Agric. Univ. SGGW-AR, Vet. Med., 11 (1983) 65.
46. J.A. Naranjo, et al., Lab. Anim., 20 (1986) 231.

121

47. R.S. Comline, L.W. Hall, J.C. Hickson, A. Murillo and R.G. Walker, J. Physiol., 204 (1969) 10P.
48. G.M. Green and K. Miyasaka, Amer. J. Physiol., 245 (1983) G394.
49. S. Ormai, M. Sasvari and E. Endroczi, Scand. J. Gastroenterol., 21 (1986) 509.
50. D.F. Magee, J. Physiol., 158 (1961) 132.
51. S.J. Konturek, P.J. Thor, J. Bilski, W. Bielański and J. Laskiewicz, Amer. J. Physiol., (1986) G570.
52. S. Kato, M. Usami and J. Ushijima, Jpn. J. Zootech. Sci., 55 (1984) 973.
53. T. Wensing and G.H.M. Counotte, The impact of the reproducibility of clinical-, biochemical- and hematological variables in diagnosing production diseases., IXth International Conference on Production Diseases in Farm Animals Free University of Berlin, 1995), pp. 61.
54. M.S. Jensen, V.M. Gabert, H. Jorgensen and R.M. Engberg, Int. J. Pancreatol., 21 (1997) 173.
55. V.M. Gabert, M.S. Jensen, B.R. Westrom and S.G. Pierzynowski, Int. J. Pancreatol., 22 (1997) 39.
56. B.P. Babkin and E. H. Starling, J. Physiol., 61 (1926) 245.
57. B. Goldstein, Z. Ges. Exp. Med., 61 (1928) 694.
58. G.L. Nardi, J.M. Greep, D.A. Chambers, C. McCrac and D.B. Skinner, Ann. Surg., 158 (1963) 830.
59. J. Hermon-Taylor, Gastroenterology, 55 (1968) 488.
60. J.F. Grenier, et al., Ann. Chir. Thrac. Cardiovasc., 8 (1969) 233.
61. M.M. Rao and R.G. Elmslie, J. Surg. Res., 10 (1970) 357.
62. D. Augier, J.P. Boucard, J.P. Pascal, A. Ribet and N. Vaysse, J. Physiol., 221 (1972) 55.
63. M.R. Eloy, J. Kachelhoffer, A. Pousse, J. Dauchel and J.F. Grenier, Eur. Surg. Res., 6 (1974) 341.
64. R.M. Case, A.A. Harper and T. Scratcherd, J. Physiol., 196 (1968) 133.
65. T. Kanno, J. Physiol., 226 (1972) 353.
66. S.L. Jensen, et al., Amer. J. Physiol., 235 (1978) E381.
67. T. Saito, Jpn. J. Pharmacol., 34 (1984) 43.
68. T. Matsumoto and T. Kanno, Peptides, 5 (1984) 285.
69. S. Teranishi and K. Okajima, Jpn. J. Surg., 9 (1979) 253.
70. S.L. Jensen, C. Kuhl, O.V. Nielsen and J.J. Holst, Scand. J. Gastroenterol. Suppl, 37 (1976) 57.
71. J.J. Holst, et al., Regul. Pept., 8 (1984) 245.
72. S. Knuhtsen, J.J. Holst, S.L. Jensen, U. Knigge and O.V. Nielsen, Amer. J. Physiol., (1985) G281.
73. J. J. Holst, T.N. Rasmussen and H. Harling, P. Schmidt, Pancreas, 8 (1993) 80.
74. T. Kanno, T. Suga and M. Yamamoto, Jpn. J. Physiol., 26 (1976) 101.
75. T. Matsumoto and T. Kanno, Amer. J. Physiol., (1988) C727.
76. T. Ishikawa and T. Kanno, Int. J. Pancreatol., 11 (1992) 75.
77. R. Tournut, A. Estival and N. Vaysse, J.P. Pascal, A. Ribet, Digestion, 15 (1977) 329.
78. F. Fichaux, J. Catala and R. Bonnafous, Diabetes Res., 13 (1990) 95.
79. K.Y. Lee, et al., Pancreas, 11 (1995) 190.
80. T. Scratcherd and R.M. Case, Gut, 14 (1973) 592.
81. R.J. Anderson, J.M. Braganza and R.M. Case, Pancreas, 5 (1990) 394.

82. Y.L. Lee, H.Y. Kwon, H.S. Park, T.H. Lee, H.J. Park, Pancreas, 12 (1996) 58-63.
83. M. Ohbo, K. Katoh and Y. Sasaki, J. Comp. Physiol. B, 166 (1996) 305.
84. A. Amsterdam, J.D. Jamieson, Proc. Natl. Acad. Sci. U.S.A., 69 (1972) 3028.
85. D. Menozzi, R.T. Jensen and J.D. Gardner, Methods Enzymol., 192 (1990) 271.
86. Y. Habara, T. Kanno, Gen. Pharmacol., 25 (1994) 843.
87. S.R. Hootman, M.E. Brown, J.A. Williams and C.D. Logsdon, Amer. J. Physiol., 251 (1986) G75.

Biology of the Pancreas in Growing Animals
S.G. Pierzynowski and R. Zabielski (Editors)

Water and electrolyte secretion, and antibacterial properties of the pancreatic juice

J.L. Valverde Piedra and T. Studziński

Department of Animal Physiology, Faculty of Veterinary Medicine,
Agricultural University of Lublin, Akademicka 12, 20-033 Lublin, Poland

The mechanisms of neural, hormonal and intracellular signal transduction in ductules and acinar pancreatic cells in the process of water and electrolyte secretion in various animal species are described.

In the pancreas, secretin has been implicated as a stimulant of ductal bicarbonate and acinar zymogen secretion, islet hormone secretion, and as a regulator of blood flow. Vagal stimulation releases several neuropeptides, which are known to stimulate pancreatic secretion. These include cholecystokinin, vasoactive intestinal peptide and pituitary adenylate cyclase activating peptide [1,2]. These peptides stimulate ductal secretion via the cAMP pathway, which is considered to be the main intracellular messenger controlling electrolyte and fluid secretion from pancreatic duct cells [3,4,5]. Exocrine acinar cells are capable of regulating fluid secretion, which is rich in Na^+ and Cl^- and has a plasma-like ionic composition. Efflux of cellular K^+ and Cl^- is thought to comprise the initial ionic movement following stimulation of exocrine acinar cells. However, in order to obtain a net K^+ and Cl^- loss from the acinar cells, it is essential that K^+ channels located in the basolateral membrane and Cl^- channels situated in the luminal area be active at the same time. These channels are activated by the agonist-induced increase in intracellular Ca^{2+} concentration. Due to the segregation of channels in the acinar plasma membrane, it is necessary for the $[Ca^{2+}]_i$ to be increased by the same amount, at the same time, throughout the cells in order to activate the channels simultaneously [4,6]. Pancreatic juice from mammalian species has been demonstrated to possess antimicrobial properties. The antibacterial activity of pancreatic juice increases with age in piglets. This change occurs soon after weaning, and might be a compensatory phenomenon in maintaining microbial homeostasis in the upper small bowel at a time when it is presented with new food-borne microorganisms and has not yet developed an effective system of defence against them [7].

1. WATER AND ELECTROLYTE SECRETION IN THE PANCREAS

Pancreatic juice collected from the intact pancreas represents a mixture of secretions originating in both ductal and acinar epithelia. The ductal epithelium of the pancreas secretes an isotonic fluid, rich in bicarbonate ions, which has several functions. First, it flushes digestive enzymes, secreted by the acinar portion of the gland, down the ductal tree towards the gut. Second, it helps to neutralise the acid chyme, which enters the duodenum from the stomach [1]. Third, pancreatic juice protects the pancreatic or pancreatico-biliary tree against ascending microbial agents [2,3,4,5].

The rate of exocrine pancreatic secretion in basal conditions is low, but it increases greatly in response to food ingestion. The postprandial pancreatic response is regulated by interacting neurohormonal factors and their influence on the acinar and ductal cells [6].

The myoelectric activity of the stomach and the duodenum also influences the exocrine activity of the pancreas. Periodic fluctuations in pancreatic juice secretion follow this myoelectric activity in dogs and calves. In conscious calves the pancreatic juice volume and the level of bicarbonate secretion change during the interdigestive period. These changes are associated with the phases of the duodenal myoelectric migrating complex (MMC) (Table 1). Bicarbonate output is highest during the phase of irregular spiking activity (ISA), lower during regular spiking activity (RSA) and lowest during the phase of no spiking activity (NSA) [7,8].

Table 1
Pancreatic juice volume and bicarbonate output in conscious calves

	ISA	RSA	NSA
Juice volume (μl.kg^{-1}. min.$^{-1}$)	7.48	5.62	3.3
Bicarbonate output (μequiv.min^{-1})	0.53	0.39	0.23

According to Zabielski *et al.*, 1994.

1.1. The role of enterohormones and neuropeptides in bicarbonate secretion

In the pancreas, secretin has been implicated as a stimulant of ductal bicarbonate and acinar zymogen secretion, islet hormone secretion, and as a regulator of blood flow [9]. In the rat, vagal stimulation releases several neuropeptides that are known to stimulate pancreatic secretion. These include cholecystokinin (CCK), vasoactive intestinal peptide (VIP), and pituitary adenylate cyclase activating peptide (PACAP) [10,11].

Secretin

The pancreatic bicarbonate response to a meal is mainly controlled by secretin, which is released by intestinal hydrochloric acid [6,9]. However, other stimulators of pancreatic bicarbonate secretion, such as amino acids, are not associated with the release of significant amounts of secretin into the circulating blood, indicating the involvement of other stimulatory mediators [12,13]. In dogs, atropine reduces the pancreatic bicarbonate response to exogenous secretin, even after truncal vagotomy, indicating that intrinsic cholinergic activity is an important modulator of the pancreatic bicarbonate response to secretin [14,13]. Secretin release experimentally induced by intraduodenal infusion of 0.05N HCl in dogs evokes a bicarbonate secretion more than ten times as high as the basal level [16] (Table 2).

In the rat, secretin is the principal hormonal stimulant of ductal bicarbonate and water secretion and a contributor to meal-stimulated acinar zymogen secretion [9,17,18,19,20]. In this species, the same secretin receptor molecule mediates the effects of secretin on both acinar and ductal cells [9,17,19,21]. Secretin binds specifically and with high affinity to membranes from isolated rat pancreatic acinar cells and activates adenylyl cyclase and phospholipase C pathways in these cells [17,22]. In isolated ducts, physiological concentrations of secretin induce intracellular cAMP generation and the opening of select chloride channels that drive bicarbonate secretion [19,21,23].

Cholecystokinin

Although CCK receptors have not been detected on pancreatic ductal and centroacinar cells, it is possible that CCK released due to intestinal stimuli causes the release of acetylcholine (ACh) close to cells secreting bicarbonates via the enteropancreatic reflex. The role of muscarinic nerve fibres ending on M_1-receptors on the one hand and of endogenously released CCK on the other hand, as mediators of the pancreatic bicarbonate response to secretin and to intestinal amino acids is not fully understood, but it has been established that there is a synergistic interaction between M-1 fibres and CCK as mediators of pancreatic bicarbonate secretion in the dog.

Table 2
Mean plasma secretin concentration and pancreatic bicarbonate output in response to intraduodenal infusion of 0.05N-HCl (ml/min) in the dog

	Basal	10 min.	20 min	30 min.
Secretin (pg/ml)	<5.0	17.40	25.14	26.46
Bicarbonate (mequiv/15min)	0.05	0.52	0.98	1.07

According to Chey et al., 1978.

CCK administered exogenously potentiates the pancreatic bicarbonate response to secretin in humans and dogs [24,25,26,27]. Telenzepine, an M_1 antagonist, and the CCK-A-receptor antagonist L-364, 718 decrease the pancreatic bicarbonate response to tryptophan duodenal loads in the dog, showing that the activation of CCK receptors is needed for an adequate bicarbonate response to stimuli. It is well known that atropine abolishes the synergistic effect of exogenous secretin and exogenous CCK on pancreatic bicarbonate secretion in humans, indicating that cholinergic nerves may be involved in the interaction between secretin and CCK [13,28,29,30]. In the dog, atropine has no effect on the bicarbonate response to secretin and caerulein, a CCK analogue. This implies that in this species, cholinergic nerves might not be responsible for the interactions between secretin and CCK as mediators of pancreatic bicarbonate secretion [13].

Somatostatin

It has been documented that cholinergic activation by vagal stimulation or cholinergic agonists induces the release of somatostatin-like immunoreactivity in the dog and the rat. Since exogenous somatostatin inhibits the pancreatic exocrine secretion stimulated both by secretin and by cholinergic agonists, it seems possible that the effects of cholinergic activation on secretin-stimulated pancreatic exocrine secretion are significantly influenced by the concomitant release of somatostatin induced by the cholinergic activation [11,31,32,33,34].

Neuropeptides

PACAP is a neuropeptide that was first isolated from the ovine hypothalamus. Two forms have been isolated: PACAP-(1–38) and the COOH-terminally truncated form, PACAP-(1–27), both of which are COOH-terminally amidated. The PACAPs show 68% sequence homology with VIP and are considered members of the VIP/glucagon/secretin family of peptides [35,36]. The PACAPs exert their actions through at least three types of receptors belonging to a subfamily of the seven transmembrane-spanning G-protein-coupled receptors. The PACAP type 1 receptor, which has been cloned for the rat, cow, human, and mouse, is a selective, high-affinity PACAP receptor, with 1 000 times lower affinity for VIP. It is abundant in the brain, pituitary gland, adrenal medulla, testes, as well as in certain tumour cell lines [35,36,37,38]. The PACAP type 2/VIP$_1$ receptor, which has been cloned for the rat and human, binds PACAP and VIP with similar affinity. The PACAP type 2/VIP$_2$ receptor has been cloned for the rat, mouse, and human and shows 50 and 51 % homology with the rat PACAP type 1 and type 2/VIP$_1$ receptors, respectively. It also binds PACAP and VIP with equal affinity [39,40,41,42]. The PACAP type 2 receptors are distributed in the brain and in various peripheral tissues, including the pancreas, in which the PACAP type 2/VIP$_2$ receptor has been found. PACAP-(1–27) and PACAP-(1–38) are widely distributed in both the central nervous system and in peripheral tissues. In the pig pancreas PACAP-(1–38), which is by far the predominant molecular form, is localised in nerve fibres and stimulates exocrine and endocrine secretion very strongly [40,42,43,44]. Similar observations have been made for other mammals, suggesting that PACAP-(1–38) may play a role in the neural control of pancreatic secretion [44,45,46,47,48].

The VIP$_1$/PACAP type 2 receptor binds and is activated by nanomolar concentrations of VIP and micromolar concentrations of secretin, suggesting that these receptors play a role in the indirect secretin stimulation of bicarbonate secretion [9,45,46]. Indeed, nerve fibres containing VIP have been localised in pancreatic islets, where VIP can stimulate glucagon secretion, and VIP has also been reported to stimulate pancreatic blood flow in the rat [9,49,50].

The stimulatory effect of VIP on pancreatic juice flow and bicarbonate output has been demonstrated in many animal species, in both *in vitro* and *in vivo* preparations. Immunohistochemical studies, using double immunohistochemical staining for PACAP and VIP, showed that the numerous ganglionic nerve cell bodies surrounded by PACAP-immunoreactive nerve fibres are mainly VIP-immunoreactive nerve cells and that the few PACAP-immunoreactive nerve cells bodies also contain immunoreactive VIP. Most nerve cell bodies in the intrapancreatic ganglia are VIP-immunoreactive. PACAP-immunoreactive nerve fibres have also been localised in relation to exocrine ducts and acini. These nerve fibres may originate from the few PACAP-immunoreactive nerve cell bodies found in the intrapancreatic ganglia. PACAP-immunoreactive nerve fibres that do not contain immunoreactive VIP have been demonstrated mainly in the exocrine parenchyma, particularly in the main pancreatic duct and around blood vessels, suggesting a function different from that of VIP [9,51,52].

PACAP stimulates pancreatic secretion mainly in terms of fluid and bicarbonates, with a lesser effect on the secretion of protein. Both PACAP and VIP evoke a substantial secretion of HCO_3^-, though not as great as the vigorous response to secretin. Bicarbonate secretion is said to arise at the level of the extralobular duct cells in the cat pancreas and is mediated through adenylate cyclase activation in isolated duct fragments in rats [52].

VIP together with secretin is reported to elevate cyclic AMP levels in duct cells. However, Ashton *et al.* reported that secretin, but not VIP, increased fluid secretion above basal levels from isolated perfused ducts of copper deficient rats without pancreatic acini [52,53].

VIP is released from the vagus nerve to the pancreas of the pig and from the chorda tympani nerve of cats and ferrets. PACAP and VIP, as well as secretin, must activate receptors on bicarbonate-secreting duct cells. In the rat, there is VIP-ergic innervation of the pancreatic duct and the role of VIP as neurotransmitter seems to be significant [51,52,54].

In preruminant calves exogenous PACAP-27, PACAP-38 and VIP increase juice flow and bicarbonate output [7,8,45,46]. PACAP-27 induces the strongest stimulation, which is comparable to that of equimolar doses of secretin, while the response is lower to PACAP-38 and lowest to VIP. However in dogs, the effect of PACAP-27 is only 1% that of secretin and very close to the stimulatory effect of VIP [7,8,55]. PACAP-38 seems to be less active than PACAP-27 in stimulating pancreatic fluid and bicarbonate secretion in the dog. A possible explanation is that the *N*-terminal, or shorter form, is important in this response, and that the *C*-terminal 28-38 sequence may reduce the potency of PACAP-38 compared to PACAP-27 [7,8,55]. Atropine blockade significantly reduces the pancreatic fluid and bicarbonate response to stimulation with 100 pmol/kg PACAP-38 and PACAP-27 in preruminant calves, but not in the dog [45,46,55]. This suggests involvement of a cholinergic pathway in the mechanism of PACAP-stimulated fluid and bicarbonate secretion in the preruminant calf. The action of PACAP-27 on bicarbonate secretion does not seem to depend on the cholinergic nerves, either in sheep or in dogs. Thus, it is suggested that PACAP-27 and VIP stimulate water and bicarbonate secretion via PACAP-27/VIP–preferring receptors on pancreatic duct cells in sheep and in dogs, and that cholinergic nerves mediate the PACAP effect on bicarbonate secretion in calves. However, the reasons for these inter-species differences are unknown [7,8,55].

1.2. The role of cholinergic stimulation in bicarbonate secretion

Fluid secretion from isolated rat pancreatic ducts can be stimulated by ACh and by bombesin, and blocked by atropine [56,57,58]. The muscarinic receptors M_2 and M_3 have been identified in isolated pancreatic ducts, and their density on the duct cell is approximately 7 times higher than on pancreatic acinar cells [1,59].

It is well established that ACh, the main parasympathetic neurotransmitter, elicits secretory responses in the exocrine pancreas through activation of cholinergic muscarinic receptors. The activation of these receptors is associated with the metabolism of membrane phosphatidylinositol 4,5-bisphosphate (PIP_2), resulting in transient elevation of inositol 1,4,5-trisphosphate (Ins $1,4,5-P_3$) and diacylglycerol (DAG) [1,59,60]. Ins $1,4,5-P_3$ in turn mobilises Ca^{2+} from intracellular pools, such as the rough endoplasmic reticulum and plasma adjacent to the cell membrane and then induces entry of Ca^{2+} from the extracellular space. Both Ca^{2+} and DAG play important regulatory roles in the activation of their respective protein kinases, which phosphorylate regulatory proteins in zymogen granular membranes, resulting in exocytosis and secretion [1,59].

1.3. Intracellular control of water and electrolyte secretion

Exocrine acinar cells are capable of regulating fluid secretion, which is rich in Na^+ and Cl^- and has a plasma-like ionic composition. Efflux of cellular K^+ and Cl^- is thought to comprise the initial ionic movements following stimulation of exocrine acinar cells. However, in order to obtain a net K^+ and Cl^- loss from the acinar cells, it is essential that K^+ channels located in the basolateral membrane and Cl^- channels situated in the luminal area be active at the same time. These channels are activated by an agonist-induced increase in intracellular Ca^{2+} concentration. Due to the segregation of channels in the acinar plasma membrane, it is necessary for the $[Ca^{2+}]_i$ to be increased at the same time throughout the cells in order to activate the channels simultaneously [61,62,64,65,66].

Several models have been proposed for electrolyte and water movement across exocrine gland cell membranes. Many of them originate in the model proposed by Silva et al. [67], which postulates that the transepithelial movement of Cl^- is the driving force for fluid secretion. This is based on the transport of Cl^- across the basolateral membrane into the cells against an electrochemical gradient driven by the combined Na^+ and Cl^- gradients as well as by Cl^- conductance in the apical membrane [62].

Petersen and Maruyama [68] have proposed a model in which the cycling of K^+ through the Ca^{2+}-activated K^+ channel and Na^+–K^+ Cl^- co-transporter allows NaCl uptake through the basolateral membrane of the cell. The rate of NaCl uptake is directly linked to the rate of transport in the cycle of K^+ release and uptake. In this model the point of regulation is the Ca^{2+} and voltage-activated K^+ channel. The Cl^- exit into the acinar lumen might be controlled by Ca^{2+}-activated Cl^- channels [62,66].

The Ca^{2+}-activated K^+ channel is regarded as a crucial regulated pathway, but in mouse and rat pancreatic acinar cells such channels have not been found. From whole-cell current recordings there is no evidence for the existence of a Ca^{2+}-activated K^+-selective conductance pathway [69]. It would appear therefore that in the mouse and rat pancreas the primary acinar fluid secretion process operates in a different way.

In these species the initial stimulant-evoked step in fluid secretion is the opening of luminal Cl^- channels due to the initial cytosolic Ca^{2+} elevation in the luminal pole of the cell [70]. Since E_{Cl} is slightly less negative than the resting potential this will lead to Cl^- exit into the lumen (push phase) [62]. The Ca^{2+} signal spreads towards the basolateral membranes where both non-selective cation and Cl^- channels are activated. The non-selective cation channel opening evokes depolarisation, which makes the membrane potential less negative than E_{Cl}, so that the opening of the Cl^- channels in the basolateral membrane causes uptake of Cl^- through the basolateral membrane (pull phase). This push-pull model depends on stimulant-evoked $[Ca^{2+}]_i$ oscillations that allow the cell to oscillate between the 'push' and 'pull' phases [62,68,70,71].

As mentioned, rodent pancreatic acinar cells are characterised by an apparent lack of the Ca^{2+}-activated K^+ channels found in other exocrine acinar cells. Patch-clamp studies have demonstrated the existence of Ca^{2+}-activated Cl^- channels and non-specific cation channels in rat pancreatic acinar cells. Moreover a voltage-sensitive K^+ current has been described in mouse pancreatic acinar cells, which is transiently activated following depolarisation of the membrane potential and therefore can act to depolarise the cell [66,69,71,72,73].

Acetylcholine and protein kinase C

In exocrine glands the primary action of stimulant neurotransmitters is not to increase the membrane Ca^{2+} permeability, allowing Ca^{2+} influx, but to release Ca^{2+} from intracellular stores into the cytoplasm. Iwatsuki and Petersen [74] obtained the first evidence for a link between receptor-activated intracellular Ca^{2+} release and the opening of ion channels. The various electrogenic transport pathways in acinar cell membranes were mapped by Petersen [75]. In many different cell types, hormones and neurotransmitters applied at submaximal concentrations evoke repetitive pulses of internal Ca^{2+} release, as in the case of stimulation of the muscarinic receptors with ACh [62,71]. Exocrine acinar cells are electrically dominated by a number of Ca^{2+}-activated ion channels [62,66].

In many systems, it has been shown that cytoplasmic Ca^{2+} signals are initiated at a particular point and then travel as waves throughout the cell or even via junctional channels throughout a cellular network [62,76]. Cytoplasmic Ca^{2+} spikes in pancreatic acinar cells are primarily generated by Ca^{2+} release from stores close to the cell membrane and reveal a role for Ca^{2+}-induced Ca^{2+} release. Ca^{2+} infusion into single cells can generate repetitive Ca^{2+} spikes near the cell membrane, similar in nature to those evoked by Ins (1,4,5) P_3 infusion or low doses of externally applied ACh. Probably ACh via Ins (1,4,5) P_3 formation evokes a steady release of Ca^{2+} that induces Ca^{2+} release from pools close to the cell membrane. Intracellular Ca^{2+} infusion evokes Ca^{2+} spikes similar to those evoked by Ins (1,4,5) P_3 infusion, not because of Ca^{2+} induced Ca^{2+} release, but by the generation of Ins (1,4,5) P_3 due to Ca^{2+} activation of phospholipase C [62,66].

ACh and its analogue carbachol both increase the intracellular free calcium concentration ($[Ca^{2+}]_i$) in duct cells and cause a marked depolarisation of the duct cell basolateral membrane potential. These changes result in a dose-dependent response of fluid secretion. Moreover, ductal fluid secretion can be stimulated by the calcium ionophore ionomycin, suggesting that an increase in $[Ca^{2+}]_i$ alone is sufficient to trigger the secretory process [1,58,77,78,79].

ACh and many other agonists evoking cellular Ca^{2+} mobilisation activate the enzyme phosphoinositidase C (phospholipase C) causing a breakdown of PIP_2 to DAG and the Ca^{2+}-releasing messenger Ins 1,4,5-P_3. ACh mobilises intracellular Ca^{2+} in duct cells via the inositol phospholipid signalling pathway and activates protein kinase C (PKC). Activation of PKC by either 12-O-tetradecanoylphorbol-13-acetate (TPA) or phorbol 12,13-dibutyrate (PDBu) inhibits ductal fluid transport stimulated by forskolin and secretin. Moreover, *in vivo* experiments show an attenuation of secretin-stimulated pancreatic juice flow by TPA [58,77,80].

ACh acting on muscarinic receptors causes a dose-dependent increase in $[Ca^{2+}]_i$ in duct cells. The $[Ca^{2+}]_i$ response to ACh is modified either by secretin or by activators of PKC [58,77,79,81,82].

Activation of the cyclic AMP pathway with secretin does not affect the ability of ACh to increase duct cell $[Ca^{2+}]_i$, which suggests that the inhibitory effect of PKC on pancreatic ductal fluid secretion cannot be explained by a reduction in $[Ca^{2+}]_i$ [1]. Moreover the inhibition of fluid secretion that results from the activation of PKC is not caused by a reduction in intracellular cyclic AMP concentration. This clearly implies that the site of PKC-mediated inhibition lies distal to intracellular messenger generation and most probably involves an effect on membrane carriers or channels involved in bicarbonate secretion [1].

In pancreatic acinar cells the activation of PKC inhibits ACh-induced chloride currents, either by down-regulating the muscarinic receptor or by disconnecting the link between the receptor and G protein [81]. In pancreatic duct cells, the inhibitory effects of PKC are clearly not mediated at the level of the stimulus-response coupling machinery, nor at the level of intracellular messenger generation [1].

There are a number of possible target sites for PKC interaction with the duct cell. The basolateral membrane contains Na^+-K^+-ATPases, Na^+-H^+ and H^+ pumps and K^+ channels. The apical membrane contains both cystic fibrosis transmembrane regulators and calcium-activated chloride channels, together with Cl^-/HCO_3^- exchangers [1,82,83].

Interaction between hormones and neurotransmitters

Cyclic AMP is widely considered to be the main intracellular messenger controlling electrolyte and fluid secretion from pancreatic duct cells. Agonists that stimulate ductal secretion via the 'cyclic AMP pathway' include the enterohormone secretin and VIP, PACAP and β-adrenergic agents. However, ductal fluid secretion can be triggered by merely a small rise in intracellular cyclic AMP [1,66,78].

Simultaneous activation of the cyclic AMP and calcium pathways in pancreatic duct cells can cause either stimulation or inhibition of fluid secretion. This depends on the doses of secretagogues employed. The inhibitory effect is mediated by PKC, which probably affects one or more of the ion transporters located in the duct cell plasma membrane. The study of Evans *et al.* clearly shows that complex interactions can occur between hormones and neurotransmitters, stimulating fluid secretion from pancreatic ducts [1].

The stimulatory effect of ACh on fluid secretion is mediated through an elevation of $[Ca^{2+}]_i$. However the stimulation of muscarinic receptors should also lead to activation of PKC [58]. Simultaneously exposing pancreatic ducts to low doses of ACh (10^{-7}M) and secretin produces a significant increase in fluid secretion. In contrast, when isolated ducts are exposed to higher doses of either secretin (10^{-10}M) or ACh (10^{-6}M), an inhibition of fluid secretion results. In addition, varying doses of another stimulant, forskolin, do not increase fluid transport under these conditions. This inhibitory response is completely reversed by atropine, indicating that it involves a specific interaction of ACh with muscarinic receptors. Moreover, the PKC inhibitors staurosporine and 1-(5-isoquinolinylsulphonyl)-2-methyl-piperazine (H-7) reverse the inhibition of fluid secretion produced by mixed doses of secretin and ACh, strongly suggesting that PKC activation mediates this inhibitory effect. In perfused rat pancreas, maximal doses of ACh and secretin have an additive effect on fluid secretion, though in the intact gland it is possible that islet hormones modify the response of the ductal epithelium to combined doses of secretin and ACh [1,62].

Although cyclic AMP can inhibit ACh-induced $[Ca^{2+}]_i$ responses in rat pancreatic acinar cells, it has been found that secretin has no effect on the $[Ca^{2+}]_i$ response to ACh in duct cells [1,77, 84,85,86]. This demonstrates that there is no interaction between the calcium and cyclic AMP pathways activated by ACh and secretin, respectively, at the level of intracellular messenger production. Secretin uses cyclic AMP as an intracellular messenger while ACh stimulates ductal fluid secretion via an increase in $[Ca^{2+}]_i$ [58,77].

Functionally distinct G-proteins can selectively couple different receptors to PIP_2 hydrolysis in the same cell. In pancreatic acinar cells, CCK and muscarinic ACh receptors are functionally coupled to phospholipase C by two different GTP-binding proteins. GTP-γ-S evokes a pattern of Ca^{2+} release more similar to that induced by CCK than by ACh. Activation of the CCK-receptor evokes PIP_2 breakdown and Ins (1,4,5) P_3 formation in pancreatic acinar cells, accompanied by significant phosphatidylcholine hydrolysis [71].

In intact mouse pancreatic acinar cells, CCK concentrations in the physiological range (5-20 p_M) evoke clear openings of the non-selective cation channels. It is therefore likely that stimulant-evoked Ca^{2+} entry in the sustained phase of secretion is mediated, at least in part, by non-selective cation channels [72,73].

In rat pancreatic duct cells, high-conductance Ca^{2+} and voltage-activated K^+ channels have been found in the basolateral membrane and the open-state probability of these channels can be regulated by cyclic AMP-dependent phosphorylation [62,71,86,87].

2. ANTIMICROBIAL PROPERTIES OF PANCREATIC JUICE

An important antibacterial factor, whose role has been clearly established, is lysozyme, which is present in human lachrymal secretions and milk [88,89]. In addition, the presence of antimicrobial factors has been demonstrated in amniotic fluid, as well as in gastric and pulmonary macrophages [90,91,92]. The regulation of intestinal microbial homeostasis is a multifactorial phenomenon and pancreatic juice may play a role in it. There are indications of the existence of a relationship between alterations in intestinal microbiota and pancreatic function [2,3,4,5,93]. The antimicrobial activity present in the pancreatic juice of many mammals is very important in the regulation of microbiota in the small bowel, apparently for the defence of the pancreas and the biliary tree against ascending infection and for the maintenance of bacterial homeostasis [2,3,4,5].

Pancreatic juice from many mammalian species has been demonstrated to possess antimicrobial properties [3,94,95]. In dog pancreatic juice the active substance has a molecular weight of less than 4000 Daltons [94], while in humans it is presumed to have a molecular weight of above 10 000 Daltons [95]. Human pancreatic juice exerts an intrinsic antimicrobial activity against gram-negative bacteria, which seems to be concentration-dependent [95].

The antibacterial action of pancreatic juice appears to be very sensitive to pH, having an optimal activity at pH 8.5 and with complete cessation of action at pH 7.0. The antimicrobial properties of pancreatic juice are independent of activation and enzymatic action. Incubation of pancreatic juice at 65°C for 15 minutes increases its antibacterial potency by about 35% on average, whereas incubation at 100°C for the same duration completely abolishes it, suggesting that the antimicrobial factor is heat-labile [2,3,4,5,94]. Dilution up to around 1:10 does not affect the antibacterial activity of pancreatic juice. Apparently the only thing that the antibacterial factor is sensitive to is pH [94], suggesting that the alkaline nature of the exocrine pancreatic secretion, brought about by a high concentration of bicarbonate ions, is not only meant for the neutralisation of gastric acid. How this delicate mechanism gets out of gear in pancreatitis is still unclear. It has been found that in patients with pancreatitis there is a significant drop in the pH of the pancreatic juice, which may pave the way for bacterial invasion since the action of the inherent antimicrobial factor is lost [4,95,96].

Pancreatic juice from almost all mammalian species is active against a whole spectrum of microorganisms. However, in the rat pancreatic juice antibacterial properties could not be confirmed. This is possibly due to the animal model used (acute experiments under anaesthesia), the secretion of antibacterial factor being inhibited by the anaesthesia; it is also possible that the rat pancreas possesses some other system of defence against ascending infection from the small bowel [4,97].

The potency of antibacterial activity during early postnatal development in the pig is independent of the flow rate of the pancreatic juice. In contrast to the developing pig, the antimicrobial activity of bovine pancreatic juice is flow-dependent.

The antibacterial activity of pancreatic juice increases with age in piglets, being weakest at 2 weeks, showing a significant increase after weaning at 4 weeks and strongest at 7-10 weeks (Table 3). A marked change occurs soon after weaning, and weaning may have a role to play in stimulating the secretion of the antimicrobial factor. This might be a compensatory phenomenon to maintain microbial homeostasis in the upper small bowel at a time when it is presented with new food-borne microorganisms and has not yet developed an effective system of defence against them. Food is the major contaminant of the small bowel, and an effective system of microbial control is necessary, especially during early postnatal development. Some of the inherent factors involved in microbial homeostasis in suckling piglets are gastric acid, secretory immunoglobulins, and milk. Milk contains immunoglobulins, lysozyme, and nonlysozyme antimicrobial factors [88,98,99,100,101].

Table 3
Antibacterial activity (ABA) of pancreatic juice in the pig during the first 10 weeks of postnatal life. One unit of ABA corresponds to 10 µg/ml neomycin

Age in weeks	Antibacterial activity (U/ ml)
2	3 ± 1
5 – 6	37 ± 15
7 –10	38 ± 30

According to Pierzynowski *et al.* 1988.

Table 4
Antibacterial activity (ABA) of pancreatic juice (U/ml) in several animal species. One unit of ABA corresponds to 10 µg/ml neomycin

Species	Sheep	Pig	Rabbit	Guinea pig
U/ml	31±9	39±17	78±15	85±18

According to Pierzynowski *et al.,* 1993.

All of these factors may have a role to play in regulating bacterial growth in the upper small intestine, a role that is taken over by pancreatic juice after weaning. The increase in the antibacterial activity of pancreatic juice seen after weaning is apparently correlated to the change from milk to a dry weaning diet. Piglet age appears to be of minor importance, since weaning at 4 or 6 weeks of age gives the same results.

The factors that bring about such a significant increase in the antibacterial potency of pancreatic juice shortly after weaning remain unknown. The answer probably lies in the breakdown products of ingested food, released as a result of bacterial action in the upper small bowel, which might be absorbed locally and cause stimulation and secretion of antibacterial factors by the exocrine pancreas.

In cattle, starvation for 48h causes a drop in the rate of secretion as well as in the antibacterial potency of pancreatic juice. It is very likely that during starvation, the system of information exchange between the upper small bowel and pancreas fails to be activated and that this results in a weak antibacterial response in the pancreatic juice. This hypothetical system postulated by Pierzynowski *et al.* may be a crucial one that signals to the pancreas when to produce more or less of the antibacterial factor [2,3,4,5].

The rate of secretion of pancreatic juice on food ingestion is regulated partly by CCK and secretin and partly by the vagus. Secretin and CCK do not potentiate antibacterial activity and this further indicates the existence of another system of control regulating the output of antibacterial factor by the pancreas [2,3,4,5,102].

In the pancreatic juice of larger animals such as pigs, sheep, and cattle the bactericidal activity seems to be weaker, while in small animals like the rabbit and the guinea pig it seems to be stronger (Table 4). This difference in bactericidal activity may be due to the fact that on small animals the experiments were carried out under general anaesthesia. It is not known whether anaesthesia has any effect on the antibacterial activity of pancreatic juice, but if it does it might be of crucial importance in human and animal gastorenterological surgery.

This difference in antibacterial activity between the larger and smaller mammals might be an index of the differences in the bacterial spectrum and populations in the upper small bowels of these animals. It may be that the broader the bacterial spectrum and the larger the population of microorganisms in the upper small bowel, the greater the requirement for strong antibacterial activity in the pancreatic juice, in order to defend the pancreas and the biliary tree from ascending infection. It is still unclear how the secretion of this so-called antibacterial factor is controlled and regulated [2,3,4,5,103].

Immunoglobulins

Studies in animal models and in humans have provided evidence that protection against microorganisms is generally correlated with levels of immunoglobulin A (IgA) antibodies in various secretions. The appearance of secretory immunoglobulin A (S-IgA) is dependent on the interaction between subendothelial plasma cells, which secrete IgA, and epithelial cells which synthesise a corresponding receptor, the poly Ig receptor [104-106].

Table 5
Concentration of IgA, secretory IgA and secretory component in the pancreatic juice of humans with chronic pancreatitis.

Author and method	SC	IgA	S-IgA
	(secretory component)		(secretory IgA)
Hayakawa *et al.*	1 - 60 µg/ml	—	—
Saito *et al.* (immunodiffusion)	—	1 - 49 µg/ml	—
Emmrich *et al.* (ELISA)	—	—	0.01 – 5.21 µg/ml

In duodenal secretions and pancreatic juice of human patients with chronic pancreatitis and pancreatic carcinoma, IgA concentrations increase and the respective levels depend on the type of pancreatic disorder [104,107-111] (Table 5).

This immunoglobulin has been shown to bind trypsin and chymotrypsin in an antibody independent manner, which inactivates the enzymes [112]. S-IgA is therefore more suitable than other immunoglobulins to protect pancreatic tissue against a variety of viral and bacterial mucosal pathogens. In humans with pancreatic disorders increased levels of immunoglobulins in pure pancreatic juice were observed [113-116]. Features characteristic of endocytotic secretory component (SC) have been detected in the pancreatic epithelium with immunofluorescence techniques, but their source has not yet been established [104,116,117].

Immunohistochemical studies have shown that SC is present in epithelial cells and in centroacinar cells, which functionally belong to the duct system of the pancreas. It has also been shown that in chronic pancreatitis, IgA and SC are expressed locally by plasma cells and epithelial cells in pancreatic tissue [104,108].

REFERENCES

1. R.L. Evans, N. Ashton, A.C. Elliott, R. Green, B.E. Argent, J. Physiol., 496 (1996) 265.
2. S.G. Pierzynowski, B.R. Weström, B.W. Karlsson, J. Svendsen, Digestive Physiology in the Pigs, Proc. 4th Int. Sem. Inst. Anim. Physiol. and Nutr., Jabłonna, Poland.(1988) 44.
3. S.G. Pierzynowski, P. Sharma, J. Sobczyk, S. Garwacki, W. Barej, Inter. J. Pancreatol., 12 (1992) 121.
4. S.G. Pierzynowski, P. Sharma, J. Sobczyk, S. Garwacki, W. Barej, B.R. Weström, Pancreas, 8 (1993) 546.
5. S.G. Pierzynowski, B.R. Weström, J. Svendsen, L. Svendsen, B.W. Karlsson, Inter. J. Pancreatol., 18 (1995) 81.
6. J. Bilski, S.J. Konturek, W. Bielański, J. Physiol. Pharmacol., 46 (1995) 447.
7. R. Zabielski, T. Onaga, H. Mineo, S.G. Pierzynowski, S. Kato, Exp. Physiol., 79 (1994) 301.
8. R. Zabielski, T. Onaga, H. Mineo, E. Okine, S. Kato, Comp. Biochem. Physiol. 109 (1) (1994) 93.
9. C.D. Ulrich II, P. Wood, E.M. Hadac, E. Kopras, D.C. Whitcomb, L.J. Miller, Amer. J. Physiol., 275 (1998) G1437.
10. H.Y. Kwon, K.Y. Lee, T.-M. Chang, W.Y. Chey, Pancreas, 13 (1996) 444.
11. H.S. Park, Y.L. Lee, H.Y. Kwon, W.Y. Chey, H.J. Park, Amer. J. Physiol., 274 (1998) G413.
12. W. Niebel, M.V. Singer, L.E. Hanssen, H. Goebell, Scand J. Gastroenterol., 18 (1983) 803.
13. E. Niebergall-Roth, S. Teyssen, M. Hartel, C. Beglinger, R.L. Riepl, M.V. Singer, Inter. J. Pancreatol., 23 (1998) 31.
14. M.V. Singer, W. Niebel, K-H. Uhde, D. Hoffmeister, H. Goebell, Amer. J. Physiol. 248 (1985) G532.
15. M.V. Singer, W. Niebel, S. Kniesburges, D. Hoffmeister, H. Goebell, Gastroenterology, 90 (1986) 355.
16. W.Y. Chey, M.S. Kim, K.Y. Lee, J. Physiol., 293 (1979) 435.
17. B.M. Bissonette, M.J. Collen, H. Adachi, R.T. Jensen, J.D. Gardner, Amer. J. Physiol. 246 (1984) G710.

18. A. Christ, B. Werth, P. Hildebrand, K. Gyr, G.A. Stadler, C. Beglinger, Gastroenterology, 94 (1988) 311.
19. M.A. Gray, J.R. Greenwell, B.E. Argent, J. Membr. Biol., 105 (1988) 131.
20. U. Rausch, P. Vasiloudes, K. Rudiger, H.F. Kern, Cell Tissue Res., 242 (1985) 633.
21. M. Otsuki, C. Sakamoto, A. Ohki, H. Yuu, S. Morita, S. Baba, Amer. J. Physiol., 241 (1981) G43.
22. E.R. Trimble, R. Bruzzone, T.J. Biden, C.J. Meehan, D. Andreu, R.B. Merrifield, Proc. Natl. Acad. Sci. USA, 84 (1987) 3146.
23. M.G. Raeder, Gastroenterology., 103 (1992) 1674.
24. C.H. You, J.M. Romiger, W.Y. Chey, Gastroenterology, 85 (1983) 40.
25. W.Y. Chey, K.Y. Lee, T. Chang, Y. Chen, L. Millikan, Amer. J. Physiol., 246 (1984) G248.
26. C. Beglinger, M.I. Grossman, T.E. Solomon, Amer. J. Physiol., 246 (1984) G173.
27. K. Gyr, C. Beglenger, M. Fried, U. Grötzinger, L. Kvasseh, G.A. Stalder, J. Girard, Amer. J. Physiol., 246 (1984) G535.
28. R.S.L. Chang and V.J. Lotti, Proc. Natl. Acad. Sci. USA, 83 (1986) 4923.
29. S. Teyssen, E. Niebergall, S.T. Chari, M.V. Singer, Pancreas, 10 (1995) 368.
30. E. Niebergall-Roth, S. Teyssen, D. Wetzel, M. Hartel, C.Beglinger, R.L. Riepl, M.V. Singer, Scand. J. Gastroenterology, 31 (1996) 723.
31. B. Ahren, T.L. Paquette, G.J. Taborsky, Jr., Amer. J. Physiol., 250 (1986) E212.
32. H. Hasegawa, Y. Okabayashi, M. Koide, Y. Kido, T. Okutani, K. Matsushita, M. Otsuki, M. Kasuga, Dig. Dis. Sci., 38 (1993) 1278.
33. K. Matsushita, Y. Okabayashi, H. Hasegawa, M. Koide, Y. Kido, T. Okutani, Y. Sugimoto, M. Kasuga, Gastroenterology, 104 (1993) 1146.
34. K. Shiratori, S. Watanabe, T. Takeuchi, Pancreas, 6 (1991) 23.
35. M. Hosoya, H. Onda, K. Ogi, Y. Masuda, Y. Miyamoto, T. Ohtaki, H. Okazaki, A. Arimura, M. Fujino, Biochem. Biophys. Res. Commun., 194 (1993) 133.
36. H. Hashimoto, T. Ishihara, R. Shigemoto, K. Mori, S. Nagata, Neuron, 11 (1993) 333.
37. J. R. Pisegna, S.A. Wank, J. Biol. Chem., 271 (1996) 17267.
38. H. Aino, H. Hashimoto, N. Ogawa, A. Nishino, K. Yamamoto, H. Nogi, S. Nagata, A. Baba, Gene, 164 (1995) 301.
39. E.M. Lutz, W.J. Sheward, K.M. West, J.A. Morrow, G. Fink, A.J. Harmar, FEBS Lett., 334 (1993) 3.
40. T.B. Usdin, T.I. Bonner, E. Mezey, Endocrinology, 135 (1994) 2662.
41. J.E. Adamou, N. Aiyar, S. Van Horn, N.A. Elshourbagy, Biochem. Biophys. Res. Commun., 209 (1995) 385.
42. N. Inagaki, H. Yoshida, M. Mizuta, N. Mizuno, Y. Fujii, T. Gonoi, J. Miyazaki, S. Seino, Proc. Natl. Acad. Sci. USA, 91 (1994) 2679.
43. A. Arimura and S. Shioda, Front. Neuroendocrinology, 16 (1995) 53.
44. K. Tornoe, J. Hannibal, M. Giezemann, P. Schmidt, J.J. Holst, Ann. NY Acad. Sci. 805 (1996) 521.
45. R. Zabielski, T. Onaga, H. Mineo, S. Kato, Biomed. Res., 13 suppl. 2 (1992) 243.
46. R. Zabielski, T. Onaga, H. Mineo, S. Kato, Exp. Physiol., 78 (1993) 675.
47. A.M. Rodriguez Lopez, I. De Dios, L.J. Garcia, M.A. Lopez, J.J. Calvo, Rev. Esp. Fisiol., 51 (1995) 29.
48. R.M. Alonso, A.M. Rodriguez, L.J. Garcia, M.A. Lopez, J.J. Calvo, Pancreas, 9 (1994) 123.
49. L. Jansson, Acta Diabetol., 31 (1994) 103.

50. P.J. Havel, B.E. Dunning, C.B. Verchere, D.G. Baskin, T. O'Dorisio, G.J. Taborsky, Regul. Pept., 71 (1997) 163.
51. J.J. Holst, Eur. J. Clin. Inv. 20, suppl. 1 (1990) S33.
52. S. Wheeler, J.E.L. Eardley, K.F. McNulty, C.P. Sutcliffe, J.D. Morrison, Exp. Physiol., 82 (1997) 729.
53. N. Ashton, B.E. Argent, R. Green, J. Physiol., 427 (1990) 471.
54. G. Tobin, J. Ekström, S.R. Bloom, A.V. Edwards, J. Physiol., 437 (1991) 327.
55. S. Naruse, T. Suzuki, T. Ozaki, Pancreas, 7 (1992) 543.
56. N. Ashton, B.E. Argent and R. Green, J. Physiol., 435 (1991) 533.
57. N. Ashton, R.L. Evans, B.E. Argent, J. Physiol., 452 (1992) 99.
58. N. Ashton, R.L. Evans, A.C. Elliott, R. Green, B.E. Argent, J. Physiol., 471 (1993) 549.
59. S.R. Hootman, J. Zukerman, S. Kovalcik, Biochem. Pharmacol., 46 (1993) 291.
60. A. Seiyama, H. Kosaka, T. Shiga, Amer. J. Physiol., 271 (1996) H1.
61. B. Nauntofte, Amer. J. Physiol., 263 (1992) G823.
62. O.H. Petersen, J. Physiol., 448 (1992) 1.
63. J. Gromada, T.D. Jørgensen, K. Tritsaris, B. Nauntofte, S. Dissing, Cell Calcium, 14 (1993) 711.
64. J. Gromada, T.D. Jørgensen, S. Dissing, Pflügers Arch., 429 (1995) 751.
65. J. Gromada, T.D. Jørgensen, S. Dissing, Pflügers Arch., 429 (1995) 578.
66. J. Gromada, N.K. Jørgensen, B. Nauntofte, S. Dissing, Acta Physiol. Scand., 159 (1997) 69.
67. P. Silva, J. Stoff, M. Field, L. Fine, J.N. Forrest, F.H. Epstein, Amer. J. Physiol., 233 (1977) F298.
68. O.H. Petersen, Y. Maruyama, Nature, 307 (1984) 693.
69. C. Randriamampita, M. Chanson, A. Trautmann, Pflügers Arch., 411 (1988) 53.
70. H. Kasai, G.J. Augustine, Nature, 348 (1990) 735.
71. Y.V. Osipchuk, M. Wakui, D.I. Yule, D.V. Gallacher, O.H. Petersen, EMBO J., 9 (1990) 697.
72. P. Thorn, O.H. Petersen, J. Gen. Physiol., 100 (1992a) 11.
73. P. Thorn, O.H. Petersen, Pflügers Arch., 428 (1992b) 288.
74. N. Iwatsuki, O.H. Petersen, Nature, 268 (1977) 147.
75. O.H. Petersen, The electrophysiology of Gland Cells. Monographs of The Physiological Society No. 36. Academic Press, London, 1980.
76. T. Meyer, Cell, 64 (1991) 675.
77. E.L. Stuenkel and S.R. Hootman, Pflügers Arch., 416 (1990) 652.
78. J. Palmer Smith, R.V. Yelamarty, S.T. Kramer, J.Y. Cheung, Amer. J. Physiol., 264 (1993) G1177.
79. M. Hug, C. Pahl, I. Novak, Pflügers Arch., 426 (1994) 412.
80. G.M. Salido, L.P. Francis, P.J. Camello, J. Singh, J.A. Madrid, J.A. Pariente, Gen. Pharmacol., 21 (1990) 465.
81. Y. Maruyama, J. Physiol. 417 (1989) 343.
82. H. Zhao, R.A. Star, S. Muallem, J. Gen. Physiol., 104 (1994) 57.
83. O. Villanger, T. Veel, M.R. Raeder, Gastroenterology, 108 (1995) 850.
84. M.A. Gray, S. Plant, B.E. Argent, Amer. J. Physiol., 264 (1993) C591.
85. M.A. Gray, J.P. Winpenny, D.J. Porteous, J.R. Dorin, B.E. Argent, Amer. J. Physiol., 266 (1994) C213.
86. H. Kase, M. Wakui, O.H. Petersen, Pflügers Arch., 419 (1991) 668.
87. M.A. Gray, J.R. Greenwell, A.J. Garton, B.E. Argent, J. Membrane Biol., 115 (1990) 203.

137

88. V. Reddy, C. Bhaskaram, N. Raghuramulu, V. Jagadessan, Acta Paediat. Scand., 66 (1977) 229.
89. M.E. Selsted, R.J. Martinez, Exp. Eye Res., 34 (1982) 305.
90. R.P. Glask, I.S. Snyder, Amer. J. Obstet. Gynecol., 106 (1970) 59.
91. H.W. Smith, J. Pathol., 91 (1966) 1.
92. R.I. Lehrer, M.E. Selsted, D. Szklarek, J. Fleischmann, J. Infect. Immun., 42 (1983) 10.
93. S. Boisen, N. Agergaard, S. Rotenberg, Z. Kragelund, Z Tierphysiol. Tierernährg Futtermittelk., 53 (1985) 245.
94. E. Rubinstein, Z. Mark, J. Haspel, G. Ben Ari, Z. Dreznik, D. Mirelman, A. Tadmor, Gastroenterology, 88 (1985) 927.
95. E. Bertazzoni Minelli, A. Benini, C. Bassi, H. Abbas, M. Falconi, F. Locatelli, R. de Marco, P. Pederzoli, Antimicrob. Agents Chemoth., 40 (1996) 2099.
96. S.K. Dutta, R.N. Russel, F.L. Iber, Am. J. Dig. Dis., 24 (1979) 529.
97. K. Gyr, O. Felsenfeld, M. Zimmerli-Ning, Amer. J. Clin. Nutr., 32 (1979) 1592.
98. F.A. Knott, Guys. Hosp. Rep., 73 (1923) 429.
99. W.A. Walker, K.J. Isslbacher, N. Engl. J. Med., 297 (1977) 767.
100. S. Ahlstedt, B. Carlsson, L.A. Hanson, R.M. Goldblum, Scand. J. Immunol., 4 (1975) 535.
101. A.S. Goldman, C.W. Smith, J. Pediat., 82 (1973) 1082.
102. J.J. Holst, O.B. Staffalitzky de Muckadell, J. Fahrenkrug, Acta Physiol. Scand., 105 (1979) 33.
103. R.K. Rao, Life Sci., 48 (1991) 1685.
104. J. Emmrich, M. Seyfarth, P. Conradi, F. Plath, G. Sparmann, M. Löhr, S. Liebe, Gut, 42 (1998) 436.
105. S. Bank, B H. Novis, E. Dowdle, Gut, 14 (1973) 723.
106. S. Liebe, E. Siegmund, W. Rehpennig, Gastroenterol. J., 50 (1990) 129.
107. J. Emmrich, P. Conradi, M. Seyfarth, Digestion, 52 (1992) 79.
108. J. Emmrich, M. Nausch, M. Seyfarth, Digestion, 54 (1993) 274.
109. F. Clemente, T. Ribeiro, E. Colomb, Biochim. Biophys. Acta, 251 (1971) 456.
110. N.J. Finkler, M. Palmer, M. Gonda, Mount. Sinai. J. Med., 46 (1979) 339.
111. M. Kilian and M.W. Russell, handbook of mucosal immunology, San Diego-New York-Boston: Academic Press, 1994.
112. B.S. Shim, Y.S. Kang, W.J. Kim, Nature, 222 (1969) 787.
113. T. Hayakawa, T. Kondo, T. Shibata, Dig. Dis. Sci., 38 (1993) 7.
114. G.W. Brasher, W.P. Dyck, F.F. Hall, Am. J. Dig. Dis., 20 (1975) 454.
115. P. Bedossa, J. Bacci, G. Lemaigre, Pancreas 5 (1990) 415.
116. H. Saito, T. Kasajima, H. Nagura, Acta Pathol. Jpn., 35 (1985) 87.
117. D.R. Tourville, R.H. Adler, J. Bienenstock, J. Exp. Med., 129 (1969) 411.

Biology of the Pancreas in Growing Animals
S.G. Pierzynowski and R. Zabielski (Editors)
© 1999 Elsevier Science B.V. All rights reserved.

139

Periodic pattern of secretion of pancreatic juice proteins in newborn calves demonstrated by SDS-page electrophoresis[*]

V. Leśniewska[a], T. Płoszaj[a], W. Barej[a] and R. Zabielski[ab]

[a]Department of Animal Physiology, Faculty of Veterinary Medicine,
Warsaw Agricultural University, Nowoursynowska 166, 02-787 Warsaw, Poland

[b]The Kielanowski Institute of Animal Physiology and Nutrition,
Polish Academy of Sciences, Instytucka 3, 05-110 Jabłonna, Poland

The aim of the present study was to examine the contribution of the periodic pancreatic secretion (PPS) associated with a duodenal three-phased migrating myoelectric complex (MMC) to the intra-animal variability in protein electrophoretical profiles of pancreatic juice. The profiles of pancreatic juice proteins in the PPS trough and the PPS peak in the preprandial period, during milk feeding, and following intravenous and intraduodenal administration of CCK-8 were studied in six 2-week-old calves surgically fitted with pancreatic duct catheters, duodenal cannulas and 2 duodenal bipolar electrodes. Duodenal MMC recording served us with precise identification of PPS cycles. Juice protein samples, adjusted to 300 ng/ml, were applied to an automated SDS-polyacrylamide gel (12.5%) electrophoresis system. Gels were silver-stained, scanned and analysed for trace density (TD; band optical density x band height) by the computer. The separations varied in the number of bands, according to the phase of the PPS. In the PPS trough 17 protein bands were detected, and at the PPS peak, 21 bands. Moreover, within the detectable bands there were significant differences in the TD between the PPS trough and peak. Following feeding and CCK-8 infusion different numbers of protein bands were observed. In conclusion, by collecting pancreatic juice strictly in phase with its natural periodic secretion and analysing the juice proteins using a computerised approach, we have shown that pancreatic secretion is apparently not uniform. The differences concern the interdigestive as well as the prandial and CCK-8-stimulated composition of pancreatic juice.

1. INTRODUCTION

Pancreatic acinar cells synthesize and secrete a large number of proteins into the pancreatic juice. The majority of these proteins are pancreatic enzymes or zymogens, e.g., serine proteases, exopeptidases, (pro)phospholipases, lipase, (pro)colipase, amylase and ribonucleases, involved in the digestive processes [1,2]. There are also pancreatic lysosomal enzymes and nonenzymatic proteins present in pancreatic juice, e.g., lithostathine [3], a

---

[*] This work was supported by grant 50102020025 from the State Committee for Scientific Research (Poland).

hypothetical protein with antibacterial activity [4], and pancreatic hormones and gut regulatory peptides in picomolar amounts [5]. Their role, however, is less documented than the role played by enzymatic proteins.

The composition of pancreatic juice has been investigated for changes in particular peptides by measurement of enzymatic activity and immunological identification, and for overall protein profiles by various means of electrophoretic and chromatographic resolution [1,2,6,7]. However, the general conclusion emerging from most of these studies is that there is a large individual, intra- and inter-species variability in the unstimulated interdigestive pancreatic protein secretion, that makes any standardization for diagnostic purposes, questionable [1]. No convincing interpretation of this physiological variability in secreted pancreatic proteins has been proposed in the available literature. On the other hand, from early studies on dogs [8] it is known that the pancreas secretes its juice in a cyclic pattern that is synchronised with changes in upper gut motility. A periodic pattern of pancreatic juice secretion (PPS), associated with the duodenal migrating myoelectric complex (MMC) has been demonstrated in several animal species, including dogs [9], pigs [10], rats [11], calves [12, 13], and humans [14]. Studies report a several-fold difference in the total protein output and enzyme activity between the asecretory phase of the PPS (associated with phase I of the MMC) and the secretory phase of the PPS (associated with phase II of the MMC). These results did not depend on pancreatic duct sphincters, since the collecting cannulas bypassed them, and the corresponding changes in concentration were significant as well. It has been suggested that neuro-hormonal regulators of pancreatic secretion that may selectively affect the composition of the juice have an important role [15, 16]. No study, however, is available concerning the possible existence of a PPS-related variability in the composition of pancreatic juice proteins.

The aim of the present study was to investigate the composition of pancreatic juice proteins in the phases of the physiological periodic fluctuations of pancreatic secretion associated with the duodenal MMC in neonatal calves. The second purpose was to investigate the effect of feeding and exogenous cholecystokinin-8 (CCK-8) on the protein composition of pancreatic juice.

2. MATERIALS AND METHODS

2.1. Animal preparation

Treatments and experiments were conducted in accordance with the European Community regulations concerning the protection of experimental animals. In six 5-day-old male Friesian calves (45 ± 2 kg body weight, BW) the pancreatic accessory duct and duodenum were catheterised and two silver bipolar electrodes were implanted in the proximal duodenum [12] (Figure 1). The pancreatic duct catheter was constructed of Silastic tubing, 2.41 x 1.57 mm in diameter (Medical Grade Tubing, Dow Corning Corp, Midland Michigan, USA) with a dead space of 0.35 ml. For surgery, the animals were premedicated with atropine (0.01 mg/kg; Atropinum Sulfuricum, Polfa, Poland) and 2% xylazine (0.15 ml/kg; Rompun, Bayer, Germany), and anaesthetised with halothane (Narkotan, Spofa, Czech).

Procaine penicillin (600,000 IU, Polfa, Poland) was administered intramuscularly for five days after the surgery. The animals recovered quickly from surgery, and the usual pancreatic juice flow, bicarbonate and protein outputs, and duodenal electrical activity (emg) were registered from the second and third post-operative days. The pancreatic duct catheter was connected to the duodenal cannula 24h after surgery. The catheter was inspected for juice flow several times a day, and once a day it was disconnected from the duodenal cannula for approximately 1h.

Calves were kept in individual cages, modified to allow free movement while ensuring sufficient restraint for the recordings. During the study, the calves received food twice daily, at 8 a.m. and 8 p.m. Liquid food, artificial milk (Pro Milk "D", crude protein 22%, crude fat 17%, ash 10%; LOL Agra International, Warsaw, Poland), was mixed with water (1:9 w/v) and given at an amount corresponding to 10% of the body weight per day from the bucket. All examined calves had a good appetite and appeared clinically healthy throughout the entire study.

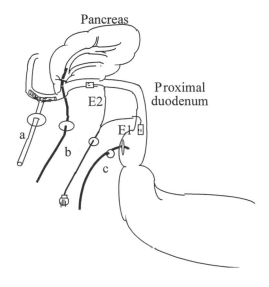

Figure 1. Surgery: six calves (2 wks old) were implanted with: (a) a duodenal T-cannula, (b) an accessory pancreatic duct catheter, (c) a duodenal bulb catheter, (E1 and E2) serosal bipolar electrodes.

2.2. Experimental protocol

The experiments were started on day 7 after surgery and repeated two or three times with a minimum of 3 days' rest between the experiments. Experiments were made on calves fasted overnight. For experiments with intravenous CCK infusions, the right external jugular vein was catheterised with a disposable polyethylene catheter 1 to 2h before the study. The indwelling electrodes were connected to an amplifier (BioAmp, ADInstruments, Australia) with high- and low-frequency cut-off filters of 50 and 3 Hz, respectively. The signals from the electrodes were recorded by means of an Apple computer-based data recording system (MacLab/4e, ADInstruments, Australia). On-line spike frequency analysis (Chart v. 3.4, ADInstruments) of the spikes exceeding a pre-set threshold amplitude ($\pm$ 40 μV) was used for visualization and analysis of migrating myoelectric complexes (MMC) in the duodenum. To observe the periodic pancreatic secretion (PPS), pancreatic juice was collected continuously at 5-min intervals during the recording of electrical activity [13]. The volume of each 5-min samples of pancreatic juice was measured, 0.2 ml of juice was taken for analysis, and the remainder was infused into the duodenum using a peristaltic pump (SJ-1211, Atto, Japan) during the next 5-min period. All samples of pancreatic juice were divided into 5 aliquots, immediately frozen, and stored at -80°C until analysis. Total protein was measured in all samples according to Lowry et al. [17]. The samples that were collected in the middle of the secretory trough (expressed as low juice flow and low protein concentration and associated with phase I of the duodenal MMC), and in the middle of the secretory peak (expressed as high juice flow and high protein concentration, associated with late phase II of the duodenal MMC) were analysed by SDS-PAGE electrophoresis.

After sampling 3 to 4 complete interdigestive pancreatic cycles as described above, the sampling procedure was continued following feeding with milk replacer or following perfusion with CCK-8 (CCK-octapeptide 26-33, sulphated form; Sigma Chemicals Co., MI, USA). Feeding (usually lasting 4-5 min), and 5-min infusion of CCK-8 (peristaltic pump with a flow rate of 1ml/min; SJ-1211, Atto, Japan) were started during late phase I when pancreatic periodic secretion was minimal (secretory trough). CCK-8 was administered either intravenously (iv; 100 pmol/kg BW) or intraduodenally (id; 300 pmol/kg BW). The samples of juice collected between 5 to 10 min and 25 to 30 min following treatment (i.e. feeding or CCK-8 administration) were analysed by SDS-PAGE electrophoresis.

The animals were killed with an overdose of pentobarbitone sodium (Nebumal Injection; Abbot, USA) after the experiment, i.e., 3 to 5 weeks after surgery. Macroscopically, the pancreas appeared normal; no distension of the accessory pancreatic duct system was observed. The major pancreatic duct was not present in the calves examined.

2.3 Sample preparation and SDS-PAGE electrophoresis

The concentration of total protein in the pancreatic juice samples was adjusted to 300 ng protein in 1 ml. Samples of pancreatic juice were mixed with a solution having a final concentration of: 2.5% SDS, 10mM Tris/HCl (pH 6.8), 5.0% b-mercaptoethanol, 1mM EDTA (pH 8.0) and 0.01% bromophenol blue. Protein standards (Low Molecular Weight [LMW] Calibration Kit, Pharmacia Biotech, Wien, Austria) were prepared in the same way.

One μl of sample was applied to each lane of 12.5% SDS-polyacrylamide gel (PhastGel[TM] homogenous 12.5, Pharmacia Biotech, Wien, Austria). Gel electrophoresis was performed using PhastSystem (PhastSystem[TM] Owner's Manual, Separation Technique File No. 111; Pharmacia Biotech, Wien, Austria). Gels were stained with a PhastGel[TM] Silver Kit (PhastSystem[TM] Owner's Manual, Development Technique File No. 210; Pharmacia Biotech). The repeatability of pancreatic juice protein resolutions was 95%.

2.4. Analysis of data

The frequency of spikes (Hz, data not shown), the duration of MMC cycles in the duodenum (min), and the indices for pancreatic juice volume (μl/kg per 5 min) and protein output (μg/kg per 5 min) were expressed as mean values and standard deviation (SD).

Distributions of secretory proteins in the samples of pancreatic juice were determined by an optical analysis of scanned silver-stained gels. Scans (scanner Sharp JX-330, Japan) were analyzed using software for scanning and optical analysis of electrophoresis bands (*pdi*, Diversity One[TM], *v.* 1.3, New York, USA). For each band, a molecular weight and a trace density (TD) were determined. TD is a quantification value equal to the optical density (OD) of the band multiplied by the height of the band in millimetres (User Guide for Diversity One™). Changes in the relative concentrations of each juice protein were determined by calculating the ratio of the TD for the juice protein relative to that of a 43 000 Da protein marker. This 43 000 Da protein marker was used as a standard because it is an external marker, and its TD, 1.16, has been found to be remarkably constant in each gel slab. Data are presented as mean values and SD.

Statistical significance in duodenal recordings, juice flow parameters and electrophoresis was determined using an ordinary or repeated measures ANOVA, followed by the Tukey-Kramer multiple comparison test and Student's t test (InStat for Macintosh v. 2.03, GraphPad Software, San Diego, California, USA), with $P < 0.05$ considered as the minimum level of significance.

3. RESULTS

The duration of MMC cycles was 36 ± 2 min, with a duration of particular phases shown in Table 1. The interdigestive pancreatic secretion fluctuated periodically in phase with the duodenal MMCs in all examined calves (Figure 2a). The lowest rate of pancreatic juice secretion (volume and protein output) was observed during phase I of the duodenal MMC. The juice secretion increased throughout early phase II, and a peak was observed during late phase II or early phase III (Table 1). The prandial periodic pancreatic cycle was significantly

Table 1
Association of minimum secretion of pancreatic juice with duodenal phase 1 of the MMC, and of maximum secretion with late phase 2 of the MMC (mean $\pm$ SD) in the pancreatic cycles during the preprandial period and following feeding

Treatment	Juice flow	Protein output
	(µl/kg/5min)	(µl/kg/5min)
Preprandial		
Minimum	8 ± 4	67.8 ± 57
Maximum	33 ± 10	350 ± 269
Feeding		
cephalic phase	$72 \pm 20^*$	$1620 \pm 1140^*$
Postprandial		
1st minimum	12 ± 5	163 ± 132
1st maximum	35 ± 13	557 ± 463
2nd minimum	8 ± 5	63 ± 56
2nd maximum	27 ± 9	310 ± 21

* Different from maximum in the preprandial period (P < 0.05).

longer than the following postprandial cycles and the control preprandial cycles (Figure 2a; Table 1). However, neither the trough nor the peak values differed significantly between the preprandial and postprandial cycles, besides a marked juice flow and protein output elevation during and just after food consumption, referred as to the cephalic phase of pancreatic secretion in preruminant calves [13, 18].

Intravenous and intraduodenal CCK-8 infusion significantly increased the pancreatic protein output per PPS cycle, by 110 and 50% respectively, but without affecting the PPS-MMC synchronicity. The response to intravenous infusion of CCK-8 was obvious within the first 5 min after the beginning of infusion, whereas the response to the intraduodenal CCK-8 started after the first 5 min of infusion (Figure 2b, Table 2).

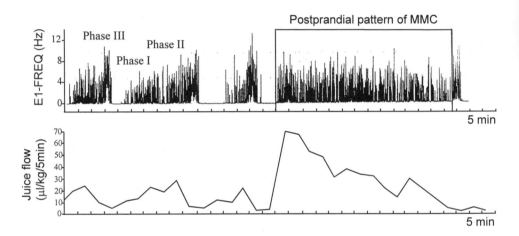

Figure 2. A representative trace showing the effect of feeding on MMC and PPS. Feeding disturbed the periodic secretory pattern and the myoelectrical activity. E1-FREQ – on-line frequency analysis of myoelectrical activity from the site near the duodenal bulb. Pancreatic juice flow collected in 5-min samples.

The composition of pancreatic secretory proteins was analysed after electrophoretic separation of pancreatic juice samples using an external protein standard. The electrophoretic patterns and the computer readings of the optical density obtained for the pancreatic juice samples taken during the secretory trough and the secretory peak of the PPS were analysed. Similar qualitative and quantitative changes were observed in the juice samples taken from all animals experimented on. The number of detectable proteins varied according to the phase of the PPS cycle (Table 2); there were 21 bands detected during the secretory peak and 17 bands detected during the secretory trough of the PPS. The number of detectable bands following feeding (cephalic phase) and. intraduodenal CCK-8 infusion was reduced compared to the preprandial protein composition. In contrast, 18 bands were detected when pancreatic secretion was stimulated by intravenous infusion of CCK-8 (Table 2), and the composition was similar to that observed 25 to 30 min after feeding (exceptor orthe 11.3 and 34.5 kDa bands).

Table 2
Relative change in secretory rates of individual secretory proteins during phases of the duodenal MMC, following feeding and id or iv CCK (mean ± SD)

Protein M.Wt.	Pancreatic secretion		Feeding		id CCK		iv CCK	
	phase 1	phase 2	5-10'	25-30'	5-10'	25-30'	5-10'	25-30'
97.0	0.11 ± 0.05^a	0.22 ± 0.08^b	0.01 ± 0.00^c	0.01 ± 0.00^c	0.09 ± 0.08^a	0.18 ± 0.05^b	$0.03^{cc} \pm 0.03^c$	0.09 ± 0.05^a
80.6	undet.	0.23 ± 0.057	undet.	undet.	undet.	undet.	undet.	undet.
76.6	0.53 ± 0.04^{ab}	0.51 ± 0.06^a	0.34 ± 0.23^{bc}	0.38 ± 0.05^c	0.12 ± 0.09^d	0.50 ± 0.14^{ab}	0.43 ± 0.13^{abc}	0.42 ± 0.14^{abc}
66.8	0.28 ± 0.03^a	0.26 ± 0.04^a	0.06 ± 0.05^b	0.02 ± 0.01^b	0.19 ± 0.05^{ac}	0.32 ± 0.10^a	0.07 ± 0.03^b	0.12 ± 0.10^{bc}
62.3	0.038 ± 0.005	0.008 ± 0.01	undet.	0.013 ± 0.015	0.01 ± 0.017	undet.	0.000 ± 0.001	0.003 ± 0.052
59.1	0.013 ± 0.019	0.04 ± 0.049	undet.	0.003 ± 0.005	0.00 ± 0.001	0.007 ± 0.121	0.025 ± 0.034	0.001 ± 0.017
56.8	0.06 ± 0.04	0.008 ± 0.020	0.005 ± 0.01	0.018 ± 0.035	undet.	0.033 ± 0.058	0.003 ± 0.006	0.000 ± 0.001
54.6	0.015 ± 0.030	0.063 ± 0.076	0.008 ± 0.015	undet.	undet.	undet.	undet.	undet.
42.4	0.51 ± 0.06^{ab}	0.49 ± 0.03^a	0.41 ± 0.10^{bc}	0.42 ± 0.04^c	0.28 ± 0.14^c	0.57 ± 0.01^a	0.54 ± 0.04^a	0.56 ± 0.00^a
36.0	0.008 ± 0.015	0.03 ± 0.038	0.005 ± 0.01	0.005 ± 0.006	undet.	undet.	0.001 ± 0.002	0.017 ± 0.015
34.5	0.018 ± 0.01	0.037 ± 0.059	0.008 ± 0.01	0.013 ± 0.01	undet.	undet.	undet.	undet.
33.0	0.013 ± 0.005	0.015 ± 0.023	undet.	0.01 ± 0.012	undet.	0.013 ± 0.023	0.012 ± 0.021	0.003 ± 0.006
27.9	1.05 ± 0.07^a	0.79 ± 0.10^b	0.50 ± 0.11^c	0.57 ± 0.05^c	0.25 ± 0.10^d	0.97 ± 0.09^a	0.86 ± 0.02^e	0.68 ± 0.10^{bc}
24.3	0.93 ± 0.03^a	0.95 ± 0.04^a	0.91 ± 0.09^a	0.76 ± 0.07^b	1.56 ± 0.08^c	1.14 ± 0.02^d	1.03 ± 1.32^{acd}	1.04 ± 0.03^d
21.6	0.043 ± 0.033	0.04 ± 0.032	0.02 ± 0.024	0.028 ± 0.022	0.003 ± 0.006	undet.	0.02 ± 0.026	0.020 ± 0.035
17.3	0.53 ± 0.05	0.46 ± 0.08	0.68 ± 0.52	0.53 ± 0.07	0.52 ± 0.01	0.74 ± 0.05	0.65 ± 0.58	0.77 ± 0.48
16.6	0.43 ± 0.19^a	0.64 ± 0.12^b	0.37 ± 0.11^a	0.55 ± 0.14^{ab}	0.07 ± 0.08^c	0.70 ± 0.08^b	0.72 ± 0.52^{ab}	0.71 ± 0.38^{ab}
14.5	0.35 ± 0.10^a	0.21 ± 0.06^b	0.33 ± 0.08^a	0.23 ± 0.12^{ab}	0.26 ± 0.01^b	0.37 ± 0.01^a	0.42 ± 0.24^a	0.42 ± 0.18^a
13.2	undet.	0.005 ± 0.008	0.003 ± 0.005	0.013 ± 0.015	undet.	undet.	0.03 ± 0.036	0.013 ± 0.023
11.3	undet.	0.018 ± 0.045	undet.	undet.	0.00 ± 0.001	0.017 ± 0.029	0.000 ± 0.001	0.027 ± 0.046
10.2	undet.	0.003 ± 0.005	undet.	0.003 ± 0.005	undet.	0.00 ± 0.001	0.000 ± 0.001	0.003 ± 0.006

undet. - undetectable protein band. Different letters in a row indicate statistical difference at $p < 0.05$ (ANOVA followed by Tukey-Kramer multiple comparison test).

Only 9 proteins, represented by 9 bands, were detected in all juice samples. These proteins had apparent molecular masses of 14.5, 16.6, 17.3, 24.3, 27.9, 42.4, 66.8, 76.6 and 97 kD.

The relative amount (expressed as a trace density, TD) of some of them changed in phase with the PPS, as evidenced by significant differences between trough and peak TD (Table 2). Comparing the quantitative composition of these 9 proteins during the trough and the peak of secretion, the TD of two proteins, 14.5 and 27.9 kDa, was significantly higher during the trough than during the peak of secretion. On the other hand, the relative amounts of another two proteins, 16.6 and 97 kDa, were significantly lower during the trough compared to the peak of PPS cycles (Table 2). The other electrophoretic bands did not show PPS-dependent periodicity. Feeding significantly reduced the TD of 66.8 and 97 kDa proteins ($p < 0.05$ and $p < 0.01$, respectively) as compared to the peak secretion during phase II in the preprandial PPS cycles (Table 2). The other proteins of these 9 that were constantly present did not change significantly following feeding. Intraduodenal administration of CCK-8 affected the TD of some of the 9 bands. The relative amounts of 7 proteins (14.5, 16.6, 17.3, 24.3, 27.9, 42.4 and 76.6 kD) were individually changed following intraduodenal infusion of CCK-8 (Table 2). Following intravenous infusion of CCK-8 no significant changes were observed with respect to control phase II (Table 2).

4. DISCUSSION

4.1. Pancreatic periodic secretion

The present study demonstrates the periodic activity of the gastrointestinal tract in neonatal calves. The duodenal MMC data are in full agreement with previous emg studies of Ruckebush and Bueno [19] and motility/emg studies of Zabielski et al.[12], that were performed in calves of the same age. On the other hand, the present pancreatic secretion data differ slightly from our previously reported kinetics of periodic pancreatic secretion [12]. This difference is due to different presentation of the data: in the present study we extracted and calculated only the extreme data. In PPS cycles in calves, the trough secretion could appear either in the first or second 5-min sample after phase III of the duodenal MMC. Similarly, the secretion peak can be observed either in the second-last or last 5-min sample before phase III, and on rare occasions during phase III. Feeding with milk replacer and stimulation with CCK produced responses similar in range to those reported elsewhere [20, 21].

4.2. Composition of pancreatic proteins in different phases of PPS

The present study demonstrates for the first time that the composition of pancreatic secretory proteins in the two phases of the PPS cycle, the secretory trough and secretory peak, is different, both in quality and in quantity. The reported phase-to-phase variability in particular pancreatic proteins was evidently greater than the in-phase animal-to-animal variability. These data suggest that for reliable analysis of pancreatic secretory protein composition the collection protocol of pancreatic juice samples must respect the natural periodic secretory activity of the exocrine pancreas. Our results obtained in conscious calves contrast sharply with the conclusion of a parallel and constantly proportional secretion of pancreatic enzymes drawn by Steer and Manabe [22]. However, the parameters of unstimulated secretions reported in their review were obtained either in *in vitro* or in acute studies, and in animal species other than the bovine. The study of Keim [23], performed on conscious rats, is also in opposition to our results, but it was performed without consideration of the natural periodic activity of the rats' GI tract [11].

We took several steps to increase the reliability of the results obtained. The chronic animal model with a pancreatic catheter implanted directly into the pancreatic duct was used to collect pure and non-activated pancreatic juice [24]. Experimental animals were clinically healthy throughout the study, and the daily monitored parameters of the interdigestive and food-stimulated duodenal MMC and of the pancreatic juice secretion (volume, bicarbonate, protein and trypsin outputs), as well as the overall periodic pattern and postprandial pattern of juice secretion did not differ from those observed previously [12, 13]. To minimise the influence of stress, collections were performed in calves well accustomed to the experimental protocol. The postmortem macroscopic inspection did not show any patho-anatomical changes in the pancreata of examined calves. For analysis, we chose SDS-PAGE electrophoresis. According to Furui et al. [25], resolution by SDS-PAGE electrophoresis, in contrast to 2-D electrophoresis, does not lead to artifactual proteolysis of pancreatic juice protein. Therefore, we think that the juice samples were collected in optimal experimental conditions, and the collections were performed under a regimen adequate to discuss the observed variability in terms of physiological fluctuations of the exocrine pancreatic secretion. Moreover, employment of an automated SDS-PAGE electrophoresis system together with a computerized band density reading system provided repeatable and objective resolution of pancreatic secretory proteins.

The present results show that during the trough of the PPS cycle the calf pancreas did not manifest the same pattern of proteins as during the peak of the PPS cycle. There were substantial differences in the relative amounts of certain proteins, besides which a certain number of proteins were not secreted (in detectable amounts). In in vitro conditions, Mroz and Lechene [26] have found that the composition of individual pancreatic zymogen granules isolated from a single animal can differ markedly; no correlation, however, between amylase and chymotrypsin activity was observed among zymogen granules in their study. In our conscious calves, the higher number of detected proteins in the peak of the PPS may suggest that certain proteins were secreted independently of zymogen granules, in response to the increased vagal activity associated with phase II of the duodenal MMC [16]. Several gut regulatory peptides, including secretin, CCK, pancreatic polypeptide and somatostatin, were found to cycle in concert with the MMC-PPS cycles in young calves [27,28]. LeBel and Beaudoin [29] suggested that the proteins released from pancreatic acinar cells without any specific stimulation could well be "washed out" by water-rich juice stimulated by secretin. However, secretin per se seems to have no effect in stimulating individual proteins [30]. This, taken together with the in vitro demonstration of individual patterns of intracellular Ca^{2+} currents in acinar cells following CCK-8 stimulation, that were not synchronous with those in the neighbouring cells in the same acinus [31] suggests a great potential for short-term variability in the composition of pancreatic secretory proteins. Consequently, the variability may result from a selective secretion of granules with different composition in particular phases of the PPS. In the study of Reseland et al. [32], pancreatic juice secretion induced by a total inhibition of tryptic activity showed a non-parallel secretion pattern, supporting the idea that specific signals (depending on CCK and/or cholinergic pathways) are required for secretion of particular enzymes. There is also increasing evidence that a proteinase-activated receptor-2 may serve as a selective trypsin sensor in the small intestinal mucosa [33].

4.3. Composition of juice proteins during and after stimulation with food and CCK

In experimental calves, the administration of food or CCK-8 produced specific changes in the composition of pancreatic juice proteins. Interestingly the immediate effect of feeding (cephalic phase) was quantitative change in the composition of the juice to similar that observed after intraduodenal CCK-8 administration, whereas the postprandial secretion (observed 25 to 30 min after feeding) was similar to that following intravenous CCK-8 administration. Thus there were distinct differences in the composition of juice proteins depending on the route of CCK-8 administration. In the secretion studies, local duodenal administration of CCK-8 needed functional vagal afferent (capsaicin-sensitive) and cholinergic atropine-sensitive pathways to be effective on the exocrine pancreas - like during cephalic phase stimulation - whereas intravenous CCK-8 did not [21,27,34]. Pharmacological blockade of mucosal CCK-A receptors by tarazepide, a specific benzodiazepine receptor antagonist, reduced both the cephalic phase of juice protein secretion and the pancreatic response to intraduodenal CCK-8 [28]. HPLC analysis of pancreatic juice proteins from anaesthetised guinea pigs demonstrated that intravenous perfusion with secretin produces a moderate increase in protein output, without changes in the composition of proteins, whereas CCK-33 and CCK-8, which increased the total protein secretion by a similar amount, apparently had different effects on individual proteins [30]. Taken together, these data suggest that the pancreatic response to feeding is not uniform at the two time points examined, and that CCK, depending on its site of action, mucosal or via the circulating blood, may evoke characteristic changes in the composition of pancreatic secretory proteins.

4.4. Implications

Although we did not identify particular pancreatic juice proteins, a remarkable variability in their composition was found in the interdigestive, and food- and CCK-stimulated conditions in the neonatal calves examined. It is suggested that the interdigestive variability is associated with the cyclic fluctuations of pancreatic juice secretion (PPS). The variability observed during and after stimulation with food and CCK may reflect the specific timing sequence of particular neuro-hormonal regulatory mechanisms. The present findings on the one hand suggest a need for standardisation of pancreatic juice sampling conditions, and on the other hand encourage further research on the consequences of this physiological phenomenon.

6. REFERENCES

1. B. Göke and V. Keim, Int. J. Pancreatol., 11 (1992) 109.
2. M.E. Lowe, L.R. Johnson (eds.), Physiology of the Gastrointestinal Tract. Raven Press, NY, (1994) 1531.
3. A. De Caro, J. Lhose and H. Sarles., Biochem. Biophys. Res. Commun., 87 (1979) 1176.
4. S.G. Pierzynowski, P. Sharma, J. Sobczyk, S. Garwacki and W. Barej, Int. J. Pancreatol., 2 (1992) 121.
5. P.M. Pour and R.E. Hauser, Int. J. Pancreatol., 2 (1987) 277.
6. C. Liebow, Pancreas, 3 (1988) 343.
7. P.J. Padfield, G.A. Scheele, V.L.W. Go et al. (eds.) The Pancreas: Biology, Pathobiology, and Disease. Raven Press, N.Y., 273 (1993) 265.
8. W. Boldyreff, Ergebnisse der Physiologie, 11 (1911) 121.

9. E.P. DiMagno, J.C. Hendricks, V.L.W. Go and R.R. Dozois, Dig. Dis. and Sci., 24 (1979) 689.
10. J. Abello, J.P. Laplace and T. Corring, Reproduction, Nutrition, Développement, 28 (1988) 953.
11. T. Onaga, R. Zabielski, H. Mineo and S. Kato, Proceedings of XXXII Congress of the International Union of Physiological Sciences, Glasgow, Great Britain, 95.1/P (1993) 83.
12. R. Zabielski, T. Onaga, H. Mineo and S. Kato, Exp. Physiol., 78 (1993) 675.
13. R. Zabielski, P. Kiela, V. Leśniewska, R. Krzemiński, M. Mikołajczyk and W. Barej, Brit. J. Nutr., 78 (1997) 427.
14. G.R. Vantrappen, T.L. Peeters and J. Janssens, Scand. J. Gastroenterol., 14 (1979) 663.
15. J.C. Dagorn, D. Paradis and J. Morisset, Digestion, 15 (1977) 110.
16. P. Layer, A.T.H. Chan, V.L.W. Go, A.R. Zinsmeister and E.P. DiMagno, Pancreas, 8 (1993) 181.
17. O.H. Lowry, N.J. Rosebrough, A.L. Farr and R.J. Randall, J. Biol. Chem., 193 (1951) 165.
18. S.G. Pierzynowski, R. Zabielski, P. Podgurniak, P. Kiela, P. Sharma, B.R. Weström, S. Kato and W. Barej, J. Anim. Physiol. Anim. Nutr., 67 (1992b) 268.
19. Y. Ruckebusch and L. Bueno, Brit. J. Nutr., 30 (1973) 491.
20. R.J. McCormick, and W.E. Stewart, J. Dairy Sci., 50 (1966) 568.
21. R. Zabielski, T. Onaga, H. Mineo, S. Kato and S.G. Pierzynowski, Int. J. Pancreatol., 17, 3 (1995) 271.
22. M.L. Steer and T. Manabe, J. Biol Chem., 254 (1979).
23. V. Keim, Ann. Nutr. Metab., 30 (1986) 104.
24. V.M. Gabert, M.S. Jensen, B.R. Weström and S.G. Pierzynowski, Int. J. Pancreatol., 22 (1997) 39.
25. T. Furui, M. Ikeda, L. Chao-Ming, K. Okita and K. Nakamura, Electrophoresis, 17 (1997) 797.
26. E.A. Mroz and C. Lechene, Science, 232 (1986) 871.
27. R. Zabielski, T. Onaga, H. Mineo, S.G. Pierzynowski, and S. Kato, Exp. Physiol., 79 (1994) 301.
28. R. Zabielski, V. Leśniewska, J. Borlak, P.C. Gregory, P. Kiela, S.G. Pierzynowski and W. Barej, Regul. Pept., 57 (1996) 278.
29. D. LeBel and A.R. Beaudoin, Biochim. Biophys. Acta, 847 (1985) 132.
30. P.J. Padfield and R.M. Case, Pancreas, 4 (1987) 439-446.
31. T. Kanno, Digestion, 58 (S2) (1997) 5.
32. J.E. Reseland, H. Holm, T. Jennsen, M.B. Jacobsen and L.E. Hanssen, Scand. J. Gastroenterol., 30 (1995) 72-80.
33. S.K. Bohm, W. Kong, D. Bromme, S.P. Smeekens, D.C. Anderson, A. Connolly, M. Kahn, N.A. Nelken, S.R. Coughlin, D.G. Payan and N.W. Bunnett, Biochem. J., 314 (1996) 1009-1016.
34. C. Owyang, Amer. J. Physiol., 271 (1996) G1.

Biology of the Pancreas in Growing Animals
S.G. Pierzynowski and R. Zabielski (Editors)
© 1999 Elsevier Science B.V. All rights reserved.

Neurohormonal regulation of the exocrine pancreas during postnatal development

R. Zabielski[ab] and S. Naruse[c]

[a]Department of Animal Physiology, Faculty of Veterinary Medicine,
Warsaw Agricultural University, Nowoursynowska 166, 02-787 Warsaw, Poland

[b]The Kielanowski Institute of Animal Physiology and Nutrition,
Polish Academy of Sciences, Instytucka 3, 05-110 Jabłonna, Poland

[c]Department of Internal Medicine II, School of Medicine, Nagoya University,
65 Tsurumai-cho, Showa-ku, Nagoya, 466-8550, Japan

The secretion of pancreatic juice in dogs, calves, pigs, rats, sheep and in humans is periodic. It works in concert with the other periodic activities in the gastrointestinal tract, e.g., gastric juice and bile secretion, gastroduodenal motility and blood flow. Studies on the secretion of pancreatic juice in conscious animals have to take this physiological variability into account. Food influences the periodic activity of the pancreas in a species- and age-specific way. Nerves, particularly the vagi, are important regulators of periodic activity, but the origin of the periodic activity of the pancreas is dependent on the extravagal cholinergic pathways located in the gastrointestinal tract. The role of the gut regulatory peptides is to modulate the already generated periodic pattern. A newly documented local duodenal mechanism regulating the pancreatic secretion via CCK is also discussed.

1. PERIODIC PANCREATIC SECRETION AS A BASIC SECRETORY PATTERN IN CONSCIOUS ANIMALS

1.1. Discovery of the periodic pancreatic secretion phenomenon

The history of research on the phenomenon of pancreatic periodic secretion (PPS) starts in the Imperial Institute of Experimental Medicine in St. Petersburg at the beginning of the 20th century. In 1911, Wassilij Von Boldyreff, chief assistant to Prof. I.P. Pavlov, published an extensive article in German, entitled "Some new features of pancreatic function" [1]. In this work of nearly 100 pages, he summarised the most important findings of his 10-year research on conscious dogs with pancreatic, gastric and Thiry-Vella fistulae [2,3]. Boldyreff demonstrated that in the preprandial or fasting condition the exocrine pancreas secretes juice in a cyclic pattern which is synchronised with other changes in gastrointestinal activity - gastric and intestinal luminal pressures and gastric and bile secretions. The secretion of pancreatic juice shows clear peaks and nadirs which coincide with the peaks and nadirs of bile secretion, respectively, as well as with the periods of alternating gastric contraction and rest. This pattern repeats itself periodically and the duration of the work-and-rest cycle in dogs is between 90 and 110 min (Figure 1). Feeding, and to a certain degree the sight and smell of the food, disrupt the periodic pattern. Boldyreff's observations of periodic changes in secretion were soon confirmed by Babkin and Ishikawa [4].

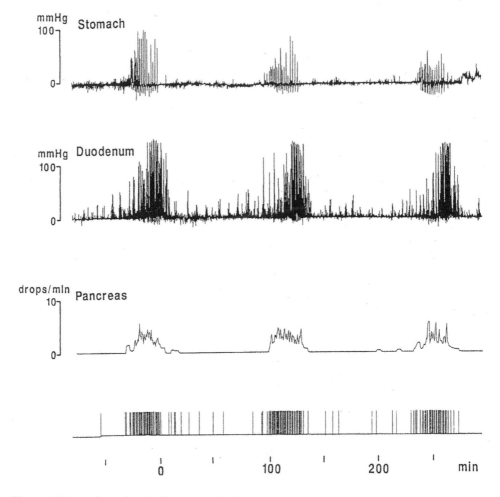

Figure 1. Recording of periodic activity in the stomach, duodenum and pancreas in the adult dog fasted for 24 h prior to the experiment. Top, luminal pressure of the stomach and duodenum. Bottom, integrated (drops/min) and raw (each vertical slash represents one drop) recording of pancreatic juice flow measured by a drop counter (S. Naruse – unpublished results).

After this, the periodic secretory pattern was forgotten (with isolated exceptions: [5]) for over 60 years, and "rediscovered" in 1979 by DiMagno et al. [6]. In the same year,

Vantrappen *et al.* [7] published similar observations made in adult men. In the following years, several groups conducted intensive research on the periodic pancreatic secretion, resulting in a better understanding of the nature of this physiological phenomenon [8,9,10, 11,12,13].

The motility cycles of the gastrointestinal tract have a history dating from 1858, when Busch [14] published his observations on fasting contractions in humans. This author was also probably the first to introduce the concept of periodic activity in the gastrointestinal tract. Since that time, there have been several waves of increased scientific interest (as periodic as the pattern they describe) in the periodic motor/electrical activity of the gastrointestinal tract. In the present chapter we refer mostly to publications concerned with the periodic activity of the pancreas. Wingate [15], Sarna [16], Davenport [17], and recently Szurszewski [18] have published extensive historical reviews concerning gastrointestinal motility cycles.

1.2. Concealment of the periodic pancreatic secretion phenomenon

As mentioned above, soon after its discovery, the phenomenon of periodic pancreatic secretion was forgotten, and remained so until the late seventies. Several questions arise; first of all, was the pattern really forgotten, or was it maybe overlooked or neglected? Probably both. It was forgotten because Boldyreff in his early scientific career did not publish his work in English, which would substantially limit the number of potential readers [15]. It was overlooked and neglected by Pavlov who did not see enough of interest in these studies and did not promote the results of his assistant [19]. It was also overlooked and neglected by the other investigators studying exocrine pancreatic function in the coming years.

The next question is *why* the PPS was forgotten. First of all, the preprandial or fasting pancreatic secretion was not as attractive a subject for investigation as was the secretion stimulated by different means (food, food components, etc). The former served "only" as a control for a certain treatment and even the words used to describe it, *basal conditions* or *basic secretion* suggested a constant process, somehow unalterable. Any alteration in basal secretion reduced the sensitivity of the test (the response to an examined stimulus was less clear), and provided problems with statistical evaluation of the experiment. Often the physiological peaks in pancreatic juice secretion seen during collection were considered an accidental problem with the juice flow in the collecting system, and the results likely to be discarded, a known, circulating anecdote but hardly to be found in scientific publications.

Secondly, pancreatic periodic secretion is a difficult pattern to demonstrate. The frequency and amplitude of peaks differ from animal to animal [10,20,21]. Several nutritional and nonnutritional factors, for example psychological factors like fear, stress, fatigue or food expectation, may influence or disturb the periodic activity. As discussed in the coming subchapters, the presence of periodic activity also depends on the health status of the experimental animal. Time limitations for the experiment could also be important - the dog, even if well trained, could only be restrained for a relatively short period of time so the period of control collection would not be long enough to convincingly register the physiological periodic pattern. To register the periodic activity in his dogs, Boldyreff conducted experiments lasting 6 to 8 hours. In the laboratories of Magee and Naruse, on each experimental day control recordings were usually made on the dog for 2 to 4 hours before any treatment was begun [10,20,22,23]. To describe a wave form, no less than 7 consecutive collections per cycle should be made; thus in experiments on dogs manifesting a periodic activity of about 2 hours it is necessary to collect the juice at 10-min intervals. From the above, it seems that successful recording of periodic activity depends more on a great deal of labour carried out by an experienced research staff, truly devoted to animal experiments, than on sophisticated laboratory equipment.

Finally, there could also be differences related to the cannulation method used. Lee et al. [24] showed that the mean length of pancreatic secretory and duodenal motility cycles in dogs with Herrera cannulas was significantly shorter than that of dogs with Thomas cannulas. The motility cycles in the latter were of normal duration, similar to those of non-cannulated dogs. Moreover, secretion of pancreatic juice (peak secretion and secretion per cycle) was higher in dogs with Herrera cannulas than in dogs fitted with Thomas cannulas, while the opposite was true for bicarbonate output. Gabert et al. [25] observed that pigs with the catheter implanted in the accessory pancreatic duct showed much larger hourly variations in the secretion of juice compared to pigs with a cannulated duodenal pouch containing the accessory pancreatic duct orifice, suggesting that the former method is more sensitive to physiological fluctuations in pancreatic secretion. It should be mentioned that there are some anatomical variations in the pancreatic duct system: in the majority of pigs and cattle the "main" pancreatic duct does not exist; its duties are taken over by the accessory pancreatic duct (for details see chapter by Kato et al.).

1.3. The pancreatic periodic secretion concept revisited

Boldyreff's finding of periodic pancreatic secretion (PPS) in association with the bile flow and duodenal motor activity [1] was revisited in the fasting dog by DiMagno et al. in 1979 [6]. In the same year it was demonstrated in humans [7], and after that confirmed in dogs [10, 12], pigs [13,26], and rats [27]. In all examined species the lowest pancreatic secretion levels occurred during phase 1 in the duodenum, i.e., the period of quiescence with no spiking activity in the duodenal migrating myoelectric complex (MMC) (Figures 1,2,3). The pancreatic secretion increased intermittently during phase 2, the period of irregular spiking activity of the duodenal MMC, and the secretion ceased just before or during phase 3, the period of regular spiking activity of the duodenal MMC. The peak volume of the PPS was only 7 % of the maximal response to exogenous secretin but the protein peak was no less than 60% of the maximal response to cholecystokinin (CCK) [20,28].

Having an idea about the pattern of periodic pancreatic secretion in monogastric animals, it became interesting to check whether such periodic oscillations could be observed in ruminant animals of different ages. One could claim that there is periodic activity in these species due to the particular flow pattern of digesta in the small intestine of ruminants as compared to monogastric animals. In adult ruminants, due to the presence of a large reservoir in the rumen and continuous delivery of digesta from the forestomach to the abomasum, the flow of digesta to the duodenum is also more continuous. Overnight fasting has little effect on the abomaso-duodenal digesta flow. In young calves, even though the forestomach is not yet developed anatomically, the flow of digesta from the abomasum to the duodenum is continuous, too. Abomasal chymosin secreted in the suckling calf leads to coagulation of ingested milk casein in the abomasum and a marked delay in the abomasal emptying rate. Milk clots are normally found in the abomasum on the day after feeding. There is a similar pattern of digesta flow in suckling piglets and human infants; thus the preruminant calf can be regarded as a good, and relatively easily handled experimental model for paediatric studies.

To investigate the periodic activity in preruminant calves, a chronic animal model was prepared on the basis of a method for cannulation of the accessory pancreatic duct in cattle

[29], with modifications [30,31,32]. This model was found suitable for monitoring pancreatic secretion for several weeks in the same animal, i.e. the calf could be observed from early life till rumination [33]. For the recording of duodenal electrical and mechanical activity, silver bipolar electrodes [34], and foil strain gauges were implanted in the duodenum and proximal jejunum [21]. In preruminant calves the duodenal MMC pattern showed regular oscillations in amplitude and spike frequency similar to those observed in adult monogastric and ruminating animals [21,35]. Three successive phases were observed: a phase of no spiking activity (phase 1), a phase of irregular spiking activity (phase 2), and a phase of regular spiking activity (phase 3). In contrast to dogs, phase 4 was usually not observed in calves and phase 3 was followed by sudden electrical quiescence. The average duration of the whole MMC cycle in 8 to 30-day-old-calves was 32-34 min. In a few calves the MMC lasted on average 40 min, and in one calf the cycle was as short as 23 min; the animals were clinically as healthy as the remaining calves in which the duration of the MMC was remarkably uniform. Less than 10% of the duodenal MMC cycles disappeared in the proximal jejunum, and the number of disappearing MMCs tended to increase with age. Pancreatic secretion fluctuated in phase with the duodenal electrical activity in the fasting state. The lowest volume concurred with electrical quiescence, phase 1 (Figure 2). The secretion increased during phase 2, reached its peak just before duodenal phase 3 and usually waned again with the onset of phase 3, although on rare occasions the zenith coincided with phase 3.

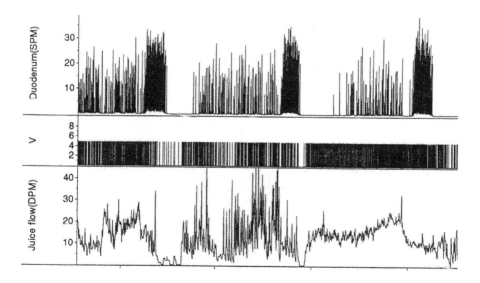

Figure 2. Recording of duodenal MMC and pancreatic juice flow in a 4-week-old preruminant calf. Top, the EMG signal was band-pass filtered (3-50 Hz) and integrated by extracting and summing up the spikes exceeding a pre-set threshold amplitude ($\pm$ 0.04 mV) over 10s periods. Bottom, flow of pancreatic juice measured by a drop counting device. The duration of MMC and PPS cycles is ca. 35 min. SPM, spikes per minute; DPM, drops per minute.

Fluctuations were quite apparent, peaks in fluid and protein secretion were usually more than 2 and 3 times greater than the trough secretion, respectively. Peak volume and protein output of PPS in examined calves were 50% and 30%, respectively, of the response to milk ingestion [21].

Pancreatic fluctuations were of the same duration as the corresponding MMCs, i.e. if an MMC was prolonged, then the respective PPS was prolonged accordingly. In adult sheep, as in monogastric animal species, the flow of pancreatic juice was lowest during phase 1 of the duodenal MMC, and the flow increased during phase 2, coinciding with the increase in duodenal spiking activity. However, there was no distinct peak of pancreatic secretion, and the amplitude of periodic activity was low compared to that in dogs and preruminant calves [36].

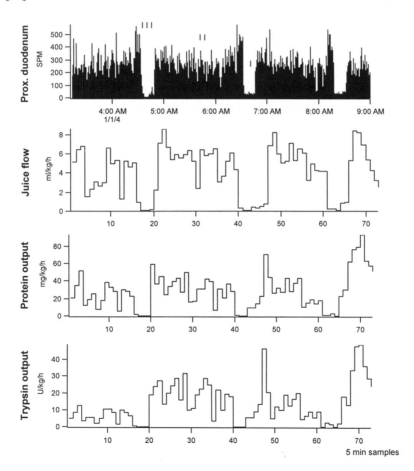

Figure 3. The duodenal MMC and pancreatic fluid, protein and trypsin outputs registered simultaneously in the 3-month-old weaned pig. SPM, spikes per minute. From doctoral thesis of P. Kiela [39].

The pig is a rather difficult animal in which to study pancreatic periodic activity; nevertheless a few trials have already been reported [37,38]. Kiela in his doctoral thesis [39], convincingly demonstrated a pancreatic periodic activity of ca. 62 min duration in juice flow, protein output and trypsin activity output in phase with the antral and duodenal myoelectric activities in weaned piglets. In precise flowmeter recordings [40], the lowest secretion was sustained during antral and duodenal phase 1 activity and it did not rise until the beginning of antral and duodenal phase 2. No clear secretion peak was observed during phase 2 (Figure 3).

Table 1
The preprandial secretion of pancreatic juice in phases of the duodenal myoelectric motor complex (MMC) in neonatal calves 10-16 days old. Mean of 9 calves $\pm$ SEM, asterisks indicate statistically significant difference to the data for phase 1 (*$P < 0.05$, **$P < 0.01$)

Measurement	Phase 1	Phase 2	Phase 3
Duration of MMC phase (min)	9.5 ± 0.3	21.0 ± 0.7**	2.0 ± 0.2
Juice flow (μl/kg/5 min)	15 ± 3	34 ± 3**	29 ± 5
Bicarbonate output (μeq/kg/5 min)	1.1 ± 0.1	2.7 ± 0.2**	1.9 ± 0.2*
Protein output (μg/kg/5 min)	60 ± 5	170 ± 20**	100 ± 15*
Amylase activity output (U/kg/5 min)	0.6 ± 0.1	1.7 ± 0.1**	1.2 ± 0.1*
Trypsin activity output (U/kg/5 min)	1.3 ± 0.2	3.7 ± 0.2**	2.7 ± 0.2**

As demonstrated, in all the species examined the flow of pancreatic juice is not constant but oscillates periodically in concert with the duodenal motor/electrical activity. The periodic pattern concerns not only the volume of the pancreatic juice but also the concentration of bicarbonate, total protein, and specific enzyme activity; thus the variations in their respective outputs in different phases of the MMC are much greater than the variation in the juice flow considered separately (Table 1, see also chapter by Leśniewska et al.). There are certain species-, age- and food-related differences in the periodic pattern in the preprandial or fasting conditions and after feeding, as discussed below.

Besides the PPS, the exocrine pancreas may exhibit other periodic activity. Thaela et al. [41] in their studies in pigs found that the secretion of pancreatic juice exhibited ultradian and circadian rhythms which were apparently associated with the feeding and lighting regimen. It was suggested that these activities underwent certain development with age, since they could not be found just after weaning. On the other hand, the daily secretion of pancreatic juice in piglets gradually increases following weaning [42], which could have interfered with the chronobiological analysis in this study.

1.4. Periodic activity of other gastrointestinal functions related to the PPS

Animal experiments show that in addition to the association between the motility of the stomach, small intestine and the secretion of pancreatic juice, the other functions of the gastrointestinal tract also manifest periodic activity which is well synchronised with the MMC and PPS. In dogs, the secretion of pepsin is strongly associated with gastric and duodenal motility but independent of changes in the secretion of gastric acid [28]. Gastric acid secretion varies from dog to dog and from cycle to cycle and the other periodic activities are not affected by alkalinization of the stomach or duodenum; thus gastric acid is probably not a driving force for the other periodic secretions in the GI tract. Similarly, in preruminant calves evacuation of the abomasal juice by an abomasal cannula did not abolish the periodic activity [43]. Bile output increases rapidly at the beginning of gastric and duodenal contractions and the peak of bile secretion in dogs precedes the duodenal motility and pancreatic secretion peaks by 30 to 40 min [28]. About 80% of bile is secreted during the peak in fasted dogs. Konturek and Thor [44] reported that the duodenal alkaline secretion fluctuates cyclically in phase with duodenal motility, being maximal during phase 2 of the duodenal MMC.

In young [21] and adult [45] ruminant animals, the duodenal motor activity was temporally co-ordinated with electrical activity, and studies with electromagnetic flow probes implanted in the duodenum showed that the duodenal MMC was well synchronised with the rate of digesta flow in preruminant calves [46]. During phase 1 of the duodenal MMC the flow of digesta came to a halt, and maximal flow was observed just before phase 3. Finally, a positive correlation between the number of spikes/phase in the duodenum and the pancreatic secretion (volume: $r = 0.73$, $P < 0.0001$, protein output: $r = 0.63$, $P < 0.001$) in MMC/PPS cycles was found in preruminant calves (Leśniewska, Zabielski, Kato - unpublished results). When phase 2 was considered in isolation, the correlation was even stronger (volume: $r = 0.87$, protein output: $r = 0.69$). Therefore, pancreatic juice seems to be secreted in harmony with duodenal function in a precisely regulated manner in preruminant calves.

An association between gastrointestinal motility and blood flow has been shown in conscious dogs, both in the stomach and in the small intestinal circulation [47,48]. During the quiescent period in the stomach of the fasting dog, an electromagnetic flowmeter implanted in the left gastric artery showed a stable blood flow of ca. 34 ml/min [47]. During the contraction period each peristaltic contraction was coupled with a rapid fall and subsequent rise in blood flow but there was a sustained elevation in blood flow coinciding with the contraction phase of the stomach. Small intestinal blood flow measured by an electromagnetic flow probe implanted on the mesenteric artery showed clear MMC-related variations in fasted dogs [48]. These relations (high blood flow during phase 2 and low blood flow during phase 1 of the jejunal MMC), however, disappeared when the intestinal content was drained out. This suggests that contact of the intestinal mucosa with the luminal fluid swept by the peristaltic movement associated with the MMC evokes a hyperaemic response. In the stomach, on the other hand, a sustained elevation of blood flow in association with periodic motor activity was observed even when gastric juice was diverted to the exterior through a gastric fistula [47]. In fact stimulation of gastric secretion by gastrin failed to increase gastric blood flow [49]. Thus, it seems that the periodic increases in blood flow in the stomach and small intestine are induced by completely different mechanisms. Cholinergic mechanisms appear to be involved in the stomach, as atropine inhibits both the periodic motility and the blood flow [47]. Feeding induced a rapid but transient increase in gastric blood flow [49] but postprandial rhythmic contractions of the stomach had little effect on left gastric arterial blood flow [47]. Periodic increases in blood flow did not appear until the next gastroduodenal MMC started. It is not known whether pancreatic blood flow exhibits periodic changes in phase with PPS as continuous measurement of pancreatic blood flow was not successful until recently [50].

The endocrine function of the gastrointestinal tract manifests periodic activity with regard to some of the gut regulatory peptides. In dogs and humans, plasma pancreatic polypeptide (PP) and motilin concentrations fluctuate in phase with the duodenal MMC [8,11,51,52,53]. The perfection in the timing of PP and motilin peaks during MMC/PPS cycles raised the question of their role in the origin and regulation of intestinal and pancreatic periodic activity. In dogs, intravenous infusion of physiological doses of motilin evoked the appearance of a PPS pattern similar to the spontaneous interdigestive PPS [11,54]. Moreover, endogenous motilin released by duodenal alkalinization had the same effect as exogenous hormone [54]. However, in studies on dogs with an autotransplanted pancreas, the coexistence of interdigestive MMC and motilin cycles but not PP cycles was found [55]. Duodenotomy in dogs did not abolish pancreatic trypsin and plasma motilin periodic activities, although the cyclic pattern in plasma PP was lost. Trypsin and motilin cycles were independent of each other in the duodenectomized dogs [56]. Similarly, in human subjects with impaired pancreatic function (chronic pancreatitis), plasma PP and pancreatic juice cycles were not co-ordinated with the interdigestive antroduodenal motility [57]. Changes in the peripheral blood plasma concentrations of PP and motilin associated with the MMC/PPS pattern were also observed in pigs [58,59], sheep [60], and calves [61]. The amplitude of preprandial fluctuations in plasma PP and motilin concentration in calves fed with milk replacer based on skim-milk powder was similar to that of the fluctuations observed in dogs [8,52,62]. In the calves, however, the plasma PP peak occurred in early phase 2 rather than late phase 2, and the motilin peak was observed during late phase 2 of the duodenal MMC [61]. Interestingly, after replacing milk protein with fish protein, the fluctuations in PP concentration were less clear, due to a high scattering of the data, while motilin fluctuations were not detected at all. Thus, the authors suggested that the synchronicity between plasma PP and motilin concentrations and duodenal and pancreatic cycles may be disrupted by "unphysiological" feeds, e.g. feed containing protein devoid of clotting activity in the abomasum and resulting in a massive inflow of digesta into the proximal duodenum immediately after feeding in preruminant calves. The physiological relevance of PP and motilin in calves needs to be clarified, although the relevance of motilin in regulation of the sheep MMC has been questioned by Plaza et al. [60].

Secretin fluctuations have been reported in pigs and calves (the plasma secretin concentration was significantly higher during phase 2 than phase 1 of the duodenal MMC) [58,63] but not in dogs [11]. Qvist et al. [53] reported that plasma secretin was slightly elevated (nonsignificant) during the duodenal phase of no spiking activity of the MMC in 3 of 7 healthy humans examined.

CCK and gastrin fluctuate in phase with the MMC and/or PPS in pigs [64], and under certain feeding conditions in preruminant calves [61, 63]. Fluctuations in plasma CCK concentration were found in calves fed with milk replacer based on skim-milk powder but not in calves fed with a milk replacer with added soya bean and fish protein. It has been shown that milk replacer containing soya bean protein elevates plasma CCK more than milk, which might nullify physiological oscillations [65]. In dogs, fluctuations in gastrin but not in CCK were registered [11,12]. Gastrin fluctuations have been explained as probably secondary to the periodic secretion of gastric juice [12].

Short (2 - 7 min) and circadian oscillations of insulin have been reviewed elsewhere [66]. In humans, 105-120-min oscillations in insulin secretion, being of very similar duration to the intestinal MMC, were shown by Shapiro *et al*. [67]. Since the endocrine and exocrine part of the pancreatic gland is strongly linked anatomically and physiologically, we were interested in the relationship between them in terms of periodic activity. In one experiment in four fasting preruminant calves, we recorded duodenal EMG, collected pancreatic juice continuously (in 5-min samples) and simultaneously sampled blood every 2 minutes from the external jugular vein. The insulin concentration in the blood showed rapid oscillations (6-8 min) which did not correspond to the timing of the fasting MMC and PPS cycles. However, after reproducing postprandial glycaemia by continuous intravenous infusion of glucose (90 - 95 mg%), the plasma insulin increased and started to fluctuate in phase with the MMC and PPS, and the timing of the duodenal and pancreatic events then became surprisingly regular (Kiela, Zabielski, Mineo and Kato, unpublished results). It is difficult to conclude which mechanism was behind the periodic changes in insulin concentration, since no other measurements were made (e.g., glucagon or pancreatic polypeptide). Nevertheless, we speculate that in calves insulin may be important in early resumption of the prandial pattern and recovery of the periodic activity of the exocrine part of the pancreas as well as of the small intestine. In calves the recovery of MMC/PPS after feeding is much faster than in adult dogs.

1.5. Effect of food on the periodic activity of the pancreas

In dogs, rats, pigs, preruminant calves, and humans feeding has a considerable stimulatory effect on pancreatic water, bicarbonate and enzyme secretion as well as on duodenal motility, while in adult sheep or cows, the prandial increase in pancreatic secretion is negligible [68, 69]. According to Pavlov's early observations the prandial pattern could be divided into 3 phases: cephalic, gastric and intestinal. The cephalic phase is related to the sight and smell of food and to the consumption of a meal (chewing, swallowing, drinking); therefore it can start well before the food is eaten. For instance, in preruminant calves kept at an experimental farm, the secretion of pancreatic juice increased 15 to 30 min before the feeding time [70], and was obviously related to the daily routine of preparing a milk replacer, feeding the other calves nearby, etc. However, under a strict feeding time regimen, but without giving the animals any possibility to see or hear the procedure of food preparation, no cephalic phase was observed *before* eating (Figure 4) [21,71]. Moreover, the pancreatic secretion increment during the cephalic phase was much higher in the former conditions than in the latter. Of the following prandial phases, the gastric phase lasts as long as food is present in the stomach, and the intestinal phase is a result of pancreatic stimulation by the digesta present in the lumen of the small intestine.

According to early observations in dogs by Boldyreff, which were later confirmed in other animal species [1,12,21,39,72], the pancreatic and gastrointestinal periodic activities disappear during food consumption or are replaced by a prandial or feeding pattern. However, there is a noticeable difference in the prandial pattern between dogs and calves. In dogs, the MMC is replaced by a continuous feeding pattern, and the pancreatic postprandial response is characterised by a complete disruption of the PPS for several hours. During the canine feeding pattern, the juice flow increases to over 10 times the peak value of the PPS; the increase in protein output is smaller. The timing of the MMC/PPS disruption depends on food composition, caloric load, and on the consistence of the meal (solid vs. liquid). Canine PPS cycles reappear together with the duodenal MMC when the stomach and intestine become empty. On the other hand, in preruminant calves the MMC and PPS cycles are disrupted postprandially for less than 2 hours, after which the usual cycles are registered again despite the presence of digesta in the abomasal and small intestinal lumen, as demonstrated in Figure 4 [21]. Also, the difference between the prandial peak (cephalic phase) and the PPS peak secretion in preruminant calves is less dramatic than in dogs. In piglets fasted overnight,

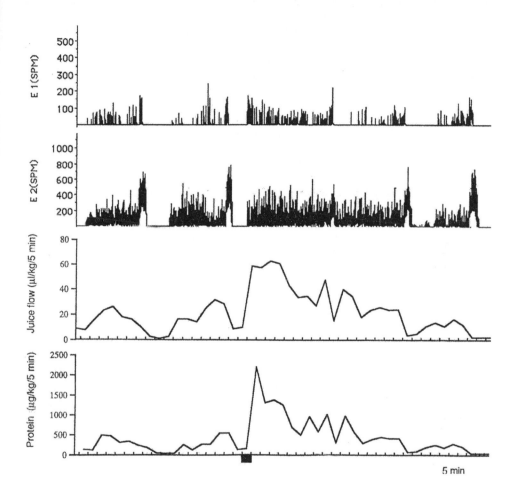

Figure 4. Effect of food on the PPS and MMC pattern in a 14-d-old calf. The calf received a morning dose of food (skim-milk based milk replacer) from a bucket, as indicated on the time scale. Upper traces represent on-line frequency analysis of the EMG signal recorded by two pairs of serosal electrodes sutured onto the duodenum 4 cm and 30 cm caudal to the pylorus. Lower traces represent juice flow and protein output in 5-min samples collected during EMG recording.

feeding does not influence the synchronisation between the PPS and MMC, and the duration of the MMC/PPS pattern remains unchanged following feeding. The pancreatic cycle during feeding is modified by a 50% elevation in protein output and a nonsignificant rise in trypsin output [39].

Moreover, in preruminant calves only a vagus-dependent cephalic phase is present; the two other phases (gastric and intestinal) are not observed [73,74,75]. The amplitude and frequency of the duodenal electrical activity are greatly increased during suckling; this characteristic event is observed only in milk-fed calves and not in ruminant calves. Concomitant with duodenal hyperactivity there is a sudden increase in pancreatic secretion, with a return to normal 25-30 min after the meal, followed by intermittent slowing of secretion as phase 3 and phase 1 migrate caudally through the duodenum. The duration of the first few postprandial PPS and MMC cycles in preruminant calves is prolonged by a few minutes [21]. To date, the postprandial characteristics of the PPS in adult ruminants have not been studied in detail. Nevertheless, electromyographical examination showed only prolonged duration of the duodenal MMC, without any disruption of the periodic fluctuations in the upper gut after feeding in cows and sheep [35]. These findings correspond well with our pancreatic studies in young ruminant calves in which food consumption prolonged the duodenal MMC in the morning by 12 min (P < 0.05) and in the evening by 3.5 min (not significant). The first six postprandial MMCs were longer by ca. 7 min than the preprandial, and modifications in the periodic activity of the pancreas were associated with the MMC duration [71]. In weaned piglets, a transient cephalic phase but no gastric or intestinal phase was observed, and the first three postprandial pancreatic cycles did not differ from the preprandial ones with regard to juice flow and trypsin activity [39]. These results imply that in young ruminants and in piglets the MMC and PPS cycles are actively involved in digestive processes, whereas in dogs they seem to play a "housekeeping" [76] role during the interdigestive period.

1.6. Development of the PPS with age

Formerly, experiments on the PPS pattern were performed only on adult animals or human volunteers, and no information was available on the characteristics of the PPS in young growing animals. Then electromyography studies by Bueno and Ruckebush [77] demonstrated the existence of species-specific patterns of small intestinal development in dog puppies and lambs, characterised by differences in the timing of the fetal, transient and "adult" MMC patterns. Using our calf model with a chronically catheterised pancreas and implanted serosal intestinal electrodes, we explored the PPS pattern in neonatal, preruminant and ruminant calves. In studies on 0 to 6-day-old calves, instead of EMG, duodenal luminal pressure was recorded. The data presented in Table 2 show that the appearance and duration of the duodenal and pancreatic periodic pattern are related to both the age of the calf and the kind of diet (liquid vs. solid).

In calves studied from the day of birth the first periodic activity of pancreatic secretion was seen on the second or third day of life [78]. This activity were associated with distinct MMC cycles that appeared in the duodenum. During the first day or two of life, however, no three-phased duodenal MMC could be recorded. Instead, a biphasic pattern resembling phase 1 (of ca. 6 min duration) and phase 2 (of ca. 12 min duration) of the MMC but without a pancreatic periodic component, was present. In older preruminant calves, the PPS pattern was obvious. The PPS displayed a shortening with age of the phase 1-related nadir secretion, with a compensatory increase in the phase 2-related peak secretion. A distinct PPS peak in ruminant calves was rare; more often the secretion was elevated during the whole of phase 2. In the adult sheep, the PPS was manifested as a temporary drop in secretion concomitant with phase 1, with no clear peak during phase 2 of the MMC [36].

Table 2
Preprandial periodic activity of the duodenum and pancreas in calves

Age (days)	Diet	Periodic activity of the duodenum	Duration of the duodenal pattern (mean ± SD, min)	Periodic activity of the pancreas
1	Colostrum	Biphasic	18 ± 3	No
2 - 3	Colostrum	Biphasic/MMC	22 ± 3	No/PPS
4 - 6	Milk replacer	MMC	27 ± 5	PPS
10 - 16	Milk replacer	MMC	32 ± 5	PPS
17 - 35	Milk replacer	MMC	35 ± 8	PPS
36 - 45	Milk replacer	MMC	40 ± 9	PPS
40 - 60	Solid food	MMC	55 ± 14	PPS
180 - 210	Solid food	MMC	69 ± 13	PPS

The cephalic phase of the pancreatic response to food decreased progressively with age, being highest during week 2 - 4 of life, lower but still significant in the second month of life and not significant thereafter when the animals only received solid food [33]. In 3 – 4-month-old ruminating calves, the cephalic phase of pancreatic secretion was not observed, either when calves were given solid food or when they were suddenly switched to cows' milk (Zabielski and Leśniewska, unpublished).

The MMC/PPS pattern which was observed in preruminant and ruminant calves and in adult sheep was short in comparison to the nearly-2-hour cycles observed in the adult dog and human. However, the motility pattern in neonatal calves was similar in duration to that recorded for human neonates [79]. We suspect that the PPS is present in children and it may undergo age- and diet-related modifications similar to those found in preruminant calves.

1.7. The importance of recognition of the PPS pattern for pancreas studies

So far the influence of the PPS on experimental treatment is still not fully appreciated in chronic pancreatic secretion studies. At best, the studies are performed on animals or human volunteers who are restrained from eating overnight, and in the materials and methods section we read that the time schedule of the experiment is rigorously kept. For instance, an experiment always starts at 8 a.m., a given number of control collections are made until 9 a.m., between 9 and 9:30 a.m. a treatment (e.g., iv infusion of examined substance) is applied,

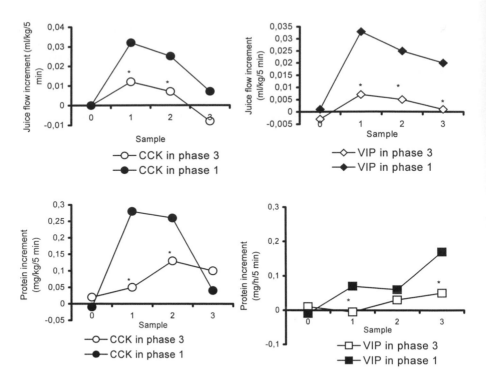

Figure 5. Pancreatic responses to intravenous infusion of CCK-8 (left) and VIP (right) during phase 3 and late phase 1 of the duodenal MMC. * Significantly different from the infusion made during late phase 1 (P < 0.05). Adapted from [80].

and pancreatic secretion is collected for another given number of hours. Such a standard protocol apparently does not take into account the periodic activity of the pancreas, meaning that on each experimental day the test substance is administered at different (arbitrary) time points, regarding the pancreatic secretory curve. Is this methodologically acceptable? It is known that the periodic activity is the result of alternating stimulation and inhibition, controlled by the enteric and vagal nerves together with a number of gut regulatory peptides (see the next subchapter). Moreover high, pharmacological doses of the test substances may disrupt the periodic activity, whereas lower doses, within the physiological range, may not interrupt it. Thus the changes evoked, especially by small doses of weak secretagogues may be overlooked if the periodic activity is not monitored. We checked in healthy preruminant calves, fasted overnight, and fitted with pancreatic catheters and duodenal electrodes, to see how much the time of drug administration can influence the results obtained. Since extended administration of exogenous peptides might elicit secondary mechanisms affecting the periodic pattern, we examined the pancreatic response to brief (5 min) infusions of CCK-8 and vasoactive intestinal polypeptide (VIP, 100 pmol/kg BW). On each experimental day either VIP or CCK-8 was given during a well-identified phase 3 of the duodenal MMC. After recording 2 to 3 PPS/MMC cycles the same dose of regulatory peptides was repeated during late phase 1 [80].

The results showed that the two regulatory peptides evoked a surprisingly different pancreatic response depending on the moment of administration (Figure 5). Both CCK-8 and VIP infused intravenously during phase 3 of the MMC resulted in much weaker pancreatic stimulation than the identical dose applied during late phase 1. Since the pancreatic response to CCK-8 and VIP was uniformly lower for the infusion during phase 3 and greater for that during phase 1, it seems that the responsiveness of exocrine pancreatic cells at different points in their periodic activity equally concerns two quite different excitatory pathways; that for CCK and that for VIP. Probable causes are the periodic changes in local blood flow, fluctuations in certain GI peptides (PP, motilin, secretin), or oscillations of neural tone [81]. Magee and Naruse [22] suggested involvement of the intrinsic pancreatic ganglia.

There is also evidence showing how much the timing is important in designing the experiment from human studies with "sham" and real meal stimulation. In humans the existence of a cephalic phase evoked by "sham" feeding depends on the moment at which it is performed [82]. Subjects fed at the beginning of phase 2 of the small intestinal MMC show a distinct elevation in pancreatic enzyme output (but not in bicarbonate output) lasting for 30 min. If the stimulation is made at other times the results are controversial. Stimulation with a meal during late phase 3 results in a 10-20 min delay in the pancreatic response, whereas the same meal eaten during late phase 1 or early phase 2 results in an immediate stimulation [83].

Since the responsiveness of the pancreas to exogenous stimuli varies during the pancreatic secretory cycle, the PPS pattern seems to be a more appropriate timekeeper for the experimental protocol than arbitrarily set hours and minutes. The PPS pattern should be monitored in all chronic studies, and the test substances should be given during a well-recognised phase of the PPS to increase the sensitivity of measurement. Indeed, using this approach we have demonstrated some fine local mechanisms of regulation of pancreatic secretion, including a mechanism originating in the duodenal mucosa [26,84,85,86].

1.8. Animal health, well-being and the PPS

The PPS as well as the duodenal MMC are sensitive indicators of animal health and well-being. The periodic activity of the pancreas in suckling calves is disturbed by diarrhoea induced by overfeeding. Depending on the severity of the diarrhoea, the PPS can either be irregular and poorly synchronised with the duodenal MMC, or indistinguishable. The duodenal MMC is also affected by the diarrhoea, seen as a shortening of the duration of phase 2 and of the entire MMC cycle. These disturbances in the PPS and MMC can be registered several hours before any clinical symptoms appear. Intraduodenal administration of enterotoxin immediately halved the pancreatic secretion in calves and transiently disrupted the PPS/MMC synchronicity, though without measurable change of rectal temperature and without clinical signs of diarrhoea (Leśniewska and Zabielski, unpublished). In chronic disease of the exocrine pancreas in human patients (chronic pancreatitis) the synchronicity between pancreatic juice cycles, antroduodenal motility and plasma PP is also disrupted [57]. The periodic activity of the pancreas and upper gut reacts to environmental stimuli. Food expectation (subchapters 1.5 and 3.1) as well as fear and stress influence the quantity of pancreatic secretion and the regularity, duration and amplitude of the PPS. Experimental animals randomly removed from their own cages and placed for recordings in a different room secrete less pancreatic juice and do not manifest a regular periodic pattern. Usually this problem disappears after a few days of training, though we have experienced the occasional piglet which did not show the PPS pattern at all. These animals, though clinically healthy, do not become accustomed to experimental conditions (connection to the extension tubing and cables) regardless of training, and manifest their discomfort immediately after the recording session is started. To minimise these influences on behaviour, young calves and pigs are experimented on in their own pen, given visual contact with other animals and with a minimum of restraint or none at all [87].

2. ORIGIN AND REGULATION OF THE PPS

2.1. Neural regulation of PPS

In 1912, Babkin and Ishikawa first demonstrated in dogs that atropine abolishes pancreatic and intestinal periodic activity and keeps the pancreatic secretion at a nadir [4]. Their findings have since been confirmed on several occasions [10,11], suggesting involvement of cholinergic pathways in the regulation of periodic activity. In preruminant calves, 1 hour of intravenous infusion of atropine (0.005 mg/kg/min) abolished the pancreatic periodic and duodenal spiking activity, and reduced pancreatic secretion to the minimum values of the usual PPS cycle. The effects of atropine, a nonselective muscarinic receptor antagonist, were similar to the effects of telenzepine (a selective M1 type muscarinic receptor antagonist) infusions in dogs [88]. In preruminant calves, single iv bolus infusion of a selective M3 type antagonist, 4-diphenylacetoxy-N-methylpiperidine-methiodide (4-DAMP, 100 nmol/kg) during phase 1 of the MMC, drastically decreased pancreatic juice flow and protein output and abolished the pancreatic cycles; this result was comparable with that of atropine (iv 0.005 mg/kg/min) (Table 3). On the other hand, the duodenal MMC persisted following 4-DAMP, but the duration of the phase 1 was prolonged and the number of spikes/min during phase 2 was reduced [89]. The effect of 4-DAMP lasted for ca. 1.5 hours, whereas that of atropine (abolition of MMC and PPS) lasted for 4 - 6 hours. However, these results are hardly conclusive, since the doses of 4-DAMP and atropine were administered differently and were not equimolar.

Pharmacological muscarinic receptor blockade by intravenous infusion is not selective in the sense of localisation of the target organs. Experiments with local reversible (cooling of vagi) or irreversible (vagotomy) blockade of vagal conductivity helped to specify the precise sites of the mechanisms. Cold blockade of the vagal nerves (to be precise, the vago-sympathetic trunks) is an interesting experimental tool. Unlike vagotomy, it allows repeated interruptions to the vagal supply of the viscera at any occasion. The adjacent sympathetic trunk at the neck level has no role in the regulation of upper gut function [90]. Blockade of vagal conductivity is complete when the mean temperature of the vagal fibres drops below $7.6°$ C, and lasts until the nerve is rewarmed [91]. Temporary blockade of the extrinsic vagal supply significantly suppressed pancreatic secretion and reduced phase 2 of the duodenal MMC in dogs and calves (Figure 6). However, phase 3 persisted and was associated with an intermittent increase in juice flow and protein output. For this reason, it has been proposed that the temporal alliance between duodenal and pancreatic activity is largely, though not exclusively, co-ordinated by extrinsic vagal information [21]. Vagotomy studies are less

Table 3
Factors affecting pancreatic secretion during the PPS cycle in preruminant calves

Treatment	Administration and dosage	Volume (µl/kg/PPS)	Bicarbonate output(µEq/kg/PPS)	Protein output (µg/kg/PPS)
Control PPS		215 ± 55	22.2 ± 6.6	1200 ± 330
Atropine[#]	iv, 5 mg/kg/min	40 ± 4.5*	1.6 ± 0.3*	140 ± 20*
4-DAMP	iv, 100 nmol/kg	25 ± 1.2*	0.9 ± 0.2*	60 ± 15*
CVB[#]	4° C	65 ± 6*	4.7 ± 0.2*	160 ± 30*
Capsaicin	id, 3nM/kg	165 ± 30	15.4 ± 3.2	990 ± 180
Lidocaine	id, 2%, 60 ml/h	190 ± 35	13.8 ± 3.1	565 ± 165*
GDCD	3 hours	130 ± 30*	8.2 ± 2.3*	510 ± 180*
DCD	3 hours	170 ± 70	13.6 ± 6.1	710 ± 270
CCK-8	iv, 120 pmol/kg/h	430 ± 115*	38.7 ± 16.7	2550 ± 680*
CCK-A	id bolus, 0.5 mg/kg	87 ± 25*	11.5 ± 3.7*	750 ± 150*
CCK-B	id, 9 nmol/kg/h	190 ± 40	Not measured	1100 ± 160
Secretin	iv, 120 pmol/kg/h	500 ± 110*	85.9 ± 24.0*	1350 ± 270
PACAP-27	iv, 120 pmol/kg/h	235 ± 90	21.9 ± 7.1	1160 ± 75
Motilin	iv, 120 pmol/kg/h	320 ± 90	28.9 ± 8.4	1650 ± 350

Atropine, 4-DAMP, lidocaine, capsaicin and GI peptides were infused for 1 hour. Mean $\pm$ SE, n = 4 to 6 calves; CVB, cold vagal blockade; GDCD, diversion of gastric and duodenal contents; DCD, diversion of duodenal contents; CCK-A receptor antagonist, Tarazepide; CCK-B receptor antagonist, PD135158; iv, intravenous; id, intraduodenal; * = significantly different from the control PPS cycle (P < 0.05). [#] When the PPS/MMC cycles were not observed (iv atropine and cold vagal blockade) the secretion was evaluated for a period of 35-min for comparison.

conclusive; contradictory results were reported for both duodenal and pancreatic activities after cutting the vagi. There are serious methodological reservations toward secondary mechanisms that may develop after surgical vagatomy, as a consequence of permanent removal of a dominating control mechanism that is normally in function [90].

Pancreas transplantation models give the possibility to investigate the secretion of pancreatic juice without the influence of extrinsic innervation. In a study in dogs, the autotransplanted pancreas retained its periodic activity, although with a shorter cycle duration (60 ± 3 min) than the duodenal MMC (125 ± 7 min).

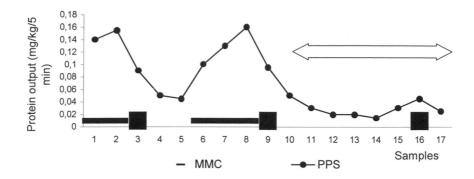

Figure 6. Effect of cold vagal blockade on the PPS in a one-month-old calf. Samples 4-5 were collected during phase 1 of the duodenal MMC; samples 10-15 and 17, during phase 1-like activity during the vagal blockade. White bar with arrows depicts the cold vagal blockade.

Plasma motilin, but not PP, cycled in phase with the duodenal MMC [55]. Malfertheiner *et al.* [56, 92] showed that the pancreas has little importance in controlling the duodenal MMC, and the adjustment of pancreatic cycles to the duodenal periodic activity is regulated primarily by a neural duodeno-pancreatic reflex. Therefore it seems that the pancreatic intrinsic nerves serve to generate pancreatic periodicity, whereas the extrinsic nerves and hormones (e.g., PP and motilin) are less relevant. Indeed, the administration of pentolinium or hexamethonium, ganglionic blockers, inhibited the periodic increase associated with the late phase of the MMC in dogs [10, 22].

Studies performed in isolated canine whole pancreas suggest the presence of insulin oscillations, presumably controlled by the pancreatic nervous system [93, 94]. Opara and Go [95] localised the pacemaker for insulin oscillations to the pancreatic islets and hypothesised that the pancreatic ganglia and the interconnecting nerves are the means of pacemaker integration. It remains unclear, however, whether this pacemaker is relevant for exocrine pancreatic activity in the preprandial or fasting conditions. On the other hand, intravenous glucose infusion to reproduce postprandial glycaemia leads to a synchronisation of insulin oscillations with juice periodic activity in preruminant calves [96]. The mean hourly secretion of pancreatic juice was unchanged during glucose infusion.

In contrast to the investigations in duodenectomized or pancreatectomized dogs [56, 92], in neonatal calves local duodenopancreatic reflexes appeared to be less relevant for the periodic activity of the pancreas. Local anaesthesia of the duodenal mucosa, by duodenal perfusion with lidocaine, did not abolish the PPS cycles but only decreased the mean secretion per cycle [43]. Diversion of the gastroduodenal contents produced similar effects although the reduction was smaller when the digesta were allowed to pass the duodenal bulb and were diverted just caudal to the duodenal bulb. The reduction in pancreatic secretion was considerably weaker than that during the cold vagal blockade described above, suggesting that in the calf either vagal tone is important for pancreatic secretion, or deeper tension receptors, within the muscle layer [97], are important in the regulation of pancreatic function via vagal or intrinsic neural pathways. These findings differed from those in the dog, in which duodenal lidocaine markedly suppressed the duodenal MMC and the level of pancreatic secretion without altering the periodicity of the PPS [52]. Perhaps, local reflexes are present but immature in preruminant calves and develop later. The limiting factor in preruminant calves could be the scanty number of duodenal chemoreceptors or the immaturity of the GI tract endocrine function [98].

Capsaicin, a neurotoxin extracted from red peppers, is used as a tool to study the involvement of sensory neurons in gastrointestinal functions. Rat studies showed that the CCK-evoked disruption of the small intestinal MMC is driven via capsaicin-sensitive vagal afferent fibres [99]. In that study, perivagal application of capsaicin was performed in rat neonates to permanently degenerate the C-fibres [100]. The effect of perivagal capsaicin on the pancreatic periodic activity was not reported, although a reduction in CCK-stimulated pancreatic secretion was [101]. In the preruminant calf model with duodenal electrodes and a pancreatic catheter, the effect of capsaicin on local afferent pathways was examined. A capsaicin bolus (3 nmol/kg BW) administered intraduodenally during early phase 2 of the MMC resulted in transient (5 min) stimulation of pancreatic secretion followed by a significant reduction of peaks and nadirs in the PPS cycles, and little shortening of the MMC/PPS cycle duration. However the secretion per PPS cycle was not significantly affected, as demonstrated in Table 3 (Zabielski, Onaga and Kato, unpublished). The results of the calf experiment should be considered cautiously, since the completeness of the blockade has not been confirmed, although the tendencies are similar to the effects of intraduodenal lidocaine and gastroduodenal content diversion.

The sympathetic system regulation of pancreatic cycles has not been investigated as intensively as that of the parasympathetic system. In preruminant calves, stimulation of an alpha$_2$-adrenergic receptors by injection of 2% xylazine (im, 0.15 ml/kg BW, Rompun, Bayer) led to an inhibition of pancreatic exocrine secretion and duodenal spiking activity (Zabielski and Guilloteau unpublished results). The effect on the pancreas and duodenum was immediate, whereas sedation of animal was only achieved 10 - 15 min after the injection. The flow of pancreatic juice was reduced by 5 and 10 times in the first and second postinjection hour, respectively. The secretion returned to control levels during the next two hours. The concentrations of total protein and trypsin activity were decreased by only 25 to 35%; thus the effect was related primarily to the inhibition of fluid secretion by the pancreas. No periodic secretion was observed for 4 to 6 hours after the injection, while the first phase 3 of the MMC appeared ca. 4 hours after xylazine injection. It is difficult to distinguish the site of a xylazine mechanism, central or peripheral, from this study. Alpha$_2$-adrenergic drugs can inhibit pancreatic secretion, both through central alpha$_2$ and peripheral alpha$_1$ and alpha$_2$ receptor mechanisms [102], though the sequence of events in studied calves, and the reduction in pancreatic secretion before sedation, may suggest the dominance of a peripheral mechanism. The localisation of the mechanism of pancreatic inhibition remains unclear. Xylazine, in addition to central activation or stimulation of alpha$_2$-adrenergic presynaptic receptors, has some alpha$_1$-adrenergic effects [103]. Thus the mechanism could be related to the activation of central adrenoreceptors, cardiovascular effects of xylazine or depression of endogenous insulin release. In preruminant calves, the latter is not a likely explanation, since insulinaemia induced by glucose infusion does not affect exocrine pancreatic secretion [96], though in adult sheep the insulo-acinar axis controls pancreatic exocrine secretion [104]. Studies with direct administration of adrenergic agonists and antagonists into the pancreatic circulation might be helpful in giving a better understanding of the role of the adrenergic system in the regulation of pancreatic periodicity.

2.2. Role of gut regulatory peptides in the control of PPS

Gut regulatory peptides produced in the gastrointestinal tract participate in the regulation of the pre- and post-prandial GI tract function; thus they are also promising candidates for the control of periodic activity. In addition, the concentration in blood of some gut peptides was found to fluctuate in phase with the gastrointestinal motility and secretion of digestive juices (subchapter 1.4.). The role of gut regulatory peptides on the pancreatic periodic activity was investigated by infusion of purified or synthetic gut regulatory peptides or their analogues as well as by administration of their specific receptor antagonists. To our knowledge, immunisation against the gut peptides has not been used for investigation of the periodic activity. Results showed that there are certain quantitative dose-related differences in the response of the pancreas to gut peptides between dogs, sheep and preruminant calves. In general, however, it seems that the gut regulatory peptides are not responsible for originating the pancreatic periodic secretion, though they may alter already generated pancreatic cycles.

2.2.1. CCK

The role of CCK-8 in canine periodic activity was studied with continuous intravenous infusion of synthetic CCK-8 in doses ranging between 22 and 175 pmol/kg/h [22]. The effect of CCK-8 was not additive to that of the PPS; with low doses of CCK-8 the peak secretion was augmented by CCK-8 whereas that of the trough was not. The interval of the PPS cycle was also prolonged by infusion of low doses of CCK-8. In contrast, high doses of CCK-8 (> 90 pmol/kg/h) disrupted the periodic activity. These results suggest that in dogs, CCK-8 can stimulate pancreatic secretion indirectly by modifying the function of a hypothetical generator of periodic activity (stimulate the onset or modulate the peaks of the cycles) but is not a generator *per se*. Indeed, the generator, wherever located, could be turned off by either muscarinic or nicotinic pharmacological blockade, and CCK-8 failed to restore the pancreatic periodic activity during blockade. Certain authors have suggested that CCK-8 acts indirectly at the level of the pancreas, via the nerves, as a neurotransmitter or neuromodulator. In preruminant calves, continuous intravenous infusion of CCK-8 (120 pmol/kg/h) led to a several-fold increase in the blood plasma CCK concentration and produced a marked increase in pancreatic protein secretion during the entire infusion period but did not disrupt the PPS pattern. Increases in volume and bicarbonate output were observed primarily at the beginning of infusion [43]. The dose of CCK-8 was 4-fold higher than that required to produce a maximal pancreatic response in humans [105] and high enough to abolish PPS cycles in conscious dogs. Intraduodenal administration of a selective CCK-A receptor antagonist, Tarazepide (Solvay Pharmaceuticals, Germany), resulted in a decrease in the preprandial and postprandial pancreatic secretion in calves, particularly in protein output [86]. It should be noted that neither the administration of exogenous CCK nor of CCK-A receptor antagonist disrupted the periodic activity of the pancreas and duodenum in examined calves. Tarazepide permeated the intestinal mucosa poorly *in vivo*. The reduction of pancreatic protein secretion was observed before any Tarazepide was detected in the blood [86], suggesting the presence of some local duodenal CCK mechanism in calves. In conscious calves, by means of infusion into the small arteries supplying the proximal duodenum with blood, it was demonstrated that CCK-8 and to some extent secretin could stimulate the exocrine pancreas indirectly, probably via the vagal pathways [106]. The intraduodenal infusion of CCK-8 in conscious preruminant calves consistently resulted in an atropine-sensitive stimulation of the exocrine pancreas [43]. Plasma CCK levels were not changed, either by the intraarterial or the intraduodenal infusion of CCK-8. These results indicated that CCK, besides having a direct receptoral effect on the pancreatic acinar cells could also stimulate the exocrine pancreas through an indirect pathway at the level of the duodenum, probably via the long vago-vagal reflexes. These suggestions are compatible with findings in pigs [26,38] and rats [101]. The local mechanism is discussed in more detail in subchapter 4.

2.2.2. Pentagastrin

Pentagastrin, like CCK-8, affected the periodic activity following intravenous infusion in fasting dogs [22]. Examined doses ranged between 62 and 1000 ng/kg/h. The length of the cycle increased with increasing doses of pentagastrin and finally the periodicity disappeared [22]. Pentagastrin was ineffective following atropine or hexamethonium infusions, suggesting mediation of a neural mechanism in the response. In contrast to dogs, intraduodenal perfusion with a CCK-B receptor antagonist (PD135158, Parke-Davies) did not disrupt the PPS cycles in preruminant calves [107].

2.2.3. Secretin

Secretin was regarded as the other gut regulatory peptide candidate, besides CCK, for control of the periodic activity of the pancreas. Moreover, in preruminant calves, plasma secretin was found to fluctuate periodically in phase with the duodenal MMC and pancreatic periodic secretion [63]. Studies in dogs and preruminant calves did not confirm its hypothetical role in generation of the PPS. In fasting dogs, the PPS was not disrupted by low doses of secretin, although the peak and nadir secretion was elevated. As the dose was increased, the intervals between peaks lengthened, the peaks became less sharp, the nadirs were raised, and finally the periodic activity was abolished. The effect of secretin in dogs was atropine-sensitive, and in part vagally-dependent [20]. In preruminant calves, continuous infusion of secretin at a pharmacological dose (iv, 120 pmol/kg/h) abolished the natural fluctuations of secretin in the blood plasma, and stimulated the mean pancreatic secretion by elevation of both peaks and nadirs of the PPS. The pancreatic cycles were not disrupted, although phase 3 of the duodenal MMC was not recorded during the infusion [43]. In contrast to dogs, in experimental calves blockade of vagal conductivity by cooling totally abolished the pancreatic response to secretin and rewarming the nerves immediately restored the pancreatic response to exogenous secretin [106].

2.2.4. PACAP

Pituitary adenylate cyclase-activating peptide (PACAP) is a regulatory peptide from the secretin family [108]. It was discovered in the ovine hypothalamus and was soon found to be widely distributed in the central nervous system and peripheral organs, including the pancreas [109]. In vitro studies with PACAP-38 and PACAP-27 show a parallel stimulation of pancreatic amylase release from the pancreatic acini and an increase in cAMP concentration in the media for both PACAPs. Naruse et al. [23] have reported that intravenously administered PACAP stimulates pancreatic juice secretion in conscious dogs. In studies on conscious calves, PACAP-27, when given as a 5-min iv infusion, had a potent stimulatory effect on the pancreatic juice volume, bicarbonate output and protein output [110]. The effect of this peptide is dose dependent and comparable to that of secretin. On the other hand, a 1-hour infusion of PACAP-27 (120 pmol/kg), aside from the stimulation seen at the beginning of infusion, does not affect the pancreatic periodic cycle [43]. PACAP-38 is a less potent stimulator of pancreatic juice secretion than PACAP-27 and secretin, but stronger than VIP in calves. The pancreatic response to the PACAPs apparently depends on a cholinergic pathway, since atropine can block the pancreatic response in dogs, calves and sheep [23,110,111]. Onaga *et al.* [112] examined the mechanism of PACAP on pancreatic periodic secretion in adult conscious sheep using a technique whereby vagal nerve conductivity is blocked by cooling. PACAP-27 and -38 were administered intravenously during early phase 2 of the duodenal MMC. In their study, the stimulatory effect of both PACAP-27 and -38 on pancreatic enzyme secretion, but not on pancreatic juice volume, was mediated mostly by the vagal cholinergic preganglionic neurons, suggesting the action of PACAPs in the central nervous system.

2.2.5. VIP

VIP did not show MMC-related fluctuations in the peripheral blood [61]. However, VIP is neuronally released, and cold vagal blockade reduces plasma VIP by 50% (Zabielski, Onaga and Kato, unpublished). VIP has a short biological half-life in the blood; thus an increase of VIP in the GI circulation by local intraarterial VIP infusion or local stimulation of endogenous VIP release does not affect the concentration of VIP in the peripheral circulation [113]. Therefore VIP was studied for possible participation in the phenomenon of periodic activity in the GI tract. In preruminant calves, it was found to be a relatively weak stimulator of pancreatic juice secretion in comparison to secretin and PACAP-27 [110]. Studies in preruminant calves showed that exogenous VIP given in a range of doses (3 - 100 pmol/kg BW) during early phase 2 of the MMC transiently modulated the peak secretion but did not disturb the pancreatic periodic activity [110]. Intravenous infusion of VIP during phase 3 of the MMC had minimal effect on the PPS [80]. Studies in weaned pigs revealed that VIP is an important secretagogue in this species [114] but its effect on the periodic activity of the pancreas was not reported.

2.2.6. PP

Basing on the observation that an increase in vagal activity was associated with PP release into the circulation, Schwartz [115] proposed that plasma PP reflects the activity of vagal tone. Indeed, plasma PP increases during eating (cephalic phase), and most interestingly, it fluctuates in phase with the MMC and PPS during the interdigestive state [11,12,52,61]. PP concentration peaks during late phase 2 of the MMC, just before a drop in pancreatic secretion. Intravenous infusion of PP in calves caused inhibition of pancreatic secretion but the doses employed were apparently pharmacological [116]. On the other hand, in calves the PPS and MMC cycles are observed soon after feeding, whereas PP cycles in the peripheral blood could not be demonstrated earlier than in the 4th or 5th MMC cycle after food consumption [61].

2.2.7. Motilin

Plasma motilin fluctuates in phase with the MMC and PPS during the interdigestive state in monogastric animals and under certain feeding conditions in calves [11,12,58,61]. In dogs, ingestion of a meat meal abolishes motilin cycles and reduces the motilin concentration in blood plasma. Motilin cycles reappear soon after the prandial pattern of duodenal motility is resumed. Administration of exogenous motilin or stimulation of endogenous motilin release shortens the interval of the canine periodic interdigestive activity but without affecting the peak and nadir values [54]. Thus the increase in overall pancreatic secretion reported previously [117] presumably reflects a higher frequency of pancreatic cycles. Similar results were obtained in preruminant calves [43]. Doses of exogenous peptide employed in these studies were calculated in such a way as to obtain a concentration equivalent to the peak values of plasma motilin. In the dog study, atropine or hexamethonium infusions totally abolished the duodenal and pancreatic cycles with and without motilin stimulation, suggesting that the interdigestive activity - even that regulated by motilin - depends primarily on neural transmission. It seems likely that circulating motilin helps to co-ordinate some of periodic events in the GI tract of monogastric animals but in preruminant calves [61] and sheep [60] it is of minor relevance.

2.3. Neurohormonal relationships

The gut regulatory peptides examined so far did not appear to be responsible for generation of the pancreatic cycles in experimental animals, although they were significant modulators of this periodic activity. Exogenous regulatory peptides given within a physiological range, affected the duration of the periodic activity, modified peak and nadir values, or changed the shape of the secretory curve. Only high, apparently pharmacological, doses of exogenous regulatory peptides were able to disrupt the PPS in dogs. In calves the effects were much less dramatic, suggesting lesser impact of gut peptides in the regulation of GI function than in dogs. Moreover, in both adult dogs and young calves, the responses to regulatory peptides given in a physiological range were greatly modulated by the spontaneous periodic activity of the nerves. In subchapter 4 more information about the relationship between CCK and the nervous system is presented.

The age of the animal and/or the stage of the GI tract development seems to be a key factor in the organisation of neurohormonal relationships. Studies with exogenous CCK in ruminants have provided some support for this hypothesis. In neonatal calves the concentration of CCK in plasma increases sharply during the first 5 days, after which the increase is minimal and there is a tendency towards a decrease after the forestomach develops [118]. CCK-A receptors in the pancreas are functional from the day of birth [119]. Normally, in 14 – 40-day-old preruminant calves, iv infusions of CCK (range 3 - 100 pmol/kg BW) cause a dose-dependent increase in pancreatic juice rich in enzymes [106]. However, iv infusion of CCK (100 pmol/kg BW) during the first week of life in calves had no effect on pancreatic secretion [78]. In an adult sheep model, Onaga et al. [36] showed that the pancreatic enzyme output hardly responds to intravenous CCK-8 infusion, compared to 1 – 2-month-old preruminant calves. However, the administration of a CCK-A receptor antagonist reduced the preprandial secretion in neonatal calves, 1 – 2-month-old calves and adult sheep.

3. REGULATION OF FOOD-STIMULATED PANCREATIC JUICE SECRETION

3.1. Regulation of the cephalic phase

The presence of a cephalic phase of pancreatic secretion has been well recognised since the days of Pavlov. In conscious dogs, sham feeding did increase pancreatic secretion, but the increases in volume and bicarbonate secretion were very small compared with those observed during the intestinal phase [120,121]. Atropine, but not antral mucosectomy, inhibited the pancreatic response to sham feeding, suggesting that acetylcholine, and not gastrin, mediates the cephalic phase response in this animal [121]. However, as the periodic aspect of fasting pancreatic secretion was not considered in these studies, the relative significance of the cephalic phase remains to be studied. The electrical stimulation of both vagi in anaesthetised dogs induced a small increase in pancreatic secretion [122]. Atropine completely inhibited the pancreatic fluid response to electrical stimulation of the vagus in dogs. This is in contrast to pigs, in which electrical stimulation of the vagus induces atropine-resistant, profuse pancreatic secretion, rich in bicarbonate [114]. The mediator for this response appears to be VIP. VIP and PHI are also released by vagal stimulation in dogs [122]. The apparent difference in sensitivity to atropine between dogs and pigs seems to be related to the relative sensitivity of duct cells to VIP in the two species. Unlike in pigs, VIP/PHI/PACAP-related peptides are not potent stimulants of pancreatic fluid and bicarbonate secretion in dogs [23]. It appears that the cephalic phase of pancreatic fluid and bicarbonate secretion is quantitatively less important in dogs than in pigs or calves, but its role in enzyme secretion and blood flow remains to be clarified.

In pigs, a distinct cephalic phase could be seen in weanlings but not in sucklings. Before weaning, piglets secrete little pancreatic juice before suckling (volume 0.5 ml; protein output 1 mg and trypsin activity output 0.2 U per kg BW/hour), and the secretion does not increase during and after suckling [75]. Though the minute kinetics of the pancreatic secretion during suckling were not observed, it could be assumed that the cephalic phase of pancreatic secretion is negligible in suckling piglets.

The overall pancreatic response to milk food in preruminant calves is short and transient compared to the responses to standard liquid or solid food in adult dogs but on the other hand is much more obvious than in suckling or weaned pigs. In preruminant calves the entire response to milk feeding is over within ca. one hour, but only during and just after the suckling is there a dramatic elevation of pancreatic secretion (volume, bicarbonate and enzyme outputs). This elevation lasts for 10 to 15 min and in terms of enzyme output it can not be reproduced by an intravenous infusion of gut regulatory peptides alone. It was successfully reproduced by injecting CCK-8 together with secretin - both in pharmacological doses [123]. In terms of juice volume, iv injection of pharmacological doses of secretin or PACAP-27 could reproduce the elevation [110]. One can question the results in calves, since examination of the cephalic phase was performed without fistulation of the oesophagus, and food in the stomach or duodenum could affect the pancreatic secretion. To clarify this, we measured pancreatic secretion and duodenal MMC in preruminant calves after putting an empty feeding bucket into the cage at the time of feeding. We observed a similar cephalic phase response to "true milk feeding" and to the empty feeding bucket (Leśniewska and Zabielski, unpublished results). Apparently the cephalic stimulation was mediated by the vagal nerves, since it could be abolished by cooling the vagi [124]. Studies with pharmacological muscarinic blockade (atropine, 4-DAMP) demonstrated the importance of a cholinergic system in the cephalic phase in calves [89,124]. Intraduodenal administration of a CCK-A receptor antagonist lowered the protein output during the cephalic phase [86], suggesting that, unlike in humans [105], a CCK component was involved in this response as well.

The cephalic phase of pancreatic secretion was present in calves fed liquid food (milk or milk replacer), and it was much more evident at the morning feeding than at the evening feeding [71]. Pancreatic secretion increments caused by cephalic stimulation showed a tendency to decrease with age. The greatest increments were observed during the first month of life; they were lower but still significant in the second month of life and not significant when the animals only received solid food [33]. In ruminant calves the continuous flow of acidic digesta through the abomasum and small intestine during the preprandial period might stimulate the exocrine pancreas continuously, to a certain degree. Therefore additional stimulation by newly ingested food would not substantially increase the secretion of juice over the already stimulated preprandial level. This was confirmed in adult sheep [125], in which the flow of digesta into the duodenum was blocked. Under these conditions the pancreatic secretion was stimulated much more by food ingestion than it was in sheep with an undisturbed flow of digesta.

3.2. Regulation of the postprandial pancreatic secretion: gastric and intestinal phase

It is generally thought that in monogastric animals, pancreatic secretion is dramatically elevated after a meal as long as there is food in the stomach and small intestine. Studies in conscious dogs have provided strong evidence to support this opinion. In calves and piglets fed twice a day, however, feeding results in a moderate increase, if any, in volume of juice and pancreatic enzyme output after the cephalic phase. The older the calves are, and the more frequently the pigs are fed, the smaller the postprandial increment. In studies exploring the periodic activity of the pancreas after a meal, distortion and not elimination of the MMC and PPS cycles, is usually seen. Zenilman et al. [126] studied the EMG signal using a time series analysis with fast Fourier transforms and found that the MMC in conscious rats does not disappear after feeding. Phase 3 of the MMC occurred early postprandially. In calf recordings, signal smoothing and frequency analysis revealed that one or two activity fronts (phase 3) of the duodenal MMC may indeed be masked by postprandial phase 2-like spiking activity, though these third phases were not followed by quiescence (phase 1). In most (but not all) recordings in calves, the duration of the prandial phase 2-like activity was a multiple of the preprandial duodenal MMC cycle (x2 or x3, on rare occasions x4) (Zabielski - unpublished results). So far, we cannot afford such precise discrimination in the pancreatic secretion pattern, though a characteristic pattern of pancreatic protein secretion has already been found in the PPS cycle and after feeding (see chapter by Leśniewska et al.).

One can ask why it is so difficult to convincingly demonstrate the presence of a gastric and an intestinal phase in calves and piglets, since food components are effective stimulants of pancreatic secretion in these animals, as demonstrated by intraduodenal infusion experiments. In the calf, the exocrine pancreas responds strongly to a soya bean extract and intraduodenal HCl infusion [32]. The pig pancreas responds specifically to a variety of organic acids, fats and proteins, as discussed in the other chapters.

The composition of milk replacer has an influence on the range of the postprandial secretion in calves. Skim-milk-based milk replacer induces a smaller pancreatic secretion increment and a shorter "postprandial pattern" than milk replacers containing additions of soya-bean protein and/or fish protein. Guilloteau et al. [127] explain this by a different abomasal emptying rate and duodenal digesta flow in these diets. Abomasal chymosin clots milk casein in calves fed with milk or skim-milk-based milk replacers. In these animals, the abomasal emptying rate is slow and causes less dramatic stimulation of pancreatic secretion. In contrast, milk replacers containing little or no casein cannot be coagulated in the abomasum as well as milk, and are evacuated from the abomasum more rapidly. A more intensive flow of nutrients into the duodenum results in more intensive stimulation of the exocrine pancreas. This effect can be modulated by the co-operation of several gut regulatory peptides, like CCK, gastrin, secretin, PP, motilin and somatostatin, as discussed above.

In contrast to the classic understanding of the regulation of prandial pancreatic secretion as being predominantly hormonal [128], there is increasing evidence for the contribution of neural controlling mechanisms. In 1995, Alder *et al.* [105] concluded their review on pancreatic regulation in humans as follows: "...it is now clear that cholinergic control is central, with hormones such as CCK or secretin modulating the response within the complex system that regulates pancreatic secretion". Results from experiments in preruminant calves correspond well with findings in humans. Data from preruminant calves indicate that the nerves, particularly the vagi, actively mediate the postprandial pancreatic secretion - the stimulatory effect of intraduodenal soya bean extract and HCl are inhibited by cold vagal blockade. Plasma CCK and secretin are not affected significantly by soya bean extract. Atropine abolishes pancreatic responses to soya-bean extract and protein responses to HCl. A part of the juice volume response to HCl is atropine resistant and this effect could be mediated by circulating CCK and secretin [32]. However, the effect of exogenous secretin is abolished and that of CCK lowered by cold vagal blockade.

3.3. The continuous prandial phase of pancreatic secretion in adult ruminants and its regulation

In cattle and sheep a cephalic phase of pancreatic secretion is usually not observed. Cows fed with grain concentrate and hay show slight variations in pancreatic secretion that are independent of feeding. No distinct gastric or intestinal phases are observed that correspond to the postprandial changes seen in canine pancreatic secretion. The average daily secretion is 13.9 ml/kg BW of pancreatic juice and 0.09 g/kg BW of total protein [69]. The range of pancreatic secretion calculated per kg of BW was similar to that observed in young ruminant calves. After enriching the cow diet with easily fermented carbohydrates (maintaining an intake and total protein energy similar to those in the standard diet), the daily exocrine flow increased to 21.9 ml/kg BW, but the protein output (0.12 g/kg BW) was not significantly affected. As in the control cows, no prandial phase was observed. The activity of pancreatic amylase, trypsin and chymotrypsin did not differ significantly between the two diets. In the other study in adult cows, fasting for 48 hours (with free access to water) decreased both the exocrine pancreatic secretion and plasma insulin concentration [129]. Following this period, a 24-hour intraduodenal infusion of glucose normalised both pancreatic functions (juice secretion and insulin concentration). The data suggest that due to the function of the forestomach, the duodenum is continuously supplied with nutrients and the pancreatic secretion is under continuous prandial stimulation.

Insulin might be one of important regulators of the exocrine pancreatic function in adult cows. This hypothesis, coming from the starvation study in cows, was supported by the results obtained in sheep with experimental diabetes induced by alloxan [104,130]. In the diabetic state, the volume of pancreatic juice decreased markedly, but returned to its initial level after insulin treatment. The daily secretion of lipase and amylase also decreased during diabetes, and insulin treatment restored the secretion of lipase but not amylase. In control sheep, vagal stimulation increased the juice flow, protein content and plasma insulin concentration. In diabetic animals, vagal stimulation had no effect on volume and resulted in only a slight increase in the exocrine protein content and plasma insulin concentration [104].

These findings suggest that vagal innervation in calves, and vagal innervation and insulin in adult ruminants are important factors for the direct regulation of exocrine pancreatic secretion.

To recap, distinct differences between the gastroduodenal flow of digesta in dogs on the one hand and cattle and pigs on the other, may explain the differences in prandial pancreatic secretion in these species. The preprandial pancreatic secretion in the latter is high compared to dogs, due to the nearly permanent presence of digesta in the stomach and small intestine.

4. DUODENAL MECHANISMS FOR LOCAL REGULATION OF PANCREATIC SECRETION

Bayliss and Starling introduced a new concept of chemical transmission in the regulation of the secretion of pancreatic juice [128]. According to their studies in dogs, a hypothetical substance - secretin - produced by the small intestinal mucosa, was released into the blood, and arrived with circulating blood in the pancreas where it stimulated the flow of pancreatic juice. This concept somehow dismissed the importance of nerves in the regulation of pancreatic secretion, revealed by Pavlov [131]. The idea of hormonal regulation developed with time, and it was strengthened by the isolation and synthesis of secretin and the other gut hormones, localisation of the endocrine cells in the gastrointestinal mucosa responsible for their production, as well as the discovery of specific receptors to gut hormones in the target organs (e.g. CCK-A receptors in the pancreas) [119]. In the meantime, Mellanby [132] proposed a compromise mechanism of dual regulation - neural in the preprandial phase, and hormonal (via secretin) in the prandial phase of pancreatic secretion. The idea of two functional regulating systems which work in concert has evolved progressively, especially in the last two decades. The term, "neurohormonal regulation" is currently used to emphasise the close functional relationship between the nervous and gut endocrine systems.

For many gut regulatory peptides the classic hormone concept can hardly be verified in animal studies. In line with the hypothesis, high doses of exogenous gut regulatory peptides produce a dose-dependent stimulation of pancreatic secretion. Simultaneously, however, these doses increase the concentration of the gut peptide in the circulating blood to a level which can not be achieved by any stimulation of endogenous release. Thus these effects have to be considered pharmacological. On the other hand, low doses of the exogenous gut peptides (keeping the increase in the circulating blood within the physiological range) hardly affect the secretion of pancreatic juice, and can not convincingly explain their role in the regulation of the postprandial pattern. Moreover, often the stimulatory effect of a low dose of gut peptide is abolished by atropine or cold blockade of the vagal nerves. Magee and Naruse [10,20,22] explained this by an interplay between the nervous and hormonal regulation systems at the level of intrapancreatic nerves and ganglions.

The mechanism of gut regulatory function, however, was still unclear. Gut peptides are produced by the endocrine cells in the intestinal mucosa as well as by the neurons in the gastrointestinal tract. Both the endocrine and neuronal release of gut peptides are localised to specific places spread throughout the gastrointestinal tract [133]. If we consider the classic hypothesis of hormonal action via the blood, we have to bear in mind that the blood plasma contains numerous deactivators of gut peptides (e.g. endopeptidases, aminopeptidases) [134].

Moreover, intestinal blood promptly transports these newly-released gut peptides to the liver – another important site of gut peptide deactivation [135]. Thus the biological half-life of gut peptides in the peripheral blood has been estimated to be only a few minutes. It seems unlikely therefore that a "very important message" generated in response to food or other local stimuli in the upper gut would be arbitrarily modified by the liver and blood plasma enzymes well before reaching the presumed target organ – the exocrine pancreas. Could it be then, that the mechanism of pancreatic juice stimulation by the regulatory peptides is located not in the pancreas, but somewhere else? Electrophysiological studies of Blackshaw and Grundy [136] resulted in an attractive idea that the mucosal afferents of the vagal nerves could be a target for duodenally released CCK. Their convincing results stimulated our efforts to search for a hypothetical local duodenal mechanism of regulation of pancreatic juice secretion. First experiments in pigs [84,137] were successful; later on a further question arose concerning the localisation of the mechanism – was it mucosal or luminal? This subchapter deals with the mechanisms of pancreatic secretion that are located in the duodenum, either in the mucosa or in the lumen, in piglets and neonatal calves.

4.1. Regulation of pancreatic secretion via CCK at the level of the duodenum

The first experimental evidence that exogenous CCK-8 can stimulate the secretion of pancreatic juice via indirect mechanism(s) located in the proximal duodenum in anaesthetised and conscious pigs was presented in 1991 at the 23rd European Pancreatic Club Meeting [84,138]. The results were soon confirmed in studies on conscious preruminant calves [80], anaesthetised and conscious pigs [26,139], and anaesthetised rats [101,140]. Similar results were obtained with VIP, but a local mechanism of secretin was less clear [106].

In situ dye infusion studies in anaesthetised pigs and calves showed that the small arterial branch(es) of the right gastroepiploic artery supplied blood to approximately the first 10 cm of the proximal duodenum and a small part of the pylorus close to the duodenal bulb, but not to the pancreas. For perfusion studies with secretagogues (CCK, VIP, secretin), a fine silicone catheter was introduced into the right gastroepiploic artery against the blood flow, with its tip placed just below the above-mentioned arterial branches. In this way the proximal duodenum and part of the pylorus could be perfused in the first pass, whereas the pancreas could only be supplied with the secretagogue from the general circulation in a "second turn"- as with classic hormones. Thus intraarterial infusions could reach part of the proximal duodenum and pylorus, and then could theoretically reach the systemic circulation via the duodenal and gastric veins, portal vein and liver. However, a CCK radioimmunoassay indicated that only a minimal part of locally administered peptide passed on to the systemic blood. Contrary to intraarterial infusions, CCK-8 and secretin given via the external jugular vein were widely distributed in the circulating blood, and thus might have reached the pancreas directly and stimulated acinar and ductal cells, released islets hormones or modified the activity of intra-pancreatic cholinergic ganglions. Perfusions were done both in acute studies under general anaesthesia as well as in chronic studies on conscious pigs and calves during monitoring of MMC and PPS. In anaesthetised pigs, the model was refined by temporary ligation of either a superior pancreatico-duodenal artery or a gastroduodenal artery, in order to perfuse the proximal duodenum or the pancreas + midduodenum, respectively (Figure 7).

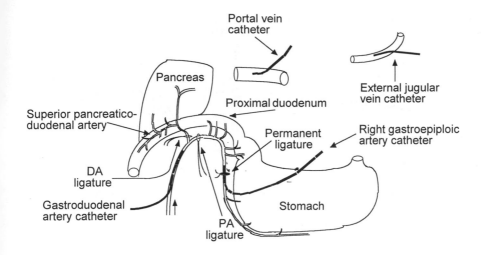

Figure 7. Model used for investigation of a local duodenal mechanism by means of local perfusions in anaesthetised pigs. To perfuse the proximal duodenum the DA ligature was temporarily closed and the infusion given through the catheter in the right gastroepiploic artery. To perfuse the pancreas and distal duodenum, the PA ligature was closed and infusion given through the gastroduodenal artery catheter. For peripheral infusions an external jugular vein was catheterised. Blood was drawn for gut peptide estimation from the portal and external jugular vein. In chronic pig and calf models, only the right gastroepiploic artery and the external jugular vein were catheterised. Pancreatic duct catheters and duodenal cannulas were present but for the sake of clarity are not shown.

In chronic studies, the secretagogues were administered during late phase 1 or early phase 2 of the duodenal MMC.

Intraarterial infusion of CCK-8 induced secretion of pancreatic juice rich in enzymes, without affecting the concentration of CCK in the peripheral blood plasma. The intraarterial stimulation was greater and had a shorter lag time than the intravenous stimulation. Cold blockade of vagal nerves diminished the effect of intraarterial CCK-8, and delayed and decreased the pancreatic response to intravenous CCK-8, suggesting that vagal reflexes are particularly important in the local duodenal mechanism (Figure 8).

Using the anaesthetised rat model, Li and Owyang [101] showed that exogenous CCK-8 infused intravenously at low concentrations may stimulate pancreatic protein secretion via vagal afferent (capsaicin-sensitive) pathways. CCK receptors, predominantly of the CCK-A type, located on the peripheral vagal afferent fibres were suggested to be a target site for this mechanism [140,141]. Gastroduodenal but not jejunal administration of capsaicin abolished the response to low doses of CCK [101], suggesting that the mechanism might originate in the gastroduodenal area.

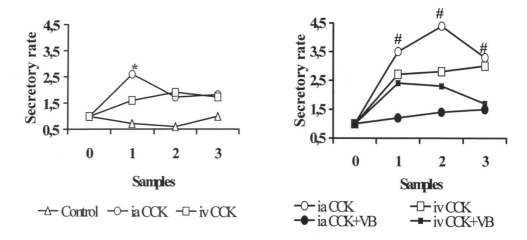

Figure 8. Pancreatic protein response to intraarterial (ia) and intravenous (iv) CCK-8. Left – result of 10 pmol/kg BW of CCK-8 and saline as control. Right - result of 100 pmol/kg BW with and without cold vagal blockade. * significantly different from the iv infusion (left), # significantly different from the respective infusion during cold vagal blockade (right). Adapted from [106].

Our intraarterial infusion studies in conscious pigs and calves gave evidence that this was so. On the other hand, high (pharmacological) doses of CCK in the rat studies, were believed to induce pancreatic secretion by acting directly on the pancreatic intrinsic nerves or the pancreatic acinar cells [140]. This point of view does not take into account any differences in the concentration of CCK in the tissues, though it sounds probable that the CCK concentration in the duodenal mucosa would be much higher than in the peripheral blood and pancreas, due to the abundance of CCK-producing cells in the duodenal mucosa. Duodenal concentrations of CCK are further increased following neural or nutritional stimulation. It is therefore doubtful that just reproducing the postprandial CCK concentration in the peripheral blood by an intravenous infusion of CCK-8 would elevate the CCK concentration in the duodenal mucosa region to a level high enough to activate a mucosal CCK-related mechanism. Blackshaw and Grundy [136] reported that 100 pmol of CCK-8 had a powerful effect on most mucosal vagal afferents in their fibre preparations. Though the threshold dose was not routinely quantified, they had only one preparation which responded to as little as 3 pmol of CCK-8. On the other hand, high doses of CCK infused intravenously may result in stimulation of complex direct and/or indirect mechanisms.

4.2. Bioactive gut regulatory peptides in the gastrointestinal lumen

Gastrin was the first gut regulatory peptide to actually be detected in the lumen of the stomach in adult humans [142]. Since then many regulatory peptides have been found in biologically active forms in the lumen of the stomach and small intestine in animals and humans. Luminal gastrin, somatostatin, secretin, CCK, substance P and polypeptide YY (PYY) originate from the endocrine cells in the intestinal mucosa [143,144,145,146].

Substantial amounts of insulin and somatostatin arrive in the duodenum together with the pancreatic juice [147]. Saliva is the main source of growth factors (EGF, IGF) and neuropeptides (substance P, neurokinin A, calcitocin gene-related peptide, neuropeptide Y, and VIP) in the GI lumen [145,148]. The peptide concentration in the gastrointestinal lumen or the calculated output into the lumen is greater than the respective venous concentration or output - both under control conditions and following stimulation [145]. *In vitro* studies revealed that despite unfavourable conditions in the stomach and gut lumen (acidic pH values, and/or abundance of proteolytic enzymes), regulatory peptides are remarkably stable. The survival of gut peptides is much better in the digestive juices collected from neonates than from adults [149,150]. The degradation rate of gastrin (G17 and G34) incubated for 20 min in the intestinal juice collected from adult pigs is between 10 and 15% [150], and that of EGF is about 20 % [149]. The addition of acid soluble or casein fractions of porcine colostrum to the intestinal fluids markedly reduces the degradation rate of gastrin and EGF. Read *et al.* [151] reported that 60 to 90% of intragastrically administered EGF reached the small intestine intact in new-born lambs. These data suggest that the biological half-life of regulatory peptides in the intestinal lumen may be much longer than in the blood plasma, which strengthens their potential physiological relevance. These data also suggest that the effects of luminal peptides, if present, may be more important in young suckling animals than in adults, due to the protective properties of colostrum and milk proteins.

4.3. Release of gut regulatory peptides into the gastrointestinal lumen

There are a few reports demonstrating how the gut regulatory peptides appear in the intestinal lumen and explaining why they could have been overlooked in previous investigations. Fujimiya *et al.* [152] showed that enterochromaffin cells actively release serotonin into the lumen of the small intestine, although the ratio of luminal content to tissue content was higher in embryonic gut compared to the gut of adult rats. Okumiya *et al.* [153], using immunelectron microscopic studies, demonstrated changes in the subcellular localisation of gastrin granules (migration from basal to apical region) and gastrin release into the small intestinal lumen induced by carbachol. This luminally oriented release of gastrin was absent in animals not pre-treated with carbachol. The above morphological studies help to explain the route by which gastrointestinal peptides appear in the intestinal lumen following stimulation, and contrast sharply with the undirectional stimulus-secretion coupling hypothesis.

Some of the luminal gut regulatory peptides have previously been shown to influence GI function. Luminal somatostatin can be reabsorbed by the intestine, circulate into the pancreas and inhibit the secretion of juice which suggests that the lumen of the intestine may be an important link in the enteropancreatic circulation of somatostatin [154]. Oral administration of insulin causes hypoglycaemia in young pigs and calves [155]. Growth factors have numerous local biological effects on the gut epithelium in neonates and sucklings, as well as peripheral effects, following their absorption from the gut into the circulating blood [151,156,157,158]. Luminal EGF and IGFs inhibit gastric secretion, and stimulate gastrointestinal epithelial cell growth and cell differentiation [159,156,160,161,162].

4.4. Luminal release of CCK

Studies in anaesthetised neonatal calves demonstrated that in a perfused closed loop of the duodenum the concentration of CCK-like immunoactivity was higher than that found in portal or jugular plasma [163]. The biliary duct and the accessory pancreatic ducts had been ligated, preventing any interference from CCK sequestered by the liver and secreted into the bile [135]. Thus the source of this CCK-like immunoactivity is presumably the duodenum - most likely the CCK-producing I cells present in the duodenal loop, although neuronal release may also contribute. This study confirms earlier findings in other species of CCK-like immunoactivity in the intestinal lumen [143]. It also adds to the findings of Sun et al. [164], showing that luminal CCK release in dogs can be stimulated by duodenal perfusion with sodium oleate and by feeding [165], by showing that luminal CCK release can also be evoked by electrical stimulation of the vagus nerves in the calf. The response to vagal stimulation was, however, only one fifth of that to oleate in dogs [164].

The importance of the vagal nerves in CCK release is presently being re-evaluated. Until now studies have mostly investigated the release of CCK into the peripheral blood plasma. Electrical stimulation of the vagus nerves has generally been reported to evoke a moderate release of CCK in dogs [166,167], pigs [168] and rats [169]. However, in one study, electrical stimulation in dogs [170] had no effect. On the other hand, truncal or selective vagotomy has generally been found to increase postprandial plasma CCK levels in man [171] and dogs [172]. In preruminant calves, cold vagal blockade halved the concentration of circulating CCK (Zabielski, Onaga, Kato - unpublished). These discrepancies may be related to species-specific regulation of CCK release, but probably are due to differences in methodology as well. It seems likely that the vagal nerves have only a minor role in controlling CCK release, i.e. in mediating the initial cephalic CCK response to feeding [167,173] and to suckling [169,174], but that the second, more protracted phase of CCK release is vagus-independent and is regulated by the presence/nature of food in the gastrointestinal tract.

CCK extracted from the lumen of the canine duodenum was biologically active [164]. Infusion of CCK-8 into the duodenal lumen was found to stimulate pancreatic exocrine secretion in conscious neonatal calves [175] and was also capable of affecting intestinal motility in the anaesthetised rabbit [144]. Whether there are CCK receptors in the duodenal lumen of calves remains unknown. However, CCK receptors as well as the expression of CCK receptor m-RNA have been found in the duodenal mucosa of the ferret and rat [136,176]. Moreover, low concentrations of CCK-8 have been reported to excite vagal afferent receptors located in the mucosa of the proximal duodenum in sheep [177], while intestinal perfusion with nutrients in the rat was found to excite vagal afferent discharge via endogenous release of CCK and activation of CCK-A receptors. Finally as discussed in the previous section, there is extensive experimental support for a duodenal, vagally-mediated action of CCK on exocrine pancreatic secretion in several animal species, and luminal CCK may contribute to this mechanism.

4.5. Luminal duodenal mechanism controlling the secretion of pancreatic juice via CCK

The physiological relevance of luminally released regulatory peptides on the function of distant organs (e.g., the pancreas) is far from being widely accepted. Studies in young suckling animals, however, have revealed numerous possibilities of local luminal regulation of the gastrointestinal structure and function. One of our aims was to examine the relationship between luminal CCK and the secretion of pancreatic juice. The administration of CCK-8 into the duodenal lumen during late phase 1 of the duodenal MMC resulted in a significant increase in juice volume and enzymes in calves [175]. The effect of id CCK appeared 5 to 10 min after the infusion, whereas the elevation of pancreatic juice after an intravenous dose usually started 2-5 min after the infusion. To clarify the site of the CCK mechanism, a poorly absorbed CCK-A receptor antagonist, Tarazepide (Solvay Pharmaceuticals, Germany) was infused intraduodenally before the id CCK [86]. The concentration of Tarazepide in the peripheral blood increased in a dose-dependent manner after intraduodenal administration. The decrease in pancreatic secretion (especially in protein output), however, started well before any Tarazepide was detected in the blood, and the absorption of the drug into the circulation was poor. The effect of intraduodenal CCK-8 on the exocrine pancreas was blocked by Tarazepide. This result clearly indicates that CCK-A receptors located at a different site than the pancreas, most likely a mucosal site, were affected by Tarazepide and these receptors were responsible for pancreatic stimulation. Furthermore, intraduodenal infusion of CCK stimulates pancreatic exocrine secretion via a cholinergic mechanism, since the secretory response could be blocked by atropine and 4-DAMP [89,175]. In contrast, cholinergic nerves play only a minor role in the pancreatic response to intravenous infusion of CCK-8 [175]. In consideration of all these points we postulate that duodenal mucosal CCK-A receptors are involved in the CCK-mediated regulation of pancreatic juice secretion (Figure 9).

Such receptors have been identified electrophysiologically in vagal afferent nerves in the duodenal mucosa of the sheep [177], ferret [136], and rat [178]. It would be expected that these receptors could be excited by luminal, paracrine or systemically released CCK and might be responsible for the physiological action of CCK on pancreatic enzyme secretion.

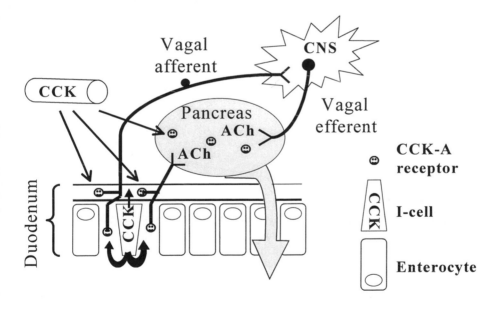

Figure 9. Schematic presentation of the peripheral and the local duodenally-mediated mechanisms controlling pancreatic secretion via CCK.

Intraduodenal Tarazepide failed to abolish pancreatic secretion in response to iv CCK-8, which could indicate that due to its poor absorption, CCK receptors other than mucosal ones were functioning, or that not only CCK-A receptors mediate the pancreatic response to iv CCK. It has recently been reported that both CCK-A and CCK-B receptors are present in the calf as well as the human pancreas [119,179], and substantial CCK-A and CCK-B gene expression has been reported in rat small intestinal mucosa [176]. Gastrin stimulates pancreatic secretion in dogs and cats [180,181] and perhaps CCK-B receptor activation also contributes to iv CCK-8-induced pancreatic secretion. Indeed, recent results with intravenous and luminal CCK and gastrin infusions and CCK-A and CCK-B receptor antagonist blockade in calves agree with this hypothesis [182,183]. In conclusion, CCK-producing cells (endocrine or neuronal) located in the mucosa of the upper gut release CCK into the intestinal lumen and into the blood, following stimulation. CCK released into the interstitial fluid and CCK released luminally can both stimulate pancreatic secretion via neural pathways involving duodenal CCK-A (and possibly CCK-B) receptors, as suggested in Figure 9.

5. CONCLUSIONS

We postulate that periodic pancreatic secretion is omnipresent in mammals, although it may be expressed differently in different species due to their dietary and digestive specificities. The PPS develops in young animals in harmony with the upper GI tract motility pattern, and it seems to be a testimony to normal function of the GI tract. The neurohormonal regulation of the exocrine pancreas function workss from the perinatal period, though the hormonal component gains in importance with age and/or the stage of GI tract development, and seems to be strongly influenced by the periodic activity. Local duodenally-mediated mechanisms regulate pancreatic secretion, at least in part by a CCK-related pathway.

REFERENCES

1. W. Boldyreff, Ergebn. Physiol., 11 (1911) 121.
2. W. Boldyreff, Gaz. Hop. Botkine., 34 (1902) 1529.
3. W. Boldyreff, Zentralbl. Physiol., 18 (1904) 489.
4. B.P. Babkin and H. Ishikawa, Pflugers Arch. Ges. Physiol., 147 (1912) 335.
5. V.B. Scott, C.C. Scott and H.J. Bugel, Amer. J. Physiol., 131 (1940) 60.
6. E.P. DiMagno, J.C. Hendricks, V.L.W. Go and R.R. Dozois, Dig. Dis. Sci., 24 (1979) 689.
7. G.R. Vantrappen, T.L. Peeters and J. Janssen, Scand. J. Gastroenterol., 14 (1979) 663.
8. F.B. Keane, E.P. DiMagno and R.R. Dozois, Gastroenterology, 78 (1980) 310.
9. F.B. Keane, E.P. DiMagno and J-R. Malagelada, Gastroenterology, 81 (1981) 726.
10. D.F. Magee and S. Naruse, J. Physiol., 344 (1983) 153.
11. K.Y. Lee, K. Shiratori, Y.F. Chen, T-M. Chang and W.Y. Chey, Amer. J. Physiol., 251 (1986) G759.

12. S.J. Konturek, P.J. Thor, J. Bilski, W. Bielański and J. Laskiewicz, Amer. J. Physiol. 250 (1986) G570.
13. J. Abello, J.P. Laplace and T. Corring, Reprod. Nutr. Developm., 28 (1988) 953.
14. W. Busch, Virchow's Arch. Pathol. Anat., 14 (1858) 140.
15. D.L. Wingate, Dig. Dis Sci., 26 (1981) 641.
16. S.K. Sarna, Gastroenterology, 89 (1985) 894.
17. H.D. Davenport, Handbook of Physiology, section 6 The Gastrointestinal System, vol 1 Motility and circulation, Oxford University Press, New York, 1989.
18. J.H. Szurszewski, Amer. J. Physiol., 274 (1998) G447.
19. A.C. Ivy, Gastroenterology, 6 (1946) 613.
20. D.F. Magee and S. Naruse, J. Physiol., 356 (1984) 391.
21. R. Zabielski, T. Onaga, H. Mineo and S. Kato, Exp. Physiol., 78 (1993) 675.
22. D.F. Magee and S. Naruse, J. Physiol., 403 (1988) 15.
23. S. Naruse, T. Suzuki and T. Ozaki, Pancreas, 7 (1992) 543.
24. K.Y. Lee, K. Shiratori, Y.F. Chen, T-M. Chang, W.Y. Chey, Amer. J. Physiol., 251 (1986) G759.
25. V.M. Gabert, M.S. Jensen, H. Jorgensen, R.M. Engberg and S.K. Jensen, J. Nutr., 126 (1996) 2076.
26. P. Kiela, R. Zabielski, P. Podgurniak, M. Midura, W. Barej, P.C. Gregory and S.G. Pierzynowski, Exp. Physiol., 81 (1996) 375.
27. T. Onaga, R. Zabielski, H. Mineo and S. Kato, Proceedings of the XXXII Congress of the International Union of Physiological Sciences, Glasgow, 1993.
28. S. Naruse and D.F. Magee, Biomed. Res., 7 (1986) 133.
29. H.C. Butler, D.C. Brinkman and P.A. Klavano, Amer. J. Vet. Res., 21 (1960) 205.
30. S.G. Pierzynowski, B.R. Weström, B.W. Karlsson, J. Svendsen and B. Nilsson, Can. J. Anim. Sci., 68 (1988) 953.
31. R. Zabielski, P. Podgurniak, S.G. Pierzynowski and W. Barej, Exp. Physiol., 75 (1990) 401.
32. R. Zabielski, S. Kato, S.G. Pierzynowski, H. Mineo, P. Podgurniak and W. Barej, Exp. Physiol., 77 (1992) 807.
33. S.G. Pierzynowski, R. Zabielski, B. Weström, M. Mikołajczyk and W. Barej, J. Anim. Physiol. Anim. Nutr., 65 (1991) 165.
34. S. Sarna, P. Northcott and L. Belbeck, Amer. J. Physiol., 242 (1982) G588.
35. Y. Ruckebush and L. Bueno, Brit. J. Nutr., 30 (1973) 491.
36. T. Onaga, H. Mineo and S. Kato, Regul. Pept., 68 (1997) 139.
37. J. Abello, J.P. Laplace and T. Corring, Reprod. Nutr. Developm., 28 (1988) 953.
38. R. Zabielski, S.G. Pierzynowski, B. Westrom, W. Barej and B. Karlsson, Digestion, 49 (1991) 60.
39. P. Kiela, Integrative role of some intestinal bioactive peptides in the regulation of pancreatic exocrine secretion and the MMC of the stomach and small intestine in piglets. Ph.D. thesis, Faculty of Veterinary Medicine, Warszawa, 1996.
40. P. Kiela, R. Zabielski, P. Podgurniak, M. Midura, W. Barej, P.C. Gregory and S.G. Pierzynowski, Exp. Physiol., 81 (1996) 375.

41. M-J. Thaela, M.S. Jensen, G. Cornelissen, F. Halberg, F. Noddegard, K. Jakobsen and
    S.G. Pierzynowski, J. Anim. Sci. 76 (1998) 1131.
42. D. Rantzer, P. Kiela, M-J. Thaela, J. Svendsen, B. Ahren, S. Karlsson and
    S.G. Pierzynowski, J. Anim. Sci., 75 (1997) 1324.
43. R. Zabielski, P. Kiela, T. Onaga, H. Mineo, P.C. Gregory and S. Kato, Can. J. Physiol.
    Pharmacol., 73 (1995) 1616.
44. S.J. Konturek and P. Thor, Amer. J. Physiol., 251 (1986) G591.
45. Y. Ruckebusch, J. Physiol., 210 (1970) 857.
46. C.L. Girard and J.W. Sissons, Can. J. Physiol. Pharmacol., 70 (1992) 1142.
47. S. Naruse, T. Takagi, T. Suzuki and T. Ozaki, J. Physiol., 446 (1992) 193.
48. J. Fioramonti and L. Bueno, Amer. J. Physiol., 264 (1984) G108.
49. M. Kato, S. Naruse, T. Takagi and S. Shionoya, Amer. J. Physiol., 258 (1989) G111.
50. O. Ito, S. Naruse, M. Kitagawa, H. Ishiguro, S. Ko, S. Nakajima and T. Hayakawa,
    Regul. Pept., 78 (1998) 105.
51. T.W. Schwartz, B. Stenquist, L. Olbe and F. Stadil, Gastroenterology, 76 (1979) 14.
52. M.H. Chen, S.N. Joffe, D.F. Magee, R.F. Murphy and S. Naruse, J. Physiol., 341 (1983)
    453.
53. N. Qvist, E. Øster-Jørgensen, L. Rasmussen, S.A. Pedersen, O. Olsen, P. Cantor and
    O.B. Schaffalitzky de Muckadell, Digestion, 45 (1990) 130.
54. D.F. Magee and S. Naruse, J. Physiol., 355 (1984) 441.
55. D.W. Zimmerman, M.G. Saar, C.D. Smith, C.P. Nicholson, R.R. Dalton, D. Baar,
    J.D. Perkins and E.P. DiMagno, Gastroenterology, 102 (1992) 1378.
56. P. Malfertheiner, M.G. Sarr, M.P. Spencer and E.P. DiMagno, Amer. J. Physiol., 257
    (1989) G415.
57. O. Pieramico, J.E. Dominguez-Muñoz, D.K. Nelson, W. Böck, M. Büchler and
    P. Malfertheiner, Gastroenterology, 109 (1995) 224.
58. J.C. Cuber, C. Bernard, J.P. Laplace and J.A. Chayvialle, Digestion, 32 (1985) 35.
59. J.C. Cuber, C. Laredo, J.P. Laplace and J.A. Chayvialle, 3rd European Symposium on
    Gastrointestinal Motility, Bruges, 1986.
60. M.A. Plaza, M.P. Arruebo and M.D. Murillo, Life Sci., 58 (1996) 2155.
61. R. Zabielski, C. Dardillat, I. Le Huerou-Luron, C. Bernard, J.A. Chayvialle and
    P. Guilloteau, Brit. J. Nutr., 79 (1998) 287.
62. S.J. Konturek, P.J. Thor, J. Bilski, W. Bielański and J. Laskiewicz, Amer. J. Physiol.,
    250 (1986) G570.
63. R. Zabielski, Y. Terui, T. Onaga, H. Mineo and S. Kato, Res. Vet. Sci., 56 (1994) 332.
64. J.C. Cuber, C. Bernard, J.P. Laplace, F. Levenez and J.A. Chayvialle, Can, J. Physiol.
    Pharmacol., 64 (1986) 45.
65. P. Guilloteau, T. Corring, J.A. Chayvialle, C. Bernard, J.W. Sissons and R. Toullec,
    Reprod. Nutr. Developm., 26 (1986) 717.
66. E. Samols, The Exocrine Pancreas, Raven Press, New York, 1991.
67. E.T. Shapiro, H.Tillil, K.S. Polonsky, V.S. Fang, A.H. Rubenstein and E.V. Cauter,
    J. Clin. Endocrinol. Metab., 67 (1988) 307.
68. W.J. Croom, L.S. Bull and I.L. Taylor, J. Nutr. 122 (1992) 191.

69. S.G. Pierzynowski, W. Barej, M. Mikołajczyk and R. Zabielski, J. Anim. Physiol. Anim. Nutr., 60 (1988) 234.
70. G. Le Drean, I. Le Huerou-Luron, J.A. Chayvialle, V. Philouze-Rome, M. Gestin, C. Bernard, R. Toullec and P. Guilloteau, Comp. Biochem. Physiol., 117 (1997) 245.
71. R. Zabielski, P. Kiela, V. Leśniewska, R. Krzemiński, M. Mikołajczyk and W. Barej, Brit. J. Nutr., 78 (1997) 427.
72. T. Onaga, R. Zabielski, H. Mineo and S. Kato, Proceedings of the XXXII Congress of the International Union of Physiological Sciences, Glasgow, 1993.
73. S.G. Pierzynowski, B.R. Weström, J. Svendsen and B.W. Karlsson, J. Pediat. Gastroenterol. Nutr., 10 (1990) 206.
74. S.G. Pierzynowski, B.R. Weström, C. Erlanson-Albertsson, B. Ahren, J. Svendsen and B. Karlsson, J. Pediat. Gastroenterol. Nutr., 16 (1993) 287.
75. S.G. Pierzynowski, B.R. Weström, J. Svendsen, L. Svendsen and B.W. Karlsson, Int. J. Pancreatol., 18 (1995) 81.
76. J.H. Szurszewski, Amer. J. Physiol., 217 (1969) 1757.
77. L. Bueno and Y. Ruckebush, Amer. J. Physiol., 6 (1979) E61.
78. R. Zabielski, P. Podgurniak, I. LeHuerou-Luron and P. Guilloteau, Digestion, 59 (1998) 253.
79. C.L. Berseth, J. Pediat., 115 (1989) 646.
80. R. Zabielski, T. Onaga, H. Mineo and S. Kato, Biomed. Res., 15 (1994) 371.
81. P. Layer, A.T.H. Chan, V.L.W. Go, A.R. Zinsmeister and E.P. DiMagno, Pancreas, 8 (1993) 181.
82. M. Katschinski, G. Dahmen, M. Reinshagen, et al. , Gastroenterology, 103 (1992) 383.
83. V.L.W. Go, E.P. DiMagno, J.D. Gardner, E. Lebenthal, H.A. Reber and G.A. Scheele (eds.), The Pancreas. Biology, Pathobiology and Disease, New York, Raven Press, 1993.
84. R. Zabielski, P. Kiela, W. Barej, S.G. Pierzynowski, B.R. Weström and B. Karlsson, Digestion, 49 (1991) 60.
85. R. Zabielski, T. Onaga, H. Mineo and S. Kato, Biomed. Res., 12 (1991) 38.
86. R. Zabielski, V. Leśniewska, J. Borlak, P.C. Gregory, P. Kiela, S.G. Pierzynowski and W. Barej, Regul. Pept., 78 (1998) 113.
87. R. Zabielski, V. Leśniewska and P. Guilloteau, Reprod. Nutr. Dev., 37 (1997) 385.
88. D.K. Nelson, G. Dahmen, J.E. Dominguez-Munoz, O. Pieramico, P. Malfertheiner and G. Adler, Gastroenterology, 104 (1993) 558.
89. V. Leśniewska, M. Ceregrzyn, S.G. Pierzynowski and R. Zabielski, Regul. Pept., 64 (1996) 108.
90. K.E. Hall, T.Y. El-Sharkawy and N.E. Diamant, Amer. J. Physiol. 243 (1982) G276.
91. A.S. Paintal, J. Physiol., 180 (1965) 1.
92. P. Malfertheiner, M.G. Saar and E.P. DiMagno, Gastroenterology, 96 (1989) 200.
93. J.L. Stagner and E. Samols, Amer. J. Physiol., 248 (1985) E516.
94. J.L. Stagner and E. Samols, Amer. J. Physiol., 248 (1985) E522.
95. E.C. Opara and V.L.W. Go, Pancreas, 6 (1991) 653.
96. P. Kiela, R. Zabielski, H. Mineo, T. Onaga, S. Kato and W. Barej, Proc. Soc. Nutr. Physiol., 3 (1994) 296.

188

97. T. Tsuda, Y. Sasaki and R. Kawashima, Physiological Aspects of Digestion and Metabolism in Ruminants, Academic Press Inc, Tokyo, 1991.

98. P. Guilloteau, J.A. Chayvialle, R. Toullec, J.F. Grognet and C. Bernard, Biol. Neonate, 61 (1992) 103.

99. Rodriguez-Membrilla and P. Vergara, Amer. J. Physiol., 272 (1997) G100.

100. S.H. Buck and T.F. Burks, Pharmacol. Rev., 38 (1986) 179.

101. Y. Li and C. Owyang, J. Clin. Invest., 92 (1993) 418.

102. J. Chariot, F. Appia, M. del Tacca, A. Tsocas and C. Rose, Pharmacol. Res. Commun., 20 (1988) 707.

103. H.R. Adams (ed.) Veterinary Pharmacology and Therapeutics, 5th edition, Iowa State University Press/AMES, Iowa, 1995.

104. S.G. Pierzynowski, P Podgurniak, M. Mikołajczyk and W. Szczesny, Q. J. Exp. Physiol., 71 (1986) 401.

105. G. Adler, D.K. Nelson, M. Katschinski and C. Beglinger, Pancreas, 10 (1995) 1.

106. R. Zabielski, T. Onaga, H. Mineo, S.G. Pierzynowski and S. Kato, Exp. Physiol., 79 (1994) 301.

107. R. Zabielski, I. Le Huerou-Luron, G. Le Drean, M. Gestin, C. Desbois, D. Gully, D. Fourmy and P. Guilloteau, Digestion, 58 (1997) 57.

108. A. Miyata, A. Arimura, R.R. Dahl, N. Minamino, A. Uehara, L. Jiang, M.D. Culler and D.H. Coy, Biochem. Biophys. Res. Commun., 164 (1989) 567.

109. A. Arimura, Reg. Pept., 37 (1992) 287.

110. R. Zabielski, T. Onaga, H. Mineo, E. Okine and S. Kato, Comp. Biochem. Physiol., 109C (1994) 93.

111. T. Onaga, M. Uchida, M. Kimura, M. Miyazaki, H. Mineo, S. Kato and R. Zabielski, Comp. Biochem. Physiol., 115C (1996) 185.

112. T. Onaga, K. Okamoto, Y.Harada, H. Mineo and S. Kato, Regul. Pept., 72 (1997) 147.

113. A.M. Reid, A. Shulkes and D.A. Titchen, J. Physiol., 396 (1988) 11.

114. J. Farenkrug, O.B. Schaffalitzky de Muckadell, J.J. Holst and S.L. Jensen, Amer. J. Physiol., 237 (1979) E525.

115. T.W. Schwartz, Gastroenterology, 85 (1983) 1411.

116. M.J. Davicco, J. Lefaivre and J.P. Barlet, Ann. Biol. Anim. Biochim. Biophys., 19 (1979) 843.

117. G.S. Konturek, A. Dembiński, R. Krol and E. Wunsh, Scand. J. Gastroenterol., 11 (1976) 57.

118. R. Toullec, J.A. Chayvialle, P. Guilloteau and C. Bernard, Comp. Biochem. Physiol., 102A (1992) 203.

119. V. Le Meuth, V. Philouze-Rome, I. Le Huerou-Luron, M. Formal, N. Vaysse, C. Gespach, P. Guilloteau and D. Fourmy, Endocrinology, 133 (1993) 1182.

120. I. Ohara, S. Otsuka and Y. Yugari, Amer. J. Physiol., 254 (1988) G424.

121. S.J. Konturek, W. Bielański and T.E. Solomon, Gastroenterology, 98 (1990) 47.

122. Yasui, S. Naruse, C. Yanaihara, et al., Amer. J. Physiol., 253 (1987) G13.

123. R. Zabielski, S.G. Pierzynowski, P. Podgurniak and W. Barej, J. Anim. Physiol. Anim. Nutr., 67 (1992) 173.

124. S.G. Pierzynowski, R. Zabielski, P. Podgurniak, P. Kiela, P. Sharma, B.R. Weström, S. Kato and W. Barej, J. Anim. Physiol. Anim. Nutr., 67 (1992) 268.
125. S. Kato, M. Usami and J. Ushijima, Jpn. J. Zootech. Sci., 55 (1984) 973.
126. M.E. Zenilman, J.E. Parodi and J.M. Becker, Amer. J. Physiol., 263 (1992) G248.
127. P. Guilloteau, I. Le Huerou-Luron, J.A. Chayvialle, R. Toullec, R. Zabielski and J.W. Blum, J. Vet. Med., A44 (1997) 1.
128. W.M. Bayliss and E.H. Starling, J. Physiol., 28 (1902) 324.
129. S.G. Pierzynowski, J. Anim Physiol. Anim. Nutr., 63 (1990) 198.
130. S.G. Pierzynowski and W. Barej, Q. J. Exp. Physiol., 69 (1984) 35.
131. I.P. Pavlov, The work of the digestive glands, Lippincott, Philadelphia, 1910.
132. J. Mellanby, J. Physiol., 60 (1925) 85.
133. J.W. Walsh and G.J. Dockray (eds.), Gut Peptides, Raven Press, New York, 1994.
134. D.R. Brown (ed.), Gastrointestinal Regulatory Peptides, Springer-Verlag, Berlin, 1993.
135. G.J. Gores, N.F. Larusso and L.J. Miller, Amer. J. Physiol., 250 (1986) G344.
136. L.A. Blackshaw and D. Grundy, J. Auton. Nerv. Syst., 31 (1990) 191.
137. S.G. Pierzynowski, H. Mortensson, B. Ahren and B.R. Westrom, Digestion, 49 (1991) 46.
138. S.G. Pierzynowski, H. Martensson, B. Ahren and B.R. Westrom, Digestion, 49 (1991) 46.
139. S.G. Pierzynowski, H. Martensson, B. Westrom, B. Ahren, K. Uvnas-Moberg and B. Karlsson, Biomed. Res., 14 (1993) 217.
140. C. Owyang, Amer. J. Physiol., 271 (1996) G1.
141. Y. Li, X.C. Zhang, L.M. Wang, E.W. Renehan, R. Fogel, and C. Owyang, Gastroenterology, 104 (1993) A837.
142. P.H. Jordan and B.S. Yip, Surgery, 72 (1972) 352.
143. G.B.G. Glass (ed.) Gastrointestinal Hormones, Raven Press, New York, 1980.
144. C.A. Sninsky, M.M. Wolfe, J.E. Guigan and J.R. Mathias, Amer. J. Physiol., 247 (1984) G724.
145. R.K. Rao, Life Sci., 48 (1991) 1685.
146. B.W. Kuvishnoff, M. Rudnicki and D.W. McFadden, J. Surg. Res., 50 (1991) 425.
147. J.M., Conlon, D. Rouiller, G. Boden and R.H. Unger, FEBS Lett., 105 (1979) 23.
148. Dawidson, M. Blom, T. Lundeberg, E. Theodorsson and B. Angmar-Mansson, Life Sci., 60 (1997) 269.
149. W.H. Shen and R-J. Xu, Life Sci., 59 (1996) 197.
150. R-J. Xu, Y.L. Mao and M.Y.W. Tso, Biol. Neonate, 70 (1996) 60.
151. A.S. Goldman, S.A. Atkinson and L.A. Hanson (eds.) Human Lactation, Plenum Press, New York, 1987.
152. M. Fujimiya, K. Okumiya and T. Maeda, Acta Cytochem. Histochem., 28 (1995) 555.
153. K. Okumiya, K. Matsubayashi, T. Maeda and M. Fujimiya, Peptides, 17 (1996) 225.
154. S.J. Konturek, J. Tasler, M. Cieszkowski, J. Jaworek, A. Arimura and A.V. Schally, Amer. J. Physiol., 241 (1981) G109.
155. L.A. Hanson (ed.), Biology of human milk: possible physiological role of hormones and hormone related substances present in milk. Nestle Nutrition Workshop Series, Vol 15, Nestle Ltd, Vevey/Raven Press, New York, 1988.

156. N. Kretchmer, E.J. Qilligan and J.D. Johnson (eds.), Prenatal and Perinatal Biology and Medicine, Vol 1, Physiology & Growth, Harwood Academic Publisher, Chru, 1987.

157. W. Thornburg, L. Matrisian, B. Magun and O. Koldovsky, Amer. J. Physiol., 246 (1984) G80.

158. W. Thornburg, R.K. Rao, L.M. Matrisian, B.E. Magun and O. Koldovsky, Amer. J. Physiol., 16 (1987) G68.

159. S.J. Konturek, M. Cieszkowski, J. Jaworek, J. Konturek, T. Brzozowski and H. Gregory, Amer. J. Physiol., 246 (1984) G580.

160. P.S. James, M.W. Smith, D.R. Tivey and T.J.G. Wilson, J. Physiol., 393 (1987) 583.

161. A.B. Lemmey, A.A. Martin, L.C. Read, F.M. Tomas, P.C. Owens and F.J. Ballard, Amer. J. Physiol., 260 (1991) E213.

162. J.A. Vanderhoof, R.H. McCusker, R. Clark, H. Mohammadpour, D.J. Blackwood, R.F. Harty and J.Y.H. Park, Gastroenterology, 102 (1992) 1949.

163. R. Zabielski, P. Kiela, P. Podgurniak, P.C. Gregory and S.G. Pierzynowski, Pol. J. Vet. Sci., 2 (1999) 13.

164. G. Sun, T.M. Chang, W. Xue, J.F.Y. Wey, K.Y. Lee and W.Y. Chey, Amer. J. Physiol., 262 (1992) G35.

165. K. Inoue, A. Ayalon, R. Yazigi, C. Watson, P.L. Rayford and J.C. Thompson, Digestion, 24 (1982) 118.

166. C.K. Kim, K.Y. Lee, T. Wang, G. Sun, T-M. Chang and W.Y. Chey, Amer. J. Physiol., 257 (1989) G944.

167. K. Uvnäs-Moberg, J. Auton. Nerv. Syst., 9 (1983) 141.

168. P. Cantor, J.J. Holst, S. Knuhtsen and J.F. Rehfeld, Scand. J. Gastroenterol., 21 (1986) 1069.

169. A. Lindén, Acta Physiol. Scand., 137 (1987) 1.

170. S. Guzman, J.A. Chayvialle, W.A. Bankes, P.L. Rayford and J.C. Thompson, Surgery, 86 (1979) 329.

171. W.P.M. Hopman, J. Jansen and C. Lamers, Ann. Surg., 200 (1984) 693.

172. F. König, H. Köhler, R. Nustede, R. Bartkowski and A. Schafmeyer, Res. Exp. Med., 192 (1992) 383.

173. A. Schafmayer, R. Nustede, A. Pompino and H. Köhler, Scand. J. Gastroenterol., 23 (1988) 315.

174. A.M.B. De Passiillé, R. Christopherson and J. Rushen, Physiol. Behav., 54 (1993) 1069.

175. R. Zabielski, T. Onaga, H. Mineo, S. Kato and S.G. Pierzynowski, Int. J. Pancreatol., 17 (1995) 271.

176. K. Miyasaka, M. Masuda, T. Kawanami and A. Funakoshi, Pancreas, 12 (1996) 272.

177. D.F. Cottrell and A. Iggo, J. Physiol., 354 (1984) 497.

178. E.S. Corp, J. McQuade, T.H. Moran and G.P. Smith, Brain Res., 623 (1993) 161.

179. Tang, I. Biemond and C.B.H.W. Lamers, Gastroenteroology, 111 (1996) 1621.

180. S.J. Konturek, J. Tasler, J.W. Konturek, M. Cieszkowski, K. Szewczyk, M. Hladij and P.S. Anderson, Gut, 30 (1989) 110.

181. S.J. Konturek, J. Bilski, M. Hladij, E. Krzyzek, R-Z. Cai and A.V. Schally, Digestion, 49 (1991) 97.

182. G. Cornou-Le Drean, La Secretion Pancreatique Exocrine Basale Et Postprandiale Chez Le Veau. Implication De La Cholecystokinine, De La Gastrine Et De Leurs Recepteurs, Ph.D. thesis, L'Universite De Rennes 1, Rennes, 1997.
183. R. Zabielski, I. Le Huerou-Luron, G. Le Drean, M. Gestin, C. Desbois, D. Gully, D. Fourmy and P. Guilloteau, Digestion, 58 (1997) 57.

Biology of the Pancreas in Growing Animals
S.G. Pierzynowski and R. Zabielski (Editors)
© 1999 Elsevier Science B.V. All rights reserved.

Role of nitric oxide in the control of pancreatic secretion

J. Bilski and S.J. Konturek

Chair of Physiology, Collegium Medicum Jagiellonian University,
Grzegórzecka 16, 31-531 Kraków, Poland

The L-arginine/nitric oxide pathway plays a key role in a number of biological processes within most organs and systems. Recently, evidence was provided that NO acts as neurotransmitter in the stomach, gut and pancreas. L-Arginine, which is a substrate for nitric oxide synthase, stimulates the release of pancreatic islet hormones but the mechanism of this stimulation is unknown. In this review we examine the role of NO in the exocrine and endocrine functions of the pancreas.

1. INTRODUCTION

1.1. Nitric oxide synthase

Nitric oxide (NO), initially described as endothelium-derived relaxing factor (EDRF) [1,2], is an unstable, fat-soluble gas formed from the terminal guanidine nitrogen atom of the amino acid L-arginine (L-Arg), through a process that incorporates molecular oxygen, by nitric oxide synthase (NOS). At least three classes of enzyme have been described, two characterized as constitutive (cNOS) forms [3-7] which are highly dependent on calcium, calmodulin, and NADPH for their activity [6-8], require no induction and are most likely involved in rapid agonist-dependent signalling responses and cellular communications [9-13]. One constitutive NO synthase isoform is present in a membrane-bound form in endothelial cells (eNOS) and the second is found in the cytosol of neural cells (iNOS). The third, inducible isoform releases large quantities of NO for a long period of time, does not require calcium for its activity and its expression in inflammatory cells, especially macrophages, can be stimulated by bacterial toxins, lipopolysaccharide and a number of cytokines [14]. This induction can be abolished by inhibitors of protein synthesis and by glucocorticoids [12]. The fact that NO diffuses easily across cell membranes enables it to act as an intracellular and intercellular messenger [15]. The physiological effects of NO are probably mediated via activation of soluble guanylate cyclase and the subsequent generation of the messenger cyclic guanosine monophosphate (cGMP) [3,16-18]. There have also been reports of some NO effects that are non-cGMP dependent; NO may activate a cytoplasmic protein, ADP-ribosyltransferase [19,20]. The biological activity of NO is short because it is rapidly oxidised to nitrite and nitrate; and its activity can be prolonged by superoxide dismutase [21].

1.2. Nitric oxide synthase inhibitors

The most effective means of inhibiting NO is by blockade of its synthesis with NOS inhibitors. The enzymatic activity of NO synthase can be inhibited by analogues of L-arginine such as N^G-monomethyl-L-arginine (L-NMMA), N^G-nitro-L-arginine (L-NNA) and N^G-nitro-L-arginine methyl ester (L-NAME) [3,22,23]. Because the NOS inhibitors are competitive, their suppression of the synthesis of NO can be overcome by addition of excess L-arginine but not its stereoisomer, D-arginine [3]. Due to the rapid disappearance of NO from tissues, the above inhibitors are often used as an indirect means of assessing the effects of NO on various bodily functions [22]. *In vitro* studies have shown that L-NNA is more potent as an inhibitor of the constitutive NOS, but less potent as an inhibitor of the inducible NOS than L-NMMA [24-26]. Some of the currently employed NOS inhibitors may well exert other actions on processes not yet well defined. A good example of this is the observation that L-NAME has affinity for muscarinic cholinergic binding sites, a property not shared by L-NNA and L-NMMA, and an action not reversed by L-arginine [27,28].

1.3. Nitric oxide in gastrointestinal physiology and pathology

The involvement of NO in an increasing variety of physiological and pathophysiological processes in many tissues, including the gastrointestinal tract, has been established [3,22,29-31]. It has become clear that the role of NO extends beyond the vasculature. The presence of NOS has been demonstrated in central and peripheral nerves [32]. Using a superfusion bioassay cascade, Bult *et al.* [33] have shown that NO-like factor may be released upon stimulation of the nonadrenergic, noncholinergic (NANC) nerves.

Nitric oxide has been implicated in neural inhibitory responses in the gastrointestinal tract, and it is now recognized as the major mediator of relaxation induced by NANC neurons [29]. Studies in animals revealed that inhibition of NOS antagonizes NANC nerve-mediated relaxation of the lower oesophageal sphincter and reduces the latency of the contraction in the oesophagus [34]. Further studies confirmed that NO mediates the mechanical and electrical response to enteric inhibitory nerve stimulation in the oesophagus and is also involved in nerve-mediated relaxation of the lower oesophagus [35-39]. Administration of L-NMMA in humans resulted in a dose-dependent reduction in the latency period between swallows and the onset of contraction, the reduction being most pronounced in the distal oesophagus. Those effects were partially reversed by addition of L-arginine to the L-NMMA infusion [40]. It has been concluded that endogenous NO is involved, at least to some extent, in the physiological regulation of the motility pattern in the distal oesophageal body. Receptive relaxation and gastric accommodation also appear to be mediated by NO [41,42], and NO regulates gastric emptying by influencing the motor activity of the pyloric sphincter [43-47]. Electrophysiological studies also support the role of NO as an enteric inhibitory neurotransmitter in the canine duodenum and jejunum [48-51]. The NO system exerts a tonic inhibitory influence on intestinal myoelectric activity by reducing the frequency of the migrating motor complex (MMC) pacesetter and by suppressing postprandial activity [52,53]. The canine ileocolonic sphincter was one of the first tissues in which the role of NO as a neurotransmitter was shown [54-56] and the presence of nitrergic innervation was demonstrated in the ileum [57,58]. NO may be also an important mediator of the inhibitory branch of the peristaltic reflex in the small and large intestine. L-NNA prevented nerve-mediated relaxation of canine colonic muscles [59-64]. Rattan *et al.* [65] have demonstrated that L-NNA causes a decrease in the reflex relaxation of the internal anal sphincter. It was recently shown that NOS inhibitors increase the gallbladder basal pressure and enhance the intensity and duration of the contractile response to CCK and bethanechol, these effects being reversible on L-arginine administration [66-68].

A number of studies have shown that NO promotes an increase in gastric mucosal blood flow during central vagal stimulation [69], pentagastrin-induced acid secretion [70], chronic renal failure [71,72] and acute normovolemic anaemia [73]. There are conflicting reports on the possible effects of NO and its inhibitors on resting mucosal blood flow [70,71,74]. Intravenous administration of NOS inhibitors did not affect either the resting or pentagastrin-stimulated acid secretion in anaesthetised rats [70], despite a substantial decrease in mucosal vasodilation associated with the acid secretory process. Similarly stimulation of acid secretion by central vagal activation was not influenced by inhibition of NO synthesis [69]. The NO inhibitor L-NAME was found to partially restore the secretory response to pentagastrin abolished by *Escherica coli* endotoxin, with complete restoration when the platelet-activating factor (PAF) receptor antagonist was concomitantly administered [75]. By contrast, in experiments on conscious dogs, the inhibition of NO synthase by L-NNA, strongly suppressed gastric acid responses to a variety of secretory stimulants (sham-feeding, ordinary feeding, urecholine, bombesin, histamine and pentagastrin) and in tests with enhanced gastrin release (sham-feeding, ordinary feeding, bombesin), L-NNA also significantly attenuated this release [76-78].

NO has been reported to promote gastric cytoprotection against various damaging agents [79-84], but the data are conflicting [71,85]. In studies in anaesthetised rats NOS inhibitors stimulated duodenal bicarbonate secretion [86-88] but on the other hand in experiments in dogs, rats and pigs, inhibition of NOS reduced the basal and stimulated alkaline secretion [89,90].

Inhibition of endogenous nitric oxide synthesis caused an increased ileal secretion of water and ions [91,92] and this response was reversed by administration of the NOS substrate L-arginine [91]. The increased NO level in the active phase of ulcerative colitis appears to revert to normal in the quiescent phase of the disease [93,94], which suggests a possible role of the substance in inflammatory bowel disease. On the other hand there are data suggesting that NO is released following gut injury and contributes to the functional process of epithelial repair [95].

2. NOS AND PANCREATIC NEURONS

A morphological basis for understanding the role of NO in the pancreas was provided by several studies on the localization and distribution of NADPH diaphorase in the pancreas. NADPH diaphorase activity was found in the neurons and vascular endothelium of the pancreas of animals and humans, and the vast majority of intrapancreatic ganglion cells coexpressed NADPH activity and VIP-immunoreactivity [96-100]. Nerve fibres with NADPH diaphorase activity were diffusely distributed in the pancreatic parenchyma, and nerve cell bodies with NADPH diaphorase activity were demonstrated in the pancreas [96,98,101-108]. Neurons that expressed NADPH diaphorase activity were found to project to the bowel and the pancreas from dorsal root ganglia [96]. NADPH diaphorase activity was seen not only in neurons of pancreatic ganglia but also in sensory and enteropancreatic neurons and most of the NADPH diaphorase-containing neurons exhibited a Dogiel type I morphology [96]. It is conceivable that at least a part of intrapancreatic nerve fibres stained for NADPH diaphorase may have originated from the intrapancreatic ganglion cells, which have been regarded as parasympathetic postganglionic. Nerve bundles in intralobular and interlobular connective tissues in different species contained numerous nonvaricose nerve fibres with NADPH diaphorase [96].

3. NO AND EXOCRINE PANCREATIC SECRETION IN ANIMALS *IN VIVO*

The observation that sodium nitroprusside, now known to release NO spontaneously, increased pancreatic secretion in dogs suggested that endogenous nitric oxide could play a role in the pancreatic response to physiological stimulants [109].

2.1. NO and basal pancreatic secretion

Several studies on conscious dogs with chronic pancreatic fistulas have been carried out. Interdigestive intestinal motility and pancreatic secretion showed synchronous cyclic changes (MMC) that were interrupted by feeding [110-112,113]. Under basal conditions, spontaneous pancreatic secretion in conscious dogs showed fluctuations with typical periodicity, in phase with the myoelectric activity of the duodenum, reaching the nadir during phase I and the peak at phase II and III. The inhibition of NOS by L-NNA decreased the phase III-related rise in pancreatic secretion, an effect that was reversed, at least in part when the L-NNA was combined with L-arginine [52].

2.2. NO in the cephalic phase of exocrine pancreatic secretion

In conscious dogs the inhibitory effect of L-NNA on exocrine pancreatic secretion was most pronounced after the cephalic-vagal stimulation of the pancreas by sham feeding [114]. L-NNA infusion resulted in a marked decrease of this pancreatic response to sham feeding and the peak protein secretion was reduced by about 74 %. When L-arginine was combined with L-NNA infusion, the increase in protein outputs during and after sham feeding were significantly higher than those observed in tests with infusion of L-NNA alone, but did not reach the rate observed in control tests with the sham feeding alone. Because the secretory effects of sham feeding are mediated mainly via vagal nerves, these results may indicate that the mechanism involving NO in pancreatic secretions is related to a vagal pathway.

Administration of insulin or 2-deoxy-D-glucose (2-DG) is used to stimulate the vagus nerve and to mimic the response to cephalic phase stimulation [115]. L-NNA infusion in conscious dogs not only significantly decreased the pancreatic response to sham feeding; the secretory response to 2-DG or insulin infusion was significantly inhibited by about 80% (Figure 1). When L-arginine was combined with L-NNA, this reduction in pancreatic secretory response was significantly attenuated (unpublished data). It is well known, however, that atropine reduces this effect only in part, while vagotomy completely abolishes it. This indicates that vagal noncholinergic efferent fibres can play an important role in the pancreatic response to sham feeding [116,118]. These afferent fibres may release various neurotransmitters besides acetylcholine, such as, GRP and VIP, in the pancreas [119]. The marked decrease in cephalic phase secretory activity caused by L-NNA in conscious dogs suggests that endogenous NO is implicated in vagal stimulation of the secretory cells.

The pancreatic response to GRP administration was characterized by a well-sustained secretion of protein that reached about 85% of the caerulein maximum. Infusion of L-NNA during the GRP-stimulated secretion resulted in a marked reduction of pancreatic output. The addition of L-arginine to iv infusion of L-NNA resulted in a significantly higher pancreatic protein secretion than that observed after infusion of L-NNA alone but lower than that obtained with GRP alone [120].

Administration of the cholinergic agonist, urecholine, caused a small but significant increase in pancreatic protein, reaching about 20% of the caerulein maximum. Infusion of L-NNA significantly decreased the urecholine-stimulated secretion and this decrease was partially reversed by addition of L-Arg to the L-NNA. L-Arg alone did not significantly change the pancreatic secretory response to urecholine [121].

These observations obtained from experiments on conscious dogs have been confirmed by studies in isolated pig pancreas prepared with an intact vagal nerve supply [122], which demonstrated that L-NNA and L-NAME reduce the secretory pancreatic response to electrical stimulation of the vagal nerve or VIP infusion. This inhibition was more effective during vagal stimulation than following VIP infusion and the effect of L-NNA was stronger than L-NAME. In that study [122] L-arginine completely restored the pancreatic secretion inhibited by L-NAME but only partially reversed the inhibition caused by L-NNA.

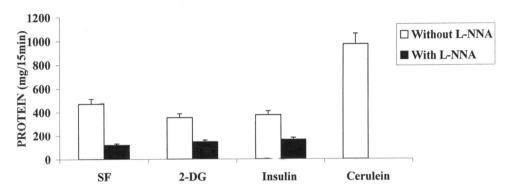

Figure 1. Effects of iv infusion of L-NNA (2.5 mg/kg + 0.5 mg/kg-h) on stimulated pancreatic protein secretion. SF, sham feeding; 2-DG, 2-deoxy-glucose. Data, shown as means ± SEM of at least six 6 tests on 6 conscious dogs, are adapted from Konturek *et al.* [114] and Konturek and Bilski (unpublished data).

3.3. NO in the pancreatic response to a meal

When chyme reaches the upper small gut, an intestinal phase of pancreatic secretion begins which is quantitatively the most important phase of the pancreatic response to a meal [123,124]. Under physiological conditions the intestinal phase acts on a pancreas which is already prestimulated by an increased blood flow and an enhanced enzyme secretion, achieved by the stimuli of the cephalic and gastric phases [124].

The pancreatic secretory response is probably mediated in part by enteropancreatic reflexes and by the release of hormones, especially CCK and secretin. In addition several regulatory peptides appear to modulate secretion, including insulin, glucagon, pancreatic polypeptide and somatostatin, all produced within the pancreas [125]. The importance of enteropancreatic reflexes as direct mediators of the pancreatic secretory response to intestinal stimulants has

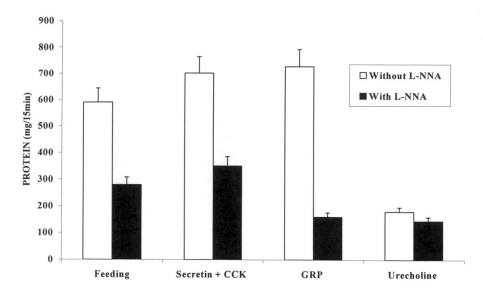

Figure 2. Effects of iv infusion of L-NNA (2.5 mg/kg + 0.5 mg/kg-h) on stimulated pancreatic protein secretion. Data, shown as means ± SEM of at least six 6 tests on 6 conscious dogs, are adapted from Konturek *et al.* [114] and Bilski *et al.* [121],

been demonstrated in several studies [126-130]. These reflexes may be critical to obtaining a rapid pancreatic response with the chyme flowing into the duodenum, and to the release of gut hormones, providing a sustained subsequent stimulus. Kirchgessner and Gershon [131] demonstrated in the rat that there are projections of enteric neurons to ganglia of the pancreas, thus providing anatomical evidence for these enteropancreatic reflexes.

When the effects of L-NNA on postprandial and hormonally stimulated pancreatic secretions were studied in dogs with chronic pancreatic fistulas [114], the pancreatic protein and bicarbonate response to a meat meal were markedly reduced (by about 70%) by L-NNA infusion. Both sham feeding and ordinary feeding caused a significant rise in the plasma gastrin level and feeding (but not sham feeding) increased plasma CCK. These increments were also significantly reduced by administration of L-NNA. The pancreatic bicarbonate and protein response to secretin plus CCK were also decreased by infusion of L-NNA, by about 50%. Glyceryl trinitrate (GTN = nitroglycerine), an NO donor, infused in graded doses caused a significant increase in protein secretion and this response was not altered by L-NNA.

Duodenal infusion of a mixed meal (carbohydrate 14%, fat 4% and protein 3.8% resulted in an increase in pancreatic protein secretion similar to that obtained with ordinary feeding. After administration of L-NNA the pancreatic secretion response was inhibited by about 75%, but when L-Arg was combined with the L-NNA, the reduction in pancreatic secretion was significantly attenuated and protein outputs were similar to those achieved with duodenal nutrient alone [120,121].

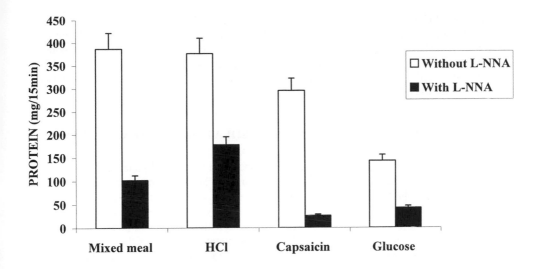

Figure 3. Effects of iv infusion of L-NNA (2.5 mg/kg + 0.5 mg/kg-h) on stimulated pancreatic protein secretion. Data, shown as means ± SEM of at least six 6 tests on 6 conscious dogs, are adapted from Bilski *et al.* [121] and Konturek and Bilski (unpublished data).

Duodenal instillation of 0.1N HCl, glucose in 10% solution and capsaicin to stimulate sensory nerves resulted in a rise in pancreatic protein secretion reaching about 31%, 16%, and 26% respectively, of the maximal response to exogenous caerulein. Administration of N^G-nitro-L-arginine significantly inhibited those pancreatic responses (unpublished data).

Studies on other animal species and/or different experimental models confirmed these observations from chronic dog studies. In rats with chronic pancreatic fistulas blockade of NO synthase by L-NNA significantly reduced the basal pancreatic protein secretion and that induced by the infusion of CCK, feeding or the diversion of pancreatic juice. This inhibitory effect was partially reversed when L-arginine was added to the L-NNA [132]. Analogously, in other study in rats, L-NAME reduced basal and caerulein-stimulated pancreatic secretion [133]. It has been demonstrated that endogenous NO plays a significant role in the regulation of secretin-stimulated pancreatic exocrine secretion, but does not influence acid-stimulated secretin release in rats [134]. In cats, L-NMMA significantly inhibited secretin- and cholecystokinin-stimulated secretion and sodium nitroprusside significantly increased pancreatic secretion [135].

3.3. NO in exocrine secretion in humans

A little is known about the role of NO in the control of pancreatic exocrine secretion in humans. A nitric oxide donor has been shown to stimulate pancreatic lipase and trypsin secretion in humans [136]. In other study, pancreatic secretion was stimulated by intravenous infusion of secretin (80 pmol/kg/h) plus caerulein (50 pmol/kg/h) and duodenal content was aspirated by gastroduodenal tube [137]. The addition of L-NMMA in graded doses (2-8 μmol/kg/h) dose-dependently reduced the secretin-caerulein stimulated pancreatic enzyme secretion without alterations of the volume flow and bicarbonate outputs. The addition of L-Arg to L-NMMA reversed the inhibitory action of L-NMMA on protein enzyme response to secretin-caerulein in these subjects. It is of interest that unlike in dogs, pigs or rats, L-NMMA in humans failed to affect water and bicarbonate secretion, but as in animals it caused a marked inhibition of protein enzyme secretion.

4. NO AND PANCREATIC SECRETION IN ISOLATED PANCREATIC ACINI

NO has been reported to influence pancreatic secretion in isolated pancreatic acini but the data remain conflicting. Studies in our laboratory on isolated rat pancreatic acini have indicated that the inhibition of NO by L-NNA does not affect basal or stimulated amylase secretion [114,132]. Only GTN, which spontaneously releases NO, was effective in stimulating basal and CCK-induced amylase secretion from the isolated pancreatic acini, but it is not clear whether similar amounts of NO are generated *in vivo* as those generated after the administration of GTN [114]. These results can be interpreted as showing that NO in the pancreatic tissue does not originate in the secretory cells but most likely in the endothelial or neural cells and that it may act, at least to some extent, directly on the secretory cells.

When pancreatic acini were obtained from rats infused for 5 h with caerulein, they showed the usual dose responses to CCK-8 added to the incubation medium in gradually increasing concentrations (10^{-12} M – 10^{-9}M). The maximal amylase secretion in caerulein-treated rats was achieved with 10^{-10} M CCK-8, whereas that in saline-infused rats occurred at 10^{-11} M. A similar „shift to the right" of the amylase response to CCK-8 was observed with acini obtained from rats infused with caerulein plus L-NNA, but the responses to all the concentrations of CCK-8 added to the incubation medium were significantly lower than those of the pancreas of rats infused with caerulein alone. Addition of L-arginine to the L-NNA infusion almost completely restored the amylase response to various concentrations of CCK [132].

In isolated pancreatic acini from the rat, L-NNA failed to affect the basal or stimulated amylase secretion in response to urecholine in graded concentrations (10^{-5} M – 10^{-3} M). However, in pancreatic slices (containing nerve fibres) urecholine dose-dependently increased enzyme secretion, and this response was abolished by L-NNA. L-Arg restored the amylase response to urecholine (unpublished data).

Molero *et al.* [133] have shown in dispersed acini, that supramaximal caerulein concentrations induced NO release, but the amylase dose-response curve was not modified by NO inhibition. In study on isolated pancreatic acini by other authors, [96] the secretion of amylase evoked by L- arginine was inhibited by L-NNA, which also inhibited VIP-stimulated secretion of amylase. However, L-NNA had no effect on amylase secretion stimulated by carbachol.

Intact pancreatic acini are much more responsive to secretory stimulation by various agonists *in vitro* than dispersed preparations of isolated acinar cells [138,139]. Integration of the activity of many neighbouring acinar cells to produce a unified overall secretory response suggests the participation of a readily diffusible paracrine substance acting across cell boundaries [138,139]. This factor could act to modulate the initial response, possibly exerting its effects through a pathway of intracellular Ca^{2+}, and NO is ideally suited for such a role in the exocrine pancreas.

A potential mechanism of action for NO in the acini is through an increase in cellular cyclic GMP. Increased cGMP has been associated with stimulation of pancreatic enzyme secretion, but its role as a mediator in this process is controversial [140-143]. It has been shown lately that cGMP can mediate the receptor-activated Ca^{2+} influx in pancreatic acinar cells [141-143]. The activation of Ca^{2+} influx is required for regulation of the free cytosolic Ca^{2+} concentration, for refilling of the internal Ca^{2+} stores, and for the secretory response in pancreatic acinar cells [144]. Carbachol-induced increase of endogenous cGMP communicates the status of internal mobilizable Ca^{2+} stores to the plasma membrane and directly modulates agonist-stimulated Ca^{2+} entry across the plasmalemma of the acinar cell [143]. In experiments by Gukovskaya and Pandol, carbachol increased both nitrite (a breakdown product of NO) levels and the production of NO, determined by conversion of ^{3}H-arginine to ^{3}H-citrulline [140]. Blocking NO production with inhibitors of NOS abolished the carbachol-induced cGMP rise and the Ca^{2+} influx in pancreatic acinar cells in a dose-dependent manner. L-NMMA also caused inhibition of the basal cGMP level, suggesting a role for NO in cGMP homeostasis in resting cells [140]. In other studies, agonist and the psigargin-activated Ca^{2+} entry and increases in cellular cGMP were blocked by specific inhibition, either of NOS (by L-NMMA) or of guanylate cyclase (by LY33583) [145]. In a study by Wren *et al.* [138], treatment of acini with L-arginine increased the nitrite level as well as the cyclic GMP and amylase release, an effect which was prevented by the nitric oxide synthase inhibitors L-NMMA and L-NNA. These nitric oxide inhibitors also blocked carbachol-induced amylase release as well as elevation of acinar cell cyclic GMP.

Treatment of rat pancreatic acinar cells with cholecystokinin-octapeptide (CCK-8) resulted in an increase in the conversion of arginine to citrulline, the amount of nitrite, the release of amylase, and the level of cGMP. Especially, CCK-8-stimulated an increase of arginine to citrulline transformation. The increase in nitrite and cGMP levels was completely counteracted by the inhibitor of NOS, L-NMMA. By contrast, the stimulated amylase release was only partially reduced. Furthermore, the L-NMMA-induced decrease in NOS activity and amylase release showed a dose-dependent pattern. The data on the time course of CCK-8-induced citrulline formation and cGMP rise indicated that NOS and guanylate cyclase were activated by treatment with CCK-8 [146].

Chanson *et al.* (147) measured the temporal changes in cytosolic free Ca^{2+} ([Ca^{2+}]i), Ca^{2+}-dependent membrane currents (Im), and gap junctional current (Ij) elicited by acetylcholine (Ach) in rat pancreatic acinar cells using digital imaging and dual perforated patch-clamp recording. Ach-induced uncoupling was prevented by blocking nitric oxide production with L-nitro-arginine and restored by exposing acinar cells to dibutyryl cGMP.

Xu *et al.* [148] examined the role of the NOS pathway in agonist-evoked (Ca^{2+})i oscillations and attempted to identify the NOS isoform most likely to regulate Ca^{2+} influx. Ca^{2+}-mobilizing agonists acting on pancreatic acinar cells, bombesin (BS) and the CCK analogue CCK-JMV-180 (CCKJ), evoked different type of (Ca^{2+})i oscillations. The bombesin-evoked (Ca^{2+})i oscillations rapidly became acutely dependent on the presence of extracellular Ca^{2+}, whereas the CCKJ-evoked oscillations continued for long periods of time in the absence of Ca^{2+} influx. Inhibitors of selective steps in the NOS pathway inhibited agonist-induced cGMP production. The inhibitors were then used to show that scavenging NO with reduced haemoglobin, inhibition of guanylyl cyclase with 1H-(1,2,4) oxadiazolo(4,3-a) quinoxaline-1-one (ODQ) and inhibition of protein kinase G with Rp-8-pCPT-cGMPS inhibited (Ca^{2+})i oscillations evoked by BS but not those evoked by CCKJ. These findings were extended to duct and acinar cells. In these cells, Ca^{2+}-mobilizing agonists stimulated a large Ca^{2+} influx, which was inhibited by all inhibitors of the NOS pathway. Western blot analysis and immunolocalization revealed that the cells did not express iNOS; eNOS was expressed only in blood vessels and capillaries, whereas nNOS was expressed at high levels next to the plasma membrane of all cells. Accordingly, the nNOS inhibitor 7-nitroindazole (7-NI) inhibited BS- but not CCKJ-evoked (Ca^{2+})i oscillations and Ca^{2+} influx into SMG acinar and duct cells.

In contrast, the results of the study by Yoshida [149] demonstrated the lack of effect of L-NAME on amylase secretion induced by various concentrations of carbachol, CCK-8 or the high-affinity CCK agonist, JMV-180, in pancreatic acini. Similarly, L-NAME did not affect the changes in Ca^{2+} spiking evoked by these secretagogues; nor was Ca^{2+} entry, refilling or oscillation altered by L-NAME. Sub- and supramaximal concentrations of these secretagogues did not change NO synthase activities compared with basal levels. Sodium nitroprusside, a NO donor, caused a 9.4-fold increase in cGMP levels compared with the basal level, and stimulated amylase secretion and Ca^{2+} transients to a level equal to 10-15% and 13-24%, respectively, of those observed with maximal concentrations of secretagogues.

5. MECHANISMS OF ACTION OF NO ON PANCREATIC EXOCRINE SECRETION

5.1. NO and the release of gut hormones

The mechanism of action of NO on pancreatic exocrine secretion is not clear. The pancreatic secretory response to feeding is mediated, at least in part, by gut hormones, especially endogenous CCK. The observation that the postprandial increments in plasma gastrin and CCK were significantly attenuated by the inhibition of NO synthase suggests that the decrease in pancreatic response to food may be due at least in part to the suppression of the gut hormones stimulating the pancreatic secretion [114]. On the other hand the pancreatic response to the combination of secretin plus CCK (producing a similar rate of exocrine secretion to that obtained with feeding) was also markedly inhibited (by about 50%) by L-NNA, suggesting that this action is independent of hormone release, maybe acting directly on the secretory cells.

The fact that NOS inhibitors caused a significant reduction in amylase release by dispersed pancreatic acini suggests that endogenous NO may be involved in the mechanism of enzyme secretion by acinar cells [133,146].

5.2. NO and pancreatic blood flow

On the other hand, the finding that L-NMMA attenuated the pancreatic blood flow in both the resting and hormonally stimulated pancreas in dogs and rats and that this effect could be reversed by the addition of L-Arg suggests that NO may affect the pancreatic secretion, at least in part, through changes in the vascular bed.

Recent results indicate that NO exerts a tonic vasorelaxing effect on the pancreatic vasculature under resting conditions and following secretory stimulation [114,150]. L-NNA caused little alteration in the pancreatic circulation in animals receiving GTN, an exogenous donor of NO, but resulted in a significant reduction in resting and hormonally stimulated total pancreatic blood flow (SPBF) and tissue blood perfusion [114]. As inhibitors of NO synthesis do not possess any inherent vasoconstrictive properties [151], the reduction in pancreatic circulation and accompanying increase in the systemic blood pressure observed in these experiments reflects an inhibition of the biosynthesis of the endogenous nitrovasodilatator in the vascular wall. This is consistent with the observation that L-arginine, which is known to restore the biosynthesis of NO in vascular tissue after its inhibition by L-NNA [152], partly prevented the inhibitory effect of L-NNA on pancreatic circulation and attenuated the increase in the systemic blood pressure caused by L-NNA [114]. Pancreatic blood flow is considered to play an important role in the control of exocrine pancreatic secretion [153]. Studies with the administration of vasopressin [153], leukotriene C [154] or PYY [155,156] showed that the decrease in the blood flow to pancreas was accompanied by a marked inhibition of the pancreatic secretory rate. However, in recent studies on isolated porcine pancreas it has been shown that the pancreatic response to vagal stimulation is independent of its vascular effect [122].

5.3. Role of NO as a neurotransmitter

NO fulfils several characteristics of a neurotransmitter in that it is released from nerves and affects the function of effector cells. However, it is not preformed or stored in presynaptic cells like other transmitters.

The inhibitory effect of L-NNA in conscious dogs was most pronounced after vagal stimulation of the pancreas by sham feeding or 2-DG-induced neuroglycopenia, which indicates that the involvement of NO in pancreatic secretion could be through a mechanism of vagal release. Since the pancreatic secretory response to ordinary feeding or duodenal perfusion with a mixed meal or capsaicin may be also mediated by duodeno-pancreatic reflexes involving vagovagal reflexes, the potent inhibitory action of L-NNA on these responses could be also attributed to the reduction in vagally-mediated release of NO in the pancreas.

6. NO IN CONTROL OF THE ENDOCRINE PANCREATIC SECRETION

Over the last few years a body of physiological evidence has accumulated that, together with earlier morphological evidence, indicates that islet hormones regulate the exocrine pancreas [157-159]. Much of this regulation is locally mediated via the islet-acinar portal vascular system [157]. For the role of physiological regulator of exocrine pancreatic functions the evidence is strongest for insulin, based on *in vivo* studies and *in vitro* studies with isolated perfused pancreas and with isolated pancreatic acini [157]. Insulin appears to have long-term effects on the regulation of the biosynthesis of pancreatic enzymes and short-term effects on the potentiation of the pancreatic secretory response to gut hormones and neurotransmitters [157]. Other islet hormones and peptides, including glucagon, somatostatin, and PP, may act as inhibitory regulators of the pancreas, although this regulation is not as well established and little is known concerning the locus of action of these peptides [157].

L-arginine mediates protein-induced insulin secretion and potentiates glucose-induced insulin release [160]. The mechanism of this process is not clearly understood and recently it was postulated that the insulinotropic action of L-arginine may be explained by the formation of NOS [161]. Islets cells were found to contain both the cNOS and iNOS isoforms [97,162,163]. The instability of NO suggests that it is unlikely to be a hormone that affects a distant target; nevertheless, the potential of insulin-containing cells to release NO is compatible with an autocrine or paracrine function of NO within the cells. NO secreted by islets cells may induce the secretion of insulin or act by increasing blood flow to the islets during periods of secretion.

It has been established that exogenous cGMP triggers insulin release and that glucose and L-arginine increase cGMP in isolated pancreatic islets [105,164,165]. Insulin release induced by glucose and L-arginine was decreased by the NOS inhibitors [161,164,166]. However, in several *in vitro* studies in isolated islets the NOS inhibitors stimulated rather than inhibited insulin release [105,162,167-180]. It is possible that low, non-toxic levels of NO released by cNOS act as signalling molecules during L-arginine or glucose-stimulated insulin secretion and that these responses are mediated by the direct activation of guanylate cyclase by NO, resulting in the formation of cGMP [164,165,176,181]. Nitric oxide produced in much larger quantities by iNOS may function as an effector molecule that mediates cytostatic and cytotoxic effects and this effect is independent of cGMP [182,183].

In studies on conscious dogs it was found that ordinary feeding, sham-feeding, 2-deoxy-D-glucose, duodenal nutrient and intravenous infusion of GRP or urecholine significantly increased insulin, glucagon and pancreatic polypeptide plasma levels. Infusion of L-NNA completely blocked the effect of sham-feeding and 2-DG on plasma glucagon insulin and PP. Increments observed in plasma glucagon, insulin and PP after ordinary feeding were significantly reduced. L-NNA markedly decreased insulin and PP but not glucagon increase after duodenal nutrient infusion. L-NNA alone also almost completely eliminated the increase in insulin and PP plasma levels seen after iv infusion of GRP and urecholine. It caused a slight but significant reduction in the glucagon increment observed after GRP but not after urecholine. These responses were partially reversed by the addition of L-arginine. Intravenous glucose solution increased the insulin plasma level and this response was significantly reduced by L-NNA alone but not in combination with L-arginine. In tests with feeding and GRP or urecholine iv infusion, L-NNA caused a small but significant rise in plasma somatostatin [120,121].

In the perfused rat pancreas the inhibition of NOS did not affect glucose-stimulated insulin release [184] and in chronic (four weeks) nitric oxide-synthase blockade with oral administration of L- NAME increases blood pressure and decreases aortic cGMP content, but does not alter insulin secretion in response to several secretagogues [185].

In the isolated perfused human pancreas, L-NMMA infusion suppressed cholinergic-stimulated insulin secretion but did not affect glucose-stimulated insulin secretion [186]. In healthy human volunteers L-NAME produced a partial but significant decrease in the insulin response to L-arginine but did not affect glucose-stimulated insulin secretion [187].

In other study in humans, secretin-caerulein infusion caused a significant increase in plasma insulin and pancreatic polypeptide levels but without changes in plasma glucagon or somatostatin levels. L-NMMA alone resulted in a significant fall in plasma insulin and pancreatic polypeptide levels, while L-Arg added to pancreatic secretagogue infusion caused a significant increase in plasma insulin and pancreatic polypeptide levels above those attained with secretagogues alone. After the addition of L-Arg to L-NMMA, both plasma insulin and pancreatic polypeptide levels rose significantly above the levels observed with L-NMMA plus secretin-caerulein stimulation [137].

As with exocrine secretion, the effect of L-NNA on endocrine secretion in conscious dogs was most pronounced after cephalic-vagal stimulation of the pancreas by sham feeding or 2-DG. In studies in mice L-NAME and L-NNA inhibited the responses of both insulin and glucagon to 2-DG. In contrast, the insulin and glucagon secretory responses to intravenous injection of arginine, glucose or the cholinergic agonist, carbachol, were not influenced by NOS inhibitors. Endocrine as well as exocrine pancreatic secretion can be markedly influenced by vagal stimulation [188,189]. Experiments in dogs with a vascularly isolated pancreas have established that the vagal drive on B-cells is direct and not mediated by hormones [190].

An interesting observation of the presence of glucoresponsive islet-innervating neurons in the pancreas was made by Kirchgessner and Liu [191]. They suggested that, in addition to a direct action on B cells, glucose also enhances pancreatic ganglionic transmission, acting postsynaptically to potentiate the effect of nicotinic stimulation. Glucose could recruit intrapancreatic secretomotor neurons to potentiates its insulinotropic response. It is possible that strong inhibition of insulin release *in vivo* by L-NNA could be in part explained by an action on this neural pathway. In addition, numerous nerves to the islets terminate around the blood vessels [192-194]. While early studies suggested that these nerve endings controlled the vascular bed, it is also likely that these neurons release secretions into the blood. In the dog, vascular neuronal endings of cholinergic, adrenergic, and peptidergic nature have been noted [194]. Moreover, Fujita speculated that these "neuroinsular complexes" may act to control the exocrine pancreas via the islet-acinar portal vascular system [194].

The decrease in pancreatic endocrine secretion observed in conscious animals, caused by L-NNA, might be at least in part be attributable to its effect on pancreatic blood flow. The pancreatic islets possess a blood flow regulation which is independent of that in the exocrine parts of the gland [195,196]. A recent study by Svensson *et al.* [197,198] has shown that inhibition of nitric oxide synthase induced a preferential decrease in pancreatic islet blood flow, when compared to the whole gland. Moldovan *et al.* have demonstrated [199] recently that hyperglycaemia resulted in an increase in islet capillary blood flow and this hyperaemia is mediated by NO. In view of these findings it seems likely that NO is an important regulator of islet blood flow. It remains to be established whether the redistribution of the blood flow to the pancreas is responsible, at least in part, for the observed inhibition of exocrine and particularly endocrine pancreatic secretion caused by the analogues of L-arginine suppressing NO biosynthesis.

REFERENCES

1. R.M.J. Palmer, A.G. Ferrige and S. Moncada, Nature, 327 (1987) 524.
2. L.J. Ignarro, G.M. Buga, K.S. Wood, R.E. Byrns and G. Chaudhuri, Proc. Natl. Acad. Sci. USA, 84 (1987) 9265.
3. S. Moncada, R.M.J. Palmer and E.A. Higgs, Pharm. Rev., 43 (1991) 109.
4. A.M. Leone, R.M.J. Palmer, R.G. Knowles, P.L. Francis, D.S. Ashton and S. Moncada, J. Biol. Chem., 266 (1991) 23790.
5. R.M.J. Palmer, D.D. Rees, D.S. Ashton, and S. Moncada, Biochem. Biophys. Res. Commun., 153 (1988) 1251.
6. M.A. Marletta, Cell, 78 (1994) 927.
7. C. Nathan and Q.W. Xie, Cell, 78 (1994) 915.

206

8.   R.M.J. Palmer and S. Moncada, Biochem. Biophys. Res. Commun., 158 (1988) 348.
9.   R.G. Knowles, M. Palacios, R.M.J. Palmer and S. Moncada, Proc. Natl. Acad. Sci. USA, 86 (1989) 5132.
10. M. Palacios, R.G. Knowles, R.M.J. Palmer and S. Moncada, Biochem. Biophys. Res. Commun., 165 (1989) 284.
11. H.H.H.W. Schmidt, P. Wilke, B. Evers and E. Bohme, Biochem. Biophys. Res. Commun., 165 (1989) 284.
12. M.W. Radomski, R.M.J. Palmer and S. Moncada, Proc. Natl. Acad. Sci. USA, 87 (1990) 10043.
13. D.S. Bredt and S.H. Snyder, Proc. Natl. Acad. Sci. USA, 87 (1990) 682.
14. M.A. Marletta, P.S. Yoon, R. Iyengar, Leaf C.D. and J.S. Wishnok, Biochemistry, 27 (1988) 8706.
15. S. Moncada, Acta Physiol Scand, 145 (1992) 201.
16. S.A. Waldman and F. Murad, Pharm. Rev., 39 (1987) 163.
17. F. Murad, C. Mittal, W.Arnold, S. Katsuki and H.Kimujra, Adv.Cyclic Nucleotide Res., 9 (1978) 145.
18. S. Katsuki, W. Arnold, C. Mittal and F. Murad, J. Cyclic. Nucleotide Res., 3 (1977) 23.
19. V. Molina, B. McDonald, B. Reep, B. Brune, M. Di Silvio, Billiar T.R. and E.G. Lapetina, J.Biol. Chem., 267 (1992) 24929.
20. K.M. Sanders, C.W. Shuttleworth and S.M. Ward In: "Advances in the innervation of the gastrointestinal tract" G.H. Holle and J.D. Wood (eds.), 285 Excerpta Medica, Amsterdam, London, New York, Tokyo, 1992.
21. R.M.J. Palmer, D.S. Ashton and S. Moncada, , Nature, 333 (1988) 664.
22. M.Guslandi, Dig. Dis., 12 (1994) 28.
23. S. Moncada, J. Lab.Clin. Med., 120 (1992) 187.
24. S.S. Gross, D.J. Stuehr, K. Aisaka, E.A. Jaffe, R. Levi, and O.W. Griffith, Biochem. Biophys. Res. Commun., 170 (1990) 96.
25. L.E. Lambert, J.P. Whitten, B.M. Baron, H.C. Cheng, N.S. Doherty, and I.A. McDonal, Life Sci., 48 (1991) 69.
26. S.S. Gross, E.A. Jaffe, R. Levi and R.G. Kilbourn, Biochem. Biophys. Res. Commun., 178 (1991) 823.
27. I.L. Buxton, D.J. Cheek, D. Exkman, D.P. Westfall, K.M. Sanders and K.D. Keef, Circ. Res., 72 (1993) 387.
28. S.M. Ward, H.H. Dalziel, M.E. Bradley, I.L. Buxton, K. Keef, D.P. Westfall and K.M. Sanders Brit. J. Pharmacol, 107 (1992) 1075.
29. M.E. Stark, and J.H. Szurszewski, Gastroenterology, 103 (1992) 1928.
30. B.J.R. Whittle, In: "Physiology of the gastrointestinal tract" L.R. Johnson, D.H. Alpers, E.H. Jacobson, J. Christensen, and J.H. Walsh (eds.), 267 Raven Press, New York, 1994.
31. S.J. Konturek and P.Ch. Konturek, Digestion, 56 (1995) 1.
32. D.S. Bredt, P.M. Hwang, and S.H. Snyder, Nature, 347 (1990) 768.
33. H. Bult, G.E. Boeckxstaens, P.A. Pelckmans, P.H. Jordaens, Y.M. Van Maercke and A.G. Herman, Nature, 345 (1990) 346.
34. J. Murray, C. Du, A. Ledlow, J.N. Bates, and J.L. Conklin, Amer. J. Physiol., 261 (1991) G401.
35. F. Christinck, J.Jury, F. Cayabyab and E.E. Daniel, Can. J. Physiol. Pharmacol., 69 (1991) 1448.

36. J.A. Murray, and E.D. Clark, Gastroenterology, 106 (1994) 1444.
37. J. Boulant, J. Fioramonti, M. Dapoigny, G. Bommelaer, and L. Bueno, Gastroenterology, 107 (1994) 1059.
38. J.L. Conklin, C. Du, J.A. Murray and J.N. Bates, Gastroenterology, 104 (1993) 1439.
39. N. Anand, and W.G. Paterson, Amer. J. Physiol., 266 (1994) G123.
40. J.W. Konturek, P. Thor, A. Lukaszyk, A. Gabryelewicz, S.J. Konturek and W. Domschke, J. Physiol. Pharmacol, 48 (1997) 201.
41. K.M. Desai, Sessa, W.C., and J.R. Vane, Nature, 351 (1991) 477.
42. G.E. Boeckxstaens, P.A. Pelckmans, J.J. Bogers, H. Butt, J.G. De Man, L. Oesterbosch, A.G. Herman and Y.M. Van Maercke, J. Pharmacol. Exp. Ther., 256 (1991) 441.
43. J.W. Konturek, P. Thor and W. Domschke, Eur. J. Gastroenterol. Hepatol., 7 (1995) 97.
44. O. Bayguinov and K.M. Sanders, Brit. J. Pharmacol., 108 (1993) 1024.
45. H.D. Allescher, G. Tougas, P. Vergara, S. Lu, and E.E. Daniel, Amer. J. Physiol., 262 (1992) G695.
46. H. Ozaki, D.P. Blondfield, M. Hori, N.G. Publicover, Kato I., and K.M. Sanders, J. Physiol. Lond., 445 (1992) 231.
47. N.B. Merchant, D.T. Dempsey, M.W. Grabowski, M. Rizzo and Ritchie, W.P.J., Surgery, 116 (1994) 419.
48. B.I. Gustafsson, and D.S. Delbro, Eur. J. Pharmacol., 257 (1994) 227.
49. M.E. Stark, A.J. Bauer, and J.H. Szurszewski, J. Physiol. Lond., 444 (1991) 743.
50. A. Calignano, B.J.R. Whittle, M. Di Rosa, and S. Moncada, Eur. J. Pharmacol., 229 (1992) 273.
51. A. Alemayehu, K.R. Lock, R.W. Coatney and C.C. Chou, Brit. J. Pharmacol., 111 (1994) 205.
52. M. Mączka, P. Thor, J. Bilski, and S.J. Konturek, J. Physiol. Pharmacol., 45 (1994) 285.
53. S.K. Sarna, M.F. Otterson, R.P. Ryan, and V.E. Cowles, Amer. J. Physiol., 265 (1993) G749.
54. S.M. Ward, E.S. McKeen, and K.M. Sanders, Brit. J. Pharmacol., 105 (1992) 776.
55. J.G. De Man, G.E. Boeckxstaens, P.P. Pelckmans, B.Y.De Winter, A.G. Herman and Van Maercke Y.M., Brit. J. Pharmacol., 110 (1993) 559.
56. M.S. Faussone Pellegrini, S. Bacci, D. Pantalone, C. Cortesini, and B. Mayer, Neurosci. Lett., 170 (1994) 261.
57. G.E. Boeckxstaens, P.A. Pelckmans, H. Bult, J.G. De Man, A.G. Herman and Y.M. Van Maercke, Brit. J. Pharmacol., 102 (1991) 434.
58. N. Dhatt and A.M. Buchan, Gastroenterology, 107 (1994) 680.
59. R. Ciccocioppo, L. Onori, E. Messori, S.M. Candura, T. Coccini and M. Tonini, J. Pharmacol. Exp. Ther., 270 (1994) 929.
60. K. Venkova and J. Krier, Amer. J. Physiol., 266 (1994) G40.
61. J.R. Grider, Amer. J. Physiol., 267 (1994) G696.
62. A.D. Medhurst, C. Greenlees, A.A. Parsons and S.J. Smith, Eur. J. Pharmacol., 256 (1994) R5.
63. G.E. Boeckxstaens, P.A. Pelckmans, A.G. Herman, and Y.M. Van Maercke, Gastroenterology, 104 (1993) 690.
64. N. Suthamnatpong, M. Hosokawa, T. Takeuchi, F. Hata and T. Takewaki Brit. J. Pharmacol., 112 (1994) 676.
65. S. Rattan and P. Thatikunta Gastroenterology, 105 (1993) 827.

66. M.L. McKirdy, H.C. McKirdy and C.D. Johnson, Gut, 35 (1994) 412.
67. M. Mourelle, F. Guarner, X. Molero, S. Moncada and J.-R. Malagelada, Gut, 34 (1993) 911.
68. M. Mourelle, F. Guarner, S. Moncada and J.-R. Malagelada, Gastroenterology, 105 (1993) 1299.
69. T. Tanaka, P. Guth and Y. Tache, Amer. J. Physiol., 264 (1993) G280.
70. J.M. Pique, J.V. Esplugues and B.J.R.Whittle, Gastroenterology, 102 (1992) 168.
71. E. Quintero and P.H. Guth, Dig Dis Sci, 37 (1992) 1324.
72. E. Quintero and P.H. Guth, Amer. J. Physiol., 263 (1992) G75.
73. J. Panes, M. Casadevall, J.M. Pique, J. Bosch, B.J.R.Whittle, and J. Teres, Gastroenterology, 103 (1992) 407.
74. B.L. Tepperman and B.J.R. Whittle, Brit. J. Pharmacol., 105 (1992) 171.
75. M.A. Martinez Cuesta, M.D. Barrachina, J.M. Pique, B.J.R. Whittle, and J.V. Esplugues, Eur. J. Pharmacol., 218 (1992) 351.
76. J. Bilski, P.Ch. Konturek, S.J. Konturek, M. Cieszkowski, and K. Czarnobilski, Regul. Pept., 53 (1994) 175.
77. J. Bilski and S.J. Konturek, In: "Gastrointestinal tract and endocrine system", M.V. Singer, R. Ziegler, and G. Rohr (eds.), 174 Kluwer Academic Publishers, Dordrecht/Boston/London, 1995.
78. J. Bilski, S.J. Konturek, M. Cieszkowski, K. Czarnobilski, and W.W. Pawlik, Biomed. Res., 15 (Suppl. 2) (1994) 63.
79. W.K. MacNaughton, G. Cirino and J.L.Wallace, Life Sci., 45 (1989) 1869.
80. T. Brzozowski, D. Drozdowicz, A. Szlachcic, J. Pytko Polończyk, Majka, J. and S.J. Konturek, Digestion, 54 (1993) 24.
81. Y. Hatakeyama, M. Matsuo, M. Tomoi, J. Mori and M. Kohsaka, Jpn. J. Pharmacol., 63 (1993) 251.
82. B.L. Tepperman, B.L. Vozzolo, and B.D. Soper, Dig Dis Sci, 38 (1993) 2056.
83. S.J. Konturek, T. Brzozowski, J. Majka, A. Szlachcic, C. Nauert and B. Slomiany, Eur. J. Pharmacol., 229 (1992) 155.
84. S.J. Konturek, T. Brzozowski, J. Majka, J. Pytko Polonczyk and J. Stachura, Eur. J. Pharmacol., 239 (1993) 215.
85. P.N. Bhandare, P.V. Rataboli, R.S. D'Souza and .VG. Dhume, Indian. J. Physiol. Pharmacol., 36 (1992) 130.
86. K. Takeuchi, T.Ohuchi, H. Miyake and S. Okabe, J. Pharmacol. Exp. Ther., 266 (1993) 1512.
87. K. Takeuchi, T.Ohuchi, H. Miyake, H.S. Sugawara and S. Okabe, Jpn. J. Pharmacol., 60 (1992) 303.
88. A. Hallgren, G. Flemström and O. Nylander, Gastroenterology, 104 (1993) A93 (Abstract).
89. J. Bilski and S.J. Konturek, J. Physiol. Pharmacol., 45 (1994) 541.
90. M. Holm, B. Johansson, A. Pettersson, and L. Fändriks, Acta Physiol Scand, 162 (1998) 461.
91. M.K. Barry, J.D. Aloisi, S.P. Pickering and C.J. Yeo, Ann. Surg., 219 (1994) 382.
92. R.K. Rao, P.J. Riviere, X. Pascaud, J.L. Junien, and F. Porreca, J. Pharmacol. Exp. Ther., 269 (1994) 626.

93. W.E.W. Roediger, M.J. Lawson, S.H. Nance and B.C. Radcliffe, Digestion, 35 (1986) 199.
94. S.J. Middleton, M. Shorthouse and J.O. Hunter, Lancet, 341 (1993) 465.
95. M.J. Miller, X.J. Zhang, H. Sadowska-Krowicka, S. Chotinaruemol, J.A. McIntyre, D.A. Clark and S.A. Bustamante, Scand. J. Gastroenterol., 28 (1993) 149.
96. A.L. Kirchgessner, M.T. Liu and M.D. Gershon, J. Comp. Neurol., 342 (1994) 115.
97. R. De Giorgio, J.E. Parodi, N.C. Brecha, F.C. Brunicardi, J.M. Becker, V.L. Goand, C. Sternini, J. Comp. Neurol., 342 (1994) 619.
98. T. Shimosegawa, T. Abe, A. Satoh, R. Abe, Y. Kikuchi, M. Koizumi and T. Toyota, Gastroenterology, 105 (1993) 999.
99. P. Kugler, D. Hofer, B. Mayer and D. Drenckhahn, J. Histochem. Cytochem., 42 (1994) 1317.
100. S.S. Tay, E.W. Moules and G. Burnstock, J. Anat., 184 (1994) 545.
101. L. Sha, S.M. Miller and J.H. Szurszewski, Neurosci. Lett., 192 (1995) 77.
102. E. Ekblad, P. Alm and F. Sundler, Neuroscience, 63 (1994) 233.
103. E. Ekblad, H. Mulder, R. Uddman, and F. Sundler, Neuropharmacology, 33 (1994) 1323.
104. H.P. Liu, S.K. Leong and S.S. Tay, J. Hirnforsch., 35 (1994) 501.
105. S.R. Vincent, Science, 258 (1992) 1376.
106. T. Shimosegawa, T. Abe, A. Satoh, T.Asakura, K.Yoshida, M. Koizumi, and T. Toyota, Neurosci. Lett., 148 (1992) 67.
107. J. Worl, M. Wies and B. Mayer, K.R. Greskotter and W.L. Neuhuber, Histochemistry, 102 (1994) 353.
108. M.T. Liu and A.L. Kirchgessner, Amer. J. Physiol, 273 (1997) G1273.
109. K. Iwatsuki, F. Iijima, F. Yamagishi and S. Chiba, Eur. J. Pharmacol., 123 (1986) 307.
110. E.P. DiMagno, J.C. Hendricks, V.L.W. Go and R.R. Dozois, Dig Dis Sci, 24 (1979) 689.
111. C. Owyang, R.R. Dozois, E.P. DiMagno and V.L.W. Go, Gastroenterology, 73 (1977) 1046.
112. G.R. Vantrappen, T.L. Peeters, and J. Janssens, Scand J. Gastroenterol, 14 (1979) 663.
113. S.J. Konturek, P.J. Thor, J. Bilski, W. Bielański, and J. Laskiewicz, Amer. J. Physiol., 250 (1986) G570.
114. S.J. Konturek, J. Bilski, P.K. Konturek, M. Cieszkowski and W. Pawlik, Gastroenterology, 104 (1993) 896.
115. S.J. Konturek, W. Bielański, and T.E. Solomon, Gastroenterology, 98 (1990) 47.
116. A. Anagnostides, V.S. Chadwick, A.C. Seldenand, P.N. Maton, , Gastroenterology, 87 (1984) 109.
117. R.S. Alphin and T.M. Lin, Amer. J. Physiol, 197 (1959) 260.
118. A. Barzilai, J.A. Medina, L. Toth, S. Konturek, and D.A. Dreiling, Mt Sinai J. Med., 54 (1987) 361.
119. J.J. Holst, In: "The pancreas: biology, pathobiology and disease", V.L.W. Go, E.P. DiMagno, J.D. Gardner, E. Lebenthal, H.A. Reber, and G.A. Scheele (eds.), 381 Raven Press, New York, 1993.
120. J.Bilski, S.J. Konturek and W. Bielański, J. Physiol. Pharmacol., 46 (1995) 447.
121. J. Bilski, J.W. Konturek, S.J. Konturek and W. Domschke, Int. J. Pancreatol, 18 (1995) 41.
122. J.J. Holst, T.N. Rasmussen and P. Schmidt, Amer. J. Physiol., 266 (1994) G206.

123. S.J. Konturek, J. Tasler, J. Bilski, de Jong, A.J. J.B.M.J. Jansen, and C.B.H.W. Lamers, Amer. J. Physiol., 250 (1986) G391.
124. T.E. Solomon, In: "Physiology of the gastrointestinal tract.", L.R. Johnson, D.H. Alpers, J. Christensen, E.H. Jacobson, and J.H. Walsh (eds.), 1499 Raven Press, New York, 1994.
125. M.V. Singer, In: "The pancreas: biology, pathobiology, and diseases", V.L.W. Go, E.P. DiMagno, J.D. Gardner, E. Lebenthal, H.A. Reber and G.A. Scheele (eds.), 425 Raven Press, New York, 1993.
126. T.E. Solomon and M.I. Grossman, Amer. J. Physiol., 236 (1979) E186.
127. M.V. Singer, T.E. Solomon, J. Wood, and M.I. Grossman, Amer. J. Physiol., 238 (1980) G23.
128. A. Barzilai, J.A. Medina, L. Toth, S.J. Konturek and D.A. Dreiling, Pancreas, 2 (1987) 159.
129. M.V. Singer, W. Niebel, J.B.M.J. Jansen, D. Hoffmeister, S. Gotthold, H. Goebell and C.B.H.W. Lamers, Gastroenterology, 96 (1989) 925.
130. M.V. Singer, J. Physiol. Lond., 339 (1983) 75.
131. A.L. Kirchgessner and M.D. Gershon, J. Neurosci., 10 (1990) 1626.
132. S.J. Konturek, A. Szlachcic, A. Dembinski, Z. Warzecha, J. Jaworek, and J. Stachura, Int. J. Pancreatol, 15 (1994) 19.
133. X. Molero, Guarner F., A. Salas, M. Mourelle, V. Puig and J.R. Malagelada, Gastroenterology, 108 (1995) 1855.
134. S. Jyotheeswaran, P. Li, T.-M. Chang, and W.Y. Chey, Gastroenterology, 106 (1994) A818 (Abstract).
135. A.G. Patel, M.T. Toyama, T.N. Nguyen, G.A. Cohen, L.J. Ignarro, H.A. Reber, and S.W. Ashley, Gastroenterology, 108 (1995) 1215.
136. F. Guarner, V. Puig, X. Molero and J.-R. Malagelada, Gastroenterology, 106 (1994) A295 (Abstract).
137. J.W. Konturek, K. Hengst, E. Kulesza, A. Gabryelewicz, S.J. Konturek, and Domschke W., Gut, 40 (1997) 86.
138. R.W. Wrenn, M.G. Currie, and L.E. Herman, Life Sci., 55 (1994) 511.
139. D. Bosco, J.V. Soriano, M. Chanson, and P. Meda, J. Cell Physiol., 160 (1994) 378.
140. A.S. Gukovskaya, and S.J. Pandol, Amer. J. Physiol., 266 (1994) G350.
141. S.J. Pandol, and M.S. Schoeffield Payne, Cell Calcium, 11 (1990) 477.
142. T.D. Bahnson, S.J. Pandol, and V.E. Dionne, J.Biol.Chem., 268 (1993) 10808.
143. S.J. Pandol and M.S. Schoeffield Payne, J. Biol. Chem., 265 (1990) 12846.
144. S. Muallem, Annu. Rev. Physiol., 51 (1989) 83.
145. X. Xu, R.A. Star, G. Tortorici, and S. Muallem, J. Biol. Chem., 269 (1994) 12645.
146. S.H. Ahn, D.W. Seo, Y.K. Ko, D.S. Sung, G.U. Bae, J.W. Yoon, S.Y. Hong, J.W. Han, and H.W. Lee, Arch. Pharm. Res., 21 (1998) 657.
147. M. Chanson, P. Mollard, P. Meda, S. Suter and H.J. Jongsma, J Biol Chem, 274 (1999) 282.
148. X. Xu, W. Zeng, J. Diaz, K.S. Lau, A.C. Gukovskaya, R.J. Brown, S.J. Pandol, and S. Muallem, Cell Calcium, 22 (1997) 217.
149. H. Yoshida, Y. Tsunoda, and C. Owyang, Pflugers Arch, 434 (1997) 25.
150. K. Klemm, J.C. Barreto, and F.G. Moody, Gastroenterology, 108 (1995) A366 (Abstract).

151. D.D. Rees, R.M.J. Palmer, H.F. Hodson, and S. Moncada, Brit. J. Pharmacol., 96 (1989) 418.
152. D.D. Rees, R.M.J. Palmer and S. Moncada, Proc. Natl. Acad. Sci. USA, 86 (1989) 3375.
153. H.J. Beijer, A.H. Maas, and G.A. Charbon, Pflugers Arch., 400 (1984) 324.
154. S.J. Konturek, W. Pawlik, K. Czarnobilski, P. Gustaw, J. Jaworek, Beck, G., and H. Jendralla, Amer. J. Physiol., 254 (1988) G849.
155. S.J. Konturek, J. Bilski, W. Pawlik, J. Taslerand W. Domschke, Gastroenterology, 94 (1988) 266.
156. K. Inoue, R. Hosotani, K. Tatemoto, Yajima, H. and T. Tobe, Dig Dis Sci, 33 (1988) 828.
157. J.A. Williams, and I.D. Goldfine, In: "The pancreas: biology,pathobiology, and disease" V.L.W. Go, E. Lebenthal, E.P. DiMagno, H.A. Reber, J.D. Gardner, and G.A. Scheele (eds.), 789 Raven Press,Ltd., New York, 1993.
158. M. Korc, In: "The pancreas: biology, pathobiology, and disease." V.L.W. Go, E.P. DiMagno, J.D. Gardner, E. Lebenthal, H.A. Reber, and G.A. Scheele (eds.), 751 Raven, New York, 1993.
159. S. Bonner-Weir, In: "The pancreas: biology, pathobiology, and disease" V.L.W. Go, E.P. DiMagno, J.D. Gardner, E. Lebenthal, H.A. Reber, and G.A. Scheele (eds.), 759 Raven Press, New York, 1993.
160. J.P. Palmer, R.M. Walter, and J.W. Ensinck, Diabetes, 31 (1978) 735.
161. H.H.H.W. Schmidt, T.D. Warner, K. Ishii, H. Sheng and F. Murad, Science, 255 (1992) 721.
162. R. Kleemann, H. Rothe, V. Kolb Bachofen, Q.W. Xie, C. Nathan, S. Martin and H. Kolb, FEBS Lett, 328 (1993) 9.
163. L. Bouwens, and G. Klöppel, Histochemistry, 101 (1994) 209.
164. S.G. Laychock, M.E. Modica, and T. Cavanaugh, Endocrinology, 129 (1991) 3043.
165. S.G. Laychock, Endocrinology, 108 (1981) 1197.
166. A.V. Edwards, M.A. Ghatei, and , S.R. Bloom, Experientia, 50 (1994) 725.
167. L.Bergmann, K.D. Kroncke, C. Suschek, H. Kolb, and Kolb V. Bachofen, FEBS Lett, 299 (1992) 103.
168. Xenos, E.S., Stevens, R.B., Gores, P.F., Casanova, D., Farney, A.C., Sutherland, D.E., and J.L. Platt, Transplant. Proc., 25 (1993) 994.
169. I.C. Green, C.A. Delaney, J.M. Cunningham, V. Karmiris and C. Southern, Diabetologia, 36 (1993) 9.
170. K.D. Kroncke, M.L. Rodriguez, H. Kolb, and V. Kolb Bachofen, Diabetologia, 36 (1993) 17.
171. G. Panagiotidis, P. Alm, and I. Lundquist, Eur. J. Pharmacol., 229 (1992) 277.
172. J.A. Corbett, J.L. Wang, J.H. Hughes, B.A. Wolf, Sweetland, M.A., Lancaster, J.R.J., and M.L. McDaniel, Biochem. J., 287 (1992) 229.
173. V. Burkart, Y. Imai, B.Kallmann and H. Kolb, FEBS Lett, 313 (1992) 56.
174. D.L. Eizirik, E. Cagliero, A. Bjorklund, and N. Welsh, FEBS Lett, 308 (1992) 249.
175. B. Kallmann, V. Burkart, K.D. Kroncke, V. Kolb Bachofen, and H. Kolb, Life Sci., 51 (1992) 671.
176. H. Kolb and V. Kolb Bachofen, Immunol. Today, 13 (1992) 157.

177. K.D. Kroncke, H.H. Brenner, M.L. Rodriguez, K. Etzkorn, E.A. Noack, H. Kolb, and Kolb Bachofen, V., Biochim.Biophys.Acta, 1182 (1993) 221.
178. W.L. Suarez Pinzon, K. Strynadka, R. Schulz, and A. Rabinovitch, Endocrinology, 134 (1994) 1006.
179. J. Turk, J.A. Corbett, S. Ramanadham, A. Bohrer, and M.L. McDaniel, Biochem. Biophys. Res. Commun., 197 (1993) 1458.
180. I.C. Green, J.M. Cunningham, C.A. Delaney, M.R. Elphick, J.G. Mabley, and M.H. Green, Biochem.Soc.Trans., 22 (1994) 30.
181. H. Kolb, and V. Kolb Bachofen, Diabetologia, 35 (1992) 796.
182. J. Radons, B. Heller, A. Burkle, B. Hartmann, M.L. Rodriguez, K.D. Kroncke, V. Burkart, and Kolb, H., Biochem.Biophys.Res.Commun., 199 (1994) 1270.
183. A.K. Nussler and T.R. Billiar, J. Leukoc. Biol., 54 (1993) 171.
184. N. Weigert, M. Dollinger, R. Schmid, and V. Schusdziarra, Diabetologia, 35 (1992) 1133.
185. M.E. Pueyo, W. Gonzalez, E. Pussard, and J.F. Arnal, Diabetologia, 37 (1994) 879.
186. A. Atiya, G. Cohen, L. Ignarro, and Brunicardi, F.C., Surgery, 120 (1996) 322.
187. V. Coiro, R. Volpi, L. Capretti, G. Speroni, G. Caffarri and P. Chiodera, Clin Endocrinol (Oxf), 46 (1997) 115.
188. J.J. Holst, In: "Nutrient regulation of insulin secretion." P.R. Flatt (Ed.), 23 Portland Press, London, 1992.
189. M.D. Gershon, A.L. Kirchgessner, and P.R. Wade, In: "Physiology of the Gastrointestinal Tract." L.R. Johnson, D.H. Alpers, E.H. Jacobson, J. Christensen, and J.H. Walsh (eds.), 381 Raven Press, New York, 1994.
190. R.N. Bergman and R.E. Miller, Amer. J. Physiol, 225 (1973) 481.
191. A.L. Kirchgessner and M.-T. Liu, Gastroenterology, 108 (1995) A365 (Abstract).
192. T.Fujita, S. Kobayashi, S. Fujii, T. Iwanaga, and Y. Serizawa, In: "Cellular basis of chemical messengers in the digestive system" M.I. Grossman, M.A.B. Brazier, and J. Lechago (eds.), 231 Academic Press, New York, 1981.
193. P.G. Legg, Z. Zellforsch., 88 (1968) 487.
194. T. Fujita, and S. Kobayashi, Arch. Histol. Jpn., 42 (1979) 277.
195. L. Jansson, Eur. Surg. Res., 24 (1992) 291.
196. L. Jansson and C. Hellerstrom, Diabetologia, 25 (1983) 45.
197. A.M. Svensson, C.G. Ostenson, S. Sandler, S. Efendic and L. Jansson, Endocrinology, 135 (1994) 849.
198. A.M. Svensson S. Sandler, and L. Jansson, Eur. J. Pharmacol., 275 (1995) 99.
199. S. Moldovan, E. Livingston, R.S. Zhang, R. Kleinman, P. Guth, and F.C. Brunicardi, Am. J. Surg., 171 (1996) 16.

Biology of the Pancreas in Growing Animals
S.G. Pierzynowski and R. Zabielski (Editors)
© 1999 Elsevier Science B.V. All rights reserved.

Effects of age and food on exocrine pancreatic function and some regulatory aspects

I. Le Huërou-Luron and P. Guilloteau

Laboratoire du Jeune Ruminant, Institut National de la Recherche Agronomique, 65 rue de St Brieuc, 35042 Rennes cedex, France

This review summarises recent advances in knowledge of the development of exocrine pancreatic function and its regulation mechanisms in response to age and ingested food in mammalian species (mainly bovine and porcine species). In the two first sections, changes are examined in relation to different situations (colostral, milk-feeding and weaned periods). The implication of some gut regulatory peptides in regulation mechanisms during these periods is discussed. For example, the plasma pattern of several gut regulatory peptides and the expression of their specific receptors could explain certain phenomena of digestive development. Recently discovered cellular and molecular aspects of the regulation of digestive enzyme production are also reported. Finally, the large differences observed between species in the pancreatic response to a meal are discussed, with reference to diet composition (milk vs. milk replacer vs. solid diet), emphasizing the decisive role played by the gastric emptying rate. In conclusion, although some phenomena are well established, it is often difficult to distinguish between age- and food-dependent events in the development of digestive function.

1. INTRODUCTION

Young animals are given liquid diets (colostrum, milk or milk replacer). Then, at weaning, the highly digestible liquid milk diet is replaced by a less digestible solid feed based on plant protein and complex carbohydrates. Before weaning, between 3 and 4 weeks of age, the amount of creep feed consumed by piglets is low, usually not exceeding 3% of total metabolizable energy intake [1]. Therefore in piglets, interrupted suckling is the general weaning procedure, and it imposes an abrupt change in both the pattern of intake and in the type of diet. In contrast, weaning is very gradual in calves, which are offered increasing amounts of solid food and declining amounts of milk over a period of weeks.

The digestive secretions play a basic part in transforming diets into nutrients absorbable in the intestine, in milk-fed as well as in weaned animals. All along the digestive tract, diets and digesta are impregnated with saliva, gastric juice, pancreatic juice, bile and intestinal juice. The main functions of these digestive secretions are to dilute the feed and facilitate its transit and luminal homogenisation, to gradually hydrolyse the dietary and endogenous substrates with various enzymes and to provide the digesta with electrolytes in order to promote hydrolysis. Furthermore, they constitute an important endogenous investment, that must be taken into account when considering the efficiency of the diet. Among these secretions, the pancreatic juice plays a major role in the digestion of nutrients flowing into the duodenum, by providing electrolytes which, together with bile, increase the pH of the digesta, and especially, by its varying and complementary enzyme content. Thus, the digestibility of nitrogen intake is more reduced (by about 50%) when the flow of the pancreatic juice is not reintroduced into the duodenum than when the abomasum is bypassed (2-4%) [Guilloteau and Le Huërou-Luron, unpublished data; 2]. Pancreatic juice from many mammalian species has also been demonstrated to contain other bioactive substances (e.g., insulin, pancreatic polypeptide (PP), somatostatin, growth factors, antibacterial activity protein, etc.) conferring other physiological properties (regulation of intestinal mucosal maturation, antibacterial activity, etc.) on pancreatic secretions [3,4].

In measurements carried out in the pancreatic gland, only amounts of enzymes present in the gland at slaughter can be assayed and secretion potential estimated. For feed digestion to be efficient, digestive secretions should enter the digestive tract at the same time as the substrates to be digested. Continuous measurement of the true secretion is made possible by using animals with a catheter in the pancreatic duct and this *in vivo* method allows chronic and acute experimentation. Different techniques for pancreatic duct cannulation (Thomas' and Routley's methods, and the duodenal pouch method) and pancreatic juice collection are used, depending on the specific animal species in question [5]. In addition, *in vitro* methods including studies on the isolated perfused pancreas, lobuli, acini or single acinar cells can lead to identification of more specific effects of a single factor, whereas cellular or sub-cellular analysis of tissue preparations can provide a more in-depth approach to the molecular mechanisms of protein synthesis. Here again, whole-animal studies are necessary to verify the physiological relevance of the results obtained *in vitro*.

This chapter describes the development of exocrine pancreatic function and the changes in plasma gut regulatory peptide concentrations that occur in response to age and ingested food, especially in calves and pigs. The underlying mechanisms regulating enzyme synthesis and secretion are discussed during different stages (colostral, milk-feeding and weaned periods) and in relation to the feeding level, the diet composition and the response to a meal.

2. CHANGES WITH AGE

2.1. Enzyme expression and secretion

The development of the pancreas starts in the prenatal period, and in general the activity of pancreatic enzymes in tissue homogenates increases with fetal age up to birth in calves and in pigs [6,7]. Pancreatic enzymes can be detected in the 2-month-old bovine fetus. Throughout the fetal period, amylase and chymotrypsin activities are very low, lipase remains almost constant, and trypsin and phospholipase A2 show a gradual increase over the gestation period [6]. Thus, in calves, most of the pancreatic enzymes are present at birth, except for amylase [8,9], while in newborn pigs enzyme activities are relatively low, except for elastase II which exhibits a maximum of activity [10,11].

Following birth, in pigs [12] and lambs [13,14], there is a positive allometry and an isometry of the pancreas, respectively, associated with age. Based on DNA and RNA measurements in pancreas, Corring *et al.* [10] ascribe the increase in pancreas weight before 4 weeks of age to a hyperplasia of pancreatic cells; subsequent increases involve both hyperplasia and hypertrophy. In preruminant lambs, the pancreas shows an extensive

215

hyperplasia without growth until day 2; its weight increases thereafter due to hypertrophy [15], as also observed in calves [9].

In addition, following birth there are major changes in the nature of the enzymes present in the pig pancreas, with the gradual appearance of chymotrypsin C, cationic trypsin and protease E [7,16]. According to these authors, elastase I does not appear until about 5 weeks of age in pigs whereas Gestin et al. [17] have detected elastase I activity as early as at birth. Trypsin undergoes some age-related modifications, as evidenced by the reduction in anodal trypsin that is independent of weaning. Generally, in pigs and calves the tissue activities of pancreatic enzymes (excluding elastase II and chymotrypsin in some studies) decrease during the two first days of life, i.e. during the colostral period, and thereafter increase to varying degrees during the first month of life. Amylase activity follows an ontogenic pattern, since amylase shows a significant increase in animals which ingest very low levels of starch or none at all [8,10,16].

In preruminant calves and in pigs, during postnatal development, the lack of parallel variations in the levels of mRNA for specific pancreatic enzymes suggests that the protein synthesis of each enzyme is specifically regulated [18]. The levels of mRNA for specific enzymes (except those for chymotrypsin) generally increase during the first months of life. These changes probably result from transcriptional control of gene expression, but variations in mRNA stability can not be excluded. In addition, translational regulation could explain the existence of enzyme levels non-proportionally related to mRNA profiles. Moreover, it would appear that the efficiency of translation differs according to the species, since the elastase II activity is higher in pigs than in calves while the number of corresponding mRNA copies is similar in both species [9].

The secretion of pancreatic juice increases with age. During the colostral period, the daily volume of pancreatic juice secreted is below 2ml/kg body weight (BW), and in 6-day- and 2-month-old calves it is 3-4- and 6-fold higher, respectively [19,20; Zabielski, Le Huërou-Luron and Guilloteau, unpublished data] (Figure 1).

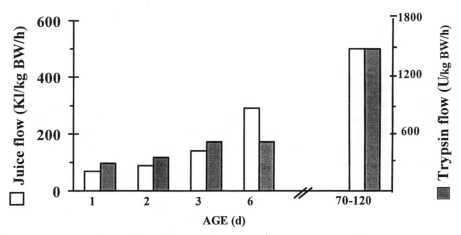

Figure 1. Mean daily pancreatic juice flow and trypsin activity in preruminant calves [20, Zabielski, Le Huërou-Luron and Guilloteau, unpublished data]. BW, body weight.

The quantity of secreted protein amounts to 80 mg/kg BW/d in 1-4-month-old calves, but the variability between individuals is very large [20]. The most prominent changes in the amount of secreted pancreatic juice, protein and trypsin outputs are observed in relation to diet composition (colostrum vs. milk vs. weaning diet). However, it is also important to mention that ontogenic changes also involve the kinetics of pancreatic secretion in response to a meal, in milk-fed calves [20]. From the age of 6 days the kinetics of the pancreatic response are similar to those observed in older preruminant calves, whereas during the first 5 days the postprandial pattern is different, since no postprandial decrease to below the basal level is recorded. In conscious suckled piglets, no effect of age between 1-2 and 4-5 weeks is observed; preprandial secretions of pancreatic juice and protein are about 0.4-1.4 ml/kg BW/h and 1-4 mg/kg BW/h, respectively [21,22]. In acute experiments performed under anaesthesia, basal pancreatic secretions seem to be lower. In 3-28-day-old suckling pigs, juice flow is 0.1-0.3 ml/kg BW/h and protein secretion averages 0.2 mg/kg BW/h [23].

Taken together, these data suggest that at birth most of the digestive enzymes are present but at varying levels. Thereafter, intake of colostrum in particular and of milk modifies the ontogenic pattern of enzyme expression. These variations are under the control of many intrinsic regulatory factors.

2.2. Regulation of pancreatic function by gut regulatory peptides

The growth of the pancreas is regulated by numerous hormones, regulatory peptides and growth factors. The development of neuro-hormonal regulation seems to parallel that of the gastrointestinal tract. In the bovine fetus, some gut regulatory peptides are synthesised and secreted as early as the third month of gestation. Moreover, plasma levels of gut regulatory peptides seem to be independent of maternal levels and are high at the end of gestation [24, 25]. Therefore, the ontogenesis of gastrointestinal and pancreatic endocrine cells (gastrin, cholecystokinin (CCK), PP, somatostatin) in porcine fetuses [26] and the high concentrations of gut regulatory peptides during gestational age in bovine fetuses [25] suggest that these peptides participate to some extent in the regulation of the growth and morphogenesis of the digestive system of endodermal origin. Somatostatin infusions in fetal lambs depress levels of plasma gastrin and PP, thereby possibly leading to decreased gut mucosal development [27]. At birth, gastrin probably enhances the growth of the digestive tract. In calves after birth there is a positive correlation between plasma PP levels and digestive organ development [8]. Since PP is considered to reflect the vagal input [28], it may also reflect a pro-trophic effect of vagal nerves on pancreatic tissue. Such a role for pancreatic development in lambs and calves has already been suggested and related to the maturation of vagal nerve function [24,29]. In addition, glucocorticoids stimulate the perinatal development of pancreatic enzymes in pigs [30].

In the newborn calf, high concentrations of CCK, gastrin and secretin parallel the storage of digestive enzymes in the pancreas at birth. High concentrations of these peptides as well as of vasoactive intestinal polypeptide (VIP), observed after the first colostrum meal, could result in a decrease in the enzymatic content of the pancreas during the first 24-h postnatal period [8,15, 31-33] by stimulating the secretion of enzymes stored at the end of the fetal period. However, according to our own recent studies in neonatal conscious calves during the first week and to those of Pierzynowski et al. [21] during the first 2 weeks in piglets, intravenous infusion of CCK does not seem to affect pancreatic secretion. In contrast, intraduodenal administration of CCK-A receptor antagonist alters intestinal mucosal morphology and regulating reduces pancreatic secretion, suggesting the involvement of some mucosal duodenal and mechanism of pancreatic secretion, [34-36]. The growth of the pancreas in the young calf and sheep and the increase of enzymatic activities [8,15,32,37,38] are parallel to the increase in CCK and PP levels [39]. There after, the slight modifications observed for most of the enzymatic activity of the pancreas in preruminant calves between the age of 4 and 17 weeks could be related to the high level of somatostatin, which could inhibit the stimulation caused by CCK.

After birth, the regulatory peptides can influence the synthesis and release of secretions because their receptors are present and functional in the digestive glands. This is the case for VIP-secretin family of receptors [41] and also for the CCK-gastrin family of receptors in the pancreas of calves [42-44] and pigs [45,46]. Furthermore, pharmacological analysis using selective agonists and antagonists indicates expression of the CCK-A receptor (high affinity for CCK and very low affinity for gastrin) at birth, whereas the CCK-B/gastrin receptor (similar affinity for CCK and gastrin) predominates at the postnatal stage. Thus there is a differential expression of CCK-A and CCK-B/gastrin receptors in the developing calf pancreas.

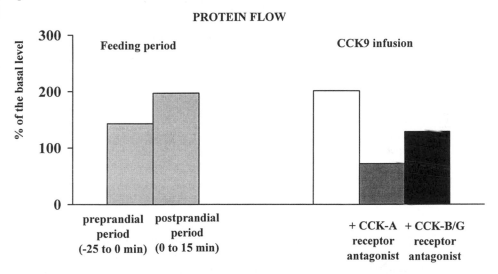

Figure 2. Effects of a morning meal and of exogenous infusion of CCK, in the presence of a specific CCK-A receptor, SR 27897, or a specific CCK-B/gastrin receptor antagonist, PD 135158, on pancreatic protein flow in 2-4 month-old preruminant calves [20, 40].

Recently, we investigated the functionality of and the biological functions mediated by these receptors *in vivo* and *in vitro*. *In vivo*, CCK-A and CCK-B/gastrin receptors, despite the low expression of the former, are involved in the exogenous stimulation of pancreatic enzyme secretion by CCK and gastrin in 2-4-month-old preruminant calves [40] (Figure 2).
However, the endogenous CCK-evoked pancreatic secretion in response to a meal is mediated by the CCK-A receptor, and not by the CCK-B/gastrin receptor [47]. The role of the CCK-B/gastrin receptor has further been studied *in vitro* using a transgenic mouse strain expressing the human CCK-B/gastrin receptor in the exocrine pancreas [48]. In mouse pancreatic acini,

gastrin modulates enzyme secretion and protein synthesis at the translational level via the CCK-B/gastrin receptor [49] (Figure 3).

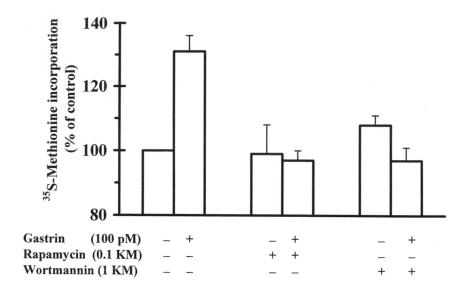

Figure 3. Inhibition of gastrin-induced protein synthesis by a specific mTOR inhibitor (rapamycin) and a specific PI3 kinase inhibitor (wortmannin) in the pancreatic acini of transgenic mice. The + and - symbols below bars indicate the presence or absence of the indicated substances, respectively [49].

The activation of the CCK-B/gastrin receptor, leading to an increase in protein synthesis, involves a PI3 kinase and an mTOR inhibitor-sensitive pathway. It is worth noting that the doses of gastrin that stimulate enzyme secretion are higher than those that elicit maximal cytosolic protein synthesis. Accordingly, a physiological role for the CCK-B/gastrin receptor in mediating protein synthesis in the exocrine pancreas in calves cannot be excluded.

Recently, a new indirect mechanism of CCK action on pancreatic juice secretion has been postulated in preruminant calves [50, 51] as well as in pigs and rats [52-54]. In preruminant calves, infusions of CCK-8 into the duodenal lumen and into the duodenal arteries markedly increase the secretion of pancreatic juice (similar results are obtained with intra-arterial infusions of secretin and VIP). The effects are blocked by both atropine and cold vagal blockade, suggesting the involvement of neural pathways in this mechanism. This local, indirect mechanism may be physiologically relevant since significant amounts of CCK are found in the duodenal lumen in calves. Furthermore, the amount of luminal CCK increases during electrical stimulation of the vagus [55,56]. The presence of CCK receptors in the small intestinal mucosa has been reported in some species [57,58] and our preliminary study suggests that they could also be expressed in calves.

3. ADAPTATION TO FOOD

3.1. Enzyme expression and secretion in relation to diet composition and weaning

Birth and weaning represent dramatic qualitative and quantitative changes in nutrition. At birth, the source of nutrients abruptly changes from a continuous supply across the placenta to an intermittent feeding of colostrum and milk. Such changes induce necessary adaptation of the digestive process to ensure survival. Then weaning implies that animals are switched to a complex solid diet at an age when most, if not all, of their nutrient intake is provided by milk. This frequently results in growth check and digestive disorders.

In newborn piglets, the growth of the pancreas is closely associated with the level of feeding [59]. In contrast, at 7 days of age, the weight of the pancreas expressed on a live-weight basis is not affected by the level of milk intake or by the diet composition (sow colostrum and milk vs. milk replacer) [60, 61]. At 7 days of age pancreatic enzyme activities surprisingly do not respond to milk restriction, whereas heavy 21-day-old pigs are reported to have higher levels of pancreatic chymotrypsin than light pigs (having ingested less milk) of the same age [62]. During the first week of life, feeding milk replacer instead of sow's milk induces a decrease in most pancreatic proteolytic activities and in lipase activity. Whereas at day 1 the quantity of fat intake has no marked effect on lipase activity [63], the low lipolytic activity measured in pigs fed with milk replacer may result from a combined effect of the quantity and the quality of fats ingested. It is worth noting that the decrease in lipase activity is parallel to a decrease in the corresponding mRNA level [60]. Therefore, as early as during the first week of life, the pancreas is ready for nutritional adaptation. Moreover, tissular lipase activity increases before weaning in suckled pigs, probably in relation to the increase in the lipid content of sow's milk during the first 3-4 weeks of lactation [64].

During the weaning period, modification of the quantity of dietary substrates ingested results in significant modifications in the outputs and tissular specific activities of pancreatic enzymes. Pancreatic amylase and protease levels undergo large increases with increasing starch and protein intake, respectively [65, 66]. However, the effects of the composition of the diet on pancreatic enzymes are rather unclear. For instance, in calves and pigs milk protein is variously found to stimulate or to decrease tissular enzyme activity compared to plant protein [11,67,68]. In calves the outflow of pancreatic fluid, protein and trypsin during the 5 hours after feeding is 40% lower, 39% higher and 82% higher, respectively, when soya bean protein is given, as compared to milk protein [69]. The level of regulation has also been studied with protein substitutes. For instance, amylase specific activity increases with pea diets but shows the opposite tendency with soya bean products [70]. Proteolytic enzyme activities in the pancreas are slightly influenced by the dietary protein source, but not as much as is claimed in the reviewed literature; the technological treatment applied to these dietary proteins could be of greater importance [70]. Specific messenger RNAs corresponding to amylase, trypsin and chymotrypsin seem to increase with soya bean diets. However, further investigations are required before any conclusions may be drawn concerning regulation levels of pancreatic adaptation to dietary protein.

The mechanisms of modulation of pancreatic development at weaning probably involve several factors, including the stage of development, feed intake and the source of dietary nutrients. As with intestinal enzymes, pancreatic enzymes are markedly reduced in the tissue during the first days after weaning in pigs. Thus, 3 to 7 days after weaning pancreatic enzymes are 30-75% depressed [65]. Activities are, however, recovered 2 weeks after weaning. In contrast, Rantzer et al. [22] report a 2.6- to 7.4-fold gradual increase in volume, protein and trypsin levels during the first 5 days after weaning in relation to the progressive increase in consumption of solid feed. These changes continue or increase 2 weeks after weaning [16]. The composition of the pancreatic juice is also modified, as indicated by variations in some enzyme:protein ratios. While elastase II and chymotrypsin are probably the predominant pancreatic proteases during the neonatal period, elastase I, trypsin and amylase are probably more specifically expressed after weaning [11]. Studies on pigs show that changes in cathodal trypsin and chymotrypsin are apparently related to the weaning time, thus the change of diet from milk to solid food could contribute to the differences [10,16]. In calves, weaning induces a large increase in all pancreatic enzyme activities. Thus, at 4 months of age, tissular chymotrypsin, carboxypeptidase A, amylase and lipase activities are 1.6- to 4-fold higher in weaned calves than in milk-fed calves. The daily pancreatic secretion, as well as the prefeeding and postfeeding secretions of fluid, protein and trypsin are also increased by 20-240% in weaned calves [20]. Larger digestive contents, a more regular flow of digesta into the duodenum with a lower pH, and different end products may be responsible for the enhancement of enzyme expression. In sharp contrast to the multiple control of protein synthesis during postnatal development in preruminant calves, weaning is found to induce increases in specific activity and in mRNA levels for amylase, lipase, trypsin, chymotrypsin and elastase I, suggesting that pretranslational modulation of gene expression is mainly, if not exclusively, concerned [9,18].

3.2. Regulation of pancreatic function by gut regulatory peptides

In the newborn calf, the ingestion of four colostrum meals during the first 22 h after birth causes a marked rise in plasma concentrations of gastrin, CCK, secretin, VIP and PP and (after the first colostrum meal) of gastric inhibitory polypeptide (GIP) as well as a decrease in motilin and somatostatin levels [71]. If the first colostrum meal is replaced by purified immunoglobulins dissolved in saline, the response of plasma gastrin, CCK, secretin, somatostatin and GIP is reduced, while that of VIP, PP, and motilin is not significantly affected [72]. The increase in GIP could be related to the high fat content of the colostrum since Martin et al. [73] have shown that the consumption of whole milk or an emulsion of milk fat but not a solution of lactose or glucose alone or an emulsion of casein plus lactose, stimulates GIP secretion in preruminant goat kids. In the same manner, gastrin and GIP increase in 1-day-old calves in response to colostrum feeding, but not when calves are fed only water or glucose [74]. The increased amounts of gastrin and CCK in circulation could have a favourable effect on gastrointestinal growth (marked hyperplasia of the pancreas observed in lambs) and on digestive functions [8,15,32].

The most important characteristics of the diet influencing plasma gut peptide concentrations are the ability of dietary protein to clot in the abomasum (consequently determining the pattern of gastric emptying), the composition and the origin of the diet and the pH of the duodenal contents. In preruminant calves and in pigs, pre-feeding and/or post-feeding plasma levels of many peptides were highly affected by diet composition [67,75,76]. In pigs, carbohydrates and fats are strong stimuli for the release of GIP and glucagon-like peptide 1-36 amide [77] and for CCK [78], and the amounts of protein ($\square$ amino nitrogen) absorbed determine gastrin, glucagon, insulin and PP release [79].

In calves progressively weaned between 28 and 56 days of age and in weaned pigs, concentrations of gastrin, CCK and PP are higher, while those of secretin and somatostatin are lower than in milk-fed animals [19,33,80,81]. Increased gastrointestinal emptying before feeding and greater distension of the stomach in milk-fed compared to weaned animals could be responsible for the differences observed. Changes in basal gastrin, CCK and somatostatin concentrations induced by weaning and especially after completion of weaning, as well as the expression of CCK-A and CCK-B/gastrin receptors [42,82] are thought to favour the development of the pancreas and to increase the secretion of some pancreatic enzymes [8, 81, 83]. Thus, G cells, producing gastrin, may be more responsive to solid than liquid feed [84]. Higher concentrations of PP possibly reflect a prolonged stimulation of the parasympathetic system [85], which could also have a trophic effect on the pancreas [27].

4. PANCREATIC SECRETION IN RESPONSE TO A MEAL AND MECHANISMS OF REGULATION

In many mammalian species, a number of integrated phases temporally associated with the regulation of pancreas exocrine response to food ingestion have been described, including the cephalic, gastric and intestinal phases. In milk-fed calves, it is difficult to differentiate between the three phases due to the shorter duration of the meal and the longer duration of gastric emptying, as compared to other species. The cephalic phase is purely a nervous reflex. The gastric and intestinal phases result from stimuli acting in the gastrointestinal tract and both nervous and hormonal regulatory mechanisms are involved as mediators.

In preruminant milk-fed calves, secretion of pancreatic fluid, protein and trypsin increases (by 40-100% compared to the basal levels) from 30-45 min before and until 15 min after the meal (Figure 4). Then outflows decrease sharply by 60-80% over a 30-min period, remain low during the next 1-4 h and return to the basal level [20,69]. Protein and trypsin concentrations are immediately increased by 60-160% after feeding. The long-lasting prefeeding increase we observed probably reflects conditioning of the animals to both a determined time for feeding and the related environmental stimulation, since the early increase in pancreatic secretion is totally inhibited when an "unexpected meal" is offered to calves (Le Dréan et al., unpublished data). There is a peak of protein secretion during and just after the meal, and this could correspond to the cephalogastric phase reported in other species [86] and in young calves reared in "laboratory" conditions [19,87]. In contrast, an "unexpected meal" does not modify the pattern of the intestinal phase, suggesting that the depression of pancreatic secretion is not due to an exhaustion of resources during the cephalic phase. In suckled piglets, pancreatic secretions are low and not affected by the meal [21]. In contrast, in weaned pigs and dogs, the postprandial secretory pattern of the pancreas consists of two peaks (an immediate peak rich in enzymes and a late increase low in enzymes but rich in bicarbonates) [88-90] (Figure 4). In humans, a solid meal induces a very prolonged stimulation of pancreatic secretion [91].

Mechanical factors play a predominant part in regulating digestion (distension of the abomasum, flow of digesta into the duodenum, intestinal transit, differential absorption of nutrients, etc.), and particularly in regulating the digestive secretions. When young calves are given whole milk or a milk replacer based on skimmed milk powder, a tough coagulum forms in the abomasum. This coagulum soon shrinks, holding back casein and lipids whose release is slow and steady. When casein is replaced by a protein substitute which cannot coagulate, all the components of the digesta leave the abomasum approximately at the same velocity and the distension period of the organ is shorter [92]. Therefore, in calves fed diets based on soya bean and whey proteins instead of milk powder, postprandial profiles of protein and trypsin outflows are similar to those observed in weaned pigs [20] (Figure 4).

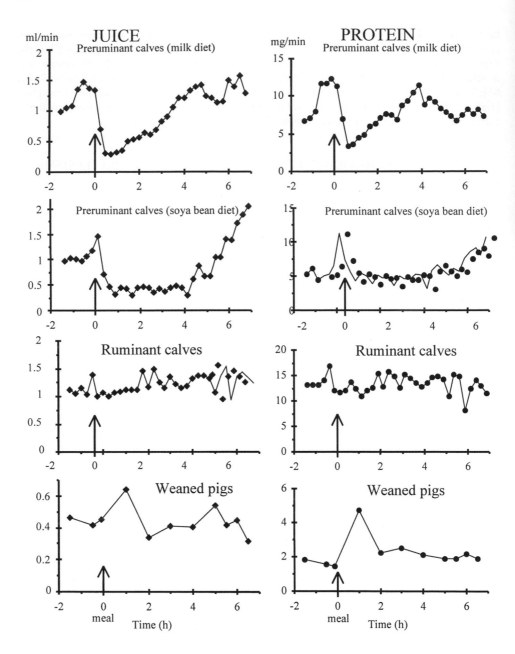

Figure 4. Profiles of the pancreatic juice and protein secretion in response to a morning meal in: 70-120-day-old preruminant calves fed a milk substitute diet mainly based either on skimmed milk (milk diet) or on alcohol-extracted soya bean concentrate (soya bean diet); in ruminant calves and in 50-60-day-old weaned pigs [20,69,90].

In suckled piglets the low and steady flow of pancreatic juice, protein and enzymes recorded compared to milk-fed calves, may be due to the frequent number of feedings during the day and to the more continuous flow of homogeneous digesta into the duodenum, resulting in a constant stimulation of the exocrine pancreas [3]. The large differences observed between species in the pancreatic response over the first 2-4 h after a meal may therefore be related to the rate of gastric emptying, which determines the intraduodenal pH, which is itself responsible for stimulation of secretin release. In preruminant calves, gastric emptying of ingested milk proteins is at a maximum over the first half-hour and then declines [93].

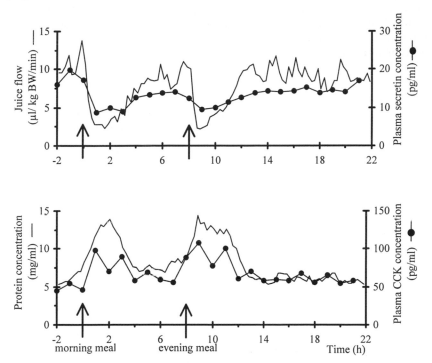

Figure 5. Circadian profiles of pancreatic juice secretion and pancreatic protein concentration as well as of plasma secretin and CCK concentrations in 70-120-day-old milk-fed calves (our unpublished data).

The pH of digesta entering the duodenum increases from 2 to 5 immediately after the morning meal and 2-3 h are required before the pH falls to below 4.5 [93]. In these conditions, secretin release is not stimulated and the decrease in plasma concentration observed in calves could be partly responsible for the depressed postfeeding pancreatic secretion. In dogs and in humans, the emptying of solid meals from the stomach takes about 4 h [94]. In dogs, the intraduodenal pH falls to below 4.5 immediately and remains there for 8 to 12 h after a meal, but a simultaneous increase in plasma secretin is not consistently described [88,95,96]. In humans and weaned pigs, the plasma secretin concentration is unchanged after feeding [97, 98]. Other mechanisms may be involved in the late phase of pancreatic stimulation in these species; for example, the arrival of nutrients in the distal ileum could release neurotensin, which is a potent stimulator of pancreatic secretion [91,99].

In milk-fed calves, parallel patterns of pancreatic juice flow and secretin as well as of protein and CCK concentrations have been found [20] (Figure 5). The role of these peptides in the regulation of pancreatic secretion is in agreement with results of Mineo et al. [100] for secretin and of Pierzynowski et al. [19] and Le Dréan et al. [40] for CCK (Figure 2) and gastrin after i.v. infusion of peptides in chronically cannulated sheep and calves. However, our recent results demonstrate that the CCK-B/gastrin receptor does not participate in the pancreatic response to a meal in the calf whereas the CCK-A subtype is involved [40,47]. Indeed, the infusion of a specific CCK-A receptor antagonist (SR 27897) completely inhibits the prefeeding and the 15 min postfeeding increases in pancreatic juice secretion. Only an increase in protein outflow persists over the first 15 min postfeeding, as observed in calves receiving an "unexpected meal". Therefore, the CCK-A receptor is implicated in the preprandial regulation of pancreatic secretion, independently of the release of CCK in to the blood. CCK may interact with the CCK-A receptor via neural pathways, at least partly in response to conditioning and environmental stimulation. The CCK-A receptor furthermore plays a major role in mediating 44 to 100% of the pancreatic secretion in response to feeding in calves. In humans and dogs, CCK-A receptor antagonists also strongly inhibit meal-stimulated pancreatic responses, and the contribution of CCK to the postfeeding enzyme secretion is around 40-75% [101-107]. In contrast, in pigs, devazepide lowered only the early postprandial peak (the first 30 min) of protein and enzymes by 30-35% [108]. The current concept suggesting that the meal-stimulated pancreatic enzyme secretion is highly dependent on cholinergic tone and that CCK modulates the enzyme-secretory response can be applied to calves, humans and dogs [103,109-112]. CCK could act directly on vagal afferents since binding sites have been evidenced on the vagal nerve [113]. However, the type of fibres involved is not yet clear [114-116].

Moreover, a noteworthy modification of the vagus-dependent cephalic phase of pancreatic secretion with a soya bean diet has been described in preruminant calves [20,87] (Figure 4). In dogs given different flavoured solutions, an important influence of taste on the pancreatic cephalic response was also demonstrated [117,118]. In preruminant calves, the higher pancreatic postprandial protein and especially trypsin concentration and trypsin outflow seen obtained with a soya bean diet as compared with a milk diet could be related to the higher basal levels of CCK [50, 69]. Similar explanations could be given for fish proteins [119]. As observed with trypsin inhibitors in rats [120], undigested soya bean protein may form a complex with duodenal trypsin that could stimulate CCK release by activation of a trypsin-sensitive CCK-releasing factor. In contrast to the results obtained in milk-fed calves, the pattern of pancreatic secretion is not modified by feeding in weaned calves [19,20,121]. This is in agreement with plasma concentrations of most gut regulatory peptides, which are not affected by feeding in weaned calves [20]. The lack of post-feeding changes could be explained by the more regular abomasal distension and digesta flow rate as well as by the stability of the duodenal pH, which is about 2.75. Therefore, in ruminant calves, the existence of a ruminal phase in relation to volatile fatty acids [122,123] is questionable.

5. CONCLUSIONS

The distinction between age- and food-dependent events in the development of digestive function is not easy. If we compare the digestive function in the piglet and the calf we may conclude that in intensive pig and dairy calf production, the pancreatic secretions follow an ontogenic pattern which is modified by ingested food. The inherited program, if allowed to continue for a prolonged period of time, can limit or slow down the rate of animal development (e.g., in the late suckling period). Moreover, it provides harmony between the development of the pancreas and of other organs. Early transition, e.g., from colostrum to artificial formula or from milk/milk replacer to solid food, may lead to serious disorders in the gastrointestinal tract. At present, the main problem is to find out how to accelerate growth and maturation of the pancreas tissue, and more generally that of the gastrointestinal tract, in order to obtain an optimum digestive secretion without producing dangerous shifts in gastrointestinal homeostasis. One approach would be to stimulate endogenous production by nutritional manipulation or to supplement the diet with additives in order to facilitate successful transitions in diet during the neonatal and weaning periods.

REFERENCES

1. J.R. Pluske, I.H. Williams and F.X. Aherne, In: M.A. Varley (ed.), The Neonatal Pig, Development and Survival, CAB International, Oxon, (1995) 187.
2. P. Guilloteau, R. Toullec, P. Patureau-Mirand and J. Prugnaud, Reprod. Nutr. Dévelop., 21 (1981) 885.
3. S.G. Pierzynowski, B.R. Weström, J. Svendsen, L. Svendsen and B.W. Karlsson, Int. J. Pancreatol., 18 (1995) 81.
4. R.K. Rao, Life Sci., 48 (1991) 1685.
5. R. Zabielski, V. Leśniewska and P. Guilloteau, Reprod. Nutr. Dev., 37 (1997) 385.
6. N.S. Track, M. Bokermann, C. Creutzfeldt, H. Schmidt and W. Creutzfeldt, Comp. Biochem. Physiol., 43B (1972) 313.
7. B.R. Weström, B. Ohlsson and B.W. Karlsson, Pancreas, 2 (1987) 589.
8. I. Le Huërou-Luron, P. Guilloteau, C. Wicker-Planquart, J.A. Chayvialle, J. Burton, A. Mouats, R. Toullec and A. Puigserver, J. Nutr., 122 (1992) 1434.
9. M. Gestin, I. Le Huërou-Luron, V. Romé, G. Le Dréan and P. Guilloteau, Pancreas, 15 (1997) 258.
10. T. Corring, A. Aumaitre and G. Durand, Nutr. Metab., 22 (1978) 231.
11. M. Gestin, I. Le Huërou-Luron, J. Peiniau, G. Le Dréan, V. Romé, A. Aumaitre and P. Guilloteau, J. Nutr., 127 (1997) 2205.
12. M.D. Lindemann, S.G. Cornelius, S.M. Elkandelgy, R.L. Moser and J.E. Pettigrew, J. Anim. Sci., 62 (1986) 1298.
13. P. Guilloteau, I. Le Huërou-Luron, M. Tallec, M. Beaufils and R. Toullec, In: J.W. Blum, T. Elsasser and P. Guilloteau (eds), Proceedings of Symposium on Growth in Ruminants: Basic aspects, theory and practice for the future, Berne, Switzerland, (1998) 287.
14. I. Le Huërou-Luron, P. Guilloteau and J.W. Blum, In: J.W. Blum, T. Elsasser and P. Guilloteau (eds), Proceedings of Symposium on Growth in Ruminants: Basic aspects, theory and practice for the future, Berne, Switzerland, (1998) 25.

226

15. P. Guilloteau, T. Corring, P. Garnot, P. Martin, R. Toullec and G. Durand, J. Dairy Sci., 66 (1983) 2373.
16. S.G. Pierzynowski, B.R. Weström, C. Erlansson-Albertsson, B. Ahren, J. Svendsen and B.W. Karlsson, J. Pediat. Gastroenterol. Nutr., 16 (1993) 287.
17. M. Gestin, I. Le Huërou-Luron, J. Peiniau, E. Thioulouse, C. Desbois, G. Le Dréan, M. Feldman, A. Aumaitre and P. Guilloteau, Dig. Dis. Sci., 42 (1997) 1302.
18. I. Le Huërou, C. Wicker, P. Guilloteau, R. Toullec and A. Puigserver, Biochim. Biophys. Acta, 1048 (1990) 257.
19. S.G. Pierzynowski, R. Zabielski, B.R. Weström, M. Mikołajczyk and W. Barej, J. Anim. Physiol. Anim. Nutr., 65 (1991) 165.
20. G. Le Dréan, I. Le Huërou-Luron, J.A. Chayvialle, V. Philouze-Romé, M. Gestin, M. Bernard, R. Toullec and P. Guilloteau, Comp. Biochem. Physiol., 117A (1997) 245.
21. S.G. Pierzynowski, B.R. Weström, J. Svendsen and B.W. Karlsson, J. Pediat. Gastroenterol. Nutr., 10 (1990) 206.
22. D. Rantzer, P. Kiela, M.J. Thaela, J. Svendsen, B. Ahren, S. Karlsson and S.G. Pierzynowski, J. Anim. Sci., 75 (1997) 1324.
23. E. Harada, H. Kiriyama, E. Kobayashi and H. Tsuchita, Comp. Biochem. Physiol., 91A (1988) 43.
24. S.N. Reddy and R.B. Elliot, Aust. J. Biol. Sci., 38 (1985) 237.
25. P. Guilloteau, I. Le Huërou-Luron, G. Le Dréan, M. Gestin, V. Philouze-Romé, Artiaga, C. Bernard and J.A. Chayvialle, Biol. Neonate, 74 (1998) 430.
26. H. Ito, Y. Hashimoto, H. Kitagawa, Y. Kon and N. Kudo, Jpn. J. Vet. Sci., 50 (1988) 99.
27. A. Shulkes and K.J. Hardy, Biol. Neonate, 42 (1982) 249.
28. T.W. Schwartz, Gastroenterology, 85 (1983) 1411.
29. A. Shulkes and K.J. Hardy, Acta Endocrinol., 100 (1982) 565.
30. P.T. Sangild, B.R. Weström, A.L. Fowden and M. Silver, J. Pediat. Gastroenterol. Nutr., 19 (1994) 204.
31. P. Guilloteau, R. Toullec, P. Garnot, P. Martin and G. Brulé, Reprod. Nutr. Dévelop., 20 (1980) 1279.
32. P. Guilloteau, T. Corring, R. Toullec and J. Robelin, Reprod. Nutr. Dévelop., 24 (1984) 315.
33. P. Guilloteau, I. Le Huërou-Luron, J.A. Chayvialle, A. Mouats, C. Bernard, J.C. Cuber, J. Burton, A. Puigserver and R. Toullec, Reprod. Nutr. Dev., 32 (1992) 285.
34. M. Biernat, P. Sysa, B. Sosak-Świderska, I. Le Huërou-Luron, R. Zabielski and P. Guilloteau, Reprod. Nutr. Dev., 1999, in press.
35. R. Zabielski, P. Podgurniak, I. Le Huërou-Luron and P. Guilloteau, Digestion, 59 (1998) 253.
36. R. Zabielski, V. Leśniewska, J. Borlak, P.C. Gregory, P. Kiela, S.G. Pierzynowski and W. Barej, Regul. Peptides, 78 (1998) 113.
37. J.H. Ternouth and H.L. Buttle, Brit. J. Nutr., 29 (1973) 387.
38. P. Guilloteau, R. Delansorne and R. Toullec, Reprod. Nutr. Dévelop., 22 (1982) 511.
39. R. Toullec, J.A. Chayvialle, P. Guilloteau and C. Bernard, Comp. Biochem. Physiol., 102A (1992) 203.
40. G. Le Dréan, I. Le Huërou-Luron, M. Gestin, C. Desbois, V. Romé, C. Bernard, M. Dufresne, L. Moroder, D. Gully, J.A. Chayvialle, D. Fourmy and P. Guilloteau, Eur. J. Physiol., (1999) in press.
41. V. Le Meuth, N. Farjaudon, W. Bawab, E. Chastre, G. Rosselin, P. Guilloteau P. and C. Gespach, Amer. J. Physiol., 260 (1991) G265.

227

42. V. Le Meuth, V. Philouze-Romé, I. Le Huërou-Luron, M. Formal, N. Vaysse, C. Gespach, P. Guilloteau and D. Fourmy, Endocrinology, 133 (1993) 1182.
43. M. Dufresne, C. Escrieut, P. Clerc, I. Le Huërou-Luron, H. Prats, V. Bertrand, V. Le Meuth, P. Guilloteau, N. Vaysse and D. Fourmy, Eur. J. Pharmacol., 297 (1996) 165.
44. C. Desbois, P. Clerc, I. Le Huërou-Luron, G. Le Dréan, M. Gestin, M. Dufresne, Fourmy and P. Guilloteau, Life Sci., 63 (1998) 2059.
45. J. Morisset, F. Levenez, T. Corring, O. Benrezzak, G. Pelletier G and E. Calvo, Amer. J. Physiol., 34 (1996) E397.
46. C. Philippe, E.F. Lhoste, M. Dufresne, L. Moroder, T. Corring and D. Fourmy, Brit. J. Pharmacol., 120 (1997) 447.
47. G. Le Dréan, I. Le Huërou-Luron, M. Gestin, C. Desbois, R. Zabielski, D. Fourmy and P. Guilloteau, Digestion, 58 (Suppl 2) (1997) 49.
48. C. Saillan-Barreau, P. Clerc, M. Adato, C. Escrieut, N. Vaysse, D. Fourmy and M. Dufresne, Gastroenterology, 115 (1998) 988.
49. C. Desbois, I. Le Huërou-Luron, A. Estival, M. Dufresne, P. Clerc, V. Romé, F. Clémente, P. Guilloteau and D. Fourmy, Proc. Nutr. Soc., (1999) in press.
50. R. Zabielski, T. Onaga, H. Mineo, S.G. Pierzynowski and S. Kato, Exp. Physiol., 79 (1994) 301.
51. R. Zabielski, T. Onaga, H. Mineo, S. Kato and S.G. Pierzynowski, Int. J. Pancreatol., 17 (1995) 271.
52. Y. Li and C. Owyang, J. Clin. Invest., 92 (1993) 418.
53. P. Kiela, R. Zabielski, P. Podgurniak, M. Midura, W. Barej, P. Gregory and S.G. Pierzynowski, Exp. Physiol., 81 (1996) 375.
54. R. Zabielski, P. Kiela, W. Barej, S.G. Pierzynowski, B.R. Weström and B. Karlsson, Digestion, 49 (Suppl 1) (1991) 60.
55. R. Zabielski, P. Kiela, T. Onaga, H. Mineo, P.C. Gregory and S. Kato, Can. J. Physiol. Pharmacol., 73 (1995) 1616.
56. R. Zabielski, P. Kiela, P. Podgurniak and S.G. Pierzynowski, Digestion 57 (1996) 278.
57. L.A. Blackshaw and D. Grundy, J. Auton. Nerv. Syst., 31 (1990) 191.
58. K. Miyasaka, M. Masuda, T. Kawanami and A. Funakoshi, Pancreas 12 (1996) 272.
59. J. Le Dividich, D. Tivey, J.W. Blum, F. Strullu and C. Louat, In J.P. Laplace, C. Février and A. Barbeau (eds), Digestive physiology in pigs, EAAP Publication, Saint-Malo, 88 (1997) 131.
60. I. Le Huërou-Luron, B. Codjo, F. Thomas, V. Romé and J. Le Dividich, 50th Annual Meeting of EAAP, Zurich, Switzerland, 1999, submitted.
61. I. Le Huërou-Luron, M. Lafuente, F. Thomas, V. Romé and J. Le Dividich, 50th Annual Meeting of EAAP, Zurich, Switzerland, 1999, submitted.
62. A.M.B. De Passille, G. Pelletier, J. Menard and J. Morisset, J. Anim. Sci., 67 (1989) 2921.
63. J. Le Dividich, P. Herpin, E. Paul and F. Strullu, J. Anim. Sci., 75 (1997b) 707.
64. F. Klobasa, E. Werhahn and J.E. Butler, J. Anim. Sci., 64 (1987) 1458.
65. P.D. Cranwell, In: M.A. Varley (ed.), The Neonatal Pig: Development and Survival, CAB International, Oxon, (1995) 99.
66. E.F. Lhoste, M. Fiszlewicz, A.M. Gueugneau, C. Wicker-Planquart, A. Puigserver and T. Corring, J. Nutr. Biochem., 4 (1993) 143.
67. P. Guilloteau, T. Corring, J.A. Chayvialle, C. Bernard, J.W. Sissons and R. Toullec, Reprod. Nutr. Dévelop., 26 (1986) 717.

228

68. J. Peiniau, W.B. Souffrant and A. Aumaitre, In: W.B. Souffrant and H. Hagemeister (eds), Digestive physiology in pigs, EAAP-Publication No 80, Dummerstorf, 1 (1994) 188.
69. Le Dréan, I. Le Huërou-Luron, M. Gestin, V. Romé, M. Plodari, C. Bernard, J.A. Chayvialle and P. Guilloteau, J. Dairy Sci., 81 (1998) 1313.
70. Le Dréan, I. Le Huërou-Luron, V. Philouze-Romé, R. Toullec and P. Guilloteau, Ann. Nutr. Metab., 39 (1995) 164.
71. P. Guilloteau, J.A. Chayvialle, R. Toullec, J.F. Grongnet and C. Bernard, Biol. Neonate, 61 (1992) 103.
72. P. Guilloteau, I. Le Huërou-Luron, J.A. Chayvialle, R. Toullec, R. Zabielski and J.W. Blum, J. Vet. Med., A 44 (1997) 1.
73. P.A. Martin, A. Faulkner and J.P. Mccarthy, J. Endocrinol., 138 (1993) 167.
74. U. Hadorn, H. Hammon, R.M. Bruckmaier and J.W. Blum, J. Nutr., 127 (1997) 2011.
75. T. Corring, A.M. Gueugneau and J.A. Chayvialle, Reprod. Nutr. Dévelop., 26 (1986) 503.
76. Le Huërou-Luron, M. Gestin, G. Le Dréan, V. Romé, C. Bernard, J.A. Chayvialle and P. Guilloteau, Comp. Biochem. Physiol., 119A (1998) 817.
77. J.M.E. Knapper, A. Heath, J.M. Fletcher, L.M. Morgan and V. Marks, Comp. Biochem. Physiol., 111C (1995) 445.
78. J.C. Cuber, C. Bernard, F. Levenez and J.A. Chayvialle, Reprod. Nutr. Dev., 30 (1990) 267.
79. A. Rérat, J.A. Chayvialle, J. Kande, P. Vaissade, P. Vaugelade and T. Bourrier, Can. J. Physiol. Pharmacol., 63 (1985) 1547.
80. C.M. Bunn, Res. Vet. Sci., 37 (1984) 362.
81. P.D. Cranwell and J. Hansky, Res. Vet. Sci., 29 (1980) 85.
82. K. Miyasaka, M. Ohta, S. Kanai, Y. Sato, M. Masuda and A. Funakoshi, Pancreas, 12 (1996) 351.
83. P. Guilloteau, I. Le Huërou-Luron, C.H. Malbert and R. Toullec, In: R. Jarrige, Y. Ruckebusch, C. Demarquilly, M.H. Farce and M. Journet (eds), Nutrition des ruminants domestiques, Inra, Paris, (1995) 489.
84. B.I. Hirschowitz, Dig. Dis. Sci., 28 (1983) 705.
85. S.R. Bloom, A.V. Edwards and R.N. Hardy, J. Physiol., 280 (1978) 37.
86. T.E. Solomon, In L.R. Johnson (ed.), Physiology of the gastrointestinal tract, third edition, Raven Press, New York, (1994) 1499.
87. S.G. Pierzynowski, R. Zabielski, P. Podgurniak, P. Kiela, P. Sharma, B.R. Weström, S. Kato and W. Barej, J. Anim. Physiol. Anim. Nutr., 67 (1992) 268.
88. Z. Itoh, R. Honda and K. Hiwatashi, Amer. J. Physiol., 238 (1980) G332.
89. J. Hee, W.C. Sauer and R. Mosenthin, Z. Tierphysiol. Tierernaehr. Futtermittelkd., 60 (1988) 249.
90. M.J. Thaela, S.G. Pierzynowski, M.S. Jensen, K. Jakobsen, B.R. Weström and B.W. Karlsson, J. Anim. Sci., 73 (1995) 3402.
91. L.Gullo, R. Pezzilli, P. Priori, F. Baldoni, F. Paparo and G. Mattiolli, Pancreas, 2 (1987) 620.
92. R. Toullec and P. Guilloteau, In: E.J. Van Weerden and J.Huisman (eds), Nutrition and digestive physiology in monogastric farm animals, Pudoc, Wageningen, (1989) 37.
93. P. Guilloteau, J.L. Paruelle, R. Toullec and C.M. Mathieu, Ann. Zootech., 24 (1975) 243.
94. J.R. Malagelada, E.P. Dimagno, W.H. Summerskill and V.L. Go, J. Clin. Invest., 58 (1976) 493.
95. K.Y. Lee, H.H. Tai and W.Y.Chey, Amer. J. Physiol., 230 (1976) 784.
96. J.R. Huertas, E. Martinez Victoria, M. Manas, M.C. Ballestra, N. Blanco and F.J. Mataix, Arch. Int. Physiol. Biochim., 99 (1991) 339.

97. M.J. Pelletier, J.A. Chayvialle and Y. Minaire, Gastroenterology, 75 (1978) 1124.
98. T. Corring and J.A. Chayvialle, Reprod. Nutr. Dev., 27 (1987) 967.
99. J.C. Cuber, C. Philippe, J. Abello, T. Corring, F. Levenez and J.A. Chayvialle, Pancreas, 5 (1990b) 306.
100. H. Mineo, T. Oyamada and S. Kato, Res. Vet. Sci., 49 (1990) 157.
101. R. Hosotani, P. Chowdhury and P.L. Rayford, Dig. Dis. Sci., 34 (1989) 462.
102. S.J. Konturek, J. Tasler, J.W. Konturek, M. Cieszkowski, K. Szewczyk, M. Hladij and P.S. Anderson, Gut, 30 (1989) 110.
103. A. Gabryelewicz, E. Kulesza and S.J. Konturek, Scand. J. Gastroenterol., 25 (1990) 731.
104. P. Hildebrand, C. Beglinger, K. Gyr, J.B.M.J. Jansen, L.C. Rovati, M. Zuercher, C.B.H.W. Lamers, I. Setnikar and G.A. Stadler, J. Clin. Invest., 85 (1990) 640.
105. G. Adler, C. Beglinger, U. Braun, M. Reinshagen, I. Koop, A. Schafmayer, L. Rovati and R. Arnold, Gastroenterology, 100 (1991) 537.
106. M. Fried, U. Erlacher, W. Schwizer, C. Lochner, J. Koerfer, C. Beglinger, J.B. Jansen, C.B. Lamers, F. Harder, A. Bischofdelaloye, G.A. Stalder and L. Rovati, Gastroenterology, 101 (1991) 503.
107. W.E. Schmidt, W. Creutzfeldt, A. Schleser, A.R. Choudhury, R. Nustede, M. Höcker, R. Nitsche, H. Sostmann, L.C. Rovati and U.R. Folsch, Amer. J. Physiol., 260 (1991) G197.
108. E.F. Lhoste, A.M. Gueugneau, A. Garofano, C. Philippe, F. Levenez and T. Corring, Pancreas, 11 (1995) 86.
109. G. Adler, Digestion, 58 (1997) 39.
110. H.C. Soudah, Y. Lu, W.L. Hasler and C. Owyang, Amer. J. Physiol., 263 (1992) G102.
111. C. Beglinger, P. Hildebrand, R. Meier, P. Bauerfeind, H. Hasslocher, N. Urscheler, Delco, A. Eberle and K. Gyr, Gastroenterology, 103 (1992) 490.
112. H. Köhler, R. Nutsede, F.E. Lüdtke, M. Barthel and A. Schafmayer, Pancreas, 7 (1992) 719.
113. E.S. Corp, J. Mcquade, T.H. Moran and G.P. Smith, Brain. Res., 623 (1993) 161.
114. D. Guan, W.T. Phillips and G.M. Green, Amer. J. Physiol., 270 (1996) G881.
115. Y. Li, Y. Hao and C. Owyang, Amer. J. Physiol., 273 (1997) G679.
116. G. Adler, D.K. Nelson, M. Katschinski and C. Beglinger, Pancreas, 10 (1995) 1.
117. I. Ohara, S. Otsuka and Y. Yugari, J. Physiol., 254 (1988) G424.
118. M.A. Powers, S.S. Schiffman, D.C. Lawson, T.N. Pappas and I.L. Taylor, Physiol. Behav., 47 (1990) 1295.
119. R. Zabielski, C. Dardillat, I. Le Huërou-Luron, C. Bernard, J.A. Chayvialle and P. Guilloteau, Brit. J. Nutr., 79 (1998) 287.
120. G. Green, H. Van Levan and R.A. Liddle, In: M. Friedman (ed.), Nutritional and Toxicological Significance of Enzyme Inhibitors in Foods, Plenum Press, New York, (1986) 123.
121. R. Zabielski, P. Kiela, V. Leśniewska, R. Krzemiński, M. Mikołajczyk and W. Barej, Brit. J. Nutr., 78 (1997) 427.
122. W.J. Croom, L.S. Bull and I.L. Taylor, J. Nutr., 122 (1992) 191.
123. S. Kato, K. Katoh and W. Barej, In: T. Tsuda, Y. Sasaki and R. Kawashima (eds), Physiological aspects of digestion and metabolism in ruminants, CA Academic Press, San Diego, 1991, pp. 89-109.

Biology of the Pancreas in Growing Animals
S.G. Pierzynowski and R. Zabielski (Editors)
© 1999 Elsevier Science B.V. All rights reserved.

Mode of exocrine pancreatic function and regulation in pigs at weaning[*]

S.G. Pierzynowski[a,b], J.F. Rehfeld[c], O. Olsen[d], S. Karlsson[e], B. Ahrén[e], M. Podgurniak[f], B.W. Karlsson[a] and B.R. Weström[a]

[a]Department of Animal Physiology, Lund University,
Helgonavägen 3 B, SE-223 62 Lund, Sweden

[b]Gramineer International AB, Ideon, S-223 70 Lund, Sweden

[c]Department of Clinical Biochemistry, Rigshospitalet, University of Copenhagen,
DK- 2100 Copenhagen, Denmark

[d]Surgical Department C, Rigshospitalet, University of Copenhagen,
DK -2100 Copenhagen, Denmark

[e]Department of Medicine, University Hospital of Malmö, Lund University,
SE-214 01 Malmö, Sweden

[f]Department of Animal Physiology, Warsaw Agricultural University,
02-766 Warsaw, Poland

The development of the mechanisms regulating pancreatic functions are still largely unknown. In an attempt to address this issue the development of the enteropancreatic reflexes regulating pancreatic secretion were followed by measuring the blood plasma levels of some essential GI hormones in young pigs from 3 weeks of age and up to a few weeks after weaning.

Exogenous secretin stimulated the exocrine pancreas before weaning, while only a slight increase in trypsin output occurred after exogenous CCK administration before weaning. The exocrine pancreas did not response to intraduodenal (id) stimulation with intact protein, amino acids or lipid, indicating that mechanisms regulating the exocrine pancreas that are based on enteropancreatic reflexes evoked by protein and fat either do not exist or are not fully developed before and directly after weaning. Moreover, the lack of any stimulation of pancreatic secretion by duodenal acidification suggests that the HCl-dependent enteropancreatic reflex does not function in pigs at the age studied. However, the increasing stimulation of pancreatic protein output seen with id infusion of oleic acid in the oldest post weaning pigs studied indicates that the stimulation of enteropancreatic reflexes evoked by

[*] This work was supported by the Swedish Council for Forestry and Agricultural Research and by the Swedish Institute (Visbyprogrammet 7391/1998(380/67). The Authors would like to thanks Inger Mattsson for efficient technical help.

fatty acids in young pigs is brought on by weaning.

The changes observed in the basal level of GI tract hormones in the blood plasma, i.e., decreased basal plasma CCK, glucagon and somatostatin levels and increased secretin and insulin levels can be related to increased pancreatic secretion around weaning.

1. INTRODUCTION

During postnatal life in mammalian neonates irreversible quantitative and qualitative developmental changes in the exocrine pancreas and its secretion occur. Three "checkpoints" in this process are critical; directly after birth when the first portion of the colostrum enters the gastrointestinal (GI) tract, around intestinal "closure" when the colostrum is replaced by milk and around weaning when milk is replaced by solid feed [1–10]. It seems that the pancreas is very well prepared for the digestion of the colostrum and milk. In contrast, at the abrupt early weaning in today pigs production the pancreas is not prepared for digestion of the solid feed.

The changes in pancreatic function that occur around weaning have been postulated to be dependent on age [2,11] but weaning-induced maturation of exocrine pancreatic secretion also has been reported and confirmed experimentally [12,13]. In pigs, at the time of weaning when the entire diet profile changes abruptly from milk to solid feed the functions of the exocrine pancreas are multiplied [10]. However, the data describing the development of the regulatory mechanisms of the exocrine pancreas are far from complete. The response of the exocrine pancreas to secretagogues seems to depend on age. In experiments on anaesthetised preweaned pigs, Harada *et al.* [14] reported an age-dependent stimulation of pancreatic secretion via exogenous CCK-8 and secretin. However, the response of pancreatic secretion provoked via duodenal acidification with HCl was not dependent on age. In long-term experiments on pigs the effect on exocrine pancreatic function of secretin and CCK-33, when administered together, was more intensive after than before weaning [15].

The main objectives of the study were to study the maturation of the enteropancreatic reflexes in pigs around weaning. The experiments were performed on the same individuals before and after weaning. To test the function and maturity of the receptors, being a part of the enteropancreatic reflexes, secretin and CCK were infused intravenously. To test complete enteropancreatic reflexes, HCl and well-defined dietary components involved in GI tract regulation were administered intraduodenally. Finally, the development of enteropancreatic reflexes was tested when whole diet, i.e., milk and homogenised feed, were loaded intraduodenally. In addition, the developmental pattern of the GI tract hormones i.e., CCK, secretin, insulin, glucagon and neurotensin in blood plasma was estimated in pigs.

2. MATERIALS AND METHODS

2.1. Animals and surgery

The experiments were performed on pure-bred Swedish Landrace pigs obtained from a herd at the Odarslöv Research Farm, Department of Agricultural Biosystems and Technology, Swedish University of Agricultural Sciences, Lund, Sweden. Animal experiments were approved by the Ethical Review Committee on Animal Experiments at Lund University.

Twenty-one 14-15-day-old suckling pigs and three 49-day-old pigs, that had been weaned at 35 days of age, were surgically prepared with catheter implantation for long-term studies of the exocrine pancreas, as previously described in detail [15,16]. Briefly, the pigs were fitted with; a) a pancreatic duct catheter for collection of pure inactivated pancreatic juice, b) a T-cannula placed in the duodenum at the orifice of the pancreatic duct, to maintain a reentrant flow of juice between the experiments and for id infusion of intestinal stimulants, and c) a jugular vein catheter for blood sampling and intravenous (iv) infusions.

After surgery and recovery from anaesthesia, usually within 12 h, the unweaned piglets were returned to their sow and littermates until weaning at 35 days of age. The sows and their litters were housed in standard farrowing crates with solid flooring, chopped straw bedding and heating lamps to ensure a good environment for the piglets. To prevent the piglets from ingesting solid feed before weaning, no supplementary (creep) feed was given, and the sows were fed in a separate pen once a day between 08.00-10.00. Visual inspection of the faeces showed, however, that the piglets occasionally consumed some straw. After weaning, the piglets were housed in individual pens in visual contact with each other and were offered solid weaning feed (Växfor, Lantmännen, Stockholm, Sweden) containing 15.5 % crude protein and 12.2 MJ metabolizable energy per kilogram, and drinking water *ad libitum*.

2.2. Experimental procedure

From 2-3 days after surgery, experiments were performed every second or third day. During the experiments, the pigs were standing/hanging in special Pavlov's slings to which they had been adapted for one week before surgery. The experiments were started around 09.00 h, 2h after the last suckling in the unweaned pigs and after an overnight fasting period in weaned pigs. Each experiment comprised 2.5 h of pancreatic juice sampling, starting with two 30-min baseline collections during id/iv infusions of vehicle (5 ml saline kg^{-1} h^{-1} id or 2 ml saline + 0.5 % bovine serum albumin (BSA, Sigma, St Louis, MI) $kg^{-1}h^{-1}iv$). After these baseline collections, 3 additional 30-min collections were performed during infusion of 3 increasing 5-10 fold doses of either hormones, HCl, feed or food constituents, according to the schedule presented in Table 1. The mid dose of the hormones/intestinal stimulants was considered to be physiological, i.e., to roughly reproduce postprandial plasma hormone levels and duodenal luminal concentrations of the nutrients fed [17].

In addition, similar experiments were performed on weaned pigs but with a single-dose id infusion with sows' milk or homogenised solid feed over 30 min (Table 1). In separate experiments, after a 60-min baseline collection unweaned pigs were allowed to suckle their dam while weaned pigs were bottle fed with 200 ml of sows' milk (during which juice was not collected), immediately followed by an additional collection period of 60 min (Table 1).

2.3. Sampling

Pancreatic juice was totally diverted and collected in plastic tubes on ice in 30-min (2 x 15 min) periods during the experiments. The volume secreted was immediately measured and the samples were stored at -20 °C until analysis.

Blood was sampled under baseline conditions (at -5 min) and at the end of the highest stimulatory dose infused (at 90 min) or at the end of the single dose load (at 30 min).

Table 1
Overview of experimental procedures. Each experiment comprised a total of 2-2.5 h of pancreatic juice collection, with 2 x 30 min before (baseline and/or during vehicle administration) and 3 x 30 min after intravenous (iv - infusion rate 2 ml/kg/h), intraduodenal (id - infusion rate 5 ml/kg/h) or oral administration of 3 doses of hormones, HCl, feed or food constituents

Time	-60' - -30'	-30' - 0'	0' - 30'	30' - 60'	60' - 90'
	Baseline	iv saline + BSA	iv secretin[I] (pmol/kg/h)		
			22	110	440
	Baseline	iv saline + BSA	iv CCK[II] (pmol/kg/h)		
			10	50	250
	Baseline	id saline	id HCl[III] (mmol/kg/h)		
			0.025	0.25	2.5
	Baseline	id saline	id ovalbumin[IV] (mg/kg/h)		
			5	50	500
	id saline	id saline	id amino acid mixture[V] (mmol/kg/h)		
			0.005	0.05	0.5
	id saline	id saline	id lipid emulsion[VI] (mg/kg/h)		
			10	100	1000
	id saline	id saline	id sodium oleate[VII] (mmol/kg/h)		
			0.005	0.05	0.5
	id saline	id saline	id milk[VIII]	id saline	id saline
			5 ml/kg/h		
	id saline	id saline	id feed[IX]	id saline	id saline
			1 g/kg/h		
Time	- 60' - 0'		0' - 60'	0' - 60'	
	Baseline		Suckling	Bottle feeding [VIII] (200 ml)	

I. Secretin (Ferring, Malmö, Sweden), II. CCK-33 (Ferring, Malmö, Sweden), III. HCl (KEBO, Stckholm, Sweden), IV. Ovalbumin (KEBO, Stockholm, Sweden), V. Mixture in equal mmol proportions of the L-amino acid, methionine, phenylalanine, tryptophan, lysine (all from Sigma), VI. Emulsified lipid mixture (Intralipid, Kabi Pharmacia, Stockholm, Sweden). VII. Oleic acid sodium salt (Sigma). VIII. Pooled milk from sows hand-milked 1-2 days after weaning during stimulation with 10 U of iv oxytocin, IX. Solid weaning feed (Växfor), 20 g homogenized in 0.9% saline to obtain 100 ml slurry.

The blood (5 ml) was mixed with 1 mg ml-1 EDTA and 500 KIU ml-1 aprotinin (Polfa, Jelenia Gora, Poland), immediately chilled on ice and centrifuged. Plasma was separated and stored at -20°C until analysis.

2.4. Analyses of pancreatic juice

Total protein was estimated with the Lowry method [18] modified to be performed on 96-well microplates, with BSA (Sigma) as standard.

Trypsin activity was measured on enterokinase-activated juice using a micro-modification of the original spectrophotometric method of Erlanger et al. [19]. Trypsin activity was expressed as units (U/l) where 1 unit is defined as the amount of enzyme that hydrolyses 1 μmol of the substrate, N-benzoyl-DL-arginine-p-nitroanilide (Sigma), per min. Intra- and interassay CV for protein determination were 3.1 and 3.6 %, and for trypsin activity determination, 2.8 and 3.2 %, respectively.

2.6. Analyses of plasma hormone levels

Insulin was determined with a radioimmunoassay (RIA) using a guinea pig anti-insulin antibody (Linco Research Inc, St. Louis, MO, USA), 125I-labelled porcine insulin as a tracer and human insulin (Linco) as standard. Intra- and interassay CV for insulin determination were 6.6 and 7.2 %, respectively.

Glucagon was determined with a RIA using a guinea-pig anti-glucagon antibody, 125I-labelled glucagon as a tracer and glucagon as standard (Linco). The bound antigen-antibody complex was precipitated by the use of an anti-IgG (goat anti-guinea pig) antibody. Intra- and interassay CV for glucagon determination were 8.5 and 9.6 %, respectively.

Plasma secretin was measured after extraction of plasma with RIA method [20]. The detection limit of the assay was 0.8 pmol/L. Intra- and interassay variation were 0.4 and 0.9 pmol/L, respectively, at a mean concentration of 6.6 pmol/L. CCK plasma analyses was performed with a RIA method [21]. Intra- and interassay CV for plasma CCK measurements were below 13%. Somatostatin analysis was performed once with a RIA developed by Dr R Ekman - intraassay CV was 10 %.

2.7. Calculations and statistics

All data were stored and preliminarily evaluated using the Excel 4.0 computer program and then transferred to the Statgraph 2.1 program for statistical evaluation with the ANOVA and Tukey range test (for significance of differences between the means of age groups) and Student's t-test (for significance of differences between basal and stimulated values). Probability of differences at the 5% level ($P<0.05$) was taken as significant and at the 1% level ($P<0.01$) as highly significant.

3. RESULTS

3.1. Exocrine pancreatic secretion
3.1.1. Response to iv secretin and CCK-33 (Table 2)

Iv infusion of increasing doses of secretin increased the volume secreted by the exocrine pancreas at intermediate (55 pM) and high (220 pM) doses, both before and after weaning

Table 2
Pancreatic juice secretion, protein output, and trypsin activity output (mean±SEM, n=7) during 30-min periods before and during iv infusion of saline (2 ml/kg/h) and during iv infusion of increasing doses of secretin and CCK (2 ml/kg/h) in pigs with chronic catheterization of the pancreatic duct 3-8 weeks of age

Age (weeks)	Baseline	iv saline + BSA	iv secretin (pmol/kg/h)		
			22	110	440
			Volume ($ml \cdot kg^{-1} \cdot h^{-1}$)		
3-4	1.2 ± 0.2^a	1.0 ± 0.2^a	1.0 ± 0.2^a	2.4 ± 0.3^{ab}	3.2 ± 0.4^b
5-6 (w)	2.9 ± 0.5^a	2.3 ± 0.5^a	2.8 ± 0.8^a	$4.5 + 0.6^{ab}$	5.9 ± 0.5^b
7-8 (w)	2.3 ± 0.4^a	2.5 ± 0.6^a	2.4 ± 0.5^a	4.1 ± 0.4^{ab}	5.8 ± 0.4^b
			Protein ($mg \cdot kg^{-1} \cdot h^{-1}$)		
3-4	2.3 ± 0.5^a	2.6 ± 0.5^a	2.4 ± 0.5^a	4.1 ± 1.1^{ab}	5.5 ± 1.5^b
5-6 (w)	$6.0 + 2.7$	4.4 ± 1.6	$3.8 + 1.1$	5.1 ± 1.6	7.3 ± 1.2
7-8 (w)	$5.2 + 0.9$	4.3 ± 0.8	5.0 ± 0.9	$4.1 + 1.6$	8.7 ± 2.0
			Trypsin ($U \cdot kg^{-1} \cdot h^{-1}$)		
3-4	0.6 ± 0.1^a	0.5 ± 0.1^a	0.4 ± 0.1^a	0.8 ± 0.2^{ab}	$1.0 + 0.3^b$
5-6 (w)	3.0 ± 1.9	2.5 ± 1.5	1.5 ± 0.7	2.0 ± 0.8	2.8 ± 0.9
7-8 (w)	3.0 ± 0.6	2.3 ± 0.6	2.8 ± 0.8	2.3 ± 1.2	4.7 ± 1.0
			iv CCK (pmol/kg/h)		
			10	50	250
		Volume ($ml \cdot kg$-1-h-1)			
3-4	0.9 ± 0.1	1.0 ± 0.3	1.2 ± 0.2	$1.4 + 0.4$	1.2 ± 0.3
5-6 (w)	2.8 ± 0.7	1.9 ± 0.4	1.4 ± 0.5	1.5 ± 0.4	2.2 ± 0.4
7-8 (w)	3.1 ± 0.5	3.3 ± 0.3	2.5 ± 0.5	2.8 ± 0.6	2.3 ± 0.4
			Protein ($mg \cdot kg^{-1} \cdot h^{-1}$)		
3-4	1.8 ± 0.6^a	2.7 ± 1.4^a	3.2 ± 1.1^{ab}	4.9 ± 2.8^b	3.7 ± 1.4^b
5-6 (w)	3.3 ± 1.1	3.0 ± 0.3	2.0 ± 0.8	2.7 ± 0.4	3.2 ± 0.6
7-8 (w)	4.3 ± 1.1	3.6 ± 0.7	3.9 ± 1.3	4.2 ± 1.4	3.2 ± 0.8
			Trypsin ($U \cdot kg^{-1} \cdot h^{-1}$)		
3-4	0.4 ± 0.1^a	0.6 ± 0.4^a	0.6 ± 0.3^a	1.1 ± 0.7^b	0.8 ± 0.4^b
5-6 (w)	1.4 ± 0.4	1.3 ± 0.2	0.6 ± 0.2	1.1 ± 0.3	1.4 ± 0.5
7-8 (w)	2.6 ± 0.9	2.1 ± 0.6	2.2 ± 0.8	$2.3 + 0.8$	1.7 ± 0.5

Differences between the treatments that were statistically significant at the $p<0.05$ level are indicated with different superscripts within each age group (tables 2 - 6), w = weaned pigs (tables 2 - 6).

(P<0.05). In contrast, the output of protein and trypsin was unaffected by secretin, except in the youngest pigs, where the highest dose, 220 pM, increased protein and trypsin activity outputs (P<0.05). Iv infusion of CCK had an effect only in the 3-4 week-old pigs, where the intermediate (25 pM) and highest (125 pM) doses increased protein and trypsin outputs, while the volume was not affected. In contrast, in 5-6-week-old pigs i.e., after weaning, CCK had no influence on exocrine pancreatic secretion (Table 2).

3.1.2. Response to intraduodenal loads of HCl and single feed constituents (Table 3 - 5)

Intraduodenal infusion of increasing doses of HCl (Table 3), the protein ovalbumin, (Table 4), and an amino acid mixture (Table 4) did not affect pancreatic secretion at any of the ages studied. Similarly, infusion of lipid emulsion did not affect pancreatic secretion (Table 5), while infusion of Na-oleate at the highest dose (0.1 M) increased protein output in the oldest pigs (Table 5). For the 3-4-week-old pigs a tendency to a decrease in the volume secreted after infusion of the intermediate (0.01 M) dose of amino acids and a tendency to a decrease in protein/trypsin outputs after the low (0.001M) dose of Na-oleate were obtained.

Table 3
Pancreatic juice secretion, protein and trypsin activity output, (mean±SEM, n=7) during 30-min periods before and during intraduodenal infusion of saline (5 ml/h/kg) and during intraduodenal infusion of increasing doses of HCl (5 ml/h/kg) in pigs with chronic catheterization of the pancreatic duct 3-8 weeks of age

Age (weeks)	Baseline	id saline	id HCl (mmol/kg/h)		
			0.025	0.25	2.5
	Volume $(ml \cdot kg^{-1} \cdot h^{-1})$				
3-4	1.4±0.3	1.7±0.2	1.1±0.1	1.4±0.4	2.0±0.4
5-6 (w)	2.8±0.4	2.9±0.6	2.3±0.6	2.7±0.6	3.8±0.3
7-8 (w)	2.2±0.5	2.6±0.6	1.8±0.7	2.2±0.6	2.8±0.4
	Protein $(mg \cdot kg^{-1} \cdot h^{-1})$				
3-4	3.1±0.6	3.7±0.9	3.0±0.7	5.0±2.4	4.3±1.4
5-6 (w)	2.8±0.4	3.2±0.7	2.2±0.6	3.0±0.5	3.3±0.4
7-8 (w)	5.1±1.7	4.2±1.6	3.0±1.1	4.0±1.3	4.1±0.8
	Trypsin $(U \cdot kg^{-1} \cdot h^{-1})$				
3-4	0.7±0.1	0.8±0.1	0.6±0.1	1.0±0.4	0.9±0.3
5-6 (w)	1.0±0.2	1.0±0.4	0.6±0.1	1.0±0.3	1.0±0.2
7-8 (w)	3.4±1.2	2.6±0.9	2.2±1.0	2.6±0.8	2.5±0.7

Table 4
Pancreatic juice secretion, protein and trypsin activity output, (mean±SEM, n=4) during 30-min periods before and during intraduodenal infusion of saline (5 ml/h/kg) and during intraduodenal infusion of increasing doses of a solution of the protein ovalbumin, or an amino acid mixture (5 ml/h/kg) in pigs with chronic catheterization of the pancreatic duct 3-8 weeks of age

Age (weeks)	Baseline	id saline	id ovalbumin (mg/kg/h)		
			5	50	500
Volume $(ml \cdot kg^{-1} \cdot h^{-1})$					
3-4	1.0 ± 0.2	1.2 ± 0.3	1.5 ± 0.3	1.2 ± 0.3	1.0 ± 0.2
5-6 (w)	2.4 ± 0.4	2.4 ± 0.5	3.5 ± 0.5	2.7 ± 0.5	2.5 ± 0.5
7-8 (w)	3.6 ± 0.5	4.9 ± 0.4	3.4 ± 0.6	3.6 ± 0.2	2.4 ± 0.6
Protein $(mg \cdot kg^{-1} \cdot h^{-1})$					
3-4	1.8 ± 0.8	1.7 ± 0.4	3.4 ± 0.9	3.2 ± 1.0	4.6 ± 1.6
5-6 (w)	5.8 ± 1.5	5.0 ± 1.3	5.6 ± 1.3	5.2 ± 1.3	4.6 ± 1.2
7-8 (w)	5.1 ± 1.6	6.5 ± 1.9	4.2 ± 1.4	4.4 ± 0.9	4.1 ± 1.1
Trypsin $(U \cdot kg^{-1} \cdot h^{-1})$					
3-4	0.6 ± 0.4	0.4 ± 0.1	1.0 ± 0.4	0.7 ± 0.2	1.1 ± 0.5
5-6 (w)	1.9 ± 0.5	1.8 ± 0.5	2.0 ± 0.5	1.9 ± 0.5	1.6 ± 0.5
7-8 (w)	3.4 ± 1.2	4.2 ± 1.2	2.8 ± 1.0	2.7 ± 0.6	2.8 ± 0.9

Age (weeks)	id saline	id saline	id amino acid mixture (mmol/kg/h)		
			0.005	0.05	0.5
Volume $(ml \cdot kg^{-1} \cdot h^{-1})$					
3-4	1.4 ± 0.6[ab]	1.5 ± 0.5[b]	1.3 ± 0.6[ab]	0.7 ± 0.5[a]	1.1 ± 0.6[ab]
5-6 (w)	1.6 ± 0.9	2.0 ± 0.6	2.4 ± 1.3	1.7 ± 0.8	1.9 ± 1.6
7-8 (w)	2.6 ± 1.6	1.5 ± 0.7	2.5 ± 1.9	1.9 ± 1.3	2.2 ± 1.7
Protein $(mg \cdot kg^{-1} \cdot h^{-1})$					
3-4	2.5 ± 1.3	2.7 ± 1.8	2.5 ± 1.9	1.7 ± 2.1	2.3 ± 1.7
5-6 (w)	2.0 ± 0.8	2.6 ± 1.2	2.4 ± 1.7	2.1 ± 1.5	2.3 ± 1.7
7-8 (w)	4.3 ± 3.0	2.9 ± 0.9	4.2 ± 2.6	3.3 ± 2.1	3.7 ± 2.7
Trypsin $(U \cdot kg^{-1} \cdot h^{-1})$					
3-4	0.5 ± 0.3	0.6 ± 0.3	0.5 ± 0.4	0.4 ± 0.5	0.5 ± 0.3
5-6 (w)	1.3 ± 0.5	1.9 ± 1.1	1.4 ± 0.9	1.4 ± 0.9	1.5 ± 1.1
7-8 (w)	3.3 ± 2.3	2.1 ± 1.0	3.1 ± 2.2	2.6 ± 2.0	2.9 ± 2.2

Table 5
Pancreatic juice secretion, protein and trypsin activity output, (mean ± SEM, n=4) during 30-min periods before and during intraduodenal infusion of saline (5 ml/h/kg) and during intraduodenal infusion of increasing doses of a lipid emulsion and sodium oleate (5 ml/h/kg) in pigs with chronic catheterization of the pancreatic duct 3-8 weeks of age

Age (weeks)	id saline	id saline	id lipid emulsion (mg/kg/h)		
			10	100	1000
	Volume (ml·kg^{-1}·h^{-1})				
3-4	1.0 ± 0.4	1.3 ± 0.6	1.2 ± 0.6	1.3 ± 0.5	1.1 ± 0.4
5-6(w)	1.7 ± 0.8	1.8 ± 0.8	1.5 ± 0.7	1.8 ± 1.4	2.2 ± 0.9
7-8 (w)	2.4 ± 1.2	3.3 ± 1.4	2.3 ± 1.4	3.5 ± 1.6	2.8 ± 1.5
	Protein (mg·kg^{-1}·h^{-1})				
3-4	1.6 ± 0.9	1.9 ± 1.2	2.0 ± 2.0	1.9 ± 1.3	2.2 ± 1.6
5-6 (w)	1.8 ± 0.4	1.9 ± 0.5	2.1 ± 1.0	2.4 ± 0.2	2.3 ± 1.1
7-8 (w)	3.5 ± 1.4	4.1 ± 2.1	4.4 ± 4.3	4.0 ± 1.6	4.2 ± 2.1
	Trypsin (U·kg^{-1}·h^{-1})				
3-4	0.3 ± 0.2	0.4 ± 0.3	0.4 ± 0.4	0.4±0.3	0.4 ± 0.3
5-6 (w)	0.9 ± 0.5	0.9 ± 0.6	1.0 ± 0.7	1.1±0.5	1.1 ± 0.9
7-8 (w)	2.3 ± 1.1	2.7 ± 1.4	2.9 ± 2.8	2.5±1.0	2.6 ± 1.3
			id sodium oleate (mmol/kg/h)		
			0.005	0.05	0.5
	Volume (ml·kg^{-1}·h^{-1})				
3-4	2.1 ± 1.3	1.9 ± 1.4	1.5 ± 0.9	1.7 ± 1.2	1.7 ± 1.8
5-6 (w)	2.1 ± 1.1	3.3 ± 1.0	2.9 ± 0.9	2.3 ± 1.6	1.6 ± 0.9
7-8 (w)	2.3 ± 1.3	2.0 ± 1.3	3.4 ± 1.3	2.2 ± 1.4	2.0 ± 0.9
	Protein (mg·kg^{-1}·h^{-1})				
3-4	3.0 ±2.3^b	2.1 ± 1.4^{ab}	1.6 ± 1.7^a	1.9 ± 1.2^{ab}	2.7 ± 2.2^{ab}
5-6 (w)	2.6 ± 1.8	3.4 ± 2.1	2.4 ± 1.5	2.2 ± 2.2	3.4 ± 1.0
7-8 (w)	3.8 ± 3.2^a	3.6 ± 2.8^a	6.0 ± 4.2^{ab}	3.4 ± 3.5^a	7.3 ± 6.7^b
	Trypsin (U·kg^{-1}·h^{-1})				
3-4	0.6 ± 0.4^b	0.4 ± 0.3^{ab}	0.3 ± 0.3^a	0.4 ± 0.3^{ab}	0.6 ± 0.4^b
5-6 (w)	1.5 ± 1.2	1.8 ± 1.4	1.4 ± 1.1	0.9 ± 0.7	1.9 ± 0.6
7-8 (w)	2.6 ± 2.1	2.5 ± 1.9	4.0 ± 3.0	2.5 ± 2.0	4.3 ± 4.5

3.1.3. Response to intraduodenal loading with feed (Table 6)

Intraduodenal infusion of sows' milk before weaning increased protein output, whereas homogenized solid feed after weaning caused a tendency to increased protein output (Table 7) and increased trypsin secretion in both groups.

Table 6
Pancreatic juice secretion, protein output and trypsin activity output (mean±SEM) during 30-min periods before and during intraduodenal infusion of saline (5 ml/h/kg) and during intraduodenal infusion of sows' milk (n = 4) or homogenized solid feed (n = 3) (5 ml/h/kg) in pigs with chronic catheterization of the pancreatic duct, 3-13 weeks of age

Age (weeks)	id saline	id saline	id milk 5 ml/kg/h	id saline	id saline
Volume (mL·kg^{-1}·h^{-1})					
3-4	0.5 + 0.2	0.6 ± 0.1	0.6 ± 0.1	0.8 ± 0.1	0.8 ± 0.2
5-8 (w)	2.0 ± 0.8	2.8 ± 0.7	3.0 ± 0.6	2.9 ± 0.8	2.2 ± 0.7
Protein (mg·kg^{-1}·h^{-1})					
3-4	2.0 ± 0.7[a]	2.8 ± 0.9[a]	4.3 ± 1.1[b]	4.7 ± 1.1[b]	3.6 ± 0.8[ab]
5-8 (w)	5.1 ± 2.3	5.5 ± 1.4	8.0 ± 2.5	7.3 ± 2.3	5.4 ± 2.1
Trypsin (U·kg^{-1}·h^{-1})					
3-4	0.6 ± 0.2[a]	1.1 ± 0.3[ab]	1.4 ± 0.4[ab]	1.7 ± 0.3[b]	1.2 ± 0.2[ab]
5-8 (w)	1.7 ± 0.8[a]	2.6 ± 0.8[ab]	3.9 ± 1.3[b]	3.2 ± 0.8[b]	2.4 ± 0.8[ab]
			id feed 1 g/kg/h	id saline	id saline
Volume (mL·kg^{-1}·h^{-1})					
7-13 (w)	2.0 ± 0.6	1.4 ± 0.4	1.6 ± 0.4	1.1 ± 0.4	1.6 ± 0.6
Protein (mg·kg^{-1}·h^{-1})					
7-13 (w)	3.9 ± 1.4[a]	5.7 ± 1.9[ab]	6.6 ± 1.5 [b]	4.0 ± 0.9[ab]	5.6 ± 1.8[ab]
Trypsin (U·kg^{-1}·h^{-1})					
7-13 (w)	2.9 ± 1.3[a]	3.1 ± 1.1[ab]	4.2 ± 1.0[b]	2.5 ± 0.7[a]	3.6 ± 1.3[ab]

3.1.4. Response to oral milk feeding (Table 7)

Natural suckling before weaning and bottle feeding with sows' milk after weaning did not significantly affect the pancreatic secretion for any variables studied.

3.2. Plasma hormone concentration

Plasma CCK levels after various stimulation (Table 8)

Intraduodenal load with sodium oleate increased plasma CCK concentrations in all age groups of piglets as compared with the basal concentrations. In addition, intraduodenal infusion of sows' milk both before (3-4 weeks of age) and immediately after weaning (5-6 weeks of age) increased CCK plasma concentrations.

241

Table 7
Pancreatic juice outflow, protein output, and trypsin activity output (mean±SEM, n=6) during 60-min periods before and after natural feeding vs. bottle feeding (200 ml) with sows' milk in pigs with chronic catheterization of the pancreatic duct, 3-13 weeks of age

Time	0' - 60'	- 60' - 0'	0' - 60'
Age (weeks)	Baseline	Suckling	Bottle feeding (200 ml)
		Volume (ml·kg^{-1}·h^{-1})	
3-4	0.7 ± 0.4	0.5 ± 1.7	-
5-13 (w)	2.2 ± 1.2	-	1.2 ± 0.5
		Protein (mg·kg^{-1}·h^{-1})	
3-4	3.6 ± 1.6	4.9 ± 1.9	-
5-13 (w)	5.0 ± 5.0	-	6.2 ± 4.3
		Trypsin (U·kg^{-1}·h^{-1})	
3-4	1.0 ± 0.8	1.2 ± 0.8	-
5-13 (w)	3.5 ± 0.4	-	4.3 ± 2.7

Table 8
Average plasma CCK concentrations (pmol/L) in pigs (means ± SD) after intravenous (iv) infusion of secretin and intraduodenal (id) infusion of different stimulants. w = weaned, Sec = secretin, AA = amino acids, Ova = ova albumin

Age (weeks)	Basal iv	Sec id	HCl id	AA id	Lipid id	Ova id	Oleate id	Milk id	Feed id	Casein id
3-4	15±7[b]	17±9	17±7[b]	12±5[b]	14±4[b]	12±5[b]	34±18[b]*	26±10[b]*	-	-
5-6 (w)	7±5[a]	11±10	8±5[a]	4±2[a]	13±5[b]	7±6[a]	25±15[ab]*	12±8[ab]*	-	-
7-8 (w)	7±5[a]	10±5	8±5[a]	6±2[a]	6±3[a]	9±4[a]	14±4[a]*	10±4[a]	-	-
7-13 (w)	4±2	-	-	-	-	-	-	-	5±3	10± 4*

Statistically significant differences between basal values and values obtained with particular treatments (horizontally) within the age group are indicated with (*); significant differences between age groups (vertically) are indicate with different superscripts (p<0.05); w = weaned pigs.

Duodenal loading both with sodium oleate and with milk increased the concentrations of plasma CCK to higher levels before weaning than after weaning. However, intraduodenal loading with HCl, ovalbumin, amino acids mixture and lipid emulsion, and iv infusion of secretin did not affect the concentrations of CCK in the plasma.

3.3. Age-dependent plasma hormone levels (Table 9)

Basal plasma levels of CCK were high in the youngest pigs but decreased progressively after weaning up to 13 weeks, whereas basal plasma secretin levels showed the opposite pattern, with increasing levels with age. Plasma insulin levels increased whereas plasma glucagon and somatostatin levels decreased after weaning.

Table 9
Average basal (preprandial) blood plasma level of secretin (pmol/L), (n = 6 and n = 5 for pigs weaned at 5 weeks of age); insulin, (mU/L); CCK (pmol/L), (n = 15 and n = 5 for pigs weaned at 5 weeks of age); (n = 4); glucagon (ng/L), (n = 4) and somatostatin (pmol/L), (n = 3) in pigs (means ± SD)

Age (weeks)	Secretin	Insulin	CCK	Glucagon	Somatostatin
3-4	3.2 ± 3.0^a	3.0 ± 2.0^a	15 ± 7^c	200 ± 57^b	32 ± 13^b
5-8 (w)	11.0 ± 7.0^b	5.0 ± 4.0^{ab}	7 ± 5^b	110 ± 38^a	17 ± 9^a
7-8 (w)	-	7.0 ± 3.0^b	7 ± 5^b	120 ± 37^a	-
7-13 (w)	10.0 ± 8.0^b	-	4 ± 2^a	-	-

Significant differences between age groups are indicated with different superscripts. $P<0.05$, w = weaned pigs.

4. DISCUSSION

These results obtained from individual pigs followed during their development strengthens findings on developmental changes. The results show that secretin stimulates the exocrine pancreas before weaning. In contrast, elevated CCK plasma concentrations after intraduodenal loading were not always followed by stimulation of the exocrine pancreas. Also, a slight increase in trypsin output occurred after exogenous CCK only before weaning. Thus, in spite of high basal concentrations in the plasma before weaning, CCK does not appear to play a role in postprandial stimulation of the exocrine pancreas in the pig.

The lack of response of the exocrine pancreas to id stimulation with protein, amino acids and lipid emulsion indicates that mechanisms regulating the exocrine pancreas that are based on enteropancreatic reflexes evoked by stimuli from protein and intact fat either do not exist or are not fully developed before and directly after weaning. Moreover, the lack of any stimulation of pancreatic juice secretion or protein output by duodenal acidification suggests that the HCl-dependent enteropancreatic reflex does not function at the age studied. However, the increasing stimulation of pancreatic protein output in the oldest pigs studied with id infusion of oleic acid indicates that stimulation of the enteropancreatic reflex by fatty acids in young pigs is brought on by weaning.

The weaning-related changes observed in the GI tract hormone pattern i.e., decreased basal CCK, glucagon and somatostatin levels and increased secretin and insulin levels in the blood, may be responsible for increased pancreatic secretion around weaning.

4.1. The secretin-mediated enteropancreatic reflex

A clear stimulatory effect of exogenous secretin on pancreatic secretion (volume, protein, trypsin) was obtained in the youngest piglets studied i.e., already before weaning, while after weaning only volume secreted was stimulated. The incremental stimulation of secretin appeared to be similar before and after weaning, when the highest values of basal pancreatic secretion were observed. Thus, the apparent maturation of the secretin stimulation seems to be due to increased basal secretion after weaning rather than to increased response. These results, obtained with conscious animals, confirm earlier results from anaesthetised pigs in acute experiments, both in young piglets, where Harada et al. [14] reported that secretin could stimulate pancreatic secretion already at the age of 3 days (although the stimulation was more potent in 28-day-old pigs), and in adolescent pigs, where Schaffalitzky de Muckadell et al. [20] found that secretin-stimulated juice secretion was dose-dependent.

In our studies duodenal acidification with HCl did not affect the exocrine pancreas in any age group. This is not consistent with earlier studies on anaesthetised young pigs by Harada et al. [14] and on adolescent pigs by Schaffalitzky de Muckadell et al. [20]. One tentative explanation for these discrepancies is that our studies were performed on conscious animals, in whom the basal pancreatic secretion previously has been shown to be considerably higher than in anaesthetised pigs [10]. During anaesthesia, pancreatic secretion and endogenous plasma levels of secretin have been shown to decrease simultaneously [22] and under such conditions id acidification may cause a limited secretin release stimulating the exocrine pancreas.

From our results it is obvious that pancreatic responsiveness to secretin is functionally developed in conscious young piglets before weaning. However, the lack of stimulation by intraduodenal HCl acidification suggests that the enteropancreatic reflex is not fully developed at this stage of development.

4.3. The CCK-mediated enteropancreatic reflex

In anaesthetised young piglets, Harada et al. [14] reported an increased secretion of the pancreas to exogenous CCK-8 with age. Also in other species, e.g., rodents and humans, CCK is known to stimulate pancreatic secretion with increasing potency during early postnatal development [23,24]. However, we could not show any effect of CCK on the exocrine pancreas in the pig, with the exception of a slight effect on the trypsin activity output, in the youngest pigs. This finding is supported by the observations of Cuber et al. [17] and Holst (personal communication) who have claimed that iv administration of CCK in physiological doses has no effect on the exocrine pancreas in the pig.

It the light of recent studies on pigs [10,25-27], calves [28-30] and rats [31,32] we therefore propose that CCK released due tu intraduodenal stimulation acts on the exocrine pancreas via a locally mediated reflex in the duodenum. CCK in a relatively high concentration of CCK at the place of its release in the intestinal wall but in amounts not influencing the peripheral blood, may activate CCK-A receptors on afferent parasympathetic nerves in the duodenum

[33] and via the CNS might stimulate the exocrine pancreas through efferent parasympathetic pathways. Circulating CCK might have roles other than stimulating exocrine pancreatic secretion, like affecting pancreatic growth [34-37] and/or constituting a satiety signal [38-40] or stimulating insulin secretion [41].

The exocrine pancreas did not respond to id administration of intact proteins or amino acid mixture. This indicates that the pig pancreas is insensitive to stimulation with proteins and protein break-down products during the age periods studied. However, intraduodenally administered oleic acid and fat-rich sows' milk (50% dry matter) stimulate pancreatic secretion, pointing to the importance of fat-induced enteropancreatic reflexes in 7-8-week-old pigs, as earlier reported for humans [42,43]. The lack of stimulation and, in fact, slightly depressive effect of id sodium oleate before weaning indicates that the enteropancreatic reflex, based on enteral stimuli by fat, is age-dependent and immature before weaning.

In addition, the release of endogenous CCK was stimulated by sodium oleate and milk loading but not by id protein and amino acid loading, and manifested as increased levels in peripheral blood.

In contrast to id loading, bottle feeding with milk did not stimulate pancreatic secretion. The reason for this difference may be that during passage through the stomach, milk loses its ability to affect the pancreatic secretion. This is supported by experiments [44] showing that the main milk component casein and hydrolysates of casein did not affect the exocrine pancreas when loaded intraduodenally. Moreover, biologically active milk components, such as insulin and cortisol, [45] have been shown to affect the exocrine pancreas during the passage of milk through the stomach and intestines. Other possible agents are ß-casomorphins which are formed in the gastrointestinal tract from casein digestion and may act inhibiting via release of somatostatin [46,47] or glucomacropeptide, the product of the chymosin degradation of k-casein, which abolishes gastric secretion [48].

4.5. CCK plasma levels during development

Higher basal plasma CCK levels were found before than after weaning. Interestingly, the high CCK plasma concentrations before weaning corresponded to a low basal (interdigestive) pancreatic secretion, indicating a low stimulatory role of CCK in suckling pigs. Instead of being an endogenous secretagogue in the pancreas, a trophic role for CCK in the pancreas is probable during this stage. In young calves, CCK-B receptors have been described [49] and recently the pig pancreas was suggested to contain mostly trophic CCK-B receptors and no secretory CCK-A receptors [50]. However, in rats stimulation of the pancreas through acinar CCK-A receptors is well documented. In humans, the stimulation of the exocrine pancreas is altered by CCK-A receptor antagonists [51-53], whose existence remains doubtful, however [54]. Thus, in some species, e.g., pigs, CCK may have little to do with direct stimulation of the exocrine pancreas.

4.6. Plasma hormone concentrations coupled to exocrine pancreatic function

Hyperglycaemia is commonly considered to be a potent inhibiting factor of exocrine pancreatic function. However, in our experiments short-term id loading of glucose (data not shown) did not affect the exocrine pancreas, in contrast to the findings of Cuber *et al.*, [55] who reported stimulatory effects of id loading of carbohydrates on CCK blood levels in the pig.

Long-term effects of carbohydrates on the exocrine pancreas via insulin and glucagon in pigs could be essential. In fasted cattle, 24 hours of id infusion of glucose was shown to stimulate the exocrine pancreas, starting 16 hours from the beginning of infusion [56], probably due to an concomitantly elevated insulin level. Insulin in turn might stimulate exocrine pancreatic secretion, as suggested by the insulo-acinar axis [57-62], where it is considered to be important in this role. An inhibitory islet/acinar axis can also be observed when somatostatin and pancreatic polypeptide suppress pancreatic secretion [63]. However, the concept of the insulo/acinar axis heve been also critically reviewed by Holst [64]. The present study showed that in pigs before weaning the basal insulin levels were lower than after weaning, while levels of glucagon and somatostatin were higher before than after weaning. Moreover, as reported earlier from our laboratory [12] milk consumption by natural suckling before weaning did not influence plasma insulin concentrations, even though the blood glucose level increased during the same time period. Thus, since insulin stimulates the exocrine pancreas while glucagon and somatostatin inhibit its function [58], this might explain the low pancreatic secretion seen during hypoinsulinaemia and parallel hyperglucagonaemia/somatostatinaemia before weaning. The sharp shift in pancreatic secretion directly after weaning may therefore be secondary to an increased insulin level and decreased glucagon and somatostatin levels. The lack of effect of suckling on the exocrine pancreas may also be explained by low insulin levels. This failure of suckling to increase plasma insulin might be related to insensitivity in the neural regulation of insulin secretion. In sheep during hypoinsulinaemia, the exocrine pancreas was found to be insensitive to parasympathetic stimulation [60], and in a recent study we have shown that neuroglycopenia (parasympathetic stimulation) induced by 2-deoxy-glucose did not stimulate the exocrine pancreas in pigs [65].

4.7. Development of hormonal patterns

The results from our study indicate a shift in the GI hormonal pattern with increasing age of the piglet. The hormonal changes appeared in connection with weaning, at 5-6 weeks of age, indicating that the hormonal shift is related to the dietary change from sows' milk to a commercial solid weaning feed. The high levels of plasma CCK in young unweaned pigs may be due to a lack of feed-back inhibition of the intestinal CCK release, due to a low pancreatic proteinase (trypsin) output, since luminal trypsin activity is thought to degrade CCK-releasing factors that stimulate intestinal CCK release. High plasma levels of CCK stimulate enzyme-rich pancreatic secretion in the adult, while in these young pigs it does not stimulate pancreatic secretion. The reason for the latter observation may be a poor co-stimulation exerted by the low plasma levels of secretin or a tonic inhibition by somatostatin and/or opioid-like milk factors, in analogy with what has been found for gastric secretion in suckling rats [47]. The low plasma secretin levels in young pigs are probably a result of low duodenal acidification caused by low gastric acid secretion and a high buffering capacity of milk, providing a poor stimulus for intestinal secretin release. Weaning is known to induce profound quantitative and qualitative changes in the GI tract, including an increased gastric acid and pancreatic enzyme secretion, thus probably explaining the reversed CCK/secretin pattern. The shift in the insulin and glucagon levels may reflect the dietary differences before and after weaning, as milk contains relatively little carbohydrate and protein, but high lipid levels, while the reverse is true for solid feed.

The results obtained confirmed our previously reported observations of a weaning-dependent developmental induction of the exocrine pancreatic function in pigs [10], where the average basal (preprandial) pancreatic secretion before weaning was lower than that after weaning. The presented data are the first showing the development of a mechanism regulating exocrine pancreatic function around weaning in conscious pigs. The observations in our presented studies indicate that hormonal changes play an important regulative role in the adaptation of the GI tract and the metabolism to the dietary change that occurs in the young piglet at weaning.

We postulate that the weaning-related changes in GI tract hormone patterns i.e., decreased basal blood CCK, glucagon and somatostatin levels and increased secretin and insulin levels, may be responsible for increased pancreatic secretion after weaning. In forthcoming studies, the development of nervous system-dependent secretion will be considered in these respects as well.

REFERENCES

1. E.M. Widdowson and D.E. Ceabb, Biol. Neonate., 28 (1976) 261.
2. T. Corring, A. Aumaitre and G. Durand, Nutr. Metab., 22 (1978) 231.
3. E. Lebenthal and P.C. Lee, Pediatrics., 66 (1980) 556.
4. P. Guilloteau, T. Corring, P. Garnot, P. Martin, R. Toullec and G. Durand, J. Dairy Sci., 66 (1983) 2373.
5. B.R. Weström, B. Ohlsson and B.W. Karlsson, Pancreas, 2 (1987) 589.
6. S.J. Henning. In: L.R. Johnson (ed.), Physiology of the Gastrointestinal Tract. Raven Press, New York, 1987.
7. K. Baintner and J. Farkas, Acta Vet. Hung., 37 (1989) 281.
8. A.-M.B. de Passillé, G. Pelletier, J. Ménard and J. Morisset, J. Anim. Sci., 67 (1989) 2921.
9. S. Githens, J. Pediatr. Gastroenterol. Nutr. 10 (1990) 160.
10. S.G. Pierzynowski, B. Weström, B. Karlsson and L. Svendsen, Int. J. Pancreat.,18 (1995) 81.
11. M.D. Lindemann, S.G. Cornelius, S.M. E. Kandelgy, R.L. Moser and J.E. Pettigrew, J. Anim. Sci., 62 (1986)1298.
12. S.G. Pierzynowski, B.R. Weström, C. Erlanson-Albertsson, B. Ahrén, J. Svendsen and B.W. Karlsson, J. Pediatr. Gastroenterol. Nutr., 16 (1993) 287.
13. D. Rantzer, P. Kiela, M-J. Thaela, J. Svendsen, B. Ahrén, S. Karlsson, and S.G. Pierzynowski, J. Anim. Sci., 75 (1997)1324.
14. E. Harada, H. Kiriyama, E. Kobayashi and H. Tsuchita, Comp. Biochem. Physiol., 91A (1988) 43.
15. S.G. Pierzynowski, B.R. Weström, B.W. Karlsson, J. Svendsen and B. Nilsson. Can. J. Anim. Sci., 68 (1988) 953.
16. M-J. Thaela, S.G. Pierzynowski, M. Skou-Jensen, K. Jakobsen, B.R. Weström and B.W. Karlsson, J. Anim. Sci., 73 (1995) 3402.
17. J.-C. Cuber, T. Corring, F. Levenez, Ch. Bernard and J.-A. Chayvialle. J. Physiol. Pharmacol., 67 (1989)1391.

18. O.H. Lowry, N. Rosebrough, A. Farr and R.J. Randall, J. Biol. Chem.,193 (1951) 265.
19. B.F. Erlanger, N. Kokowski, and W. Cohen. 1961, Arch. Biochem. Biophys., 95 (1961) 271.
20. O.B. Schafalitzky de Muckadel, J Fahrenkrug and J.J. Holst, Scand. J. Gastroent., 12 (1977) 267.
21. P. Cantor and J.F. Rehfeld, J. Immun. Met., 82 (1985) 146.
22. S.G. Pierzynowski, P. Podgurniak, O. Olsen., B. Weström and B. Karlsson, In: W.B. Soufrant and H. Hagemeister, eds., Forschugsinstitut fur die Biologie landwirtschaftlicher Nutztiere (FBN), Schriftenreihe 3,4. Dummerstorf, Bad Doberan, Germany, II (1994) 408.
23. C.M. Doyle and J.D. Jamieson. Dev. Biol., 65 (1978) 11.
24. E. Lebenthal and Y.K. Leung. J. Pediatr. Gastroenterol., Nutr., 5 (1986) 1.
25. S.G. Pierzynowski, H. Mårtensson, B. Ahrén and B.R. Weström, Digestion, 49/1 (1991) 46.
26. S.G. Pierzynowski, H. Mårtensson, B. Weström, B. Ahrén, K. Uvnäs-Möberg and B. Karlsson, Biomed. Res., 14 (1993) 217.
27. P. Kiela, R. Zabielski, P. Podgurniak, M. Midura, P.C. Gregory, W. Barej, and S.G. Pierzynowski, Exp. Physiol., 81 (1996) 375.
28. R. Zabielski, T. Onaga, H. Mineo, S.G. Pierzynowski and S. Kato, Exp. Physiol., 79 (1994) 301.
29. R. Zabielski, T. Onaga, H. Mineo, S. Kato and S.G. Pierzynowski, Int. J. Pancreat., 17 (1995).
30. R. Zabielski, V. Leśniewska, J. Borlak, P.C. Gregory, P. Kiela, S.G. Pierzynowski and W Barej, Reg. Pep., 78 (1998) 113.
31. Y. Li and Ch. Owyang, Gastroenterol., 107 (1994) 525.
32. Ch. Owyang, Amer. J. Physiol., 34 (1996) G1.
33. L.A. Blackshaw and D. Grudy, J. Auton. Nerv. Syst., 31 (1990) 191.
34. J. Morisset, Biom. Res., 1 (1980) 405.
35. U.R. Folsh, Clin. Gastroenterol., 13 (1984) 679.
36. A.G. Nylander, D. Chen, I. Ihse, J.F. Rehfeld and R. Håkanson, Scand. J. Gastroenterol., 27 (1992) 743.
37. D. Chen, A.G. Nylander, J.F. Rehfeld, J. Axelson, I. Ihse and Håkanson, Scand. J. Gastroenterol., 27 (1992) 606.
38. J.C. Pekas and W.E. Trout, Growth Develop. Aging, 54 (1990) 51.
39. J.C. Pekas and W.E. Trout,J. Anim. Sci., 71 (1993) 2499.
40. J.N. Crawley and R.L. Corwing, Pept., 15 (1994) 731.
41. S. Karlsson and B. Ahrén, Scand. Gastroenterol. 27 (1992) 161.
42. O.B. Schaffalitzky de Muckadell, O. Olsen P. Cantor and E. Magid, Pancreas, 1 (1986) 636.
43. O. Olsen, O.B. Schaffalitzky de Muckadell and P. Cantor, Int. J. Pancreat., 1 (1986) 363.
44. S.G. Pierzynowski, M.-J. Thaela, B.W. Karlsson, J. Rehfeld, J. Svendsen and B.R. Weström, In: W.B. Soufrant, H. Hagemeister (eds.), Forschugsinstitut fur die Biologie landwirtschaftlicher Nutztiere (FBN), Schriftenreihe 3,4. Dummerstorf, Bad Doberan, Germany, I (1994) 192.
45. N.F. Sheard and W.A. Walker, Nutr. Rev., 46 (1988) 1.

248

46. V. Schusdziarra, R. Schick, A. de la Fuente, A. Holland, V. Brantl and E.F. Pfeiffer, Endocrinology, 112 (1983) 1948.
47. R.K. Rao, S. Pepperl and F. Porreca, Amer. J. Physiol., 269 (1995) G721.
48. L.S. Vasilevskaya, Y. Stan, M.P. Chernikov and G.K. Shlygin, Vopr. Pitan., 4 (1977) 21.
49. V. Le Meuth, V. Philouze-Rome, I. Le Huerou-Luron, M. Formal, N. Vaysse, Ch. Gespach, P Guilloteau and D. Fourmy, Endocrinology, 133 (1993) 1182.
50. E.F. Lhoste, A.M. Gueugneau, A Garofano, C Phillippe, F. Levenez and T. Corring. Pancreas, 11 (1995) 86.
51. A. Gabryelewicz, E. Kulesza and S.J. Konturek, Scand. J. Gastroenterol., 25 (1990) 731.
52. G. Adler, C. Beglinger, U. Braun, et al. Gastroenteology, 100 (1991) 537.
53. W.E. Schmidt, W Creutfeldt, A. Schelser, et al. Amer. J. Physiol., 260 (1991) G197.
54. C. Susini, A Estival, J.L. Scemama, et al., Pancreas, 1 (1986) 124.
55. J.C. Cuber, F. Vulas, N. Charles, C. Bernard and J.A. Chayvialle, In: J.P. Bali and J. Martinez, eds., Gastrin and cholecystokinin chemistry, physiology and pharmacology. Elsevier, Amsterdam, (1987) 195.
56. S.G. Pierzynowski., J. Anim. Physiol. a. Anim. Nutr. 63 (1990) 198.
57. T. Kanno, N. Ueda and A. Saito, In: T. Fujita (ed.), Endocrine gut and pancreas. Elsevier, Amsterdam, (1976) 335.
58. J.R. Henderson, P.M. Daniel and P.A. Fraser. Gut. 22 (1981) 158.
59. S.G. Pierzynowski and W. Barej, Q. J. Exp. Physiol., 69 (1984) 35.
60. S.G. Pierzynowski, P. Podgurniak, M. Mikołajczyk, W. Szczesny. Q. J. Exp. Physiol., 71 (1986) 401.
61. C. Alvarez and M.A. Lòpez, Int. J. Pancreat. 5 (1989) 229.
62. K.Y. Lee, L. Zhou, X.S. Ren, T.-M. Chang and W.Y.Chey, Amer. J. Physiol. 258 (1990) G268.
63. A. Nakagawa, J.I. Stagner and E Samols, Gastroenterology. 105 (1993) 868.
64. J.J. Holst. Pancreas. 2 (1987) 613.
65. S. Karlsson, S.G. Pierzynowski, B.R. Weström, M.-J. Theala, B. Ahrén and B.W. Karlsson. Pancreas. 11(1995) 271.

Biology of the Pancreas in Growing Animals
S.G. Pierzynowski and R. Zabielski (Editors)

249

Feedback regulation of pancreatic secretion

T. Fushiki[a], S. Tsuzuki[a] and S.G. Pierzynowski[b]

[a]Laboratory of Nutrition Chemistry, Division of Applied Life Sciences,
Graduate School of Agriculture, Kyoto University,
Kyoto 606-8502, Japan

[b]Department of Animal Physiology, Lund University,
Helgonavagen 3B, SE-223 62 Lund, Sweden

We review the mechanisms underlying the feedback regulation of pancreatic enzyme secretion in response to a meal. Pancreatic enzyme secretion in animals is known to be regulated by a negative feedback mechanism mediated by intestinal proteases such as trypsin and chymotrypsin. The presence of these enzymes in the small intestine suppresses pancreatic enzyme secretion, whereas their removal increases it. This mechanism has also been noted in humans. Two novel peptides have been proposed to account for the stimulation of pancreatic enzyme secretion seen in response to feeding of a trypsin inhibitor; one present in rat pancreatic juice and the other spontaneously secreted by the rat small intestine. In both cases, trypsin and trypsin inhibitors do not interact directly with the luminal surface of the small intestine, but their actions are mediated by a trypsin-sensitive, cholecystokinin-releasing peptide. This is an explanation for the well-known stimulation of pancreatic enzyme secretion seen in response to dietary protein intake.

1. DISCOVERY OF THE FEEDBACK REGULATION OF PANCREATIC ENZYME SECRETION

It is well established that dietary trypsin inhibitors evoke increased pancreatic enzyme secretion in rats and chicks. Green and Lyman [1] first proposed that the presence of trypsin, chymotrypsin, or a mixture of bile and pancreatic juice in the small intestine controls enzyme secretion from the pancreas. In rats, the bile duct is joined by numerous ducts from the pancreas; in humans it is joined by a single main pancreatic duct. Green and Lyman [1] collected a mixture of bile and pancreatic juice from the common bilary-pancreatic duct that opens into the duodenum. Removal of proteolytic activity from the intestine, by exclusion of bile-pancreatic juice through ligation of the common biliary-pancreatic duct as well as by intestinal infusion of soya bean trypsin inhibitors, markedly increased pancreatic enzyme output. This indicates that this negative feedback control of pancreatic enzyme secretion could be the mechanism by which dietary trypsin inhibitors increase pancreatic enzyme secretion in rats.

This idea was extended to dietary protein; that is, in the course of digestion, soya bean trypsin inhibitor (SBTI) or another protein bind to proteolytic enzymes in effect removing them from the small intestine, thereby abolishing their negative feedback on pancreatic enzyme secretion [2,3]. Ihse *et al.* [4] and many other investigators have confirmed the relationship between the intraduodenal pancreatic enzyme milieu and pancreatic secretion in rats.

Cholecystokinin (CCK) has been suggested to mediate the negative feedback control over pancreatic enzyme secretion. CCK is a well-known hormone that is found in the gut and brain [5]. In visceral tissues it plays an important role in the control of pancreatic secretion, gallbladder contraction, and gut motility [6]. The specific radioimmunoassay and bioassay for CCK were developed and established in the 1980s [7,8]. Since the plasma CCK concentration is increased by bile-pancreatic juice diversion and by administration of trypsin inhibitor, it has been concluded that CCK is the major candidate for mediating feedback regulation [9-11].

2. FEEDBACK REGULATION IN VARIOUS ANIMAL SPECIES

Similar negative feedback regulation has been observed in pigs, calves, and hamsters [12-14]. In pigs, diversion of pancreatic juice from the intestine caused an increase in pancreatic enzyme secretion [15,16]. The increase was suppressed by returning the pancreatic juice to the intestine but not by infusion of NaCl-NaHCO$_3$. Therefore, a pancreatic regulatory mechanism similar to that in the rat appears to exist in the pig. Fukuoka *et al.* [17] showed that intestinal infusion of 50 mg of SBTI markedly stimulated pancreatic enzyme secretion only when the pancreatic juice was returned to the pig duodenum throughout the experiments. Without return of the pancreatic juice to the duodenum, SBTI had no stimulatory effect. The requirement of its presence for stimulation by SBTI suggests the importance of pancreatic juice in the pancreatic response to SBTI.

In the dog, negative feedback regulation of pancreatic enzyme secretion by trypsin has not been demonstrated. In acute and chronic experiments on dogs Sale *et al.* [18], found no evidence of exocrine pancreatic feedback regulation. According to Cooke *et al.* [19], the pancreatic enzyme response to feeding was the same whether the pancreatic juice was drained or returned. However, Imamura *et al.* [20] recently reported that postprandial pancreatic secretion was regulated by feedback regulation, and its mediator was secretin. Nustede *et al.* [21] reported that the inhibition of intraduodenal trypsin activity by a protease inhibitor caused a significant increase in basal pancreatic secretion in dogs. The reason for these discrepancies is not apparent.

Mayer and Kelly [22] demonstrated that intestinal perfusion of intact bovine serum albumin, egg albumin, casein, and haemoglobin in the dog did not evoke more pancreatic secretion than saline, although after peptide digestion of the same proteins the resulting polypeptides were potent stimulants of pancreatic enzyme secretion. Indeed, dietary amino acids were the most potent stimulants of pancreatic enzyme secretion in the dog [23]. Mayer and Kelly suggested that enzyme secretion from the dog pancreas is triggered by receptors in the mucosa of the small intestine that are responsive to free or amino-terminal aromatic amino acids [23]. Why are amino acids major stimulants for pancreatic enzyme secretion in the dog but not in the rat? The dog is basically a carnivore, eating food that contains many free amino acids, whereas rats and pigs are omnivorous animals. The latter generally eat storage proteins in seeds, beans, and grain, which contain fewer free amino acids than meat. These obvious differences in dietary intake may in part account for the pancreatic response to dietary amino acids.

3. FEEDBACK CONTROL OF PANCREATIC ENZYMES IN HUMANS

The control mechanism for exocrine pancreatic secretion in humans is still not fully elucidated, with conflicting results from different studies. The existence of a feedback regulation of pancreatic secretion in humans was first described by Ihse et al. in 1977 [24]. Several studies have since revealed a feedback inhibition of pancreatic secretion in humans, regulated by trypsin [25-28]; intraduodenal instillation of trypsin and a number of other proteases caused a significant suppression of pancreatic enzyme secretion, which could be reversed by instillation of protease inhibitors. This effect is supposed to be mediated by CCK [29-32], but it remains unclear whether pancreatic proteases have a direct or an indirect effect on CCK release.

However, other studies have failed to show any stimulation of pancreatic secretion by inhibition of trypsin, and the involvement of CCK in feedback regulation has not yet been confirmed [33-36]. Furthermore, the normal baseline and postprandial plasma concentration of CCK in patients with severe pancreatic insufficiency and the resulting low intraduodenal trypsin activity suggest that in humans, unlike in animals, the hormonal feedback regulation of pancreatic enzyme secretion does not play an essential role. These data are supported by a recent investigation in which application of 1200 mg Camostate for 120 min intraduodenally showed no effect on CCK release. Liener et al. [37], however, demonstrated that the Bowman-Birk trypsin inhibitor, an inhibitor of chymotrypsin and elastase, markedly stimulated pancreatic enzyme secretion in humans. Friess et al. [38] claimed that such short-term experiments do not show the physiological consequences that may accompany long-term protease inhibitor treatment [38]. They investigated the long-term effects of oral protease inhibition on exocrine pancreatic function and pancreatic morphology in humans. Duodenal trypsin output after secretion stimulation was significantly increased and duodenal bicarbonate output decreased after 4 weeks of Camostate application. The size of the pancreatic head had increased at week 4 and had decreased to pre-treatment values 2 weeks after the end of treatment. CCK plasma levels 15 min after application of a standard test meal increased. It was concluded that the human pancreas adapts to oral application of the proteinase inhibitor Camostate and that feedback control of the exocrine pancreas does existin humans. Further studies are needed to confirm this.

4. EVIDENCE FOR THE PRESENCE OF A CCK-RELEASING PEPTIDE

The active site of trypsin is necessary for the suppression of pancreatic enzyme secretion. The effect of trypsin treated with diisopropyl fluorophosphate (DFP), which blocks the active site, was compared with that of the same amount of active trypsin. The active trypsin suppressed the secretion, but the DFP-treated trypsin had no such effect, and neither did DFP-treated chymotrypsin [39]. Trypsin inactivated by heat treatment showed no suppressive activity, while trypsin derived from other species did suppress secretion [40]. An intestinal infusion of pronase E, which is a mixture of proteases from Streptomyces griseus, as well as bovine pancreatic trypsin [39], suppressed rat pancreatic enzyme secretion. Pronase E contains about 10% of a trypsin-like enzyme that shows no molecular homology to pancreatic trypsin or chymotrypsin. The results indicate that for the suppression of pancreatic enzyme secretion, not the trypsin molecule itself but its enzymatic activity is needed.

Trypsin inhibitors evoke increased enzyme secretion indirectly, by counteracting the suppression due to trypsin. Fushiki and co-workers demonstrated that SBTI [41], egg white trypsin inhibitor, and dietary protein [42], which are potent stimulants of CCK and pancreatic enzyme secretion, had no effect when they were introduced into well-washed, protease-free rat small intestine. Stimulation of pancreatic enzyme secretion occurred only when the enzyme was infused into the upper third of the intestine [39]. Also, the increase in enzyme secretion on trypsin inhibitor administration did not occur in rats after resection of the duodenum and jejunum [43]. The proximal small intestine is a suitable area for receiving a signal that regulates the pancreatic enzyme secretion in response to a meal. Dietary protein is rapidly digested and absorbed within the upper small intestine, so the signal receptor site for feedback control, if present in the intestine, must be located in its proximal part. The gut hormone CCK, which is believed to be the major hormonal regulator of pancreatic enzyme secretion, is produced in the endocrine cells of the proximal small intestine [44]. However, no evidence has been obtained for a direct interaction between trypsin and CCK-producing cells. The proximal small intestine releases CCK into the blood when it receives the signal that trypsin and/or chymotrypsin activity is relatively decreased. It is clear that a specific peptide sequence in these enzyme molecules is not concerned in the system, since only their activity is needed for the regulation. Thus, there must be unknown factors in the proximal small intestine that convert the decrease in trypsin and chymotrypsin activity into a CCK release signal; for example, a trypsin-sensitive, CCK-releasing factor. Alternatively, the proximal small intestine may have one or more special receptor sites that react with trypsin, chymotrypsin, and elastase and respond to a decrease in the activities of these proteases.

5. TRYPSIN-SENSITIVE, CCK-RELEASING FACTOR IN THE SMALL INTESTINE

Miyasaka *et al.* [45] suggested that the spontaneous pancreatic hypersecretion that occurs in the absence of luminal trypsin is caused by a trypsin-sensitive polypeptide that is spontaneously secreted by the small intestine into the lumen and, once there, stimulates pancreatic enzyme secretion. They examined whether the hypersecretion that occurs during diversion of bile-pancreatic juice from the intestine could be inhibited by a rapid washout of the proximal small intestine with buffer. Rapid perfusion of the proximal small intestine with phosphate buffer caused, at maximum, 40% inhibition of pancreatic protein secretion. This was reversed by perfusion with the pooled concentrated perfusate, an effect that was not abolished by boiling for 10 min but was abolished by incubation with trypsin. They concluded that trypsin regulated pancreatic enzyme secretion through inactivation of the trypsin-sensitive polypeptide that is secreted into the lumen. Lu *et al.* [46] confirmed the above observations. Perfusion of the duodenum with buffer under the same conditions as those of Miyasaka and Green [45] lowered the plasma CCK level. The concentrated perfusate increased the plasma CCK level. The putative peptide was heat-stable and trypsin-ensitive. The results of Sephadex molecular sieving showed that its molecular weight was not greater than 3000 Da. The release of the peptide was blocked by atropine treatment. Whether these two peptides are identical remains to be elucidated.

5.1 Luminal cholecystokinin releasing factor (LCRF)

Recently Green *et al.* [47] purified a CCK-releasing peptide from rat intestinal perfusate, and named it luminal CCK-releasing factor (LCRF). Amino acid analysis and mass spectrometric analysis showed that the purified peptide is composed of 70-75 amino acid residues and has a mass of 8136 Da. Microsequence analysis of LCRF yielded an amino acid sequence for 41 residues. When infused intraduodenally, the purified peptide stimulated pancreatic protein and fluid secretion in a dose-related manner in conscious rats and significantly elevated plasma CCK levels. The study demonstrated the first chemical characterisation of a luminally secreted enteric peptide functioning as an intraluminal regulator of intestinal hormone release (Figure 1).

An amino-terminal fragment of LCRF, LCRF-(1-35), was synthesised and its stimulatory effect on pancreatic exocrine secretion in conscious rats was examined [48,49]. Intraduodenal injection of the LCRF fragment increased fluid and protein secretion. The response was biphasic, as observed in a study using purified LCRF. The distribution and localisation of LCRF in the gastrointestinal tract and pancreas of the rat was examined [50]. Radioimmunoassay analysis revealed LCRF immunoreactivity throughout the gut, including the pancreas, stomach, duodenum, jejunum, ileum, and colon, with the highest levels in the small intestine. Extracts of the duodenum and an intestinal lumen perfusate gave dose-dependent inhibition curves that were parallel to the synthetic LCRF standard. Immuno-histochemical analysis revealed LCRF immunoreactivity staining in intestinal villi, Brunner's glands of the duodenum, the duodenal myenteric plexus, gastric pits, pancreatic ductules, and pancreatic islets. These results demonstrated the potential sources of the secretagogue-stimulated release of luminal LCRF and supported the hypothesis that LCRF is secreted into the intestinal lumen to stimulate CCK release from mucosal CCK cells. However, LCRF-(1-35) stimulated pancreatic protein secretion and fluid secretion when given intravenously during the return of pancreatic juice and bile to the duodenum, suggesting that the LCRF fragment stimulates CCK release by occupying receptors on the basolateral border, rather than the apical border, of intestinal cells [51]. Studies to localise the putative LCRF receptor will be necessary to validate this hypothesis.

5.2 Diazepam-binding inhibitor (DBI)

Herzig et al. [52] isolated a trypsin-sensitive peptide that is secreted intraduodenally, releases CCK, and stimulates pancreatic enzyme secretion in rats. This peptide was shown to be identical to the porcine diazepam binding inhibitor (DBI) by peptide sequencing and mass spectrometric analysis. DBI had no sequence similarity with LCRF. Intraduodenal infusion of the synthetic DBI1-86 in rats stimulated pancreatic amylase output. Infusion of the CCK antagonist MK329 completely blocked the DBI-stimulated amylase secretion. Luminal secretion of DBI immunoreactivity has been detected in intestinal washing from rats, following the diversion of bile-pancreatic juice. The secretion of this peptide was inhibited by atropine. However, it is still unclear whether DBI is identical to the peptide found by Lu et al. [46].

5.3 Other intraluminal releasing factors

Secretin release may also be increased after exclusion of pancreatic juice from the intestine and is under negative feedback control [53]. In a manner similar to that for CCK, diversion of pancreatic juice from the duodenum has been shown to significantly increase plasma secretin levels. This increase coincided with an increase in both volume and bicarbonate output of pancreatic secretion, and could be inhibited by intraduodenal reinstillation of pancreatic juice. The release of secretin is stimulated by fatty acids such as sodium oleate, but the regulation of secretin and its releasing factor differs from that of the CCK-releasing factor, since secretin release is also increased by HCl [54,55]. The secretin-releasing factor in the intestinal lumen that mediates these effects has been shown to be a heat-stable, trypsin-sensitive peptide, between 1000 and 4000 Da in size [56]. Its existence underscores the significance of bioactive factors within the lumen of the gut and indicates that regulation of gut hormone secretion by intraluminal releasing factors may be a general phenomenon, applying also to other gastrointestinal hormones.

6. TRYPSIN-SENSITIVE, CCK-RELEASING FACTOR IN PANCREATIC JUICE

A hypothesis was regarding the molecural background for a feedback control of the pancreatic secretion. Fushiki *et al.* [41] found a trypsin-sensitive, CCK-releasing peptide in rat pancreatic juice. The pancreatic juice was separated into three fractions: mol wt 10,000 Da, mol wt 1000 Da, and intermediate fractions. The 10,000 Da fraction was rich in proteases, which inhibited pancreatic enzyme secretion. In contrast, the intermediate fraction markedly enhanced pancreatic enzyme secretion. The effect was not abolished on incubation at 80°C for 40 min. Brief digestion of the intermediate fraction with rat trypsin or rat chymotrypsin decreased its stimulatory activity. The factor was purified using its trypsin inhibitor activity as an index. On reverse phase HPLC, the trypsin inhibitory activity was separated into four peaks. The predominant peak had the shortest retention time and was further purified. The other three peak materials were not purified and their CCK-releasing activity was not studied.

The amino acid sequence of the 61-residue peptide was determined [57]. Sequence 24-33 closely resembled that of a highly conserved region in pancreatic secretory trypsin inhibitors (PSTIs; Kazal-type inhibitors), that is, -Ile-Tyr-Asp-Pro-Val-Cys-Gly-Thr-Asn-Gly-. Duodenal infusion of 10 μg of the purified peptide, which is approximately the amount in 1 ml of rat bile-pancreatic juice, stimulated pancreatic enzyme secretion in rats, to the accompaniment of a significant increase in plasma CCK concentration [58]. An immunochemical study using a peptide-specific antibody confirmed that the peptide is involved in the mechanism underlying the pancreatic enzyme secretion seen in response to intraduodenal infusion of a trypsin inhibitor.

6.1. The monitor peptide hypothesis

Figure 1 shows our model for the mechanism underlying pancreatic enzyme secretion in response to trypsin inhibitor or food protein intake. During the postabsorptive state, the bioactive peptide secreted from the rat pancreas is easily hydrolysed by digestion. If excess food protein or trypsin inhibitor enters the lumen, in the postprandial state, for example, the protease is so engaged that the peptide survives intact, and in turn causes release of CCK into the circulation. Accordingly, the peptide from the pancreas is able to monitor the intraduodenal environment for protein digestion, and has been designated a monitor peptide. This model explains the pancreatic response to trypsin inhibitor administration. The monitor peptide is also known as PSTI-61 and is distinct from a 56-amino acid PSTI known as PSTI-II (PSTI-56), which shares 66% sequence homology with the monitor peptide [59]. The biological activities of the monitor peptide and PSTI-56 were compared on the basis of their ability to stimulate pancreatic secretion and CCK release in rats [60]. On an equimolar basis, the monitor peptide (PSTI-61) was substantially more potent than PSTI-56, providing

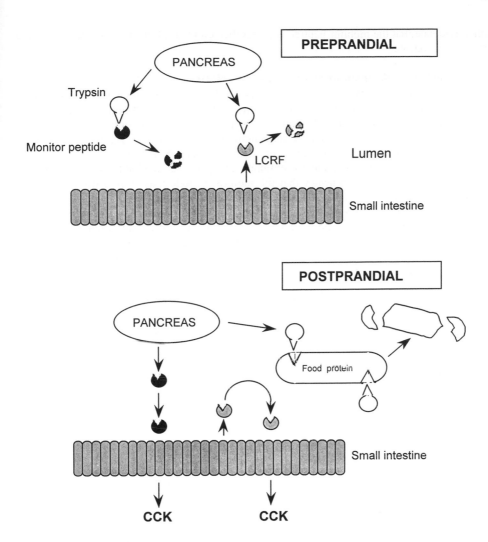

Figure 1. Schematic model of the mechanism underlying the pancreatic enzyme secretion mediated by CCK-releasing peptides. During the preprandial phase, the peptides are hydrolyzed by trypsin. Therefore, no stimulatory effect on pancreatic enzyme secretion is observed. When food protein enters the lumen, in the postprandial phase, the trypsin is engaged in hydrolysing food or is inhibited, so the CCK-releasing peptides survive intact. The intact peptides stimulate the release of CCK into the circulation.

further evidence that the monitor peptide is a specific stimulant of intestinal CCK release and pancreatic secretion.

6.2 Direct effects of the monitor peptide on CCK release

Since the structure of the monitor peptide is similar to that of other pancreatic trypsin inhibitors, its ability to stimulate CCK release might be related to inhibition of intraluminal protease activity. Miyasaka *et al.* [61] instilled the protease inhibitor aprotinin and the monitor peptide, separately and together, into the duodenum of rats. The monitor peptide together with aprotinin stimulated pancreatic secretion more markedly than did aprotinin alone, suggesting that the ability of monitor peptide to stimulate the pancreas was not due to its trypsin inhibitor-like property. This indicates that the monitor peptide may have a direct effect on epithelial cells of the intestine. In the vascularly perfused intestine, Cuber *et al.* [62] demonstrated that the monitor peptide stimulated CCK release. Because pancreatic proteases were excluded from this preparation, the monitor peptide must affect intestinal cells directly rather than protecting an endogenously produced CCK-releasing factor from enzymatic degradation. The direct effects of monitor peptide on CCK release were also examined in vitro in a preparation of isolated rat intestinal mucosal cells [63, 64]. The monitor peptide stimulated CCK release and this release required the presence of extracellular calcium, indicating that calcium may serve as an intracellular messenger in monitor peptide-mediated CCK release.

Yamanishi *et al.* [65] examined the specific binding of monitor peptide to dispersed intestinal mucosal cells of the rat jejunum *in vitro*. The monitor peptide was shown to bind in a reversible, temperature- and pH-dependent manner, consistent with receptor binding. The specific binding site has a trypsin-like specificity. In addition, the monitor peptide stimulated calcium efflux in the isolated cells, suggesting that the monitor peptide binding has some physiological function in CCK release. This study provides strong evidence that the monitor peptide binds directly to cell surface receptors on the small intestine to stimulate CCK release.

7. COMPARISON BETWEEN LCRF AND MONITOR PEPTIDE

The essential mechanism of LCRF and the monitor peptide is the same; when the luminal protease activity decreases below a certain threshold due to ingestion of a dietary protein or a trypsin inhibitor, CCK-releasing peptides survive proteolytic inactivation and elicit CCK release (Figure 1). Iwai et al. have demonstrated in reconstitution experiments in rats [66] that the characteristic pattern of pancreatic enzyme secretion in response to food protein intake can be reproduced by infusing only three components: food proteins, porcine trypsin, and the monitor peptide. The small intestinal peptides are not involved in the mechanism since the small intestine of the rat was thoroughly washed out with saline in this experiment. Miyasaka and Funakoshi claimed [67] that the monitor peptide could not be responsible for CCK release induced by bile-pancreatic juice diversion because it was excluded from the intestinal lumen and therefore absent from the intestinal secretion. They suggested that the monitor peptide acts as a CCK-releasing peptide only during pancreatic juice return. Recently, it has been reported that pancreatic secretory trypsin inhibitor is expressed in the small intestine of humans [68-70] and is secreted into the lumen [71]. CCK release induced during bile-pancreatic juice diversion can be accounted for both by monitor peptide secreted from the intestine and by LCRF. In other words, it is possible that the monitor peptide secreted by the intestine reinforces the CCK release stimulated by LCRF during bile-pancreatic juice diversion. Expression of the monitor peptide in the intestine of rats should be demonstrated.

Miyasaka *et al.* [49] and Spannagel *et al.* [48] compared the bioactivities of the LCRF fragment and the monitor peptide in stimulating pancreatic secretion. The maximal secretion induced by the LCRF fragment was about 60% of that induced by the monitor peptide. The LCRF fragment was more potent than the monitor peptide at the same molar ratio [49]. At present it is not possible to distinguish which of these peptides is the most important in regulating CCK release under physiological conditions.

REFERENCES

1. G.M. Green and R.L. Lyman., Proc. Soc. Exp. Biol. Med., 140 (1972) 6.
2. G.M. Green, B.A. Olds, G. Matthews and R. L. Lyman, Proc. Soc. Exp. Biol. Med., 142 (1973) 1162.
3. B.O. Schneeman, I. Chang, L.B. Smith and R.L. Lyman, J. Nutr., 107 (1977) 281.
4. I. Ihse, P. Lilja and I. Lundquist, Scand. J. Gastroenterol., 14 (1979) 873.
5. J.F. Rehfeld, J. Biol. Chem., 253 (1978) 4022.
6. J.H. Walsh, L.R. Johnson (eds.), Physiology of the gastrointestinal tract. vol. 1 Raven Press, New York, (1981) 60.
7. E. Hashimura, F. Shimizu, T. Nishino, K. Imagawa, K. Tateishi and T. Hamaoka, J. Immunol. Methods., 55 (1982) 375
8. R.A. Liddle, I.D. Goldfine and J.A. Williams, Gastroenterology, 87 (1984) 542.
9. D.S. Louie, D. May, P. Miller and C. Owyang, Amer. J. Physiol., (1986) G252.
10. U.R. Folsch, P. Cantor, H.M. Wilms, A. Schafmayer, H.D. Becker and W. Creutzfeldt, Gastroenterology, 92 (1987) 449.
11. R. Nakamura, K. Miyasaka, A. Funakoshi and K. Kitani, Proc. Soc. Exp. Biol. Med., 192 (1989) 182.
12. T. Corring, J.A. Chayvialle, N.C. Simoes and J. Abello, Reprod. Nutr. Dev., 25 (1985) 439.
13. M.J. Davicco, J. Lefaivre, P. Thivend and J.P. Barlet, Ann. Rech. Vet., 10 (1979) 428.
14. S.A. Andren and I. Ihse, Scand. J. Gastroenterol., 18 (1983) 697.
15. T. Corring and D. Bourdon, J. Nutr., 107 (1977) 1216.
16. I. Ihse and P. Lilja. Scand, J. Gastroenterol., 14 (1979) 1009.
17. S. Fukuoka, M. Tsujikawa, T. Fushiki and K. Iwai, Agric. Biol. Chem., 50 (1986) 2795.
18. J.K. Sale, D.M. Goldberg, A.N. Fawcett and K.G. Wormsley, Digestion, 15 (1977) 540.
19. A.R. Cooke, D.L. Nahrwold and M.I. Grossman, Amer. J. Physiol., 213 (1967) 637.
20. M. Imamura, K.Y. Lee, Y. Song, M. Moriyasu, T.M. Chang and W.Y. Chey, Gastroenterology, 105 (1993) 548.
21. R. Nustede, W.E. Schmidt, M. Jager, F. Stockmann, H. Kohler, U.R. Folsch and H.J. Peiper, Int. J. Pancreatol., 15 (1994) 209.
22. J.H. Meyer and G.A. Kelly, Amer. J. Physiol., 231 (1976) 682.
23. J.H. Meyer, G.A. Kelly, L.J. Spingola and R.S. Jones, Amer. J. Physiol., 231 (1976) 669.
24. I. Ihse, P. Lilja and I. Lundquist, Digestion, 15 (1977) 303.
25. C. Owyang. J. Nutr., (1994) 1321.
26. J.H. Meyer, J. Elashoff, F.V. Porter, J. Dressman and G.L. Amidon, Gastroenterology, 94 (1988) 1315.
27. J. Mossner, R. Secknus, J. Meyer, C. Niederau and G. Adler, Digestion, 53 (1992) 54.

28. J. Slaff, D. Jacobson, C.R. Tillman, C. Curington and P. Toskes, Gastroenterology, 87 (1984) 44.
29. C. Owyang, D.S. Louie and D. Tatum, J. Clin. Invest., 77 (1986) 2042.
30. C. Owyang, D. May and D.S. Louie, Gastroenterology, 91 (1986) 637.
31. J.I. Slaff, M.M. Wolfe and P.P. Toskes, J. Lab. Clin. Med., 105 (1985) 282.
32. G. Adler, C. Beglinger, U. Braun, M. Reinshagen, I. Koop, A. Schafmayer, L. Rovati and R. Arnold, Gastroenterology, 100 (1991) 537.
33. J. Dlugosz, U.R. Folsch and W. Creutzfeldt, Digestion, 26 (1983) 197.
34. B.R. Krawisz, L.J. Miller, E.P. DiMagno and V.L. Go, J. Lab. Clin. Med., 95 (1980) 13.
35. G. Adler, A. Mullenhoff, T. Bozkurt, B. Goke, I. Koop and R. Arnold, Scand. J. Gastroenterol., 23 (1988) 158.
36. G. Adler, A. Mullenhoff, I. Koop, T. Bozkurt, B. Goke, C. Beglinger and R. Arnold, Eur. J. Clin. Invest., 18 (1988) 98.
37. I.E. Liener, R.L. Goodale, A. Deshmukh, T.L. Satterberg, G. Ward, C.M. DiPietro, P.E. Bankey and J. W. Borner, Gastroenterology, 94 (1988) 419.
38. H. Friess, J. Kleeff, R. Isenmann, P. Malfertheiner and M.W. Buchler, Gastroenterology, 115 (1998) 388.
39. B.O. Schneeman and R.L. Lyman, Proc. Soc. Exp. Biol. Med., 148 (1975) 897.
40. T. Fushiki, S. Fukuoka and K. Iwai, Agric. Biol. Chem., 48 (1984) 1867.
41. T. Fushiki, S. Fukuoka and K. Iwai, Biochem. Biophys. Res. Commun., 118 (1984) 532.
42. S. Fukuoka, M. Tsujikawa, T. Fushiki and K. Iwai, J. Nutr., 116 (1986) 1540.
43. I. Ihse, Scand. J. Gastroenterol., 11 (1976) 11.
44. J. F. Rehfeld. J. Biol. Chem., 253 (1978) 4016.
45. K. Miyasaka, D.F. Guan, R.A. Liddle and G.M. Green, Amer. J. Physiol., (1989) G175.
46. L. Lu, D. Louie and C. Owyang, Amer. J. Physiol., (1989) G430.
47. A.W. Spannagel, G.M. Green, D. Guan, R.A. Liddle, K. Faull and J.J. Reeve, Proc. Natl. Acad. Sci. USA., 93 (1996) 4415.
48. A.W. Spannagel, J.J. Reeve, R.A. Liddle, D. Guan and G.M. Green, Amer. J. Physiol., (1997) G754.
49. K. Miyasaka and A. Funakoshi, Pancreas, 15 (1997) 310.
50. N. Tarasova, A.W. Spannagel, G.M. Green, G. Gomez, J.T. Reed, J.C. Thompson, M.R. Hellmich, J.J. Reeve, R.A. Liddle and G.J. Greeley, Endocrinology, 138 (1997) 5550.
51. A.W. Spannagel, J.J. Reeve, G.J. Greeley, N. Yanaihara, R.A. Liddle and G.M. Green, Regul. Pept., 73 (1998) 161.
52. K.H. Herzig, I. Schon, K. Tatemoto, Y. Ohe, Y. Li, U.R. Folsch and C. Owyang, Proc. Natl. Acad. Sci. USA., 93 (1996) 7927.
53. G. Sun, K.Y. Lee, T.M. Chang and W.Y. Chey, Gastroenterology, 96 (1989) 1173.
54. P. Li, K.Y. Lee, T.M. Chang and W.Y. Chey, Amer. J. Physiol., (1990) G960.
55. P. Li, K.Y. Lee, X.S. Ren, T.M. Chang and W.Y. Chey, Gastroenterology, 98 (1990) 1642.
56. P. Li, K.Y. Lee, T.M. Chang and W.Y. Chey, J. Clin. Invest., 86 (1990) 1474.
57. K. Iwai, S. Fukuoka, T. Fushiki, M. Tsujikawa, M. Hirose, S. Tsunasawa and F. Sakiyama, J. Biol. Chem., 262 (1987) 8956.
58. K. Iwai, S. Fukuoka, T. Fushiki, T. Kodaira and N. Ikei, Biochem. Biophys. Res. Commun., 136 (1986) 701.
59. A. Horii, N. Tomita, H. Yokouchi, S. Doi, K. Uda, M. Ogawa, T. Mori and K. Matsubara, Biochem. Biophys. Res. Commun., 162 (1989) 151.

60. K. Miyasaka, A. Funakoshi, R. Nakamura, K. Kitani, K. Uda, A. Murata and M. Ogawa, Jpn. J. Physiol., 39 (1989) 891.
61. K. Miyasaka, R. Nakamura, A. Funakoshi and K. Kitani, Pancreas, 4 (1989) 139.
62. J.C. Cuber, G. Bernard, T. Fushiki, C. Bernard, R. Yamanishi, E. Sugimoto and J.A. Chayvialle, Amer. J. Physiol., (1990) G191.
63. E.P. Bouras, M.A. Misukonis and R.A. Liddle, Amer. J. Physiol., (1992) G791.
64. R.A. Liddle, Amer. J. Physiol., (1995) G319.
65. R. Yamanishi, J. Kotera, T. Fushiki, T. Soneda, T. Saitoh, T. Oomori, T. Satoh and E. Sugimoto, Biochem. J., (1993) 57.
66. T. Fushiki, H. Kajiura, S. Fukuoka, K. Kido, T. Semba and K. Iwai, J. Nutr., 119 (1989) 622.
67. K. Miyasaka and A. Funakoshi, Pancreas, 16 (1998) 277.
68. M. Fukayama, Y. Hayashi, M. Koike, M. Ogawa and G. Kosaki, J. Histochem. Cytochem., 34 (1986) 227.
69. H. Bohe, M. Bohe, C. Lindstrom and K. Ohlsson, J. Gastroenterol., 30 (1995) 90.
70. T. Marchbank, R. Chinery, A.M. Hanby, R. Poulsom, G. Elia and R.J. Playford, Amer. J. Pathol., 148 (1996) 715.
71. H. Bohe, M. Bohe, E. Lundberg, A. Polling and K. Ohlsson, J. Gastroenterol., 32 (1997) 623.

Biology of the Pancreas in Growing Animals
S.G. Pierzynowski and R. Zabielski (Editors)
© 1999 Elsevier Science B.V. All rights reserved.

261

Possible feedback mechanisms involved in exocrine pancreatic secretion in pigs and rats[*]

S.G. Pierzynowski [ab], S. Jakob[a+], K.H. Erlwanger[a#], S. Tsuzuki[c], T. Fushiki[c], P.C. Gregory[d], J.A.M. Botermans[e] and B.W. Weström[a]

[a]Dept of Animal Physiology, Lund University,
Helgonavägen 3B, SE-223 62, Lund, Sweden

[b]Gramineer International AB, Ideon, SE-223 70 Lund, Sweden

[c]Laboratory of Nutrition Chemistry, Division of Applied Life Sciences,
Graduate School of Agriculture, Kyoto University, Kyoto 606-8502, Japan

[d]Department of Pharmacology Research, Solvay Pharmaceuticals GmbH,
Hans-Böckler-Allee 20, D-30173 Hannover, Germany

[e]Department of Agricultural Biosystems and Technology, Swedish University of Agricultural
Sciences, P.O. Box 59, 230 53 Alnarp, Sweden

This paper presents the results of a series of experiments undertaken to test the hypothesis of the existence of unrecognised elements of regulatory feedback for the exocrine pancreas of pigs and rats.

In pigs, the preprandial pancreatic juice secretion was not affected by juice diversion or intraduodenal juice loading.The prandial secretion was reduced by intraduodenal and intraileal administration of non-activated juice and bile. Intravenous administration of trypsin significantly reduced the prandial protein and trypsin outputs in pigs and the effectiveness of exogenous CCK-33 in rats. One group of rats was infused with a constant dose of CCK-33 and the second group with a constant dose of secretin, 150 pmol in both cases, during 2 h. At the same time, the first group was infused with secretin (150 pmol) and the second group with CCK-33 (150 pmol) in increasing doses in the proportion 0:1:10:100, every 30 min. Total protein and trypsin activity outputs were higher in the second group.

There is a proved existence of feedback regulation of prandial pancreatic secretion in conscious pigs at the duodenal and ileal levels. The inhibition of pancreatic secretion in pigs

[*]This work was supported by the Swedish Council for Forestry and Agricultural Research and by the Swedish Institute (Visbyprogrammet 7391/1998(380/67). Current addresses: [+]Inst. Animal Nutrition, Hohenheim University, Stuttgart, Germany, [#]Department of Preclinical Veterinary Studies, University of Zimbabwe, Harare, Zimbabwe.

and desensitisation of pancreatic secretion to exogenous CCK-33 in rats by exogenous elevation of plasma trypsin concentrations indicate the presence of a trypsin-related feedback mechanism in the plasma, regulating the exocrine pancreas.

The results obtained from experiments on both rats and pigs encouraged us to speculate that the concerted action of the volume secreted and protein concentration of the pancreatic juice are factors governing the pancreatic protein outflow. However, it seems the volume of pancreatic juice secreted is the driving force in this process.

1. INTRODUCTION

A great number of experiments, often quite sophisticated, have confirmed the existence of feedback mechanisms controlling the exocrine pancreas in mammals. Studies on humans [1, 2,3,4,5] and on different animal models, including the pig [6,7,8], rat [9,10,11,12], calf [13], and dog [14,15,16] have been carried out.

It has been postulated that trypsin in the lumen of the proximal small intestinal exerts the discovered negative feedback mechanism [17,18]. There is strong evidence that this mechanism is linked with the release of cholecystokinin (CCK). Several have shown [9,12,19] that the diversion of pancreatic juice from the duodenum causes an increase in concentrations of CCK and pancreatic enzyme. In addition, if the trypsin activity is inhibited by aprotinin or soya bean trypsin inhibitors, the CCK level increases [9,12,20]. This explains why rats with exocrine pancreatic insufficiency and low protease concentrations have a 2.5-fold higher CCK level than control animals [21].

Fushiki et al. [22] and Miyasaka et al. [23] proposed that trypsin and trypsin inhibitors do not interact directly with the luminal surface of the small intestine, but that their actions are mediated by a trypsin-sensitive, CCK-releasing peptide originating in the pancreatic juice. Feedback regulation via CCK-releasing peptides has been described by a number of authors. Miyasaka et al. [24] described the purification of two different kinds of releasing peptides: the monitor peptide (MP) and the luminal CCK-releasing factor (LCRF).

A trypsin-sensitive CCK-releasing peptide was discovered and purified in rat pancreatic juice by Iwai et al. [25]. The authors showed that this "monitor peptide" has stimulatory activity on pancreatic secretion and postulated that it was a mediator of pancreatic enzyme secretion in response to dietary protein intake, playing an important role in the feedback control of the pancreas. During the preprandial phase, the peptide is hydrolysed by trypsin, and therefore no stimulatory effect on pancreatic enzyme secretion is observed. When food protein enters the lumen, in the postprandial phase, for instance, the trypsin is engaged in hydrolysing food or is inhibited, so the monitor peptide remains intact. The intact peptide stimulates the release of CCK into the circulation.

Another approach to this subject is feedback regulation via a peptide known as the intestinal releasing peptide. It is postulated that, like the monitor peptide, it stimulates CCK release. A CCK-releasing factor has been found which stimulates CCK secretion after protein or fat ingestion. Ingestion of trypsin inhibitors into the duodenum and diversion of the bile-pancreatic juice from the upper small bowel [5,27] abolished this effect. Moreover, Herzig [28] showed that somatostatin blocks CCK release by inhibiting the secretion and action of the CCK-releasing peptide. He isolated and characterised a CCK-releasing peptide identical to the porcine diazepam-binding inhibitor [29]. Intraduodenal infusion of this peptide stimulated amylase output and CCK release in rats, while the infusion of a CCK antagonist (MK-329) blocked the amylase output induced by the diazepam-binding inhibitor. Moreover, the authors showed that atropine administration blocked the secretion of this peptide in rats where it was previously found in the intestine.

In the last few years it has been shown that there are other hormones besides CCK involved in the feedback mechanism of exocrine pancreatic secretion. Chey *et al.* [30] and Herzig [31] suggest, on the basis of experimental evidence, the existence of a secretin-releasing peptide acting on pancreatic secretion. Guan *et al.* [32] showed that Peptide YY (PYY), whose release is stimulated by nutrients in the proximal and distal intestine and which inhibits pancreatic secretion, also plays an important role in the negative feedback control of pancreatic secretion. The authors stimulated the pancreatic secretion of rats by diversion of the pancreatic juice, resulting in a significant increase of PYY in the blood. This increase was paralleled by the pancreatic protein and fluid output.

Yet another mechanism of feedback regulation of the exocrine pancreas was proposed by Erlanson-Albertsson *et al.* [33], based on the luminal action of enterostatin. Enterostatin is a pentapeptide released during procolipase activation by trypsin, and probably exerts its inhibitory effect on pancreatic secretion from the distal intestine, since the lag time of enterostatin action after duodenal administration in conscious pigs is always about 0.5 h.

Finally, there are the gastric acid and bile secretion-related feedback mechanisms regulating the exocrine pancreas, described a long time ago [34,35]. They are very often ignored as important mechanisms affecting and modifying other classic feedback mechanisms related to pancreatic juice enzymes.

The question arises of whether there are further as-yet unrecognised feedback mechanisms controlling the exocrine pancreatic secretion. The main aim of the series of studies performed in our lab was to search for other such mechanisms.

2. RESULTS OF RECENT EXPERIMENTS IN OUR LABORATORY

2.1. Duodenal, ileal and blood-born feedback mechanisms controlling pancreatic secretion in pigs

Studies were performed with 10 crossbred 2–3-month-old (Swedish Landrace x Yorkshire x Hampshire) barrows weighing 15 ± 5 kg at surgery. The pigs were weaned at an age of 4 wk. and from the operation day they were adapted to live under 12h L/12h D cycles (lights on from approximately 08:00 to 20:00). During the dark period, lamps providing light with an intensity of 6 lux (at the eye level of the pigs) were used. The pigs were fed *ad libitum* between 10:00 – 11:00 and 13:00 – 17:00 hours daily with a standard diet for growing-finishing pigs (Slaktfoder, Läntmännen, Sweden, metabolizable energy, 12.6 MJ/kg; crude protein, 14.0 %; and lysine 8.5 g/kg).

Pigs were sedated with azaperone (Stresnil, LEO, Helsingborg, Sweden; 2 mg/kg BW, im), and anaesthetised with ketamine (Ketalar, Parke-Davis, Barcelona, Spain; 10 to 20 mg/kg BW, im) and pentobarbital (Mebumal, Nordvacc, Stockholm, Sweden; 5 to 10 mg/kg BW, iv). Surgery was performed under aseptic conditions.

Seven days after surgery, starting at 09:00 daily, 3-hour collections of pancreatic juice were made in overnight-fasted, freely-moving pigs. Each pig was subjected to two sessions of treatment. Two x 30 min preprandial collections, followed by 2 x 30 min prandial collections and 2 x 30 min. postprandial collections were made. During the prandial collection (between 10:00 and 11:00 h), food was offered *ad libitum*, and the amount of food consumed was measured. During prandial collections intraduodenal or intraileal infusions of the test substances (pancreatic juice, bile, saline) were given in two bolus portions of 7.5 ml/kg BW The first infusion was given directly after the food was offered, and the second 30 min later. The infusates were administered (manually by syringe) in two boluses, each lasting for approx. 5 min. The amount of the infusates per kg BW per hour was calculated to be not larger than twice the prandial pancreatic secretion obtained in our laboratory in previous experiments. After all experimental treatment with intestinal infusions had been completed, an iv bolus infusion of trypsin (Novo, Beagsvered, Denmark) diluted in saline was given (100 U/kg BW = 100 μg/kg BW, 2U/ml - expected to elevate the prandial blood trypsin level by 2-3 times) at the beginning of the prandial period in a similar experimental design as for id/il treatments.

After measurement of the volume, approximately 1.5 ml of the pancreatic juice was stored at -20°C for further analysis, while the remainder was pooled and saved.

To examine the differences between respective treatments, the integral (incremental) responses to certain treatments were calculated (e.g., the value from 1 h prandial minus the control value from 1 h preprandial secretion). The results were then evaluated with the unpaired Student t-test, or if the data came from populations with different SDs the nonparametric Wilcoxon test was used instead. The differences were recognised as significant when $P<0.05$. For statistical analysis InStat for Macintosh (version 2.03, GraphPad Software, San Diego, CA, USA) software was used.

Incremental/integral responses to feeding showed that food ingestion did not stimulate an increase in the volume of pancreatic juice, whereas it significantly stimulated the protein output and trypsin output in experiments with pigs. The differences between the incremental secretion during food ingestion (0.84 ml/kg/h) vs. food ingestion with intraduodenal (id) (1.66 ml/kg/h) or intraileal (il) (1.24 ml/kg/h) saline infusions were not statistically significant. However, there were significant differences between incremental prandial responses to id vs. il saline administration, with a higher prandial protein output int the letter (12.3 and 24.4 mg/kg/h, respectively).

The incremental trypsin response to food and ongoing id or il loading of pancreatic juice was lower; (1.6 and 8.8 U/kg/h) than the incremental response to food plus id/il NaCl; (10.3 and 15.2 U/kg/h respectively), while the decrease in incremental protein response was significantly lower after the id loading (12.3 vs. 3.5 mg/kg/h) and tended to be lower (24.4 vs. 11.4 mg/kg/h) after il loading of pancreatic juice.

The incremental pancreatic secretion showed that id bile did not affect feeding-stimulated volume, protein or trypsin secretion. Ileal bile administration significantly reduced prandial incremental secretion (0.03 ml/kg/h) as compared to prandial secretion during ileal saline administration. Comparison of the increments after il vs. id bile administration demonstrated a significantly lower trypsin response to food stimulation for il administration (5.6 vs. 18.0 U/kg/h).

Intravenous (iv) infusion of trypsin diminished the pancreatic response to food. Generally, the protein and trypsin output increments following iv trypsin infusion were significantly smaller compared to food ingestion or id/il saline administration (Table 1).

Table 1
Incremental prandial protein output and volume after iv trypsin infusion during food ingestion in pigs in comparison to id or il saline infusion (own, unpublished data)

	Protein output, mg/kg/h	Trypsin output, U/kg/h
Food vs. Trypsin iv	$15.9 > 4.5$, $p = 0.027$	$0.9 = 1.0$, $p = 0.097$
NaCl id vs. Trypsin iv	$12.3 > 4.5$, $p = 0.050$	$1.7 > 1.0$, $p = 0.020$
NaCl il vs. Trypsin iv	$24.4 > 4.5$, $p = 0.010$	$1.2 > 1.0$, $p = 0.020$

2.2. Preprandial, prandial and postprandial relations between volume and protein concentration in pancreatic juice

Studies were performed with 8 crossbred 2-3-month-old (Danish Landrace x Yorkshire x Hampshire and Swedish Landrace x Yorkshire x Hampshire) barrows weighing 14 ± 1 kg at surgery. The pigs were weaned at an age of 4 wk. and from the operation day they were adapted to live under 12h L/12h D cycles (lights on from approximately 07:00 to 19:00). During the dark period, lamps providing light with an intensity of 6 lux (at eye level for the pigs) were used. The pigs were fed *ad libitum* between 09:30 – 10:30 and 16:30 – 17:30 daily with a standard diet for growing-finishing pigs; metabolizable energy, 12.6 MJ/kg; crude protein, 14.0 % and lysine 8.5 g/kg.

Pigs were sedated with azaperone (Stresnil, LEO, Helsingborg, Sweden; 2 mg/kg BW, im), and anaesthetised with ketamine (Ketalar, Parke-Davis, Barcelona, Spain; 10 to 20 mg/kg BW, im) and pentobarbital (Mebumal, Nordvacc, Stockholm, Sweden; 5 to 10 mg/kg BW, iv). Surgery was performed under aseptic conditions.

Seven days after surgery, starting at 07:00 daily, 11-hour collections of pancreatic juice were made on freely-moving pigs. Pancreatic juice was collected at 1h intervals, except between 1.5 hours before and 1 hour after morning and evening feeding, when the interval was changed to 30 min. After the volume had been measured, 2 ml of pancreatic juice was removed and frozen for further analysis, while the rest was reintroduced into the duodenum at the rate of secretion, using syringe pumps.

As illustrated in Figure 1, the exocrine pancreatic secretion followed a specific pattern: the protein output (mg/h) increased immediately after consumption of the diet, resulting in a postprandial peak, and within 1.5 to 2 h it approached preprandial values again. However, when the volume outflow and the protein concentration (mg/ml) in the pancreatic juice were compared, a different rhythmic pattern could be observed. The volume outflow reached its maximum value 30 min after feed consumption, while the protein concentration reached its highest value 1.5 h after food intake, when the volume already had declined to an intermediate level or to even to the lowest level of secretion. The picture changed once more 2 to 3 h preprandially. Now the protein concentration was at its lowest level, while the volume outflow reached its highest peak. This relationship between the volume of pancreatic juice secreted and the concentration of pancreatic juice proteins/enzymes we named the "low-high, high-high and high-low" principle (Table 3).

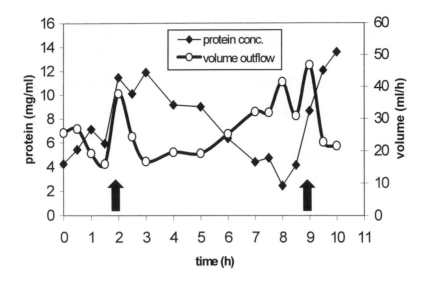

Figure 1. Rhythmic pattern of pancreatic juice protein concentration and volume outflow; arrows indicate feeding (Pierzynowski, unpublished).

2. 3. Relationship between blood trypsin and pancreatic juice secretion after stimulation with exogenous CCK and secretin in rats

Two groups (2 x 6) of male Sprague Dawley rats (350 - 380 g) were fasted overnight, anaesthetised (ketamine/azoperone) and fitted with jugular vein catheters (for trypsin and/or CCK + secretin infusions, each at 50 pmol/kg/h, Ferring) and common pancreatic-biliary duct catheters. The bile duct was ligated near the liver. After 30 min of stabilisation, both groups received the respective iv infusions and pancreatic juice was collected and not reintroduced to the duodenum in respective intervals: group I - 1 hour iv infusion of trypsin (500 mg/kg/h) + saline (always with 0.5 % BSA) followed by 1 hour infusion of trypsin + CCK-33/secretin; group II - 1 hour infusion of saline + saline, followed by 1 hour infusion of saline + CCK/secretin. The results were then evaluated with the unpaired Student t-test, or if the data came from populations with different SDs then the nonparametric Wilcoxon test was used instead. The differences were recognised as significant when $P<0.05$. For statistical analysis InStat for Macintosh (ver. 2.03, GraphPad Software, San Diego, CA, USA) software was used. Different letters indicate statistically significant differences, where $p<0.05$.

As shown in Table 2, there were no significant differences in protein output in rats after iv infusion of trypsin + saline or trypsin + CCK-33/secretin, or after the infusion of saline + saline. However, a significant ($p < 0.05$) increase in protein output of 45% above the control value was seen after iv saline + CCK/secretin.

With CCK-33/secretin infusion there was a significant ($p < 0.05$) increase in volume outflow compared to the control value, both after iv infusion of trypsin + CCK-33/secretin and after iv infusion of saline + CCK-33/secretin.

Table 2
Pancreatic protein output and volume secreted in anaesthetised rats during iv trypsin and CCK-33/secretin infusion (Pierzynowski, unpublished)

	Trypsin iv infusion group I		Saline iv infusion group II	
	1h	1h	1h	1h
	Saline + BSA	CCK/Secretin	Saline + BSA	CCK/Secretin
Protein output, mg/kg/h	129 ± 28^a	126 ± 36^a	120 ± 15^a	175 ± 17^b
Volume outflow, ml/kg/h	0.76 ± 0.13^a	1.20 ± 0.20^b	0.88 ± 0.11^{ab}	1.70 ± 0.18^c

2. 4. Concerted action of CCK-33 and secretin on the exocrine pancreas in rats - intrapancreatic feedback

Two groups (2 x 6) of male Sprague Dawley rats (250 – 270 g) were fasted overnight, anaesthetised (ketamine/azoperone) and fitted with jugular and common pancreatic-biliary duct catheters. The bile duct was ligated near the liver. After 30 min of stabilisation, the following treatment was given.

Both groups received equal doses of CCK-33 (150 pmol/kg), and secretin (150 pmol/kg), but applied in different manner. The first group was infused over a period of 2 hours with a constant dose of CCK-33 and the second group with a constant dose of secretin (75 pmol/kg/h). At the same time, the first group was infused with secretin and the second group with CCK-33 in increasing doses (0, 2.75, 27.5 and 275 pmol/kg/h) every 30 min. Pancreatic juice was collected and not reintroduced to the duodenum during 2 h of infusion plus 30 min postinfusion period. Stimulation of the exocrine pancreas with a steady infusion of CCK-33 and gradually increasing doses of secretin caused a mean protein output rate of 4.0 ± 0.5 mg/kg/h (mean $\pm$ SD) and mean trypsin activity output rate of 0.6 ± 0.09 U/kg/h. In experiments with steady infusion of secretin and increasing doses of CCK-33, the mean protein and trypsin output rates were 6.1 ± 1.4 mg/kg/h and 1.3 ± 0.3 U/kg/h, respectively.

The mean protein output rate was higher with steady infusion of secretin ($p < 0.05$). The mean trypsin activity output rate was also higher in this group ($p < 0.05$).

3. HYPOTHESIS

A number of different feedback mechanisms regulating exocrine pancreatic secretion have been described in different animal species. The presence of pancreatic juice in the intestine inhibits the exocrine pancreas via different kinds of monitor or releasing peptides [24, 25]. Most of these mechanisms are localized to the upper small bowel; few of them are found in the distal part of the small intestine (ileal brake) [27,40]. However, as stressed before, all of them are based on the presence of pancreatic juice (enzymes or electrolytes) in the intestinal lumen [5,22]. The mystery of pancreatic feedback begins when the pathways of enzyme/electrolyte action are examined individually.

Our studies were designed to explore the existence of unknown feedback mechanisms regulating the exocrine pancreas. We proved the existence of a prandial pancreatic juice-related feedback, both on the duodenal and ileal level, in pigs (valid also for bile). However, we could not prove the existence of a protein (trypsin/enzyme)-dependent interdigestive feedback in pigs.

On looking more closely at our data from long-term experiments on pigs and considering both volume and protein concentration in pancreatic juice in pigs, we discovered intriguing patterns of secretion. It seems that volume secretion and protein concentration in pigs, and especially the relationship between them, are extremely important, acting as an overall control mechanism, providing a stable protein output during the interdigestive phase and protecting the pancreas from oversecretion during the prandial phase (Table 3).

Table 3
Pattern of pancreatic protein concentration and volume outflow in pigs in long-term experiments

| | Preprandial | Prandial | Postprandial | Preprandial |
	2 - 3 h	0.5 - 1 h	3 - 4 h	2 – 3 h
Protein output	constant	stimulated	constant	constant
Protein conc.	low	high	high	low
Volume outflow	high	high	low	high

All the above indicates that there is a principle of precise regulation, with a stimulated protein/enzyme output at the time of food ingestion and a constant, reduced output during the interdigestive period. We can speculate that this type of regulation protects the pancreas from unnecessary enzyme secretion and the gastrointestinal tract from protein losses, and can probably only exist when the feeding frequency is optimal. The described principle of so-called intrapancreatic feedback was confirmed in acute experiments on rats. There we showed that infusion of the same amounts of hormones can result in different pancreatic secretion, depending on the administration scheme. The difference in protein output and trypsin activity output between the groups supports the hypothesis that animals given a constant high dose of secretin will not experience intrapancreatic inhibition of enzyme secretion from acinar cells, since the lumen will continuously be washed out by a secretin-induced flow of juice. Animals initially not given secretin experience a lower flow of juice, and consequently (compare with the high-low hypothesis in pigs) the concentration of protein in the lumen (or of specific inhibitory factors) will rise to levels inhibiting further enzyme secretion. The larger the dose of CCK infused, the less protein will be secreted per pmol of infused CCK. Our results support this postulation, and intrapancreatic feedback as a possible explanation for this phenomenon.

It is speculated that the output of protein was negatively affected by the high concentration of protein in the pancreatic juice. It could be that a specific protein is secreted into the pancreatic juice as soon as a threshold protein/enzyme concentration is reached in the pancreatic acini. The mechanism behind this is probably similar to that for the recently described protein [41] controlling milk production in the mammary gland - feedback inhibitor of lactation (FIL). FIL is synthesised in the epithelial cells of the mammary gland and acts as an autocrine inhibitor, blocking constitutive secretion in a concentration-dependent, reversible manner [42,43]. The concentration of protein *per se* can also inhibit protein secretion (inhibition via substrate). The volume of the pancreatic secretion can also be the limiting factor for protein secretion, by preparing a so-called diluting space for proteins secreted into the acinar cavity or via washout effects. The "high-low" mechanism in pigs and that now discussed in rats are probably of the same nature, based on intrapancreatic feedback. However, in the case of "high-low" regulation, neuro-hormonal signals from the intestinal lumen can play a trigger role.

Observations of blood-borne feedback regulatory mechanisms for the exocrine pancreas are more controversial, including the inhibition of prandial secretion in pigs by iv trypsin, and the stimulation of pancreatic secretion by infusion of exogenous hormones in rats. A possible explanation is the so-called "circulatory shock" and a reduction in pancreatic secretion caused by a reduction in the blood supply to the pancreas. However, we should remember that in the conscious pig, iv doses of trypsin were on a physiological level, only doubling the postprandial natural trypsin level in the blood and not effecting preprandial secretion (data not shown). Another possible explanation for how iv trypsin reduces pancreatic secretion is given indirectly by Fölsch [9] in his *in vitro* studies on a CCK assay. He postulated that in order to increase the sensitivity of the CCK assay, the CCK-33 released from the duodenum (intestine) needed to be converted to CCK-8 by trypsin. We need to consider that CCK-8 is the most powerful stimulant of the exocrine pancreas of the whole CCK family, via pancreatic CCK-A receptors. However, CCK-8 is not able to pass the liver to reach the pancreas, where it acts (CCK-33: 70% passes, CCK-8: less than 3% passes the liver). In this situation the trypsin degrades the natural or exogenously administered CCK-33 to CCK-8, which in turn is more quickly eliminated via the liver, resulting in weak effects on CCK-A receptors or none at all. Moreover, CCK-33 is a potent stimulator of afferent pathways of the vagal system according to the recently postulated local - intestinal action [44,45] on the exocrine pancreas, while CCK-8 is not (unpublished data). In favour of all this speculation, it is a fact that secretin action remained unchanged in the rats treated with trypsin. The above is not consistent with the recent [46] interpretation of a vagal dependency of the action of physiological doses of CCK on the exocrine pancreas. The postulation that physiological doses of CCK act via CCK-A receptors on vagal afferent pathways starting in the duodenum, while pharmacological doses act via CCK-A receptors in the pancreas, in synergy with local intrapancreatic cholinergic pathways, needs to be generally re-evaluated. Both doses affect levels of CCK equally, both in the pancreas and in the duodenum. One should consider the concentration of different forms of CCK in the place where they are formed, i.e. the duodenum, and factors e.g. trypsin, which can modify the relationship between them.

4. IMPLICATIONS

There are a number of different types of feedback mechanisms regulating the exocrine pancreas. As described above, these mechanisms can be of a complicated nature.

There is no doubt of the existence of a mechanism localised to the luminal side, and of a pancreatic juice and bile-dependent mechanism. However, intrapancreatic and blood-borne feedback mechanisms - probably pancreatic trypsin (protein)-dependent feedback mechanisms, also regulate exocrine pancreatic secretion, and can be of importance when the physiological role of CCK on the pancreas is discussed i.e. the complicated mechanism of a local, vagus-dependent effect vs. a systemic CCK-A receptor-mediated effect of CCK on the exocrine pancreas.

REFERENCES

1. G. Adler, A.G, Mullenhoff, A. Koop, T. Bozkurt, B. Goke, C. Beglinger and R. Arnold, Eur. J. Clin. Invest.,18 (1988) 98.
2. G. Adler, M. Reinshagen, I. Koop, B. Goke, A. Schafmayer, L.C. Rovati and R. Arnold, Gastroenterol., 96 (1989) 1158.
3. P. Layer, J.B. Jansen, L. Cherian, C.B. Lamers and H. Goebell, Gastroenterol., 98 (1990)1311.
4. C. Owyang, D.S. Louie and D.J. Tatum, Clin. Invest., 77 (1986) 2042.
5. C. Owyang. J. Nutr., 124 (1994) 1321S.
6. T. Houe, S.S. Saetre, P. Svendsen, O. Olsen, J.F. Rehfeld and O.B. Schaffalitzky de Muckadell, Sand. J. Gastroenterol., 32 (1997) 374.
7. T. Corring, J.A. Chayvialle, S.C. Nunes and J. Abello, Reprod. Nutr. Dev., 25 (1985) 439.
8. T. Corring, A.M. Gueugneau, J.A. Chayvialle, Reprod. Nutr. Dev., 26 (1986) 503.
9. U.R. Fölsch, P. Cantor, H.M. Wilms, A. Schafmayer, H.D. Becker and W. Creutzfeldt, Gastroenterol., 92 (1987) 449.
10. U.R. Fölsch, Eur. J. Clin. Invest., 20 Suppl 1 (1990) S40.
11. K. Kataoka, Gastroenterol. Jpn., 23 (1988) 292.
12. D.S. Louie, D. May, P. Miller, C. Owyang, Amer. J. Physiol., 250 (1986) G252.
13. R. Zabielski, S. Kato, S.G. Pierzynowski, H. Mineo, P. Podgurniak and W. Barej, Exp. Physiol., 77 (1992) 807.
14. M. Imamura, K.Y. Lee, Y. Song, M. Moriyasu, T.M. Chang and W.Y. Chey, Gastroenterology, 105 (1993)548
15. A. Schafmayer, R. Nustede and H. Kohler, Pancreas, 8 (1993) 627.
16. K. Shiratori K, Y.H. Jo, K.Y. Lee, T.M. Chang and W.Y. Chey, Gastroenterology, 96 (1989) 1330.
17. I. Ihse, P. Lilja and I. Lundquist, Scand, J. Gastroenterol., 14 (1979) 873.
18. A. Czajkowski and J. Długosz, Acta. Physiol. Pol., 40 (1989) 486.
19. A. Pusztai, G. Grant, S. Bardocz, K. Baintner, E. Gelencser and S.W. Ewen, Amer. J. Physiol., 272 (1997) G340.
20. J.E. Reseland, H. Holm, T. Jenssen, M.B. Jacobsen and L.E. Hanssen, Scand. J. Gastroenterol., 30 (1995) 72.
21. U.R. Fölsch, A. Schafmayer, R. Ebert, H.D. Becker and W. Creutzfeldt, Digestion, 29 (1984) 60.
22. T. Fushiki and K. Iwai, FASEB J., 3 (1989) 121.
23. K. Miyasaka, D.F. Guan, R.A. Liddle and G.M. Green, Amer. J. Physiol., 257 (1989) G175.

24. K. Miyasaka and A. Funakoshi, Pancreas, 16 (1998) 277.
25. K. Iwai, S. Fukuoka, T. Fushiki T.M. Tsujikawa, M. Hirose, S. Tsunasawa, and F. Sakiyama. J. Biol. Chem., 262 (1987) 8956.
26. T. Kinouchi, S. Tsuzuki, C. Minami, Y. Hayashi, E. Sugimoto and T. Fushiki, Amer. J. Physiol., 272 (1997) G794.
27. R.A. Liddle, Amer. J. Physiol., 269 (1995) G319.
28. K.H. Herzig, D.S. Louie and C. Owyang, Amer. J. Physiol., 266 (1994) G1156.
29. K.H. Herzig, I. Schon, K. Tatemoto, Y. Ohe, Y. Li, U.R. Folsch, and C. Owyang [published erratum appears in Proc. Natl. Acad. Sci.,93 (1996) 14214]. Proc. Natl. Acad. Sci., 93 (1996) 7927.
30. W.Y. Chey, P. Li, H. Jin, Y.K. Lee and T.M. Chang, Biomed. Res., 15 (1994)151.
31. K.H. Herzig, Reg. Pep., 73 (1998) 89.
32. D. Guan, I.L. Maouyo, A. Taylor, T.W. Gettys, G.H. Greeley, Jr. and J. Morisset, Endocrinol., 128 (1991) 911.
33. C. Erlanson-Albertsson, B.R. Weström, S.G. Pierzynowski, S. Karlsson and B. Ahren. Pancreas, 16 (1991)619.
34. G. Gomez, F. Lluis, Y.S. Guo, G.H. Greeley, Jr., C.M. Townsend, Jr. and J.C. Thompson, Surgery, 100 (1986) 363.
35. G. Gomez, J.R. Upp, Jr., F. Lluis, R. W. Alexander, G. J. Poston, G.H. Greeley, Jr. and J.C. Thompson, Gastroenterology, 94 (1988)1036.
36. S.G. Pierzynowski, B.-R. Weström, B.W. Karlsson, J. Svendsen and B. Nilsson, Can. J. Anim. Sci., 68 (1988) 953.
37. M.-J. Thaela, S.G. Pierzynowski, M.S. Jensen, K. Jakobsen, B.W. Weström and B.W. Karlson, J. Anim. Sci., 73 (1995) 3402.
38. O.H. Lowry, N. Rosenbrough, A. Farr and R.J. Randall, J. Biol. Chem., 265 (1951) 265.
39. S.G. Pierzynowski, J. Anim. Physiol. Anim. Nutr., 63 (1990) 198.
40. H.C. Lin, X.T. Zhao and L. Wang, Dig. Dis. Sci., 42 (1997) 19.
41. C.J. Wilde, C.V. Addey, L.M. Boddy and M. Peaker, Biochem. J., 305 (1995) 51.
42. M.E. Rennison, M. Kerr, C.V. Addey, S. E. Handel, M.D. Turner, C.J. Wilde, and R.D. Burgoyne, J. Cell Sci.,106 (1993) 641.
43. C.J. Wilde, L.H. Quarrie, E.Tonner, D.J. Flint and M. Peaker, Livest. Prod. Sci., 50 (1997) 29.
44. S.G. Pierzynowski, H. Mårtensson, B.W. Weström, B. Ahrén, K.Uvnäs-Möberg and B.W. Karlsson, Biomed. Res., 14 (1993) 217.
45. P. Kiela, R. Zabielski, P. Podgurniak, M. Midura, P.C. Gregory, W. Barej, and S.G. Pierzynowski, Exp. Physiol., 81 (1996) 375.
46. C. Owyang, Amer. J. Physiol., 34 (1996) G1.

Biology of the Pancreas in Growing Animals
S.G. Pierzynowski and R. Zabielski (Editors)

273

Phytohaemagglutinin stimulates pancreatic enzyme secretion in rats by a combination of cholecystokinin- and noncholecystokinin-linked pathways

A. Pusztai*

The Rowett Research Institute, Bucksburn, Aberdeen, AB21 9SB, Scotland, UK

Kidney bean (*Phaseolus vulgaris*) E_2L_2 lectin (PHA) given orally to rats or continually infused into the duodenum of both anaesthetised and conscious rats stimulated the secretion of cholecystokinin (CCK) from gut enteroendocrine (I) cells and of digestive enzymes from the pancreas. PHA also stimulated the release of CCK from duodenal I cells *in vitro*. The pancreatic secretory response to PHA in the early stages was mainly independent of CCK mediation. At later stages, additional mechanisms, not directly involving CCK, also appeared to play a role in modulating exocrine pancreatic responses to PHA. In addition to its effects of CCK-secreting I cells, PHA could stimulate or inhibit the release of other gut hormones which are important in overall regulation of exocrine pancreatic metabolism. As a result the PHA-induced CCK release and pancreatic growth could be effectively uncoupled from the synthesis of digestive enzymes in the pancreas and their secretion into the duodenum. In addition, systemically absorbed PHA may also have some slight role in directly triggering enzyme secretion from pancreatic acini. All these PHA effects were in contrast to the known CCK-mediated stimulatory effects of soya bean trypsin inhibitors, which were fully abolished after treatment with L-364718.

1. INTRODUCTION

The primary responses of the rat pancreas to food proteins in rats are mediated via the hormone cholecystokinin (CCK) which is produced by entero/neuroendocrine (I) cells in the gastrointestinal tract [1,2]. CCK is secreted into the circulation by the I cells when undigested nutrients or other dietary stimulating factors are present in the small intestine. The hormone binds to pancreatic and/or neural receptors and triggers the release of pancreatic pro-enzymes and enzymes into the duodenal lumen. Once the food is digested, secretion of CCK and pancreatic enzymes returns to basal levels. These responses are therefore usually rapid and transient. In contrast, some bioactive components of plant-based foodstuffs such as lectins, inhibitors of proteases and other proteinaceous factors can trigger the release of gut regulatory peptides, including CCK, in a more direct and sustained fashion as a result of their interaction

---

* *Present address: 6 Ashley Park North, Aberdeen AB10 6SF; Phone/fax: 44-1224-594954.
This work was supported by the Scottish Office Agriculture, Environment and Fisheries Department and was part of the COST 98 European Programme.

with the gut epithelium and/or luminal enzymes [3-5].

The powerful CCK-mediated trophic effects of trypsin/chymotrypsin inhibitors incorporated into the diet on the pancreas and their interference with the regulatory control of CCK secretion have been studied extensively [4,6-8]. Thus, protease inhibitors [4] or their protease complexes [8] induce rapid CCK-mediated pancreatic enlargement and hypersecretion of proenzymes and enzymes from pancreatic acini, but no gut growth [8,9]. More recently some lectins were shown to be trophic for the acinar pancreas [for references see 7]. Thus, feeding rats on diets containing such lectins for 10 days significantly enlarged their pancreas. As this effect was apparently abolished by pre-treatment of the rats with CCK-A receptor antagonists it was suggested that stimulation of the growth of the pancreas by lectins is possibly CCK-mediated, in contrast to that of the gut which is apparently not [10]. The acute duodenal administration of lectins from soya bean (*Glycine max*), wheat (*Triticum vulgare*) germ and peanut (*Arachis hypogeae*) was also shown to induce the release of CCK and increase protein secretion by the pancreas in anaesthetised rats [11,12]. This secretory response was abolished by L-364718. Similarly, kidney bean (*Phaseolus vulgaris*) phytohaemagglutinin (PHA) induced the release of CCK from duodenal I cells both *in vitro* and *in vivo* [10] and in rats fed diets containing PHA there was a highly significant enlargement of the acinar pancreas. Moreover, the trophic effects of PHA on the rat pancreas were significantly reduced by simultaneous treatment of the rats with a CCK-A receptor antagonist. Although the growth of the pancreas was only inhibited by 72% at the dose of L-364718 used (0.18 mg/kg body weight), this was in agreement with published data [13]. Moreover, the inhibition was comparable to that obtained with rats given soya (Kunitz) trypsin inhibitor (69%) as a positive control group [10]. It was therefore concluded that the stimulatory effects of lectins on exocrine pancreatic metabolism were mainly if not exclusively mediated via a CCK-dependent pathway. Furthermore, the PHA effect in pancreatic duct cannulated conscious rats was also abolished by the CCK-A receptor antagonist L-346718 [14], supporting the idea that under normal physiological conditions CCK-mediation might indeed be the major, and possibly the only pathway for the mediation of the PHA stimulus. In the light of this the recently published evidence that the acute pancreatic stimulatory effects of PHA and the release of trypsinogen, chymotrypsinogen and α-amylase from the pancreas in halothane-anaesthetised rats were not fully abolished by L-346718 [15] suggested that in anaesthetised rats the PHA effect and its inhibition by CCK-A receptor analogues might be critically dependent on the anaesthetics used. That this was indeed so was supported by the finding that, in contrast to halothane anaesthesia, in urethane-anaesthetised rats in which the negative feed-back mechanism did not operate, PHA did not induce pancreatic secretion [14]. Therefore in the present review these and other data are critically examined together with some recently obtained new data on stimulation of CCK secretion from duodenal I cells *in vitro* and on the acute *in vivo* effects of pure PHA E2L2 lectin, and discussed in comparison with the similar effects of soya bean Kunitz (trypsin) inhibitor, KTI.

2. MATERIALS AND METHODS

Cholecystokinin-8, rabbit anti-CCK-8 antibody, bovine trypsin, bovine chymotrypsin, porcine pancreatic α-amylase, bovine enterokinase, N-α-benzoyl-DL-arginine-p-nitroanilide (BAPNA), glutaryl-L-phenylalanine-p-nitroanilide (GAPNA) and soluble potato starch were purchased from Sigma Aldrich (Poole, Dorset, UK) and ^{125}I labelled CCK-8 from Amersham International

(Little Chalfont, Buckinghamshire, UK). Kidney bean E_2L_2 lectin and soya bean Kunitz (trypsin) inhibitor were prepared as before [16,17] and α-amylase inhibitor was purified from kidney beans [18]. The CCK-A receptor antagonist L-364718 was a gift from Merck Sharp and Dohme (West Point, DA, USA).

2.1. Animal experiments

All management and experimental procedures were in strict accordance with the requirements of the UK Animals (Scientific Procedures) Act 1986.

Experiment 1

Pancreatic secretion studies with anaesthetised male Hooded-Lister rats (150-200 g) were carried out essentially as before [8]. After feeding the rats on a lactalbumin (LA) control diet for 4 days, they were fasted overnight and anaesthetised with Halothane (Rhone Merieux, Dublin). The abdominal cavity was opened, and the pancreatic duct cannulated close to its junction with the duodenum, approximately 1.5 cm below the pylorus. Body temperature was monitored and maintained at 36-37°C and, to keep the peritoneal cavity moist, 1.5 ml of saline was injected at hourly intervals. The pancreatic/bile juice was not returned to the intestine. Instead, a bile acid/trypsin solution (50 mM $NaHCO_3$, 78 μM Na taurocholate and 0.5 mg trypsin/ml) [19] was infused into the duodenum at a rate of 0.7 ml/h. After a 1 h basal period, bile acid/trypsin solution containing soya bean Kunitz (trypsin) inhibitor (KTI) or kidney bean E_2L_2 lectin (PHA) was infused into the duodenum at a rate of 0.7 ml/h for 2.5 h. Stock solutions of KTI and PHA were prepared so that the total amount administered was: KTI, 1.5 mg/h and PHA, 0.5 mg/h, 1.0 mg/h, 2.0 mg/h or 4.0 mg/h. Secretions were collected on ice in preweighed tubes over 30-min intervals during the basal and test periods. Rats treated with the CCK-A receptor antagonist L-364718 were subcutaneously injected with 1 ml of a methyl cellulose suspension (5 mg/ml) containing 200 μg of the antagonist 30 min before commencement of the test infusions. Controls were injected with 1 ml of the carrier.

Experiment 2

Male Hooded-Lister rats (80-85 g) were fed a control diet for 4 days. The amount of food provided was 7 g/rat d^{-1} divided into 3 feeds. On the fourth day, half the rats were given 100 μg of L-364718 mixed in the 7 g of diet. Next morning, these rats were injected subcutaneously with 1 ml of a methyl cellulose suspension (5 mg/ml) containing 50 μg of the antagonist. The remaining rats were injected with 1 ml of the carrier. Thirty min later the rats were given 1 ml of saline (9 g NaCl/l) containing 5 mg of bovine gamma globulin, KTI or PHA by gavage. After 2 h, the rats were killed by halothane overdose and exsanguination, the stomach and small intestine were removed and their contents flushed out with ice-cold saline and snap frozen. The pancreas was also removed, snap frozen and extracted as before [8]. Trypsin, chymotrypsin and α-amylase levels in pancreatic extracts, intestinal washes and pancreatic secretions were estimated using BAPNA, GAPNA and soluble potato starch, respectively, as substrates and bovine trypsin, bovine chymotrypsin and porcine pancreatic α-amylase as standards [8,18]. Enzyme activities were expressed as mg enzyme per total intestinal content or per pancreas and as μg enzyme secreted per 30 min. Trypsinogen and chymotrypsinogen were activated with enterokinase (6 g/l in 50 mM sodium citrate buffer pH 5.8; zymogen:enterokinase, 1:3 (v/v) for pancreatic extracts and 1:20 (v/v) for pancreatic secretions) at 37°C for 30 or 60 min respectively [8].

Experiment 3

Groups of rats (5 rats per group) were fed a lactalbumin control diet or a control diet into which PHA or KTI or α-amylase inhibitor was incorporated at the level of 0.7% w/w of the diet. Rats were pair-fed for 10 days with 6 g of these diets, ensuring that the daily intake of PHA or KTI or α-amylase inhibitor was 42 mg. Rats were blood sampled before the start and at the end of the experiment for CCK determination. After killing and dissection the gut contents were washed out with saline; the washings and the pancreas were immediately frozen and used for estimating trypsinogen, chymotrypsinogen and α-amylase content

Experiment 4

Male Hooded-Lister rats (85-90 g) were given a control diet (7 g/rat d^{-1}) for 4 days. Next morning, the rats were given 1 ml of saline containing 5 mg of bovine gamma globulin, KTI or PHA by gavage. Exactly 2 h later the rats were killed by halothane overdose and exsanguination, the small intestine was removed, the contents flushed out with ice-cold saline and 20 cm of tissue (5-25 cm from the pylorus) was snap frozen. CCK was extracted from small intestine tissues with a water and acetic acid extraction procedure [20] and determined by a bioassay procedure using dispersed pancreatic acini prepared from the pancreas of female Hooded-Lister rats [21] or by radioimmunoassay [22] using rabbit anti-CCK-8 antibody.

Experiment 5

Male Hooded-Lister rats (150 g) were fed a control diet (15 g diet/rat d^{-1}) for 4 days and then fasted overnight. Four rats were killed by halothane overdose and exsanguination, 40 cm of small intestine removed from each (0-40 cm from the pylorus) and the contents flushed out with saline. Each intestinal piece was cut open and a mucosal scraping collected and incubated in 60 ml oxygenated Krebs-Henseleit bicarbonate buffer containing mixed amino acids and 2.5 mM EDTA [23] for 10 min at 37°C. The preparation was centrifuged (350 g x 3 min) and the supernatant discarded. The pellet was resuspended in 8 ml of an oxygenated HEPES buffer [23], separated into 1 ml aliquots and incubated at 37°C for 15 min. The preparations were recentrifuged (350 g x 3 min) and the supernatants discarded.

The pellets were resuspended in 1 ml of oxygenated HEPES buffer or in buffer containing PHA, PHA + fetuin, or KCl, incubated for 30 min at 37°C and centrifuged (350 g x 3 min). The supernatants were collected and snap frozen. The pellets were resuspended in 1 ml of buffer, incubated for 30 min at 37°C, centrifuged (350 g x 3 min), and the supernatants collected and frozen.

3.2. Statistical analysis

For statistical evaluation, one-way analysis of variance in combination with the Tukey test was carried out using the Instat Statistical Package (GraphPad Software Inc, San Diego, California).

4. RESULTS

Kidney bean E$_2$L$_2$ lectin (PHA) infused into the duodenum of anaesthetised rats induced a dose- and time-dependent secretion of pancreatic digestive enzymes (Figure 1). Rats were fitted with duodenal and bile/pancreatic duct cannulae to allow administration of PHA and collection

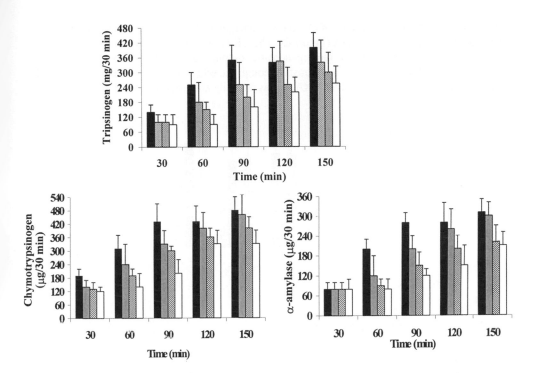

Figure 1. Pancreatic enzyme outputs by anaesthetised rats given kidney bean lectin (PHA) by infusion into the duodenum. Filled bars, PHA 4.0 mg/h; hatched bars, PHA 2.0 mg/h; cross-hatched bars, PHA 1.0 mg/h; open bars, 0.5 mg PHA/h.

of secretions. Trypsinogen and chymotrypsinogen were activated with enterokinase.

Thus, α-amylase, trypsinogen and chymotrypsinogen outputs by rats given 4.0 mg PHA/h was maximal at 90 min, almost 260% above basal rates, and remained at this level. In rats infused with 2.0, 1.0 or 0.5 mg PHA/h the secretion of α-amylase (and the two proteases) was less extensive, approximately 163%, 88% and 37% above the basal rate, respectively, at the same time point. However, in these rats secretion increased further with time; at 1 and 2 mg PHA/h it was close to maximal (240-260% above basal rate) at 120 and 150 min. Even at the lowest PHA dose (0.5 mg/h), which had no effect on pancreatic enzyme secretion at 60 min and only a limited effect at 90 min (37% above basal value), trypsinogen, chymotrypsinogen and α-amylase outputs had increased to around 160% above basal rates by 150 min after duodenal infusion of PHA. Soya bean trypsin inhibitor (KTI) infused at a rate of 1.5 mg/h into the duodenum of anaesthetised rats induced the secretion of pancreatic digestive enzymes (Figure 2). Secretion was maximal after 90 min and persisted at this level for the remainder of the study.

Pre-treatment of rats with the CCK-A receptor antagonist L-364718 had varying effects on pancreatic responses to KTI or PHA (Figure 2). Thus, KTI did not stimulate pancreatic secretion in rats given the antagonist. In fact, pancreatic outputs by these rats were lower than basal values at 120 and 150 min. In contrast, although the rate of enzyme secretion was greatly reduced by the antagonist in rats given PHA, it was not fully abolished.

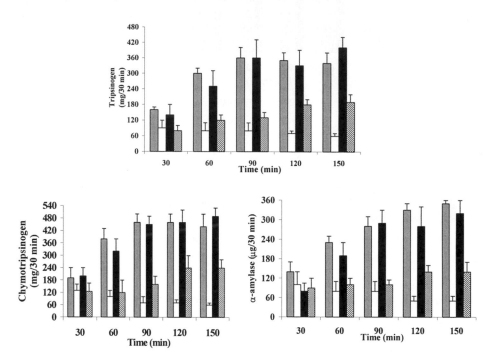

Figure 2. Pancreatic enzyme outputs by anaesthetised rats duodenally infused with kidney bean lectin (PHA; 4.0 mg/h) or soya bean Kunitz (trypsin) inhibitor (KTI; 1.5 mg/h), with or without pre-treatment with the CCK-A receptor antagonist L-364718. Secretions were collected via a bile/pancreatic duct cannula. Trypsinogen and chymotrypsinogen were activated with enterokinase. Hatched bars, KTI; open bars, KTI + L-364718; solid bars, PHA; cross-hatched bars, PHA + L-364718.

Trypsin and α-amylase levels in the lumen of the small intestine were significantly elevated 2 h after rats had been given a single oral dose of PHA or KTI (Experiment 2; Table 1). Intestinal chymotrypsin levels were also increased on KTI administration but reduced in rats which had been given PHA. There was no change in duodenal enzyme levels in rats gavaged with α-amylase inhibitor. PHA or KTI did not affect the amounts of trypsinogen and chymotrypsinogen in the pancreas (Table 1). However, PHA-treatment did cause a reduction in pancreatic α-amylase, even after 2 h of treatment, probably mirroring its high rate of secretion into the intestine. KTI did not significantly alter pancreatic α-amylase levels.

The amounts of trypsin, chymotrypsin and α-amylase detected in the intestinal contents of rats given PHA by gavage were not significantly altered by pre-treatment of the animals with L-364718 (Experiment 2; Table 1). In contrast, intestinal enzyme levels in those dosed with KTI were significantly reduced by prior administration of the antagonist and not significantly different from those in unstimulated controls with or without L-364718 (Table 1).

Table 1
Pancreatic and small intestine enzyme levels (mg/small intestine) in rats 2 h after being given a single oral dose of saline (1 ml) containing 5 mg bovine gamma globulin (control), kidney bean lectin (PHA) or soya bean Kunitz trypsin inhibitor alone or in combination with the CCK A-receptor antagonist L-364718 given by intraperitoneal injection.

	Control		PHA		KTI	
	-*	+	-	+	-	+
Small intestine						
Trypsin	0.8 ± 0.1^a	0.8 ± 0.1^a	1.3 ± 0.2^b	1.1 ± 0.1^b	1.1 ± 0.2^b	0.6 ± 0.3^a
Chymotrypsin	1.0 ± 0.1^a	0.9 ± 0.1^a	0.4 ± 0.1^b	0.4 ± 0.1^b	1.8 ± 0.3^c	1.2 ± 0.2^a
Amylase	0.03 ± 0.0^a	0.04 ± 0.03^a	0.7 ± 0.2^b	0.5 ± 0.1^b	0.3 ± 0.1^c	0.01 ± 0.0^a
Pancreas						
Trypsinogen	2.5 ± 0.3^a	2.4 ± 0.1^a	2.3 ± 0.2^a	2.3 ± 0.1^a	2.3 ± 0.1^a	2.2 ± 0.2^a
Chymo-Trypsinogen	9.3 ± 0.3^a	9.6 ± 0.3^a	9.5 ± 0.4^a	9.4 ± 0.4^a	8.9 ± 0.3^a	9.0 ± 0.1^a
Amylase	2.0 ± 0.3^a	1.6 ± 0.4^a	1.1 ± 0.3^b	1.3 ± 0.4^{ab}	1.5 ± 0.3^a	2.2 ± 0.3^a

Values in a horizontal row with distinct superscripts differ significantly ($P<0.05$).
* Without or with L-364718

After 10 days' dietary exposure (Experiment 3) both PHA and KTI but not α-amylase inhibitor significantly increased the weight of the pancreas and its protein and DNA contents (Figure 3) and, as previously, plasma CCK levels were elevated (results not given). Pancreatic growth was abolished by L-364718. Similar to the significant elevation in duodenal enzyme levels after a single acute dose of KTI, the concentration of pancreatic enzymes in the duodenum remained high even after 10 days on diets containing KTI in comparison with control rats. The increase in pancreatic weight and protein content induced by KTI was also reflected in the significantly increased amounts of chymotrypsinogen and trypsinogen but not α-amylase in the pancreas of rats exposed to

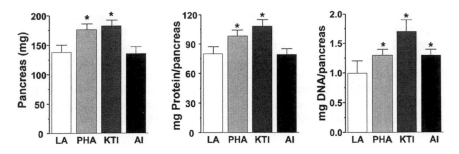

Figure 3. Dry weight, protein and DNA contents of the pancreas of rats fed a control (LA) diet or a control diet containing 0.7% PHA, KTI or α-amylase inhibitor (αAI) for 10 days.

KTI in the diet for 10 days (Figure 4). In contrast, with PHA in the diet both duodenal and pancreatic enzyme levels returned to control values after feeding for 10days, or in the case of α-amylase, amounts in the pancreas decreased to well below that of control rats. Pancreatic enzyme levels, except the increase in trypsin levels, were not significantly affected by feeding rats on diets containing our preparation of α-amylase inhibitor. However, as this sample contained 7% w/w trypsin inhibitor [18] the elevation in trypsin was probably due to this contamination. Jejunal tissue (20 cm) from control rats contained 58 ± 9 pmoles of CCK. This was reduced to 36 ± 7 pmoles CCK in rats dosed with PHA and 39 ± 6 pmoles CCK in rats given KTI (Experiment 4).

Table 2
Secretion of CCK (fmoles/30 min) from jejunal mucosa cell preparations treated with PHA, PHA + fetuin or KCl

	Treatment	
	Stimulus or buffer	Buffer
	0-30 min	30-60 min
Basal	70 ± 20^{a}	78 ± 23^{a}
PHA (10 ng)	113 ± 25^{a}	160 ± 38^{b}
PHA (100 ng)	140 ± 30^{a}	232 ± 37^{b}
PHA (100 ng)+fetuin (1μg)	92 ± 20^{a}	89 ± 30^{a}
KCl (4 mg)	188 ± 35^{b}	100 ± 25^{a}

Values in a vertical row with distinct superscripts differ significantly (P<0.05).

PHA stimulated the secretion of CCK from intestinal cells *in vitro* (Experiment 5; Table 2). The response was dose-dependent and could be fully inhibited by inclusion of fetuin in the medium. CCK-release persisted when the cells were subsequently incubated with buffer alone. In contrast, CCK-secretion by KCl rapidly diminished in the absence of the stimulus (Table 2).

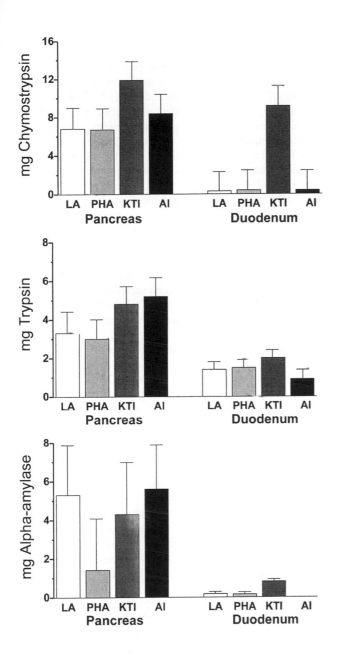

Figure 4. Chymotrypsin, trypsin and α-amylase content of pancreas and duodenum of rats fed control (LA) diet or control diet containing 0.7% PHA, KTI or α-amylase inhibitor (αAI) for 10 days.

5. DISCUSSION

Chronic (10-day) feeding of rats with diets containing PHA has previously been shown to result in increased levels of CCK in the blood and rapid hypertrophic and hyperplastic growth of the pancreas [3,10,17] both of which were abolished by L-364718. This was confirmed in the present work, indicating that, similar to the effect of KTI, the trophic effect of PHA in conscious rats fed on diets containing this lectin and under normal physiological conditions was mediated via a CCK-related mechanism. This received further, albeit indirect, support from the finding that even on first-time exposure, within 2 h of the administration of PHA by gavage into the duodenum of conscious rats, the CCK content of the proximal gut tissue was significantly reduced, raising the possibility that the ensuing hypersecretion of digestive enzymes from the exocrine pancreas may indeed have been caused by CCK [15]. Direct experimental evidence for the involvement of CCK as the main, if not the only, mediator of pancreatic enzyme secretion was also provided by the fact that L-364178 also abolished this secretion in conscious rats stimulated by oral PHA [14].

The CCK-mediation of the lectin effect on the pancreas was further supported by the recent findings that lectins from soya bean (SBA), wheat germ (WGA) and peanut (PNA) also increased the levels of CCK in circulation and stimulated pancreatic secretion of proteins when administered on a short-term basis to rats; and that this effect was abolished by pre-treatment with L-364718 [11,12]. It is thus possible that lectins may all act on the pancreas by a similar CCK-dependent mechanism.

The results of measurement of enzyme levels in the pancreas or in the duodenum of rats stimulated by short-term or long-term dietary exposure to PHA, however, could not easily be fitted into the above mechanism, particularly when compared with those in KTI-stimulated rats which are strictly CCK-dependent. Thus, in agreement with what is generally found, duodenal enzyme levels were found to have increased, both on acute exposure and after 10 days' feeding with diets containing KTI in the present work. Moreover, the increase could be abolished by pre-administration of L-364718. Enzyme levels in the pancreas were not affected in the short term but were significantly increased after 10 days' feeding with KTI and this could also be blocked by the CCK-A receptor antagonist.

On acute exposure to PHA, as with rats stimulated by KTI, the levels of trypsin and α-amylase but not of chymotrypsin in the duodenum were increased over those in control rats. The α-amylase content of the duodenum was particularly high. As a result, after 2 h exposure to PHA, α-amylase levels (but not levels of the other enzymes) in the pancreas were significantly reduced, probably mirroring the high secretion rate of this enzyme in PHA-stimulated rats. As none of these alterations in enzyme levels were affected by the CCK-A receptor analogue, the early stages of the PHA stimulation were apparently not mediated by CCK but some other unknown mechanism.

Further complications arose when diets containing PHA were fed to rats for 10 days. In contrast to the situation in KTI stimulation, the total trypsinogen and chymotrypsinogen contents of the pancreas remained similar to those in control, unstimulated rats. Moreover, the α-amylase content of the pancreas after 10 days' dietary exposure to PHA was severely reduced - so much so that the α-amylase band became undetectable by SDS-gel electrophoresis in the duodenum of these rats [Pusztai, unpublished]. Thus, although PHA was able to stimulate pancreatic growth and increase its protein and DNA contents, and that this was abolished by L-364718, in contrast to that found with KTI, PHA did not stimulate the synthesis and accretion of digestive enzymes in the pancreas. On the contrary, their concentration was in fact reduced after 10 days on PHA in the diet, particularly that of the α-amylase. This suggests that although PHA induces a short-lived and non-CCK-mediated increase in the concentration of digestive enzymes in the duodenum on acute exposure, this lectin does not stimulate the secretion of pancreatic enzymes in the long term. Whether this is due to the observed slight inhibition of the synthesis of the pancreatic proteases or a more extensive blocking of the synthesis of α-amylase, or whether it is due to direct/indirect interference by PHA with the secretion process (mediated by gut regulatory peptides other than CCK), is unclear. However, the complexity of all these possible mechanisms makes it difficult, at least for the time being, to confirm or reject any CCK mediation in the changes in enzyme levels induced by PHA, particularly on long-term dietary exposure to this lectin.

In anaesthetised rats the involvement of CCK as mediator of the PHA stimulus was also complex, particularly in relation to the effect of KTI. Thus, pre-treatment of rats with the CCK-A receptor antagonist, L-364718, reduced but did not abolish the stimulatory effects of PHA on pancreatic digestive enzyme output in halothane-anaesthetised rats (Figure 2; [15]), whereas, as before [8], it fully inhibited the secretory response of the rat pancreas to soya bean KTI. This again suggests that the acute exocrine pancreatic responses to PHA, unlike those to KTI, are probably mediated only in part by CCK in halothane-anaesthetised rats. However, as the extent of stimulation of pancreatic enzyme secretion in anaesthetised rats is dependent on the anaesthetics used, the results of such studies need to be interpreted with caution. This was clearly shown; in rats anaesthetised with urethane, which is known to abolish the negative feed-back mechanism, instead of halothane, PHA did not stimulate pancreatic secretion [14].

CCK release from neuroendocrine (I) cells appears to be triggered through a number of different mechanisms, depending on the nature of food components in the gut lumen [1,2]. I cell responses to proteins are thought to be induced by trypsin-sensitive CCK-releasing peptides which are continuously released from the intestine and pancreas [6,24,25], bind to receptors on the I cells and stimulate CCK release. It has often been suggested that in the absence of protein in the duodenum, the CCK-releasing peptides are rapidly degraded by luminal trypsin and therefore the I cells are not stimulated in the absence of food in the duodenum. Thus, protease inhibitors, such as KTI, working through a negative feedback system are generally believed to interfere with this regulation of CCK release by preventing degradation of the CCK-releasing peptides by trypsin [6,25]. As a result prolonged secretion of CCK occurs. However, an alternative or concurrent mechanism is also possible. Recent studies have suggested that it is trypsin/chymotrypsin bound by the membranes of I cells that triggers the secretion of CCK, after these enzymes are neutralised by association with exogenous or endogenous protease inhibitors. Such a mechanism was clearly supported by the finding that trypsin:trypsin inhibitor complexes were as effective in CCK release as the free trypsin inhibitors [8].

In contrast to the relative simplicity of the two alternative mechanisms for the stimulation by protease inhibitors of CCK release and the consequent pancreatic enzyme secretion, the mechanism of PHA stimulation is far more complex. As PHA does not inhibit trypsin it cannot act through the negative feedback loop. However, PHA is highly resistant to proteolytic degradation *in vivo* [3,7] and binds to all epithelial cells of the intestines which express the appropriate membrane glycoconjugates on their luminal surface [3,7,9]. These include the membrane glycans of I cells *in vivo* and PHA triggers the secretion of CCK through these by an unknown hormone-like membrane signalling mechanism. This mode of action is supported by the finding that PHA [10] (Table 2) induced the release of CCK from isolated intestinal cell preparations *in vitro* and that this was fully abolished by fetuin, a hapten of PHA. Furthermore, the PHA-induced CCK-secretion persisted even in the absence of PHA in the medium (Table 2), suggesting that the lectin attached to intestinal cells is not removed in the same manner as receptor-bound hormones or hormonal-releasing factors but probably remains bound to the cells for a prolonged period. As a result, by its direct effects on the I cells, PHA may provide long-term stimulation of CCK-release.

High levels of PHA (4 mg/h) infused into the duodenum induced a progressive and rapid increase in pancreatic enzyme secretion which reached a maximum by 90 min. This rate was comparable to that induced by 1.5 mg/h KTI, even though on a molar basis this amount of KTI was twice that of the PHA. It is not surprising that low amounts of PHA (0.5-1.0 mg/h) appeared to have little or no effect on enzyme output for up to 60 min but were later able to induce very high rates of enzyme output (Figure 1). Clearly maximal CCK secretion will only occur when all possible receptors are saturated. As cell-bound PHA remains attached to cell membranes for considerable periods of time, the total amount of lectin bound to I cells throughout the upper small intestine would have steadily increased with time since the animals were infused continuously with PHA throughout the test period.

In the light of the results presented in this work some of the reasons for the complexity of the PHA effect may have become a little clearer. Thus, there is little reason to doubt that PHA is at least as effective as, if not more effective than KTI as a hormone-like stimulant of CCK release from duodenal I cells *in vitro* in cell cultures and *in vivo* in conscious rats, both in the short- and long-term perspective. However, their mechanism of action is totally different. Clearly, unlike KTI, PHA first has to displace the endogenous ligand, be it the CCK-releasing peptide or trypsin/chymotrypsin, from the I cell receptor before it can send the signal for CCK release to internal parts of the cell signalling system. Thus, there must inevitably be some delay in CCK secretion, particularly at low PHA concentrations and in the short term. Moreover, as the PHA-induced increase in duodenal digestive enzyme concentration was unaffected by L-364718 treatment, it is likely that, at least in part, the stimulation was not directly mediated by CCK. However, as the exocrine pancreas is regulated through a number of neural and hormonal pathways in the gastrointestinal tract [1,2] it is not surprising that at this early stage PHA may act through other pathways than CCK. Thus, it is known that secretin stimulates pancreatic secretion whilst others, such as somatostatin and peptide YY, inhibit pancreatic output in rats [1,2]. It may be relevant that secretin has been shown to stimulate pancreatic protein output in rats and to potentiate the stimulatory effects of CCK on the pancreas [26-28]. As the secretin-secreting endocrine cells are also mostly located in the upper jejunum of rats [29] it is not surprising that PHA binds to them and stimulates their secretion of secretin [15].

There is also some evidence that although the PHA-induced release of CCK is followed by growth of the pancreas and an increase in its protein and DNA contents, this trophic effect on the pancreas is uncoupled by some unknown mechanism from the synthesis of digestive enzymes in and their secretion from the pancreas, particularly in the long term. This may again be the result of an indiscriminate effect of PHA on all intestinal cells, including all gut regulatory peptide-releasing cells, which carry the particular carbohydrate structures which PHA can specifically bind to. Accordingly, the resulting effect of PHA on CCK-release, pancreatic growth, pancreatic enzyme synthesis and the secretion of enzymes into the duodenum may be due to a combination of the additive, synergistic and/or inhibitory effects of the individual hormones released together by PHA signalling. It is therefore unprofitable to attempt to find a single mechanism, such as CCK-mediation, to explain the diverse effects of PHA on gut and pancreatic metabolism.

A number of lectins have been found to interact with pancreatic acinar cells *in vitro* [30,31]. In particular, PHA and SBA have recently been shown to trigger the secretion of digestive enzymes *in vitro* [32]. Furthermore, in addition to binding to the epithelial surface of the small intestine *in vivo*, PHA and other lectins can be taken up into enterocytes by endocytosis, traverse the cells and be released systemically in an intact and fully reactive form *in vivo* [3,33]. Indeed, up to 5% of orally administered PHA reaches the bloodstream and remains, , in circulation for up to 3 h, bound to blood glycoproteins [33]. A small amount of this systemically absorbed PHA associates with the pancreas and other tissues *in vivo* [33]. It is thus possible the PHA binds directly to acinar, or possibly neural, hormone-receptors and thereby stimulates secretion of digestive enzymes *in vivo*.

6. CONCLUSIONS

Kidney bean lectin (E_2L_2; PHA) can trigger the release of CCK from the small intestine and induce hypersecretion of pancreatic digestive enzymes following its short-term administration, by gavage or duodenal infusion. In the early stages the pancreatic secretory response to PHA appears to be largely independent of CCK mediation. At later stages, additional mechanisms, not directly involving CCK, appeared to play a role in modulating exocrine pancreatic responses to PHA. In addition to its effects on CCK-secreting I cells, PHA may stimulate or inhibit the release of other gut hormones which are important in the overall regulation of exocrine pancreatic metabolism. As a result the PHA-induced CCK release and pancreatic growth could be effectively uncoupled from the synthesis of digestive enzymes in the pancreas and their secretion into the duodenum. In addition, the systemically absorbed PHA may also have some slight role in directly triggering enzyme secretion from pancreatic acini.

REFERENCES

1. M.V. Singer, In: The Pancreas, Biology, Pathobiology and Disease, V.L.W. Go (ed.), Raven Press Ltd, New York. (1993) 425.
2. T.E. Solomon, In: Physiology of the Gastrointestinal Tract, L.R. Johnson (ed.), Raven Press Ltd, New York. (1994) 1499.
3. A. Pusztai, Plant Lectins, Cambridge University Press, Cambridge, UK 1991.
4. 1.I.E. Liener, J. Nutr. 125, (1995) 744S.
5. G. Grant, S.W.B. Ewen, S, Bardocz and A. Pusztai, In: Effects of Antinutrients on the Nutritional Value of Legume Diets, Volume I, S. Bardocz, E. Gelencsér and A. Pusztai A (eds.), European Commission, Brussels, (1996) 60.
6. T. Fushiki and K. Iwai, FASEB J., 3 (1989) 121.
7. A. Pusztai, G. Grant, D.S. Brown, S. Bardocz, S.W.B. Ewen, K. Baintner, W.J. Peumans, E.J.M. Van Damme, In: Lectins: Biomedical Perspectives, A. Pusztai and S. Bardocz (eds.), Taylor AND Francis, London (1995) 141.
8. A. Pusztai, G. Grant, S. Bardocz, K. Baintner, E. Gelencser and S.W.B. Ewen, Am. J. Physiol., 272 (1997) G340.
9. A. Pusztai, S.W.B. Ewen, G, Grant, W.J. Peumans, E.J.M. Van Damme, L. Rubio, and S. Bardocz, Digestion, 46 (suppl. 2) (1990) 308.

10. K. Herzig, S. Bardocz, G. Grant, R. Nustede, U.R. Folsch and A. Pusztai, Gut, 41 (1997) 333.
11. M. Jordinson, P.H. Deprez, R.J. Playford, S. Heal, T.C. Freeman, M. Alison and J. Calam, J. Am. J. Physiol., 270 (1996) G653.
12. M. Jordinson, R.J. Playford and J. Calam, Am. J. Physiol., 273 (1997) G946.
13. W.E. Schmidt, A. Roy Choudhury, E.G. Siegel, C. Löser, J.M. Conjon and U.R. Fölsch, Regul. Pept., 24 (1989) 64.
14. K. Kordas, B. Burghardt, K. Kisfalvi, S. Bardocz, A. Pusztai and G. Varga, J. Physiol. (1999), in press.
15. G. Grant, J.E. Edwards, E.C. Ewan, S. Murray, T. Atkinson, D.A.H. Farningham and A. Pusztai, Pancreas, (1999), in press.
16. A. Pusztai, W.B. Watt and J.C. Stewart, J. Agric. Food Chem., 39 (1991) 862.
17. S. Bardocz, G. Grant, A. Pusztai, M.F. Franklin and A. de F.F.U. Carvalho, Br. J. Nutr., 76 (1996) 613.
18. A. Pusztai, G. Grant, T.J. Duguid, D.S. Brown, W.J. Peumans, E.J.M. Van Damme and S. Bardocz, J. Nutr., 125 (1995) 1554.
19. K. Herzig, G. Brunke, I. Schon, M. Schaffer and U.R. Fölsch, Gut, 34 (1993) 1616.
20. S.J. Brand and R.G.H. Morgan, J. Physiol. Lond., 319 (1981) 325.
21. G. Grant, J.E. Edwards and A. Pusztai, J. Sci. Food Agric., 67 (1995) 235.
22. K. Beardshall, P. Deprez, R.J. Playford, M. Alexander and J. Calam, Regul. Pept., 40 (1992) 1.
23. E.P. Bouras, M.A. Misukonis and R.A. Liddle, Am. J. Physiol., 262 (1992) G791.
24. T. Fushiki, S. Fukuako, and K. Iwai, Biochem. Biophys. Res. Commun., 118 (1984) 532.
25. A.W. Spannagel, G.M. Green, D. Guan, R.A. Liddle, K. Faull and J.R.J. Reeve, Proc. Natl. Acad. Sci., 93 (1996) 4415.
26. Y. Moriyoshi, K. Shiratori, S. Watanabe and T. Takeuchi, Pancreas, 6 (1991) 603.
27. S. Alcon, J.A. Rosado, L.J. Garcia, J.A. Pariente, G.M. Salido and M.J. Pozo, Can. J. Physiol. Pharmacol., 74 (1996) 1342.
28. Y.L. Lee, H.Y. Kwon, H.S. Park, T.H. Lee and H.J. Park, Pancreas, 12 (1996) 58.
29. F. Sundler, E. Ekblad and R. Hakanson, In: Gastrointestinal Regulatory Peptides, D.R. Brown (ed.), Springer-Verlag, New York (1993) 1.
30. L. Jonas, G. Fulda, I. Damm, B. Nebe and J. Rychly, Acta. Histochem., 97 (1995) 81.
31. C. Wirth, J. Schwuchow and L. Jonas, Acta. Histochem., 98 (1996) 165.
32. G. Grant, L.T. Henderson, J.E. Edwards, E.C. Ewan, S. Bardocz and A. Pusztai, Life Sci., 60 (1997) 1589.
33. A. Pusztai, F. Greer and G. Grant, Biochem. Soc. Trans., 17 (1989) 481.

Biology of the Pancreas in Growing Animals
S.G. Pierzynowski and R. Zabielski (Editors)

287

Appetite regulation and pancreas

C. Erlanson-Albertsson

Dept of Cell and Molecular Biology, Medical Faculty, University of Lund,
P. O. Box 94, SE-221 00 Lund, Sweden[*]

Appetite regulation and feeding behaviour are critical for survival. Through appetite regulation the proper amounts of fat, carbohydrate and protein are provided, as well as the proper amounts of micronutrients. The signals involved in appetite regulation occur at several sites in the body, including the gastrointestinal tract, pancreas, liver and adipose tissue. These signals affect not only feeding behaviour, but also energy metabolism. The pancreas is important for appetite regulation in various ways. First, it provides digestive enzymes whose insufficiency in the intestinal lumen severely reduces appetite. Second, although feeding is necessary to provide energy, it also leads to severe perturbations in the homeostasis of the body. To help the body maintain homeostasis various pre-meal events occur, like the cephalic phase of pancreatic secretion. Third, the pancreas itself produces peptides that restrict feeding. The role of the pancreas is thus to provide energy for the body, at the same time maintaining homeostasis. This review focuses on the molecular signals that modulate food intake and energy metabolism and the specific role of the pancreas in this process.

1. WHY DO ANIMALS EAT?

Animals and humans eat for a variety of reasons, the most obvious being energy deficiency. Other reasons for eating involve palatability/reward, stress, social setting and in the case of humans, the availability of food at little or no cost. The various situations involve different signals and molecular mechanisms (Figure 1).

2. ENERGY DEFICIENCY FEEDING

Historically, the first studies of appetite regulation had as a working model that feeding was initiated by food deprivation or food restriction. The underlying concept was that the body continually sensed the amount of energy available; hence a deprivation of food would trigger the onset of feeding. According to Mayers´ glucostatic theory, a small decline in blood

[*]My thanks go to the Swedish Medical Research Council, (K99-03X-07904-13B), Dr A. Påhlssons Foundation and M. Bergwalls Foundation, who have allowed me to do active research within the field of appetite regulation and pancreas and penetrate this fascinating area.

glucose would trigger the initiation of a meal [1]. These studies were supported by Louis-Sylvestre and Le Magnen [2], who showed that all meals were preceded by a 6 to 8 % fall in blood glucose levels, starting 5 to 6 min prior to meal onset. Campfield and Smith [3] likewise demonstrated that a transitory decrease in blood glucose levels, obtained by injection of insulin, caused the initiation of meal. Under normal conditions an overnight fast leads to a lowering of blood glucose, which would therefore be a natural signal for initiating the first meal of the day.

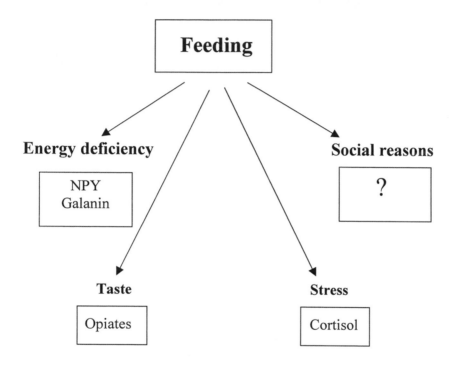

Figure 1. Feeding occurs for various reasons, including energy deficiency following fasting or physical exercise, taste when the animal is presented with palatable food, stress following isolation of pain and social reasons. The signals and mechanisms regulating feeding in the various situations are different and starting to become clear.

In an analogous way, a lipostatic model was proposed by Kennedy [4], stating that appetite regulation and feeding were closely related to the amount of fat stored in the adipose tissue. Experimentally a depletion of adipose tissue was found to increase food intake [5]. That this relationship is not as straightforward and simple as for carbohydrates is obvious, with the increasing prevalence of obesity and overweight seen in humans in modern affluent society.

2.1. Molecular signals during energy deficiency

Which then are the signals involved in initiating feeding during caloric restriction? In order for a signal to be physiologically relevant for such a function it must be shown to stimulate appetite, and increased amounts of this substance must occur following food deprivation. Conversely, levels of the same signal should decrease during overfeeding. There are a couple of signals fulfilling these criteria, notably neuropeptide Y and galanin.

2.2. Neuropeptide Y

Neuropeptide Y (NPY) is a potent appetite-stimulating signal, fulfilling the above requirements. It is a 36-amino acid neuromodulator that is distributed throughout the nervous system [6,7]. For appetite regulation the presence of NPY in the hypothalamus is of interest. In this organ the arcuate nucleus has the greatest density of cell bodies expressing NPY, with primary projections of the cell bodies into the paraventricular nucleus. NPY belongs to the pancreatic polypeptide family and has considerable sequence homology both with pancreatic polypeptide and peptide YY [8].

Central infusion of NPY has shown that this peptide promotes food intake in the rat [9,10]. In a macronutrient choice between carbohydrate, fat and protein, NPY is furthermore effective in specifically stimulating carbohydrate intake [11], although background preference has some importance for selectivity. The ability of NPY to specifically stimulate carbohydrate intake may be important in re-establishing the energy balance after an overnight fast, the storage of carbohydrate as energy substrate being highly limited. This hypothesis is supported by the demonstration of a diurnal variation in NPY levels [12]. Thus, in the rat the endogenous levels of NPY in the arcuate nucleus of the hypothalamus were demonstrated to reach peak levels at the onset of darkness, i.e. prior to the onset of feeding [12]. Analyses of natural behaviour show carbohydrates to be the preferred macronutrient at this time [13].

NPY, however, affects not only feeding behaviour, but also energy metabolism. On central infusion it was found to suppress energy expenditure in brown adipose tissue [14]. This effect may be explained by a suppression of the sympathetic nervous system activity in the innervation of brown fat [15], the sympathetic activity being crucial for raising the energy expenditure in brown adipose tissue. The ability of NPY to promote body weight gain at a rate greater than can be accounted for by enhanced food intake is consistent with the observed metabolic effects of NPY in the suppression of energy expenditure. In addition, NPY was found to decrease the insulin-stimulated glucose uptake in skeletal muscle, at the same time increasing the insulin-mediated glucose uptake in adipose tissue [16]. Such a divergent effect of NPY on glucose utilisation means that the carbohydrate consumed after NPY stimulation is directed to white adipose tissue, where it is stored in the form of neutral fat. This process is further enhanced by the ability of NPY to increase lipogenic enzymatic activity, both in the liver and in white adipose tissue [16]. NPY also stimulates the pituitary-adrenal axis, increasing the circulating levels of corticosterone [17]. This release of corticosterone may provide a partial explanation for the reduction in energy expenditure seen in the NPY-treated animal.

That NPY is important for feeding behaviour in a state of energy deficiency has been suggested by several groups demonstrating increased levels of NPY mRNA following food restriction or food deprivation [18-20]. Food restriction also increases levels of NPY in the paraventricular nucleus [21]. Likewise other manipulations that lead to an energy deficit also increase the gene expression of NPY or the peptide levels. NPY mRNA levels are thus increased in the arcuate nucleus of lactating rats [22]. Other energy-consuming activities, like intense running in rats, have also been found to increase NPY levels in the hypothalamus in a similar way to food restriction [23], providing evidence that NPY has a role in energy-deficiency feeding.

In NPY-deficient mice (NPY -/-) obtained by gene targeting, the animals were found to grow and reproduce at a normal rate, with no abnormality in food intake or body weight [24]. This probably reflects the abundance of mechanisms and factors involved in appetite regulation. The animals exhibited an increased level of anxiety, however, with an increased sensitivity to seizures and an increased ethanol consumption [24]. Thus one function of NPY would be to protect neural circuits from excessive stimulation. The normal anxiolytic effect of NPY would in these animals be temporarily replaced by that of ethanol.

2.3. Galanin

The peptide galanin, first isolated from porcine intestine [25], has been shown to exist in high concentrations in the brain as well as in the pancreas [26, 27]. It consists in most species of a 29-amino acid chain that is amidated at the C-terminal end. Galanin in man is not amidated but has 30 amino acids instead [28].

Like NPY, galanin has a stimulatory effect on feeding behaviour [29]. Direct hypothalamic injection of the peptide strongly increases food intake in satiated rats. The activity resides in the sixteen N-terminal amino acids, which are also needed for binding of galanin to its receptor [30]. In investigations where animals were served separate macronutrient diets of carbohydrate, fat and protein as a free choice, galanin was found to specifically stimulate fat intake [31]. If the animals were served a choice of only two diets, carbohydrate and protein, galanin stimulated carbohydrate intake instead [31]. The macronutrient choice of the animal following galanin infusion is, however, not only dependent on the availability of the macronutrient, but also on the background preference of the animal strain. In the rat, galanin was recently shown to stimulate carbohydrate intake rather than fat intake [32].

To discern whether galanin has a physiological function in feeding behaviour, peptide levels and messenger RNA levels have been measured both within the diurnal cycle and during development, when energy demands are excessive and the animal is dependent on dietary fat consumption. Akabayashi et al. [33] found galanin to display a clear light/dark rhythm, with a peak activity in the middle of the dark feeding cycle, in the rat. Such a rise in galanin in the middle of the dark period correlates with the period of fat ingestion, which is generally low in the first part of the feeding period, to rise sharply during the second half. The diurnal rhythm of galanin is thus strikingly different from that of NPY, both peptides acting to stimulate feeding. Whereas NPY is released prior to the onset of feeding and specifically stimulates carbohydrate intake, galanin is released in the middle to end phase of the feeding period, stimulating fat intake.

In further studies using rats with different voluntary fat intake, a positive correlation between 24-hour fat intake and galanin levels in the paraventricular nucleus of the hypothalamus was found [34], whereas no relationship was found between galanin and ingestion of carbohydrate or protein. These studies support a role for hypothalamic galanin in voluntary fat intake. A relationship was also established between galanin values in the hypothalamus and body weight, the dietary fat in fact being a primary contributor to body weight gain.

In addition to its appetite-regulating properties, galanin affects energy expenditure and energy metabolism. On central injection galanin was recently found to depress sympathetic nervous system activity [35], which is most likely the explanation for the observed reduction in energy expenditure [36]. The importance of galanin in establishing obesity is, however, still under debate, mainly since repeated injections of galanin fail to increase body weight [37]. One reason for this may be its insulin-lowering effect [38], insulin levels in all species being positively correlated to body weight gain. A reduction of insulin secretion during fat intake may be important to maintain constant blood glucose levels during the process of fat absorption.

Being a peptide responsible for the stimulation of feeding, one would expect galanin values to rise during starvation. Fasting for 24 hours or 48 hours gave, however, no change in hypothalamic expression of mRNA for galanin in rats, in contrast to NPY expression which was significantly raised following food deprivation [39]. Further studies are needed to establish the role of galanin in long-term feeding behaviour.

3. TASTE FEEDING

Not only humans overeat as a result of readily available palatable foods. This is true also for animals. A highly palatable diet may induce a positive energy balance, the animal eating in excess of its requirements. The main difference between energy-deficit feeding and taste feeding is thus that the latter occurs even if the animal is in energy balance. Taste feeding is dependent on the species of animal, certain strains of rat maintaining an energy balance even on palatable diets. Several different neuroregulatory pathways have been described for the perception of taste, with endogenous opioids seemingly having a crucial role.

3. 1. Endogenous opioids

The possibility that the endogenous opiates may be important in the perception of taste and reward during feeding is an attractive hypothesis and was suggested several years ago [40,41]. In these and later studies it was found that opioids increase food intake, and if given a choice the animals overeat of high-fat food rather than low-fat food [42]. They also prefer sweet food to non-sweet food under the influence of opiate agonists [43]. Evidence that opioids are involved in the palatability/reward aspect of feeding behaviour is in part based on studies using naloxone, which causes a blockade of opioid receptors. Using naltrexone, for instance, it was found that the hedonic properties of sucrose-containing solutions were significantly reduced in rats [44].

Rats in energy deficit will also choose a palatable diet. In various experiments to evaluate the interaction between reward and deprivation, Weldon et al. [45] found that opiate-induced feeding was not only related to taste but also to the state of energy deprivation. Rats were served three different diets that differed only in the type of carbohydrate included, the carbohydrates being starch, sucrose or polycose. In rats fed ad libitum, naloxone reduced the intake of all three diets, indicating that under normal conditions the endogenous opiates are involved in the drive to eat all three carbohydrates.

However, in animals with chronic food restriction, naloxone had no effect on the consumption of starch, whereas an inhibitory effect on feeding was observed for the sucrose as well as for the polycose diet [45]. These experiments may be interpreted to show that during energy deficiency, opiates are less important for feeding behaviour; they are important only with tasty and highly palatable food and when the animals are in a state of energy balance and satiated. Thus during food deprivation, opiates are less important in the drive to eat, although there is still a small opiate-driven search for very tasty food, such as that which has a high fat content. Thus endogenous opiates are involved in the rewarding properties of food rather than the energy content of the food [46].

On analysis of feeding behaviour during opiate-induced feeding, it is known from several studies that opiates prolong feeding without changing the time for onset of feeding. Such a pattern is consistent with a substance affected by palatability and taste rather than energy deficiency or hunger [47].

Another point of interest is the regulation of synthesis of the opiate peptides. Levels of mRNA for prodynorphin in the paraventricular nucleus of the hypothalamus were found to be increased following consumption of a high-fat diet [48]. A similar increase in prodynorphin mRNA was found after consumption of a high-fat and high-sucrose diet [49]. Thus it may be concluded that the synthesis and expression of prodynorphin in the brain is in part due to the consumption of energy-dense and tasty food like fat and sucrose. This correlates with the increased production of beta-endorphin and dynorphin found in the hypothalamus of the hyperphagic ob/ob mouse [50].

In contrast to the overproduction seen during overfeeding, endogenous opioids have been shown to be decreased during fasting or food restriction [52], as well as in situations of increased energy demand, such as lactation [51].The prodynorphin levels in the hypothalamus were thus significantly reduced after 24 hours of fasting in rat; a similar reduction was observed after chronic food restriction. The significance of these findings is that reward/palatability eating is dependent on a steady food intake, food restriction gradually leading to a loss of reward eating or taste feeding.

4. STRESS-INDUCED FEEDING

That stress is a factor leading to a generalised physiological reaction in the body is well known. That stress also affects feeding behaviour, both in man and animals, is a more recent finding. In man, stress responses include bulimic behaviour and hyperphagia. In animals there is also a change in feeding behaviour following stressful events like loud sounds, isolation and tail pinching [53].

There is not a uniform stress reaction regarding feeding behaviour, the reaction being related to the specific type of stress. Physical restraint in animals will decrease feeding [54], whereas tail pinching in rats will increase feeding [55]. The chemical signals mediating the feeding behaviour response to stress are consequently difficult to describe.

The first system to be associated with stress reactions is the CRH-ACTH-cortisol system. The system is complicated since corticotropin-releasing factor (CRH) essentially has an anorectic effect on feeding behaviour, whereas cortisol has a stimulatory effect on food intake. The anorectic effect of CRF is controlled by a CRF-binding protein, inactivating the effects on ingestion of this and related peptides, like urocortin. A dissociation of CRF from its binding protein by synthetic peptides was found to hamper weight gain in the genetically obese Zucker rat [56], pointing to a physiological role of CRF and its binding protein in body weight regulation. That CRF is released during stress could be concluded from experiments carried out on animals in physical restraint, where the decrease in food intake could be reversed with a CHF-antagonist, consisting of a partial CRF-peptide [54].

One important role of CRH is the increased expression of proopiomelanocortin, which in turn serves as a precursor for several hormones in the hypothalamic-pituitary axis, among them melanocyte-stimulating hormone and ACTH. The melanocortin peptides have an inhibitory effect on feeding [57].

Another important system involved in stress-induced feeding is the endogenous opioid system. The stress-induced feeding following tail pinching in rats is blocked by naloxone, suggesting the involvement of endogenous opioids [58]. The opioid genes form part of the proopiomelanocortin gene.

The stress situation in humans is easier to define than in animals [59]. This may hamper more systematic investigation of stress and neuropeptide expression in animals, aimed at relating various situations with specific signals.

5. WHEN DO ANIMALS STOP EATING?

The physiological mechanisms that produce satiety after food intake cover an array of regulatory systems, including pre-absorptive, absorptive and post-absorptive mechanisms. The pre-absorptive signals include the peptides produced in the gastrointestinal tract after the arrival of food products in the intestine. One example of these hormones is cholecystokinin (CCK) [60], in this review interesting since it also stimulates pancreatic exocrine secretion. Another pre-absorptive signal is enterostatin, which is an exocrine pancreatic protein product [61]. This peptide is interesting because it specifically inhibits fat intake [61].

The absorptive stimuli consist of digestive products like fatty acids and glucose and their metabolites. Since these are end products of the digestion of dietary macromolecules, optimal function of the exocrine pancreas is a prerequisite for absorptive appetite regulation. Rats with a pancreatic exocrine fistula draining pancreatic juice become severely hyperphagic [64], most probably due to failure in the digestion of dietary macromolecules and hence of their absorption and metabolism in the liver. In a similar way animals treated with inhibitors of pancreatic enzymes become severely hyperphagic [64]. The exocrine pancreas is thus important not only for pre-absorptive satiety mechanisms but also for the absorptive satiety system.

The post-absorptive signals are those that maintain a constant long-term energy balance in the body. Critical factors in this control system are leptin and insulin, being secreted in proportion to body adiposity. Leptin is a secretory product of the adipose tissue [65], whereas insulin, a product of the pancreatic beta cells, is secreted into the circulation in proportion to the size of the adipose tissue [66]. As described below these two factors work in a co-ordinated way. Thus the pancreas is also deeply involved in the post-absorptive or long-term regulation of the energy balance in the body.

6. PRE-ABSORPTIVE SATIETY SIGNALS

Several gastrointestinal signals have been described that elicit satiety, shortening the meal. These peptides are produced along the gastrointestinal tract, and include cholecystokinin, glucagon-like peptide, somatostatin and enterostatin. Since cholecystokinin was the first peptide described and since it also affects pancreatic secretion it will be described in more detail.

6.1. Cholecystokinin (CCK)

Ever since CCK was discovered to be a satiety peptide regulating meal size [60], investigations have been undertaken to examine its role as a physiological regulator of food intake, both in animals [67-69] and in man [70]. The role of CCK as a meal-terminating signal initially generated some controversy, essentially since bolus injection of CCK by intraperitoneal, intravenous or subcutaneous routes does not imitate physiological conditions. Reidelberger et al. [69] found that the doses of CCK needed to inhibit feeding were five times larger than those needed to maximally stimulate pancreatic secretion or to ensure gallbladder contraction.

One way of answering the question of whether CCK has a physiological role in appetite regulation has been the use of CCK-receptor antagonists. With the use of a selective receptor antagonist, L364,718, an increased food intake was observed in rats [71], suggesting that there may indeed be a physiological role for CCK in meal termination. Using the same CCK-A receptor antagonist these results were confirmed in non-fasted rats, whereas no effect on food intake was observed in fasted rats [72]. This behaviour suggests that the energy balance of the animal is critical for the effect of CCK, its action being suppressed during starvation. One explanation for the failure of CCK to inhibit food intake during short-term fasting may be the absence of insulin and/or leptin signalling, since both these hormones have been reported to potentiate the effect of CCK in reducing meal size [73,74].

Since CCK release from its site of production is above all dependent on contact with dietary fat and its digestive products, a hypothesis was formulated that endogenous CCK had a role in fat-induced satiety [75]. There was no effect on the pattern of response in man following infusion of fat in the presence of loxiglumide, a specific CCK-A receptor antagonist [75]. The conclusion was drawn that CCK has a general inhibitory effect on food intake, without any macronutrient specificity.

Although the injection of CCK prior to a meal can alter the size of an individual meal, repeated administration has no influence on the body weight of the animal [76]. The CCK-treated animals compensate for the reduced size of each meal by increasing the number of meals, in order to maintain a constant body weight. That CCK still is important for body weight regulation is clear from studies on Otsuka Long-Evans Tokushima Fatty rats, which do not express CCK-A receptors and develop hyperphagia and obesity [77].

CCK not only stimulates pancreatic secretion, it also causes pancreatic growth. Flo et al. [78] found that CCK administration induced pancreatic hypertrophy together with an increased brown adipose tissue weight and an increased energy metabolism, which in turn reduced the growth of the rats. This effect was only seen in food-restricted animals, receiving 65 % of normal food intake. Thus CCK under certain conditions will affect energy metabolism and thermogenesis, which is a general property of appetite-regulating signals.

The effects of CCK on appetite and metabolism have been demonstrated for several animal species, including the sheep and dog, with similar findings to those in the rat. The peptide analogue ARL 1429 was recently shown to induce satiety both in the rat and in the dog [79]. This compound, which is a high-affinity ligand for CCK-A receptors (Ki = 0,034 nM), gave a significantly prolonged inhibition of feeding during five hours instead of the one hour obtained with CCK-8, and the frequency of emesis was lower in the animals tested. This demonstrates the importance of the degradation of peptides in the normal appetite-regulating effect.

Regarding the mechanism of action for CCK, there is now considerable evidence that both afferent and efferent vagal pathways are involved [80]. Moran and his research group found that CCK increased the discharge rate of vagal afferent fibres situated in the duodenum. In subsequent work a subdiaphragmatic deafferentation was shown to cause a loss of sensitivity to CCK-effects on feeding behaviour, whereas a vagal deefferentation resulted in lower levels of basal food intake and a truncation of the inhibitory actions of CCK on feeding [80]. These results tell us that the circulating levels of CCK may be less important in determining the role of CCK on meal termination, making the previously observed discrepancy between the measured endogenous plasma levels of CCK and those needed to inhibit food intake less relevant [69].

6.2 Enterostatin - an exocrine pancreatic peptide

In the regulation of food intake we have so far discussed regulation of the size and frequency of the meal. There is also regulation of the composition of the meal [81,82], documented in studies showing that overfeeding with one macronutrient will lead to a reduced intake of that particular macronutrient, while the intake of others is unaffected [83,84].

The molecular mechanisms underlying macronutrient selection are starting to emerge. A number of peptides and neurotransmitters have been shown to selectively regulate the intake of specific macronutrients. Carbohydrate intake is specifically stimulated by NPY as mentioned above, as well as by noradrenaline through alpha-2-receptors [85]. Galanin has been shown to stimulate fat intake (see page 3), but will stimulate carbohydrate intake in carbohydrate-preferring rats, the effect thus being dependent on the background preference of the animal [86]. It has been claimed that protein intake is regulated through the peptide glucagon [82], suggesting the involvement of the pancreas in the intake of this macronutrient. Enterostatin is a peptide that has been found to selectively inhibit fat intake [61].

Enterostatin is the N-terminal pentapeptide formed through the tryptic cleavage of pancreatic procolipase [87,88]. The resulting colipase molecule forms a complex with pancreatic lipase, this complex being the enzymatically active form responsible for the hydrolysis of dietary triacylglycerol mixed with bile salt in the intestine. For unknown reasons the ratio between lipase and colipase varies with animal species. In the pig there is an excess of colipase relative to lipase, whereas in the rat and mouse there is a deficit of colipase [89]. In man the ratio between lipase and colipase is approximately one to one [90].

The first studies on enterostatin demonstrated a general reduction in food intake in the rat upon peripheral or central administration [91,92]. Using a three-choice macronutrient selection between carbohydrate, fat and protein, Okada *et al.* [93] were the first to observe a selective inhibition of the intake of fat by enterostatin. In a two-choice paradigm with a high-fat and a low-fat diet also, the animals selectively reduced their intake of the high-fat diet after being injected with enterostatin [94].

For enterostatin to inhibit feeding, chronic ingestion of dietary fat during a period of three weeks was a prerequisite [95]. The identity of the signal appearing within these three weeks is not clear. Fat feeding will increase the synthesis of pancreatic procolipase, the precursor of enterostatin [88]. It is possible that increased secretion of enterostatin leads to the up-regulation of enterostatin signalling pathways. This is true for the SK-N-MC-cell, a neuroblastoma target cell for enterostatin, where the binding of enterostatin [96] is up-regulated through long-term enterostatin treatment (K. Berger, unpublished observation). Another hypothesis is that corticosterone secretion may be a prerequisite for enterostatin to have any effect on feeding behaviour [95], since corticosterone has been shown to promote the feeding response to enterostatin [97]. A third possibility is that leptin provides a permissive signal, allowing enterostatin to be active in regulating fat intake. Leptin production and secretion from adipose tissue increases when animals are fed a high-fat diet [98]. The Zucker rat (fa/fa), however, which has a mutated leptin receptor, is very sensitive to enterostatin [99], making such a signal unlikely.

When inhibiting fat intake, enterostatin has been shown to induce early satiety, and the time of resting and sleeping is significantly increased [100]. The effect of enterostatin occurs within 30 minutes of administration, except after intravenous administration, which gives a delay of 60 to 90 minutes [101]. The potency of action of enterostatin is reflected in its long duration of action, up to 6 hours after a single injection. The reduced intake of dietary fat was not compensated for by an increase in the intake of other macronutrients.

Among the various effects of enterostatin the effects on pancreatic secretion and gastrointestinal motility are of special interest. In pigs provided with cannulae for collection of pancreatic juice it was found that intraintestinal infusion of enterostatin caused a significant inhibition of pancreatic secretion after stimulation with CCK [102]. Such an inhibition might result in a postprandial arrest of digestive secretion, designed to allow a renewed build-up of the secretory products of the pancreas.

Coupled to this inhibitory effect on pancreatic secretion there was also an inhibition of gastrointestinal motility after intraduodenal infusion of enterostatin [103]. This inhibition was not observed after intravenous injection of enterostatin, nor was it observed in vitro on isolated intestinal segments [104]. The conclusion that may be drawn from these experiments is that secretion from the pancreas and the motility of the intestine may be co-ordinated by enterostatin. Further experiments are needed to confirm such a relationship.

It has also been noted that on intraintestinal infusion together with Intralipid, enterostatin inhibits insulin secretion [105]. This inhibition may be important in preventing blood glucose from dropping to dangerously low levels during fat intake.

6.3. Enterostatin - an anti-taste compound?

In the search for its mechanism of action, enterostatin was found to inhibit a kappa-opioid pathway that promotes the ingestion of dietary fat [106]. In these experiments enterostatin affected feeding behaviour in the rat in a similar way to the synthetic kappa-opioid antagonist nor-BNI, inhibiting the intake of a high-fat diet in a two-choice situation between a low-fat and high-fat diet [106]. Using sub-threshold doses of the two compounds, enterostatin and nor-BNI were found to act synergistically. The finding that the kappa-opioid agonist U50,488 selectively stimulated fat intake [106] was further proof of the involvement of a kappa-opioid pathway in fat feeding.

More direct proof of an opioid component in the mechanism of action of enterostatin was the finding that the opiate peptides met-enkephalin and leu-enkephalin compete with enterostatin for binding sites on its target cell, the SK-N-MC-cell [96]. At high concentrations these peptides displaced enterostatin from its binding sites. Such experiments suggest that fat intake really involves a competition between enterostatin and the opiate peptides for signal transduction. With an excess of opiates a stimulation of fat intake will occur, and with an excess of enterostatin fat intake will be inhibited. Using beta-casomorphin, Lin *et al.* [107] indeed found that intake of dietary fat was stimulated in rats and that central injection of enterostatin inhibited this fat intake. Beta-casomorphins are released from beta-casein during digestion of milk and are absorbed in small quantities from the intestine in young lambs and pigs [108]. They may also pass directly from breast parenchymal cells into the plasma and reach the central nervous system. A variety of biological effects have been ascribed to the beta-casomorphins, including stimulation of gastric motility [109]. A stimulation of fat intake by the casomorphins may be important for the stimulation of feeding during infancy, milk being rich in fat and the newborn in great need of calories. During this period the activities of pancreatic enzymes, including pancreatic procolipase, are low [110], and do not increase until after weaning. It may therefore be important to keep the enterostatin levels low as well, to allow a large ingestion of fat.

How does the biological activity of enterostatin fit with its postulated function as an anti-opiate factor? Opiates act by increasing taste and thus prolonging feeding. With enterostatin the meals are shortened, which is what would be expected of opiate antagonist [61].

Another property of opiates is that they are particularly active in stimulating the intake of tasty food, like high-fat diets. The specific inhibitory effect of enterostatin on intake of high-fat diets could act through an "anti-taste" effect. A third property of opiates is that they disappear during fasting [52]. During fasting in the rat, pancreatic procolipase levels are first decreased, followed by an increase [61]. In man, fat has been shown to decrease the taste for fat [111]. It may be that this diminished taste for fat is linked to high levels of endogenously produced procolipase/enterostatin, a hypothesis still waiting to be tested.

These studies indicate that the body not only has a system involving taste mechanisms but also anti-taste mechanisms. Some of the satiety peptides like CCK have adverse effects at high doses and responses associated with the emetic reflex [112]. There seems to be a continuous line from satiety to aversion. It may also be significant that of the three macronutrients fat, carbohydrate and protein, fat is the nutrient with the shortest way to malaise and aversion.

7. ABSORPTIVE SIGNALS

Since energy balance is mainly regulated through changes in food intake, it is likely that a food digestive product or a metabolite is involved in the control of feeding. In experimental animal models the administration of metabolites has been shown to give a short-term reduction in food intake [113,114]. The food inhibition may not fully compensate for the administered energy, the reduction in food intake corresponding to 40-70 % of the administered energy. One important factor is the composition of the infusate, glucose and amino acids being more effective than lipids as "satiety" agents [115].

In the metabolic control of food intake, glucose and free fatty acids are the most important substrates, the digestive enzymes of the exocrine pancreas being of paramount importance for such regulation to occur.

7.1. The role of glucose in satiety

Evidence for the role of glucose in the metabolic control of feeding is provided by experiments with infusion of glucose, which will inhibit feeding [3]. Campfield *et al.* [116] found, for instance, that infusion of glucose prior to a meal delayed the onset of feeding in the rat. The experiments were taken as proof of the importance of a decline in blood glucose concentration as a signal for starting the meal. The other line of evidence for metabolic control of feeding behaviour is the stimulation of feeding seen with metabolic inhibitors of glucose, for instance 2-deoxy-D-glucose [115].

Metabolic signals are thought to be important during and after a meal. The clearest effects are thus observed when the infusion of glucose occurs concomitant with carbohydrate intake [117]. This suggests that intravenous glucose is more satiating at a time when other satiety signals are acting, such as during a meal. A simultaneous infusion of insulin significantly augmented the satiating power of the glucose infusion [118], pointing to an interaction between insulin and the glucose-sensing mechanisms for satiety.

The mechanism for the detection of glucose in the control of feeding involves both central glucose-sensitive neurons in the lateral hypothalamus [119] and glucosensors in the liver [115]. The identity of the glucose-sensing mechanism in the liver is still not known. One important factor is the ability of glucose to increase the spike frequency in vagal afferent nerves, the glucose-sensing mechanism for regulation of food intake being blocked by hepatic branch vagotomy [115].

7.2. The role of fatty acids in satiety

Fatty acids are known to suppress hunger, both at a pre-absorptive site and at an absorptive site. The evidence for a pre-absorptive action comes from studies where Intralipid was infused intraduodenally into the rat, leading to satiety behaviour as little as 15 min after intraintestinal infusion [120]. Fatty acids, however, also act as satiety signals after their intestinal absorption. First, it has been reported that infusion of lipids will significantly reduce food intake, a phenomenon which has been demonstrated in several animal species, including the monkey [121]. A second type of evidence is the increased hunger and food intake demonstrated upon inhibition of fatty acid oxidation [122,123]. This increased food intake is particularly marked when the animals are fed a high-fat diet. The inhibitors used for blocking fatty acid oxidation can either act directly on the beta-oxidation, for instance mercaptoacetate which blocks acyl CoA dehydrogenase; or they can block the transport of fatty acids into the mitochondrial matrix, for instance methyl palmoxirate, which blocks carnitin-palmitoyltransferase. After injection of these inhibitors the animals start to eat earlier than expected, indicating that fatty acid oxidation is the main factor involved in intermeal satiety.

Sensors for fatty acid oxidation have been localized in the liver using a mechanism involving hepatic branches of vagal afferent nerves [124,125]. The sensor mechanisms for fatty acids and glucose are, however, not identical, since capsaicin treatment abolished the lipoprivic response, (that is the increased feeding observed after blocking of fatty acid oxidation), but not the glucoprivic response [125]. It is unlikely that fatty acids are sensed directly by vagal afferents. Ketone bodies have been discussed as possible mediators, these metabolites being transiently increased in plasma after a fat-rich meal [126]. It has been suggested that an elevation of cytosolic ATP following oxidation of fatty acids may stimulate the activity of the Na/K-pump, causing an enhancement of the membrane potential of hepatic vagal afferents to signal satiety. In conclusion strong evidence indicates that hepatic fatty acid oxidation contributes to the control of food intake, but the exact sensing mechanism still needs to be identified.

8. POST-ABSORPTIVE SIGNALS

Whereas both the pre-absorptive and the absorptive signals are related to the intake of a meal, the post-absorptive signals are those that reside over long periods of time and emanate from or are closely related to the adipose tissue. Two important signals, leptin and insulin, will be described below.

8.1. Leptin

No discovery in the modern history of energy metabolism has generated so much excitement as the cloning of the leptin gene in 1994 [65]. Leptin is a 167-amino-acid protein, produced and secreted by the adipose tissue [65]. The protein was discovered due to a mutation in the corresponding gene, the ob-gene, introducing a stop codon at amino acid 105. As a result the animals carrying this mutated gene became severely hyperphagic and obese, the obesity being corrected by the addition of leptin [127].

Leptin is, however, not only a product of the adipocyte. More recent publications have revealed the existence of leptin in the placenta [128] as well as in the stomach [129]. The production of leptin in the stomach was localised to chief cells in the fundus region, to which procolipase has also been localised [130]. The secretory chief cell of the stomach thus produces not only pepsinogen, but also other energy-balance-controlling factors like leptin and procolipase, the precursor of enterostatin. The physiological function of this source of leptin is unknown. However, both feeding and administration of CCK-8 were found to result in a rapid and large decrease in the leptin content of the fundic epithelium, with a concomitant increase in the concentration of leptin in plasma [129].

Soon after the discovery of leptin the receptor for leptin was cloned [131]. Somewhat surprisingly, the receptor for leptin proved to be a class I cytokine receptor, most similar to the interleukin-6-receptor [131]. The receptor has been shown to exist in at least six different forms, obtained by alternative splicing. One of these, the so-called long form receptor, is probably the one that mediates the inhibitory effects of leptin on food intake, as illustrated by a mutation in the obese db/db mouse [132]. The leptin receptor is expressed at high levels in the hypothalamic areas important in the control of food intake, the brain thus being a primary target organ for the anorectic effect of leptin. The entry of leptin from the circulating blood into the brain appears to occur through a receptor-mediated process, and the efficiency of this transport decreases with increasing amounts of leptin in the circulating blood [133].

When leptin was injected into the ob/ob mice, not only did the animals eat less, but there was also an elevation in body temperature and an increase in locomotor activity [127]. Thus leptin also stimulates energy metabolism, in a similar way to other anorectic peptides [82]. In addition insulin, glucose and cholesterol levels in the plasma were reduced [134]. Thus leptin, like many of the appetite regulating peptides, has a broad range of activities within energy metabolism.

What is the mechanism of action by which leptin regulates appetite and the energy balance of the body? One important mechanism through which it diminishes appetite is by the inhibition of NPY synthesis [135]. This effect was demonstrated in ob/ob mice, who were at the same time deficient in the NPY gene through a targeted gene knockout [135]. These animals had a reduced hyperphagia and a reduced body weight compared to the normal ob/ob mice.

Regarding the role of leptin in the development of obesity, it has been found that leptin mRNA in adipose tissue and plasma levels of leptin are elevated in all rat and mouse models of obesity investigated, both genetically inbred species and animals made obese by feeding with a highly palatable high-fat diet [136]. This is true also for man [137], suggesting that obesity, whether in humans or laboratory animals, is due to overconsumption of highly palatable food and unrelated to signals controlling the energy balance, like leptin. Eating is continued in spite of an energy balance. The importance of leptin in achieving an energy balance is demonstrated by the severe overeating seen in association with inborn mutated forms of leptin [138].

8.2. Leptin and insulin

Leptin and insulin are both adiposity signals. Leptin is secreted by the adipose tissue and although insulin is secreted by the pancreatic beta cell, its concentration in the circulating blood is proportional to the adipose mass [139].

The appetite-regulating effects of insulin are known to be mediated by central receptors; thus insulin like leptin needs to enter the brain from the peripheral circulation. A receptor-mediated uptake of insulin has been described [140] and the receptors for insulin are located in the same hypothalamic areas as for leptin [141]. When administered centrally, insulin has similar properties to leptin in reducing body weight. This reduction in body weight cannot be accounted for by a reduction in food intake only, but has to be explained by an activation of the sympathetic nervous system. It thus appears that leptin and insulin under certain conditions induce a response that leads to the loss of body fat.

Given peripherally, insulin has the opposite action of leptin, i.e. enhancing fat storage and decreasing blood glucose levels. The peripheral receptors for insulin thus trigger an anabolic response. The mutual importance of peripheral and central insulin therefore needs to be clarified. It has also been shown that the synthesis of insulin is inhibited by leptin [142], indicating that there is an opposite regulation of leptin/insulin synthesis.

At the cellular level, leptin has been found to modulate insulin activity. Thus in isolated cell cultures leptin was found to down-regulate the insulin-dependent tyrosine phosphorylation of the insulin receptor substrate IRS-1 [143]. This is a key step in the insulin receptor cascade and it therefore seems that leptin attenuates some of the insulin-induced signals. One could speculate that the high levels of leptin in obese individuals might favour the development of insulin resistance. Further studies are obviously needed to understand the interaction between leptin and insulin in the regulation of energy balance.

9. THE IMPORTANCE OF PANCREATIC JUICE SECRETION FOR APPETITE REGULATION

Food selection represents a major challenge for omnivorous species. A variety of potential food stuffs being available, most of these beneficial and some deleterious, the omnivorous animal must decide which food to eat and which to reject. In this selection process the taste and texture of the food is particularly important. The animal can readily distinguish between a sweet taste, leading to a selection reaction, and a bitter taste, causing an aversion reaction. These stimuli, named pre-ingestive stimuli, have an important influence on pancreatic secretion, well-tasting food strongly stimulating pancreatic secretion, and bitter-tasting food giving weak stimulation [144].

With experience animals select food on the basis of the post-ingestive consequences of eating it, involving the digestion, absorption and processing of the food component [145]. For this selection the secretion of pancreatic juice with its digestive enzymes is of paramount importance. A low secretion of pancreatic juice in relation to a certain food component leads to the rejection of that particular food [146].

Strong preferences for certain foods can also be explained by the learning of a positive nutritive effect, for instance in the preference for energy-dense foods like lipids. The exocrine pancreas and its synthesis and secretion of digestive enzymes is thus involved in various ways in the choice of and appetite for food components.

9.1. Pre-ingestive stimuli

Digestive secretion is classified into three phases, cephalic, gastric and intestinal. The importance of taste and smell for the stimulation of digestive secretions is revealed in the cephalic phase. The digestive stimulation triggered by the cephalic phase is in the same direction as that triggered by the gastric and intestinal phases, and although smaller in magnitude and shorter in duration than the other two phases, it is important for the efficiency of the digestion and for the nutritional wellbeing of the animal.

In studying the cephalic phase of digestive secretion sham feeding is used, in which ingested food is swallowed and then diverted through an oesophageal fistula to the exterior. In humans, a modified procedure is used where the food is ingested and chewed, followed by expectoration. The act of swallowing is thus omitted, and thereby the detection mechanisms of the pharynx and oesophagus in the cephalic phase of digestive secretion.

9.2. Taste and gastric secretion

The observation that the cephalic phase affects gastric secretion was experimentally described by Pavlov, who called these effects "psychic effects" [147]. In his studies Pavlov also noted the importance of taste for the secretion of gastric juice. He observed that the majority of dogs preferred flesh to bread, and that less gastric juice was produced on sham feeding with bread compared to flesh. However, he also noted that some dogs actually preferred bread to flesh, and in these dogs gastric juice production was higher on sham feeding with bread than with flesh.

The basic concept of an increased stimulation of digestive secretion by a preferred food has been further documented since this initial observation by Pavlov [147]. In the choice between three meals, in humans, - a cereal gruel, a standard hospital diet and a meal composed by the subject - it was found that the freely composed meal led to higher levels of acid secretion than the cereal gruel [148]. As a consequence of the taste-induced stimulus a greater response of gastric juice secretion was noted in evening meals than in morning meals, even when both meals were preceded by 12-hour food deprivation. The conclusion was that evening meals were composed more according to the subjects' preferences than the morning meal.

Another important factor in the cephalic phase of secretion is the texture of the meal. Thus a greater response of gastric secretion was observed after a solid meal than after a homogenised meal of identical composition, probably due to prolongation of the operations of tasting, smelling, masticating and swallowing during a solid meal [149].

In an attempt to quantify the response of gastric secretion following the selection of a favourite meal, Moore and Motoki [150] observed that the response amounted to 55 % of the normal pentagastrin response. This figure gives an idea of the importance of taste in the stimulation of gastric secretion.

9.3. Taste and pancreatic secretion

The cephalic-phase response of exocrine pancreatic flow has been a well-established phenomenon since the days of its discovery by Pavlov [147], but the mechanism and cause behind cephalic phase secretion are still debated. One theory holds that it is due to the entry of gastric acid into the duodenum and subsequent release of secretin [144]. Another theory is that there is a direct stimulation of pancreatic exocrine secretion through the vagal nerve. Pavlov noted, however, that the secretion of pancreatic juice had a very short lag period of three minutes, a time insufficient for indirect stimulation of pancreatic juice secretion [147]. In achlorhydric human subjects pancreatic secretion was stimulated following modified sham feeding, suggesting that the cephalic phase of pancreatic secretion is primarily due to vagal stimulation [151].

In assaying the importance of taste and smell Sarles et al. [152] found that a familiar breakfast caused a significantly higher pancreatic flow, and bicarbonate and lipase activity compared with a less typical breakfast, such as a steak. Chewing of the less-preferred breakfast, on the other hand, caused a greater pancreatic secretion compared to just seeing and smelling it [152]. The extent of secretion was also dependent on the time of the day, early morning being the period with the lowest secretion.

The cephalic phase of pancreatic secretion thus is dependent on the taste, the chewing and the time of the day. In further studies on the importance of the palatability of the diet with the addition of either acceptable or aversive taste stimuli to a basal diet, it was found that the animals showed a greater pancreatic response to the palatable diets compared to those with aversive taste [153].

In the choice between sodium chloride, sucrose and monosodium glutamate it was found that sucrose was a better stimulus for pancreatic secretion than monosodium glutamate in conscious dogs, while sodium chloride gave the lowest stimulation of exocrine pancreatic secretion [154]. The pancreatic secretory response was thus found to vary with the type of taste stimulus in a graded way.

As with the stimulation of gastric juice, the secretion of pancreatic juice is dependent on the texture of the food [155]. With a solid-liquid meal a prolonged pancreatic and biliary response was obtained compared to the response for a homogenised meal of identical composition. One reason could be that the solid meal entered the duodenum at a considerably slower rate than the homogenised food [155].

That the act of chewing and swallowing is important for the taste stimuli of pancreatic secretion was demonstrated in studies by Naim *et al.* [156]. Dogs were prepared with pancreatic fistulae. Taste stimuli were applied using cotton swabs soaked with three test solutions: sucrose, quinine sulphate and citric acid. Oral stimulation lasting six minutes produced a significant increase in pancreatic secretion, that of sucrose being larger than that of either quinine sulphate or citric acid. After 45 minutes, application of the taste stimuli was repeated [156], but this time there was no exocrine secretion at all, indicating that the dogs associated the initial taste stimulation with no food forthcoming. This phenomenon of reduced response following repeated stimulation is true also for taste stimuli and probably occurs through a central mechanism.

In conclusion, pancreatic juice secretion occurs in response to the stimulus of the taste and smell of food. Palatable food gives a better stimulation than non-palatable food, solid food a better stimulation than liquid food. Another factor that is important is the time of the day, the morning being associated with a low secretion profile. An appetite for certain food components thus goes hand in hand with a strong stimulus for pancreatic secretion, leading to a positive post-ingestive effect of that particular food item.

9.4. Stress and pancreatic secretion

It is generally accepted that psychological stress causes disturbances in the function of the stomach and the motility of the upper small intestine. It is less well known that the release of pancreatic enzymes is also affected by stress [157]. In one investigation male volunteers were subjected to acute psychological stress induced by solving mental arithmetic for a financial reward during 60 minutes. The test significantly increased the scores of anger and excitement according to a self-reported questionnaire. The pancreatic secretion was unchanged during the initial 30 minutes of the stress period. However, during the second 30-minute period of mental stress a significant increase in pancreatic protein secretion was observed, diminishing again during the post-stress period [157]. The arterial blood pressure and heart rate were significantly increased. It is thus apparent that the pancreas also reacts to acute mental stress. The increased appetite observed during stress may be related to the increased secretory response in the exocrine pancreas.

9.5. Appetite loss and pancreatic function

While investigating the relationship between appetite and pancreatic secretion Sarles *et al.* [152] identified anorectic patients in whom the sight and smell of a meal completely failed to stimulate pancreatic secretion. The taste aversion in these patients may thus have a functional link to the inability to produce digestive secretions.

A more direct approach to understanding the role of the digestive enzymes of the pancreas is the use of enzyme inhibitors. One such inhibitor, tetrahydrolipstatin, has been shown to reduce fat digestion and fat absorption in several animal species, including mice, rats, dogs, monkeys and humans [158, 159]. Tetrahydrolipstatin is an inhibitor of pancreatic lipase as well as of pancreatic carboxylester hydrolase. Through an inhibition of dietary fat digestion, fat absorption is impaired, leading to steatorrhoea.

One interesting consequence of treatment with tetrahydrolipstatin was the avoidance of fat in studies using a self-selection diet [146]. In these studies the rats being treated with tetrahydrolipstatin reduced their absolute and proportional fat intake and increased their protein and carbohydrate intake instead. Given the opportunity to select non-fat foods during tetrahydrolipstatin treatment, weight losses were minimal. These findings are in contrast with the increased fat consumption and drastic weight loss observed in rats fed a high-fat diet as a single choice after treatment with tetrahydrolipstatin [159]. Clearly, the feeding pattern following maldigestion of fat is related to the food choice available. If a choice is available the animal shifts from a fat energy source to a non-fat energy source.

The reason for avoiding fat could either be that it acquires an aversive flavour because of the drug or it could be the drug-induced malabsorption. Using conditioned stimulus tests Ackroff and Sclafani [146] found that the reduction of fat intake following tetrahydrolipstatin treatment was primarily due to the postingestive effects of the drug rather than its orosensory effects.

The conclusion to be drawn from these experiments is that post-ingestive feedback signals contribute to the appetite for fat. A disturbance of these signals through inhibition of fat digestion and fat absorption will lead to a decreased appetite for fat.

10. THE ROLE OF BODY TEMPERATURE IN APPETITE REGULATION

By regulating appetite, body temperature is one factor controlling feeding behaviour. Several arguments are in favour of such a control. As a general rule a high body temperature will inhibit feeding, whereas a low body temperature will stimulate feeding [160].

DeVries *et al.* [161] found that when the liver of rats had reached a critical temperature of $39.1°C$, the animals stopped eating, as if they could not tolerate any higher temperatures. This temperature is near the temperature at which damage occurs to vital organs. Since heat is created during feeding by the process of diet-induced thermogenesis, food consumption is significantly reduced when the body temperature is elevated, as it is during infectious disease. Various cytokines mediate a reduction of appetite during these conditions [162]. Generally, animals stop all activities to avoid hyperthermia.

The stimulation of feeding cause by low body temperature is illustrated by the ob/ob mice, who have a body temperature of $34.8°C$ instead of the normal $37.0°C$ [127]. These animals are hyperphagic, one reason for this being to raise the body temperature. Correction of the body temperature to a normal level by the injection of leptin stops the hyperphagia.

During the meal itself there are various changes in body temperature. The rise in body temperature that occurs prior to a meal may be an anticipatory event aimed at maintaining homeostasis during the meal.

11. PRE-MEAL EVENTS DESIGNED TO MAINTAIN HOMEOSTASIS

Meals are events that although necessary for the supply of nutrients to the body lead to undesirable perturbations in homeostasis. There are several strategies to minimise these homeostatic disturbances. One is the digestive secretion occurring during the cephalic phase, which begins when the animal understands that food is coming, as mentioned above. This anticipatory response starts a long time before the meal itself and is probably important in preserving homeostasis even when the meal is large. It is interesting to note that if this cephalic response is prevented, the animals will consume less [164].

Another strategy for the preservation of homeostasis is the elevation of body temperature prior to the onset of meals [163]. Body temperature, in addition to having a circadian rhythm, changes with feeding. The pre-meal rise in temperature may represent an anticipatory response, preparing the animal for feeding. The temperature increases relatively steadily before the meal starts, increases even further during the meal and rapidly declines after the meal has ended. The decline in temperature soon after the meal may be a safety mechanism to allow the animal to engage in other activities that produce heat, like physical activity.

The mechanism for the pre-meal rise in body temperature is not known. Such a rise in temperature probably facilitates critical processes involved in ingestion, digestion and the passage of food through the intestine. The influence of temperature on digestibility and intestinal transit time can be illustrated by comparing exothermic animals with endothermic animals. While food retention time in many herbivorous mammals of less than 3 kg is between 2 and 18 hours, the food passage time through the intestine of herbivorous lizards amounts to several days [165]. This is an extreme example and there may be other explanations for the more rapid transit time in mammals, for instance a greater capacity for food digestion as well as a greater intestinal surface area. That body temperature itself still has an influence upon food digestion and intestinal transit time was demonstrated in experiments on the lizard *Iguana Iguana*, an exothermic herbivore [166]. In these animals an increase in body temperature from 30.0°C to 36.1°C induced a significant curvilinear decrease in food transit time from ten days to three days. Dry-matter digestibility was affected only to a minor degree by the change in body temperature [166].

A third strategy for maintenance of homeostasis during a meal is the drop in blood glucose levels that occurs prior to the onset of the meal [163]. This should minimise the postprandial elevation of blood glucose caused by absorption of carbohydrate. The cephalic secretion of insulin also leads to more stable blood glucose levels during the meal-taking.

12. ENERGY METABOLISM AND UNCOUPLING PROTEINS

The production of heat in the body occurs in either of two ways, through a rise in metabolic activity or through an uncoupling of ATP synthesis from electron transport in the mitochondria. Since heat itself acts as a satiety agent, uncoupling mechanisms of the body are important for appetite regulation.

A number of proteins, recently cloned and characterised [167], are responsible for the uncoupling mechanism. They are named uncoupling proteins 1-4. The first, UCP1, was described as early as in 1985, and is a protein produced in the brown adipose tissue of rodents [168,169]. It contributes to the maintenance of a constant body temperature in a cold environment in rodents, its expression being up-regulated during exposure to cold. Since ablation of brown adipose tissue leads to hyperphagia and increased body weight, UCP1 through its uncoupling and heat-producing activity may act as a satiety agent. Lack of UCP1-mediated thermogenesis in knock-out mice does not in itself cause hyperphagia [170]. Himms-Hagen [171] therefore has suggested that a satiety factor is produced in brown adipose tissue in inverse relation to ambient temperature. The identity of this factor is unknown.

Several observations led to the hypothesis that uncoupling proteins could exist in tissues other than the brown adipose tissue. It has been reported that heat is produced in muscle tissue in response to catecholamine administration without any physical activity. In addition mitochondrial proton leaks have been observed in tissues other than the brown adipose tissue [167]. In 1997 two new uncoupling proteins were discovered, UCP2 [172] and UCP3 [173], and in 1998 a fourth, UCP4 [174].

The discovery of UCP2 caused great excitement [172]. One reason was the finding that the gene was expressed in several different tissues, including the brain, muscle, adipose tissue and lymphoid tissues, but also the gastrointestinal tract. The gene is also expressed in the pancreas [R. Denis, unpublished observation]. In the gastrointestinal tract the UCP2 gene is expressed at the highest level in the pylorus-antrum region of the stomach, the expression gradually diminishing in the distal parts of the intestine. Another reason for the great excitement caused by UCP2 was the report that a high-fat diet caused increased expression in adipose tissue [172]. This up-regulation occurred in A/J-mice, who remained thin upon high-fat feeding in contrast to the C57 mice, who became obese upon high-fat feeding and in whom the UCP2 gene was not up-regulated at a similar rate. Such a pattern suggests that UCP2 has a role in burning excess fat. Whether this is true in other animals or in man is not known. Somewhat paradoxically the gene was found to be up-regulated during starvation [175]. The reason could be that the body has to maintain its core temperature, and when totally deprived of food, heat is produced by up-regulation of the UCP2 gene.

UCP3 has properties similar to those of UCP2, but in addition to brown adipose tissue it is expressed mainly in muscle. High-fat feeding has given conflicting results, with either an up-regulation or no effect at all [167]. As for UCP2, the UCP3 gene has been found to increase during fasting [167]. The exact role of these uncoupling proteins is not known.

UCP4, the fourth uncoupling protein discovered, is uniquely expressed in the brain [174]. The gene resembles that of other mitochondrial carrier proteins. The role of this protein may be to protect the brain from oxygen free radicals by the consumption of oxygen through

307

uncoupling. This would protect the tissue from oxidative damage and apoptosis, for example during inflammation.

The discovery of uncoupling proteins in a variety of tissues has created a new tool for understanding energy balance and the importance of heat production in its regulation. The uncoupling activity in the pancreas may be important to prevent the tissue from oxidative damage. It could be speculated that the rapid damage to the tissue that occurs during pancreatitis may in part be due to an inefficient uncoupling, since it has been claimed that oxygen free radicals are involved in causing pancreatitis.

13. CONCLUSIONS

Appetite regulation and energy metabolism are two tightly regulated systems that govern feeding behaviour and body weight in animals. An understanding of these systems is of crucial importance for optimisation of the conditions for growth and homeostasis in the animals under various conditions.

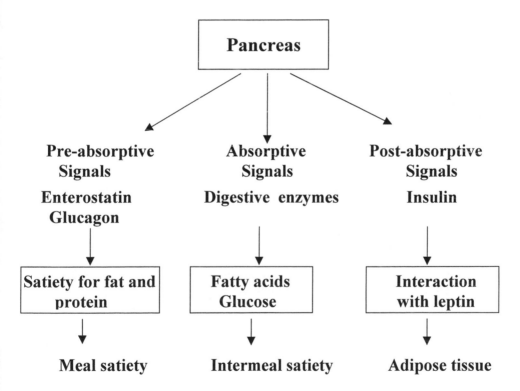

Figure 2. The pancreas and appetite regulation. The pancreas is heavily involved in appetite regulation, primarily through production of satiety signals (pre-absorptive, absorptive and post-absorptive).

That the pancreas has a fundamental role in various aspects of appetite regulation is obvious. Through the pre-meal secretion of enzymes food intake is stimulated and the handling of food optimised. A low secretion or inhibition of the pancreatic enzymes leads to a reduction of appetite in a macronutrient-selective way. Through the production of regulatory peptides the pancreas is also involved in the handling of nutrient substrates and their oxidation, as summarized in Figure 2. These interrelationships await further studies.

REFERENCES

1. J. Mayer and D.W. Thomas, Science, 156 (1967) 328.
2. J. Louis-Sylvestre and J. Le Magnen, Neurosci. Biobehav. Rev., 4, Suppl. 1 (1980) 13.
3. L.A. Campfield and F.J. Smith, Int. J. Obes., 14, Suppl. 3 (1990) 15.
4. G.C. Kennedy, Proc. R. Soc. London B Biol. Sci., 140 (1953) 578.
5. J.H. Strubbe and J. Gorrisen, Physiol. Behav., 25 (1980) 775.
6. W.F. Colmer and C. Wahlestedt. The biology of neuropeptide Y and related peptides, Humana, Totowa, NJ, 1993.
7. Y. Dumont, J.C. Martel, A. Fournier, S. St Pierre and R. Quirion, Prog. Neurobiol., 38 (1992) 125.
8. K. Tatemoto, M. Carlqvist and V. Mutt, Nature, 296 (1982) 659.
9. J.T. Clark, P.S. Kalra, W.R. Crowley and S.P. Kalra, Endocrinology, 115 (1984) 427.
10. B.G. Stanley and S.F. Leibowitz, Life Sci., 35 (1984) 2635.
11. B.G. Stanley, D.R. Daniel, A.S. Chin and S.F. Leibowitz, Peptides, 6 (1985) 1205.
12. M. Jhanwar-Uniyal, B. Beck, C. Burlet and S.F. Leibowitz, Brain Res., 536 (1990) 331.
13. C. Larue-Achagiotis, C. Martin, R. Verger and J. Louis-Sylvestre, Physiol. Behav., 51 (1992) 995.
14. C.J. Billington, J.E. Briggs, S. Harker, M. Grace and A.S. Levine, Amer. J. Physiol., 266 (1994) R1765.
15. M. Egawa, H. Yoshimatsu and G.A. Bray, Amer. J. Physiol., 260 (1991) R238.
16. N. Zarjevski, I. Cusin, R. Vettor, F. Rohner-Jeanrenaud and B. Jeanrenaud, Diabetes, 43 (1994) 764.
17. C. Wahlestedt, G. Skagerberg, R. Ekman, M. Heilig, F. Sundler and R. Håkanson, Brain Res., 417 (1987) 33.
18. L.S. Brady, M.A. Smith, P.W. Gold and M. Erkenham, Neuroendocrinology, 52 (1990) 441.
19. S.C. Chua, A.W. Brown, J.Kim, K.L. Hennessey, R.L. Leibel and J. Hirsch, Brain Res. Mol. Brain Res., 11 (1991) 291.
20. L. Davies and J.L. Marks, Amer. J. Physiol., 266 (1994) R1687.
21. A. Sahu, P.S. Kalra and S.P. Kalra, Peptides, 9 (1988) 83.
22. C. Li, P. Chen and M.S. Smith, Brain Res., 824 (1999) 267.
23. D.E. Lewis, L. Shellard, D.G. Koeslag, D.E. Boer and H.D. McCarthy et al., Amer. J. Physiol., 264 (1993) E279.
24. T.E. Thiele, D. J. Marsh, L. S. Marie, I. L. Bernstein and R.D. Palmiter, Nature, 396 (1998) 366.

25. K. Tatemoto, A. Rokaeus, H. Jörnvall, T.J. McDonald and V. Mutt, FEBS Lett., 164 (1983) 124.
26. T. Melander, T. Hokfelt and A. Rokaeus, J. Comp. Neurol., 248 (1986) 475.
27. E. Adhegate, Z. Ember, T. Donath, D.J. Pallot and J. Singh, Peptides, 17 (1996) 503.
28. M. Bersani, A.H.Johnsen, P. Hojrup, B.E. Dunning, J.J. Andreasen and J.J. Holst, FEBS Lett., 283 (1991) 189.
29. S.E. Kyrkouli, B.G. Stanley, R.D. Seirafi and S.F. Leibowitz, Peptides, 11 (1990) 995.
30. J.N. Crawley, M.C. Austin, S.M. Fiske, B. Martin, S. Consolo, M. Berthold, U. Langel, G. Fisone and T. Bartfai, J. Neurosci., 10 (1990) 3695.
31. D.L. Tempel, K.J. Leibowitz and S.F. Leibowitz, Peptides, 9 (1988) 309.
32. B.K. Smith, D.A. York and G.A. Bray, Brain Res. Bull., 39 (1996) 149.
33. A. Akabayashi, C.T.B.V. Zaia, J.I. Koenig, S.M. Gabriel, I. Silva and S.F. Leibowitz, Peptides, 15 (1994) 1437.
34. A. Akabayashi, J.I. Koenig, Y. Watanabe, J.T. Alexander and S.F. Leibowitz, Proc. Natl. Acad. Sci. USA, 91 (1994) 10375.
35. H. Nagase, G.A. Bray and D.A.York, Brain Res., 709 (1996) 44.
36. J.A. Menendez, D.M. Atrens and S. F. Leibowitz, Peptides, 13 (1992) 323.
37. B.K. Smith, D.A. York and G.A. Bray, Peptides, 15 (1994) 1267.
38. D.L. Tempel and S.F. Leibowitz, Brain Res., 536 (1990) 353.
39. M.W. Schwartz, A.J. Sipols, C.E. Grubin and D.G. Baskin. Brain Res. Bull., 31 (1993) 361.
40. J.E. Morley, A.S.Levine, G.K.Yim and M.T. Lowy, Neurosci. BioBehav. Rev., 7 (1983) 281.
41. L.D. Reid, Amer. J. Clin. Nutr., 42 (1985) 1099.
42. C. Barton, L. Lin, D.A. York and G.A. Bray, Brain Res.,702 (1995) 55.
43. A. Drewnovski, D.D. Krahn, M.A.Demitrack, K. Nairn and B.A. Gosnell, Physiol. Behav., 51 (1992) 371.
44. L.A. Parker, S. Maier, M. Rennie and J. Crebolder, Behav. Neurosci., 106 (1992) 999.
45. D.T. Weldon, E. O'Hare, J. Cleary, C.J. Billington and A.S. Levine, Amer. J. Physiol., 39 (1996) R1183.
46. M.J. Glass, M. Grace, J.P. Cleary, C.J. Billington and A.S. Levine, Amer. J. Physiol., 271 (1996) R217.
47. T.C. Kirkham and J.E. Blundell, Pharmacol. Biochem. Behav., 26 (1987) 515.
48. G. Brennan, S.E. Bachus and M. Jhanwar-Uniyal, J. Neurosci., 20 (1994) 818.
49. C.C. Welch, E.M. Kim, M.K. Grace, C.J. Billington and A.S. Levine, Brain Res., 721 (1996) 126.
50. X.Z. Khawaja, A.K. Chattopadhyay and I.C. Green, Brain Res., 555 (1991) 164.
51. E.M. Kim, C.M. Kotz, C.C. Welch, M.K. Grace, C.J. Billington and A.S. Levine, Brain Res., 769 (1997) 303.
52. E.M. Kim, C.C. Welch, M.K. Grace, C.J. Billington and A.S. Levine, Amer. J. Physiol., 270 (1996) R1019.
53. A.S. Levine and C.J. Billington, Clin. Appl. Nutr., 1 (1991) 33.
54. D.D. Krahn, B.A. Gosnell, M.Grace and A.S. Levine, Brain Res. Bull., 17 (1986) 285.
55. J. Junquera, G. Lanzagorta and M. Russek. Appetite, 9 (1987) 113.
56. S.C. Heinrichs, J. Lapsabsky, D.P. Behanm R.K, Chanm, P.E Sawchenko, M. Lorang et al., Proc. Natl. Acad. Sci. USA, 93 (1996) 15475.
57. B.A. Boston, K.M. Blaydon, J. Varnerin, and R.D. Cone, Science, 278 (1997) 1641.

310

58. J.E. Morley and A.S. Levine, Science, 209 (1980) 1259.
59. T. Rutledge and W. Linden, J. Behav. Med., 21 (1998) 221.
60. J. Gibbs, R.C. Youngs and G.P. Smith, Nature, 245 (1973) 323.
61. C. Erlanson-Albertsson and D.A. York, Obes. Res., 5 (1997) 360.
62. M.I. Friedman, Proc. Nutr. Soc., 56 (1997) 41.
63. W. Langhans, Proc. Nutr. Soc., 55 (1996) 497.
64. U.R. Fölsch, N. Grieb, W.F. Caspary and W. Creutzfeldt, Digestion, 21 (1981) 74.
65. Y. Zhang et al., Nature, 372 (1994) 425.
66. K.S. Polonsky, B.D. Given, E. Van Cauter, J. Clin. Invest., 81 (1988) 442.
67. R.D. Reidelberger, T.J. Kalogeris and T.E. Solomon, Amer. J. Physiol., 256 (1989) R1148.
68. C.A. Baile, C.L. McLaughin and M.A. Della-Fera, Physiol. Rev., 66 (1986) 172.
69. R.D. Reidelberger and T.E. Solomon, Amer. J. Physiol., 251 (1986) R97.
70. H.R. Kissileif, F.X. Pi-Sunyer, J. Thornton and G.P. Smith, Amer. J. Clin. Nutr., 34 (1981) 154.
71. G. Hewson, G.E. Leighton, R.G. Hill and J. Hughes, Brit. J. Pharmacol., 93 (1988) 79.
72. S. Khosla and J.N. Crawley, Life Sci., 42 (1988) 153.
73. C.A. Riedy, M. Chavez, D.P. Figliwicz and S.C. Woods; Physiol. Behav., 58 (1995) 755.
74. M.D. Barrachina, V. Martinez, L. Wang, J.Y. Wei and Y.Tache, Proc. Natl. Acad. Sci. USA, 94 (1997) 10455.
75. J. Drewe, A. Gradient, L.C. Rovati and C. Beglinger, Gastroenterology, 102 (1992) 1654.
76. J.N. Crawley and M.C. Beinfeld, Nature, 302 (1983) 703.
77. T.H. Moran, L.F. Katz, C.R. Plata-Salaman and G.J. Schwartz. Amer. J. Physiol., 274 (1998) R618.
78. G. Flo, S. Vermant, M. van Boven, P. Daeneus, J. Buyse, E. Decuypere, E. Kuhn and M. Cokelane, Horm. Metab. Res., 30 (1998) 504.
79. R.D. Simmonds, F.C. Kaiser, M.E. Pierson and J.R. Rosamund, Pharmacol. Biochem. Behav., 59 (1998) 439.
80. T.H. Moran, A.R. Baldessarini, C.F. Salorio, T. Lowery and G.J. Schwartz, Amer. J. Physiol., 272 (1997) R1245.
81. J. Blundell, Trends Pharmacol. Sci., 12 (19919 147.
82. G.A. Bray, Am. J. Clin. Nutr., 55 (1992) 2655.
83. S.F. Leibowitz, Ann. NY Acad. Sci., 739 (1994) 12.
84. J.M. Van Amelsvoort, P. Van Straum, J.H. Kraal, R.N. Lussenberg and V.M.T. Houtsmuller, Brit. J. Nutr., 61 (1988) 267.
85. S.F. Leibowitz, Neurosci. Biobehav. Rev., 12 (1988) 101.
86. B.K. Smith, D.A. York and G.A. Bray, Brain Res. Bull., 39 (1996) 149.
87. C. Erlanson-Albertsson. Biochim. Biophys. Acta, 1125 (1992) 1.
88. J. Mei, R.C. Bowyer, A.M.T. Jehanli, G. Patel and C. Erlanson-Albertsson, Pancreas, 8 (1993) 488.
89. C. Rippe and C. Erlanson-Albertsson, Nutr. Neuroscience, 1 (1998) 111.
90. C. Erlanson-Albertsson, Pancreatic lipase, colipase and enterostatin - a lipolytic triad. In: Esterases, lipases and phospholipases: From Structure to Clinical Significance, M.I. Mackness and M. Clerc, (eds.), Plenum Press, New York, 1994.
91. C. Erlanson-Albertsson and A. Larsson, Biochimie, 70 (1988) 1245.

92. N.S. Shargill, S. Tsujii, G.A. Bray and C. Erlanson-Albertsson, Brain Res., 544 (1991) 137.
93. S. Okada, D.A. York, G.A. Bray and C. Erlanson-Albertsson, Physiol. Behav., 49 (1991) 1185.
94. S. Okada, D.A. York, G.A. Bray, J. Mei and C. Erlanson-Albertsson, Amer. J. Physiol., 262 (1992) R1111.
95. L. Lin and D.A. York, Amer. J. Physiol., 275 (1998) R619.
96. K. Berger, M. Sörhede-Winzell and C. Erlanson-Albertsson, Peptides, 19 (1998) 1525.
97. H. Mizuma, J. Abadie and C. Prasad, Peptides, 15 (1994) 447.
98. B. Ahren, S. Mansson, R.L. Gingerich and P.J. Havel, Amer. J. Physiol., 273 (1997) R113.
99. S. Okada, T. Onai, G. Kilroy, D.A. York and G.A. Bray, Amer. J. Physiol., 265 (1993) R21.
100. L. Lin, S. McClanahan, D.A. York and G.A. Bray, Physiol. Behav., 53 (1993) 789.
101. J. Mei and C. Erlanson-Albertsson, Regul. Pept., 41 (1992) 209.
102. C. Erlanson-Albertsson, B. Weström, S.C. Pierzynowski, S. Karlsson and B. Ahrén, Pancreas, 6 (1991) 619.
103. S.C. Pierzynowski, C.Erlanson-Albertsson, P. Podgurniak, P. Kiela and B. Weström, Biomed. Res., 15, Suppl.2 (1994) 257.
104. P. Kiela, S C. Pierzynowski, T. Oldak, M. Ceregrzyn, C. Erlanson-Albertsson, M. Wiechetek and S. Garwacki, Biomed. Res., 15, Suppl.2 (1994) 303.
105. J. Mei, M. Bourras and C. Erlanson-Albertsson, Peptides, 18 (1997) 651.
106. K. Ookuma, C. Barton, D.A. York and G.A. Bray, Peptides, 18 (1997) 785.
107. L. Lin, M. Umahara, D.A. York and G.A. Bray, Peptides, 19 (1998) 325.
108. L.C. Read, A.P.D. Lord, V. Brantl and G. Koch, Amer. J. Physiol., 259 (1990) G443.
109. H. Daniel, M. Vohwinkel and G. Rehner, J. Nutr., 120 (1990) 252.
110. S.C. Pierzynowski, B. Weström, C. Erlanson-Albertsson, B. Ahrén, J. Svendsen and B. Karlsson, J. Pediatr. Gastroenterol. Nutr., 16 (1992) 287.
111. M. Krotkievsky and B. Carlsson, Int. J. Obesity, 22, Suppl. 3 (1998) S8.
112. J.G. Verbalis, D.W. Richardson and E. M. Stricker, Amer. J. Physiol., 252 (1987) R749.
113. W. Langhans, U. Damaske and E. Scharrer, Appetite, 6 (1985) 143.
114. M.G. Tordoff and M.I. Friedman, Amer. J. Physiol., 254 (1988) R969.
115. W. Langhans, Proc. Nutr. Soc., 55 (1996) 497.
116. L.A. Campfield, F.J. Smith and P. Brandon, Brain Res. Bull., 14 (1985) 605.
117. D. Novin, K. Robinson, L.A. Culbreth and M.G. Tordoff, Amer. J. Clin. Nutr., 42 (1985) 1050.
118. P. Even and S. Nicolaidis, Brain Res. Bull., 17 (1986) 621.
119. S. Ritter and T.T. Dinh, Brain Res., 641 (1994) 111.
120. D. Greenberg, G.P. Smith and J. Gibbs. Amer. J. Physiol., 259 (1990) R110.
121. S.C. Woods, L.J. Stein, L.D. McKay and D. Porte, Amer. J. Physiol., 247 (1984) R393.
122. E. Scharrer and W. Langhans, Am. J. Physiol., 250 (1986) R1003.
123. M.I. Friedman, I. Ramirez, C.R. Bowden and M.G. Tordoff, Amer. J. Physiol., 258 (1990) R216.
124. W. Langhans and . E. Scharrer, J. Auton. Nerv. Syst., 18 (1987) 13.
125. S. Ritter and J.S. Taylor, Amer. J. Physiol., 258 (1990) R1395.

312

126. M. Senn, S. Gross-Lüem and W. Langhans, Proc. Soc. Nutr. Physiol., 4 (1995) 64.
127. L.A. Campfield, F.J. Smith, Y. Guisez, R. Devos and P. Burn, Science, 269 (1995) 546.
128. H. Masuzaki, Nature Med., 3 (1997) 1029.
129. A.Bado, S. Levasseur, S. Attoub, S. Kermorgant, J-P. Laigneau, M-N. Bortoluzzi, L. Moizo et a.l, Nature, 394 (1998) 790.
130. M. Sörhede, H. Mulder, J. Mei, F. Sundler and C. Erlanson-Albertsson, Biochim. Biophys. Acta, 1301 (1996) 207.
131. L.A. Tartaglia et al., Cell, 83 (1995) 1263.
132. Chen et al., Cell, 84 (1996) 491.
133. M.W. Schwartz, E. Peskind, M. Raskind, E.J. Boyko and D. Porte, Nat. Med., 2 (1996) 589.
134. M.A. Pelleymounter et al., Science, 269 (1995) 540.
135. J.C. Erickson et al., Nature, 381 (1996) 415.
136. R.C. Frederich, B. Lollmann, A. Hamann, A. Napolitano-Rosen, B.B. Kah, B.B. Lowell and J.S. Flier, J. Clin. Invest., 96 (1995) 1658.
137. M. Maffei, J. Halaas, E. Ravussin et al., Nat. Med., 1 (1995) 1155.
138. C.T. Montague, I.S. Farooqi, J.P. Whitehead, M.A. Soos et al., Nature 387 (1997) 903.
139. J.D. Bagdade, E.L. Bierman and D. Porte, J.Clin. Invest., 46 (1967) 1549.
140. D. Wu, J. Yang amd W.M. Pardridge, , J.Clin. Invest., 100 (1997) 1804.
141. J.W. Unger and M. Betz, Histol. Histopathol., 13 (1998) 1215.
142. J. Seufert, T.J. Kieffer and J.F. Habener, Proc. Natl. Acad. Sci. USA, 96 (1999) 674.
143. B. Cohen, D. Novick and M. Rubinstein, Science, 274 (1996) 1185.
144. J.G. Brand, R.H. Cagan and M. Naim, Ann. Rev. Nutr., 2 (1982) 249.
145. A. Sclafani, Proc. Nutr. Soc., 54 (1995) 419.
146. K. Ackroff and A. Sclafani, Amer. J. Physiol., 271 (1996) R48.
147. I.P. Pavlov, The work of the digestive glands, London, Charles Griffin, 1902.
148. H.D. Janowitz, F. Hollander,D. Orringer, M.H. Levy, A. Winkelstein, M.R. Kaufmann and S.G. Margolin, Gastroenterology, 16 (1950) 104.
149. C.T. Richardson, J.H. Walsh, K.A. Kooper, M. Feldman and J.S. Fordtran, J. Clin. Invest., 60 (1977) 435.
150. J.G. Moore and D. Motoki, Gastroenterology, 76 (1979) 71.
151. B.H. Novis, S. Bank and I.N. Marks, Scand. J. Gastroenterol., 6 (1971) 417.
152. H. Sarles, R. Dani, G. Prezelin, C. Souville and C. Figarella, Gut, 9 (1968) 214.
153. H.R. Behrman and M.R. Kare, Proc. Soc. Exp. Biol. Med., 129 (1968) 343.
154. I. Ohara, S. Otsuka and Y.Yugari, J. Nutr. 109 (1979) 2098.
155. J.R. Malagelada, V.L.W Go and W.H. J. Summerskill, Dig. Dis. Sci., 24 (1979) 101.
156. M. Naim, M. R. Kare and A.M. Merritt, Physiol. Behav., 20 (1978) 563.
157. G. Holtmann, M.V. Singer, R. Kriebel, K.H. Stäcker and H. Goebell, Dig. Dis. Sci., 34 (1989) 1701.
158. M.L. Drent and E.A. van der Veen, Int. J. Obes., 17 (1993) 241.
159. S. Hogan, A. Fleury, P. Hadvary, H. Lengsfeld, M.K. Meier, J. Triscari and A.C. Sullivan, Int. J. Obes., 11, Suppl.3 (1987) 35.
160. A. Adachi, M. Funahashi and J. Ohga, Brain Res. Bull., 27 (1991) 529.
161. J. DeVries, J.H. Strubbe, W.C. Wildering, J.A. Gorter and A.J.A. Prins, Physiol. Behav., 53 (1993) 229.

162. W. Langhans, Nutrition, 12 (1996) 303.

163. S.C. Woods and J.H. Strubbe, Psychonomic Bulletin and Review, 1 (1994) 141.

164. J. Louis-Sylvestre, I. Giachetti and J. Le Magnen, Appetite, 4 (1983) 295.

165. W.H. Karasov and J.M. Diamond, Science, 228 (1985) 202.

166. W.D. van Marken Lichtenbelt, Physiol. Zool., 65 (1992) 649.

167. O. Boss, P. Muzzin and J-P Giacobino, Eur. J. Endocrinol., 139 (1998) 1.

168. D. Cannon and J. Nedergaard, Essays Biochem., 20 (1985) 111.

169. D. Ricquier, F. Bouillard, P. Toumelin, G. Mory, , R. Bazin, J. Arch and L. Penicaud, J. Biol. Chem., 261 (1986) 13905.

170. S. Enerbäck, A. Jacobsson, E. Simpson, C. Guerra, H. Yamashita, M. Harper and L.P. Kozak, Nature, 387 (1997) 90.

171. J. Himms-Hagen, Int. J. Obesity 22, Suppl. 3, (1998) S2.

172. C. Fleury, M. Neverova, S. Collins, S. Raimbault, O. Champigny, C. Levi-Meyrueis, Bouillard, M.F. Seldin, R.S. Surwit, D. Ricquier and C.H. Warden, Nature Gen., 15 (1997) 269.

173. O. Boss, S. Samec, A. Paoloni-Giacobino, C. Rossier, A. Dulloo, J. Seydoux, J. Muzzin and J.P. Giacobino, FEBS Lett., 408 (1997) 39.

174. D. Sanchis, C. Fleury, N. Chomiki, M. Goubern, Q. Huang et al., J. Biol. Chem., 273 (1998) 34611.

175. O. Boss, S. Samec, A. Dulloo, J. Seydoux, J. Muzzin and J.P. Giacobino, FEBS Lett., 412 (1997) 111.

Biology of the Pancreas in Growing Animals
S.G. Pierzynowski and R. Zabielski (Editors)

Role of the endocrine pancreas in animal metabolism, growth and performance

S.S. Donkin

Department of Animal Sciences, 1151 Lilly Hall, Purdue University,
West Lafayette, IN, 47097, USA

The endocrine pancreas acts as a sensor to glucose supply and demand and integrates these signals to release hormones that modulate metabolism in order to maintain blood glucose concentrations within physiological limits. In so doing, the hormones of the endocrine pancreas co-ordinate the availability of glucose for growth, adipose tissue deposition and milk production. The purpose of this review is to highlight some recent advances in our understanding of the actions of the hormones of the endocrine pancreas, primarily insulin and glucagon, with particular reference to their actions in domestic livestock and their impact on whole animal performance. Understanding the actions of these hormones will provide a basis for concepts that will advance the ability to better predict and manipulate animal growth, well-being, and performance.

1. INTRODUCTION

The primary function of the endocrine cells of the pancreas, located within the islets of Langerhans, is to synthesise and secrete insulin, glucagon and somatostatin. The centrality of these hormones to control of metabolism is evident by the disease states that are precipitated by aberrant control of their synthesis, release and action. The vast literature exploring the *in vivo* and *in vitro* mechanism of their actions underscores the commonalities yet the subtle difference, across species and physiological states.

Circulating glucose concentration is a function of glucose production rate and the rate of glucose removal. Too often changes in circulating glucose concentrations are interpreted as increases in glucose production by liver cells and/or increased glucose absorption. Insulin and glucagon mediate the balance between glucose removal and glucose production and absorption. Glucagon stimulates the production of glucose by the liver and the breakdown of glucose stores, such as glycogen. Insulin acutely opposes the action of glucagon by increasing the removal of glucose by adipose tissue and muscle. Insulin-mediated changes in muscle protein synthesis and amino acid availability may indirectly impact hepatic glucose synthesis. More prolonged changes in metabolism evoked by insulin and glucagon are mediated through changes in receptor numbers, receptor sensitivity and other endocrine factors which transmodulate the responsiveness of target tissues. These homeorrhetic adaptations often involve changes in expression of key genes in glucose production and glucose disposal, alterations in receptor numbers and activity, and are mediated by hormones and metabolites.

In considering the role of the endocrine pancreas in relation to growth and metabolism the acute and chronic effects of insulin, glucagon and to a lesser extent somatostatin will be discussed with particular regard to control of glucose synthesis and disposal.

2. HORMONE SECRETION AND REMOVAL

Circulating hormonal concentrations are a function of secretion and removal rate yet in livestock they are influenced more by secretion rates than by clearance rates [1]. Net portal insulin appearance in cattle is 419 ug/h [2] and represents insulin release from the pancreas minus insulin removal by the portal drained visceral (PDV) tissue. The rate of insulin secretion is inhibited in catabolic states such as prolonged cold exposure, exercise or early lactation [3] and is increased by feeding and the absorbed products of digestion in ruminants [4]. A temporal pattern of insulin secretion is evident in response to feeding pattern in cattle and frequent feeding removes the large postprandial insulin increases in dairy steers [5] and lactating dairy cattle [6]. Portal drained visceral flux of insulin was not statistically different between lactating and nonlactating cattle despite a 3-fold higher mean portal insulin appearance rate in nonlactating animals [7]. The net portal insulin appearance rate was similar in lactating cattle at 4 weeks and 8 weeks postpartum [8]. These data suggest that insulin secretion is responsive to physiological state but may not be the only factor regulating peripheral insulin concentrations.

Under normal conditions, insulin and glucagon are secreted by the pancreas into the portal vein and travel first to the liver. The liver is not only one of the primary target organs for pancreatic hormones but is also an important site for their clearance [9]. The liver and kidneys are the main sites of insulin removal, with the liver accounting for the majority of insulin clearance [10]. Hepatic extraction of insulin, as a percentage of portal insulin flux, is only 8% in nonlactating sheep and 13% in lactating cattle [2]. Hepatic extraction, as a percentage of net portal insulin appearance, is 50% in sheep [10] and 66% in cattle [2]. The sum of liver and kidney insulin extraction accounts for 88% of total pancreatic production [10].

The liver plays an important role in determining the concentrations of insulin and glucagon in peripheral blood in nonruminants and may contribute to diurnal variations in peripheral insulin concentrations [11]. Also, peripheral glucagon concentrations during fasting are relatively constant, despite elevated portal glucagon concentrations [11]. The effect of the liver to alter the ratio of insulin to glucagon in favour of high insulin during feeding [11] acts to promote postprandial glucose utilisation by peripheral tissue.

Quantitative data for glucagon secretion and clearance in livestock is lacking. Peripheral plasma concentrations are increased after feeding and increase in response to ruminal and intravascular volatile fatty acids (VFA) infusions in goats [4]. Net removal of glucagon by the liver accounts for 31% of net PDV production in sheep [12] and 13.1% in cattle [2].

Insulin is released from the β-cells of the pancreas in response to elevated blood glucose concentrations by emicytosis. In ruminants, the physiological relevance and implication of the effects of volatile fatty acids on insulin release remains controversial [4]. Observations that insulin secretion from bovine islets is more sensitive to propionate and less sensitive to glucose than secretion from human or pig pancreatic islets [13] suggests species differences in energy sensing by the pancreas. These inherent differences cannot be ignored, particularly in light of the conflicting reports on the effects of glucose on insulin status in lactating cows and sheep [14,15,16].

3. MODULATION OF GLUCONEOGENESIS

Gluconeogenesis is the process by which glucose is produced from noncarbohydrate precursors such as lactate, amino acids, glycerol, and propionate. The latter is especially important in ruminants where more than 50% of glucose carbon can originate from propionate [17]. The importance of hepatic gluconeogenesis in dairy cattle during lactation is highlighted by the fact that hypoglycaemia, ketosis, and related metabolic disorders are often observed when gluconeogenic capacity fails to adapt to the increased demands of lactose synthesis and mammary metabolism.

Hepatic gluconeogenesis accounts for most of the glucose synthesised in the body and is regulated by substrate availability and a number of hormones. Insulin and glucagon are the primary regulators of gluconeogenesis in pigs, chickens, and cattle, although the impact of these hormones on specific substrate utilisation differs across species. There are distinct phases during the life cycle of livestock that underscore the importance of gluconeogenesis: 1) adaptations in the neonate to extrauterine life 2) the transition from preruminant to ruminant state 3) the transition to lactation and 4) adaptation to nutrient imbalance or shortage. The ability of insulin and glucagon to regulate gluconeogenesis during these periods is modulated by other hormones as well as by the supply and profile of gluconeogenic precursors.

3.1. Gluconeogenesis and substrate metabolism *in vivo*

The effects of insulin and glucagon on specific gluconeogenic substrates have been investigated using trans-hepatic balance measurements in conjunction with portal infusions of these hormones and (^{14}C)gluconeogenic precursors [18]. Determining gluconeogenesis by transfer quotient methods, in those experiments, assumes that the underestimation errors associated with the technique are constant when hormonal conditions are perturbed [19]. Inhibitory effects of insulin on hepatic glucose output have also been demonstrated using the euglycaemic hyperinsulinaemic clamp technique [3,18,20], but changes in glucose output determined by this model reflect a general effect of insulin on hepatic gluconeogenesis.

Insulin *in vivo* acts to decrease net hepatic uptake of lactate, alanine, glutamine and glycerol [21] and to decrease lactate conversion to glucose in sheep [22]. Insulin had no effect on the rate of propionate conversion to glucose but increased gluconeogenesis from propionate [23]. The slight increase in gluconeogenesis from propionate in these experiments may reflect insulin effects to decrease glucose output from all other glucogenic substrates by 26% [23]. These results indicate that insulin effects on gluconeogenesis are specific for lactate, alanine, glutamine and glycerol and result in decreased hepatic extraction of these substrates [22].

The effects of glucagon on hepatic gluconeogenesis oppose the effects of insulin described above. Glucagon stimulates glycogenolysis [10,24] and gluconeogenesis in sheep liver [10]. Gluconeogenesis from (U-^{14}C)alanine was increased from 1.68 to 2.79 mmol/h by portal infusion of glucagon in fed sheep which corresponds to a doubling, from 15 to 30%, of alanine use for glucose synthesis [10]. The effects of glucagon to increase gluconeogenesis from alanine are matched by increased hepatic uptake of alanine [10,25]. Hepatic uptake of glycine, glutamine, arginine, asparagine, threonine, and serine are also increased by glucagon and contribute to increased hepatic glucose production [25]. Similar changes are observed during the transition to lactation in dairy cattle when gluconeogenesis from lactate is increased [26]. It has been proposed that glucagon, in addition to promoting hepatic gluconeogenesis, regulates the availability of amino acids for extrahepatic tissue metabolism by altering hepatic extraction of amino acids [22].

Gluconeogenesis from propionate in fed sheep is unchanged by somatostatin-imposed glucagon insufficiency or by elevated portal glucagon concentrations achieved through glucagon infusions [24]. Hepatic propionate removal is 90% efficient [27] and propionate accounts for 63% of glucose synthesis [24]. Complete use of propionate for glucose synthesis under basal conditions, when there is adequate reserve capacity for propionate metabolism [28], would explain the lack of glucagon effects on propionate metabolism. The lack of effect on propionate and the apparent specific effect on alanine metabolism suggest regulation of flux through pyruvate carboxylase (PC) by glucagon [22], an enzyme not directly involved in the metabolism of propionate to glucose. The PC enzyme is not acutely regulated by glucagon via phosphorylation [29] as are other substrate cycle enzymes which regulate flux from propionate and lactate to glucose, therefore suggesting alternative regulation.

3.2. Gluconeogenesis and metabolic zonation of liver tissue

The functional unit of the liver is a cluster of hepatocytes known as a lobule, where blood flows through sinusoids that branch from the portal vein to the central vein. Usually there is only one layer of hepatocytes between sinusoids so that the contact area between plasma and hepatocyte is very large. The diffuse blood flow through the liver results in histological and anatomical uniformity of lobules. Adaptations to hormonal, metabolite, and oxygen gradients across the liver lobule are partly responsible for metabolic heterogeneity of the liver *in vivo* [30]. Hepatocytes immediately adjacent to the portal veins (periportal hepatocytes) display higher activities of the key gluconeogenic enzymes phosphoenolpyruvate carboxykinase (PEPCK) [31,32], fructose-1,6-bisphosphatase [33], and glucose 6-phosphatase [34] and have higher rates of gluconeogenesis [35]. Chronic incubation of cells in the presence of glucagon or insulin respectively invokes them to acquire periportal-like and perivenous-like characteristics [36].

Substrate antagonisms may impact the effects of hormones on net hepatic gluconeogenesis. Experiments using isolated cultured hepatocytes indicate that propionate inhibits gluconeogenesis from lactate in the bovine [37]. Given that propionate is mostly removed during the first pass through the ruminant liver, any increase in the gluconeogenic capacity of periportal hepatocytes will result in a steeper gradient of propionate removal across the liver lobule and decrease the antagonistic effects of propionate on gluconeogenesis from lactate. Conversely, shifting propionate metabolism towards the pericentral cells would decrease gluconeogenesis from lactate with little effect on gluconeogenesis from propionate. The observed lack of glucagon effects on gluconeogenesis from 2-(^{14}C)propionate [24] but increased hepatic extraction of lactate *in vivo* [22] support this model.

In vitro data demonstrate that gluconeogenesis from both propionate and lactate are responsive to glucagon [37,38,39] and dibutyryl cAMP [38,40] and conflict with *in vivo* data demonstrating lack of effects of glucagon on gluconeogenesis from propionate [24]. Direct regulation of gluconeogenesis by insulin also conflicts with *in vivo* data and indicates that insulin decreases gluconeogenesis from propionate but not lactate or glycerol [37]. Differences between *in vivo* and *in vitro* data may reflect the shortcoming of each system to account for the substrate interactions and hormonal effects that occur within the liver microstructure.

The decreased portal concentration of insulin observed early in lactation [7] coupled with unchanged glucagon secretion rate [41], may favour recruitment of hepatocytes closer to the central vein in order to support an increase in hepatic glucose output. *In vitro* experiments using bovine hepatocyte monolayer cultures suggest that low circulating insulin concentrations would favour gluconeogenesis from lactate and enhance the ability of glucagon to increase that flux [37].

3.3. Regulation of expression of genes encoding gluconeogenic enzymes

Long-term regulation of gluconeogenesis in *nonruminants* has been characterised by changes in the expression of genes encoding glucoregulatory enzymes, mainly PEPCK and pyruvate kinase [42]. It is well established that insulin represses whereas glucagon (or cAMP) and glucocorticoids induce PEPCK activity by directly regulating expression of the gene [43]. Lactate use for glucose synthesis is distributed between pyruvate kinase and the reactions involving PC and PEPCK. [44]. Glucocorticoids and glucagon have little effect on flux through the PK catalysed reaction; therefore, an increase in gluconeogenesis from lactate in glucocorticoid treated rats or hepatocytes is mainly due to the combined increases in flux through reactions catalysed by PC and PEPCK [45].

Regulation of PEPCK expression has been extensively studied in the liver of rodents as well as rat and human hepatoma cell lines. Glucagon acting in the presence of dexamethasone is one of the primary stimulators of PEPCK gene expression. Control of PEPCK activity is largely exerted through activation of basal, tissue-specific, and hormone-dependent transcription factors and binding to promoter elements within the 5' region of the PEPCK gene. Crucial liver control elements are located within -460 to +73 of the promoter and 6 primary protein binding sites have been characterized by DNAse I footprinting. These six sites contain docking sites for at least 15 separate transcription factors.

The cAMP response element CRE-I acting synergistically with P3 and P4 is primarily responsible for the cAMP-mediated increase in PEPCK transcription. Insulin counteracts the effects of cAMP by repressing the promoter, perhaps by blocking the ability of glucocorticoids to promote the activity of accessory factor-2. Although the PEPCK gene is transcriptionally controlled there is also regulation through stability of the PEPCK mRNA which is mediated by a 3' noncoding sequence [46]. There is some indication that PEPCK expression may be inhibited directly by glucose as well, which is also the case with other insulin-responsive genes. This is particularly intriguing in ruminants based on the observation that glucokinase is lacking in the ruminant liver [47] but may represent a evolutionary advantage considering the continual need for gluconeogenesis in ruminants.

Bovine somatotropin (bST) increases hepatic glucose output in cattle [48]. Hepatocytes isolated from sheep treated with somatotropin had higher rates of $(2-{}^{14}C)$propionate incorporation into glucose [49]. The ability of liver slices to fix ${}^{14}CO_2$ into glucose is increased and labelling of the pyruvate pool is decreased in liver slices from cattle treated with bST [50]. The latter is indicative of increased flux through PC and PEPCK relative to PK and suggests up-regulation of either or both of these enzymes. A portion of the effect of bST may be mediated by the insulin antagonistic effects [51] although this has not been evaluated directly for bovine liver.

In cattle and sheep the activity of PC, an enzyme unique to lactate and alanine metabolism to glucose, is responsive to nutritional and physiological states which impose the greatest demands for endogenous glucose production, such as lactation and feed deprivation [52]. In contrast, the activity of PEPCK is relatively invariant between different nutritional and physiological states in ruminants, diabetes being the exception. Recent data from the author's laboratory [53] indicate that expression of PC mRNA is dramatically increased across the transition to lactation whereas PEPCK is relatively unchanged during this period. Increased expression of PEPCK lags the increase in PC expression and increases up to 56 days in milk. The differential expression of these genes suggests a regulation that may be related to differences in hormonal profile, sensitivity to hormones, and/or nutrient availability in the peripartum dairy cow.

4. REGULATION OF GLUCOSE DISPOSAL

4.1. Glucose transport

The initial step in the metabolism of glucose by any tissue is transport into the cell. With the exception of active transport of glucose from the lumen of the small intestine and proximal tubule of the kidney, the transport of glucose occurs by facilitated diffusion across cell membranes through the action of the family of glucose transporter (GLUT) proteins. Adipose tissue and muscle express GLUT4 and GLUT1 whereas liver expresses GLUT2 [54]. In adipose tissue and muscle the translocation of GLUT4 from intracellular vesicles to the plasma membrane, in response to activation of the insulin receptor, enhances the capacity of cells to transport glucose across the plasma membrane. Although GLUT1 is not acutely regulated by insulin the prolonged exposure of adipose cells to insulin preferentially increases GLUT1 through changes in gene expression to impact basal glucose transport [55].

Despite extensive characterisation of the GLUT proteins in humans and experimental models of diabetes there is limited information on their regulation in livestock. A partial sequence of porcine GLUT4 (246 base pairs) revealed a 78% sequence identity with human GLUT4 exon 4a and the remainder contains 91% identity with human GLUT4 exon 4b [56]. The importance of GLUT4 in pig adipose tissue is highlighted by the fact that one of the insulin antagonistic effects of somatotropin is a decrease in glucose transport in pig adipose tissue [57]. A portion of the 20-60% decrease in adipose tissue in pigs treated with somatotropin [51] appears to be mediated by changes in GLUT4 gene expression [58].

Bovine GLUT4 [59] is greater than 90% similar to human GLUT4 and bovine GLUT1 is 89 % similar to human GLUT1 [60]. The expression of GLUT4 in bovine adipose tissue is approximately one-tenth that found in muscle, which coupled with the fact that GLUT4 mRNA is undetected in bovine adipocyte cell lines after differentiation suggests a limited role for GLUT4 in lipogenesis in the bovine. Lower glucose clearance in ruminants, relative to nonruminants, in response to insulin infusions further suggests that GLUT4 is less abundant in ruminant species [61]. However, the acute stimulation of lipogenesis in adipose tissue explant cultures by insulin [62] suggests involvement of GLUT4 in insulin-regulated glucose transport in the bovine.

Insulin also facilitates glucose uptake in muscle in livestock [63] presumably by activation of the GLUT4 transporter, described above. Insulin-mediated glucose uptake in lactating cattle is only 8% [64] compared with 18% in non-lactating sheep [65]. Comparable measures in nonruminants indicate that 15-30% of glucose uptake is mediated by the acute actions of insulin [66,67]. Presumably differences in the distribution of GLUT1 and GLUT4 in muscle and adipose tissue of ruminants compared with nonruminants account for some of these differences.

The greater activity of hexokinase relative to glucose uptake by bovine muscle strips indicates that transport is rate limiting for glucose metabolism in cattle and sheep muscle, [61] as is the case in nonruminant muscle. The low level of mRNA for GLUT1 relative to GLUT4 suggests that GLUT4 is the major glucose transporter isoform in ruminant muscle and adipose tissue [61]. Differences also exist between muscle fibre types relative to the distribution of glucose transporters [61]. The decline in insulin-mediated glucose uptake with age in growing steers [68] may reflect an age-related decrease in GLUT4 [69] or changes in muscle fibre types [61]. Conversely, differences reflect an adaptation of ruminant muscle to use of acetate and ketones as energy substrates.

The hepatocyte glucose transporter, GLUT2, and glucose-6-phosphatase act in concert to control the release of glucose from the liver in response to glycogenolysis or gluconeogenesis. The symmetry of GLUT2 enables the transport of glucose into or out of the hepatocyte and the directionality depends only on the concentration differential between intracellular free glucose and blood glucose [70]. Glucose-6 phosphate, formed through gluconeogenesis or glycogenolysis, must be dephosphorylated through the action of glucose-6-phosphatase, and enzyme which is contained within the endoplasmic reticulum in order to release glucose from the hepatocyte. The endoplasmic glucose transporter GLUT7 facilitates the transport of G-6-P to the endoplasmic reticulum where glucose-6-phosphatase acts to release free glucose into the cytoplasm [70]. The lack of appreciable glucokinase activity in the ruminant liver [47] suggests that release of glucose may be controlled by the combined activities of GLUT7 and glucose-6-phosphatase. The cDNAs corresponding to bovine GLUT2 have been cloned and correspond to transcripts of 6.3, 3.8, 2.2 and 1.6 kb which are most abundant in liver, and less abundant in the kidney and duodenum [71]. The effects of GLUT2 in the proximal jejunum of the suckling pig have been characterised, where an increase in glucose oxidation is observed in response to fasting [72]; however there is little additional information on GLUT2 in domestic livestock.

4.2. Lipogenesis and lipolysis

The storage of excess dietary energy as glycogen and lipid is essential for survival and normal function in all animals. Despite several commonalities in the processes of lipogenesis between livestock the main sites of fatty acid synthesis differ greatly across species. Lipogenesis in the chicken occurs almost exclusively in the liver [73] whereas lipogenesis in cattle, sheep and pigs occurs mainly in adipose tissue. Furthermore acetate, and to a lesser extent lactate are the primary lipogenic substrates in ruminants whereas glucose is the primary substrate for fatty acid synthesis in swine [74].

During growth, in meat animals, the proportion of energy stored as adipose tissue becomes the predominant component of body energy gain [75]. Insulin, in addition to affecting glucose transport, also acts to increase the activity of acetyl-CoA carboxylase (ACC) and fatty acid synthase (FAS), two key lipogenic enzymes, primarily through stimulating transcription of the genes for these enzymes. Regulation of lipogenesis in cattle, pigs and poultry is linked to changes in expression of genes encoding these enzymes.

Triglyceride content of adipocytes is the balance of the reciprocal regulation of lipogenesis and lipolysis [76]. A shift in this balance towards net hydrolysis of triglyceride and release of fatty acids and glycerol is precipitated through activation of hormone sensitive lipase by a number of endocrine and paracrine factors. As discussed below insulin promotes further metabolism of glucose in lipogenesis through activation of ACC and FAS, key reaction sequences in the storage of glucose as lipid.

ACC catalyses the ATP-dependent carboxylation of acetyl-CoA in the synthesis of long-chain fatty acids [77]. Short-term changes in the activity of ACC are mediated by allosteric and covalent modifications [77]. Long-term regulation of ACC activity due to feed intake and diet composition is partly mediated by insulin.

The structure of the ACC gene indicates the presence of five different 5'-untranslated regions that are the product of two different promoters and differential splicing of the primary transcripts [77]. These transcripts, although they contain the same coding region, display differential translation efficiency [78]. In rats, the promoter I (PI) isoform of ACC mRNA contains a 12-base-pair positive-acting insulin response element. The promoter II (PII) isoform also contains an insulin response element, that is activated by insulin only after it is acted upon by cAMP [77]. The cDNAs for ovine [79] and chicken ACC [80] have been cloned and show considerable homology to rat ACC. Ovine adipose tissue, unlike rat adipose tissue, expresses the PI and PII forms of ACC mRNA although only the PI form is altered during lactation [81], a period marked by adipose tissue mobilisation due to decreased lipogenesis and elevated lipolysis.

FAS, a multi-enzyme complex, plays a central role in *de novo* lipogenesis in liver, adipose and mammary tissue, by catalysing the elongation of malonyl-CoA by the sequential addition of two carbons units from acetyl-CoA. Allosteric effectors or covalent modifications do not regulate the activity of the FAS. Changes in the activity of FAS, instead, are due to alterations in the rate of transcription of the FAS gene [82]. Insulin activation of FAS transcription is mediated through activation of the FAS insulin response sequence (IRS) in the proximal promoter region of the gene [82]. The rate of lipogenesis in swine adipose tissue is closely linked to FAS expression and suppression of lipogenesis by somatotropin in growing pigs is reflected in a dose-dependent decrease in expression of FAS [83]

Lipolysis, the co-ordinated breakdown of triglyceride in the adipocyte to yield fatty acids and glycerol, is initiated upon activation of hormone sensitive lipase in response to elevated intracellular cAMP. Glucagon receptors have been characterised in intact rat adipocytes and adipocyte membranes, providing a mechanism for lipolysis during fasting [84]. However controversy exits, as to whether glucagon has any physiological effect on lipolysis in humans and other monogastrics [85]. Glucagon is a major lipolytic hormone in poultry. It increases the release of glycerol and free fatty acids from chicken adipose tissue explants and increases free fatty acid release *in vivo* in chickens and turkeys [74]. Glucagon does not appear to play a role in lipolysis in bovine adipose tissue [86].

4.3. Mammary glucose metabolism

Glucose uptake in the mammary gland is a rate-limiting step for lactose synthesis. Mammary tissue does not express GLUT4 but expresses relatively high levels of GLUT1 [71] which is consistent with a lack of acute insulin effect on glucose uptake by the mammary gland [87]. Experiments with lactating goats suggest that mammary uptake of glucose is determined primarily by mammary glucose metabolism, not glucose supply [88]. Consequently the regulation of glucose removal by mammary tissue may be regulated by the expression of GLUT1 and/or intracellular glucose metabolism. The GLUT1 transporter is elevated in response to chronically elevated insulin [89]; therefore prolonged stimulation by insulin may indirectly increase mammary glucose removal.

5. RECEPTORS AND SECOND MESSENGERS

Insulin elicits its biological effects by first binding to its cell surface receptor. The receptor is composed of two subunits: an extracellular α-chain that binds insulin, and a β chain that is partially extracellular but primarily intracellular. The β–chain contains intrinsic tyrosine autophosphorylase activity that is activated when insulin occupies the receptor binding pocket. Several endogenous substrates for the insulin receptor tyrosine kinase have been identified over the past decade. Much effort has focused on determining the role of insulin receptor substrate (IRS), IRS-1 and IRS-2 in the insulin signal cascade [90]. Insulin receptor activation and autophosphorylation promotes tyrosine phosphorylation of IRS-1. Tyrosine phosphorylated IRS-1 then associates with the SH-2 containing GREB-2 which is linked to the ras activator sevenless (SOS) protein. Binding of SOS and GREB-2 to IRS-1 activates SOS through displacement of GDP with GTP. Active SOS then activates ras which ultimately activates mitogen activated protein (MAP) kinase and its downstream effectors [90] to alter cellular events [91].

A second, less well-characterised, substrate for the IRS proteins is the membrane-associated phosphatidylinositide (PI) 3-kinase an enzyme that converts phosphatidylinositide 4,5 bisphosphate (PI-4,5 P2) to phosphatidylinositide 3, 4, 5 triphosphate (PI-3,4,5 P3) [91]. Activation of IRS-1 and −2 permits docking and activation of PI 3-kinase [92]. One of the proposed substrates for the resulting PI-3,4,5 P3 is protein kinase B (PKB) which phosphorylates glycogen synthase kinase-3, phosphofructokinase 2 and activates translocation of the glucose transporter GLUT4 to the cell membrane [91].

Studies using sheep adipose and skeletal muscle indicate the presence of both second messenger systems and their downstream regulation as part of the development of insulin resistance during lactation in ruminants [93]. The effects of wortmanin, an inhibitor of PI 3-kinase, in decreasing acetyl CoA carboxylase activity indicate involvement of PI 3-kinase signalling as part of the insulin cascade in sheep adipose tissue [93].

The glucagon receptor is a 485-amino-acid g-protein-coupled protein with 7 transmembrane spanning domains [84]. Activation of the glucagon receptor stimulates at least two intracellular signalling systems: 1) the adenylyl cyclase system, to increase intracellular cyclic AMP and the protein kinase A cascade or 2) the system whereby intracellular free calcium is increased through phosphatidylinositol turnover to activate protein kinase C [84]. In liver tissue the cAMP cascade is the dominant signal in response to glucagon binding [84]. Prolonged stimulation of cells with glucagon decreases adenylyl cyclase activation by glucagon which may be linked to transient phosphorylation of the receptor by protein kinase C [94]. Similar desensitisation to glucagon has been observed in chicken adipose tissue [95,96].

6. PROTEIN SYNTHESIS AND CATABOLISM

The importance of insulin in protein synthesis is demonstrated by the loss of body protein during uncontrolled insulin-dependent diabetes mellitus. A cardinal effect of insulin is the stimulation of protein synthesis through promotion of the rate of transcription and translation of specific proteins. Conversely insulin also decreases the rate of catabolism of proteins by the liver and of amino acid release by muscle.

Insulin status is primarily regulated by energy supply [97]. Changes in insulin concentrations with lactation may reflect energy sufficiency relative to demand and are subject to regulation by other endocrine factors such as growth hormone and glucocorticoids. Insulin concentrations in plasma are sensitive to amino acid supply [98] and insulin infusions decrease plasma amino acid concentrations [99]. Insulin infusion in lactating dairy cattle decreased plasma amino acids, primarily through changes in branched chain amino acids, and increased milk protein synthesis [100]. The effect of insulin on milk protein synthesis appears to be mediated, at least in part, by changes in insulin-like growth factors and their binding proteins [100]. Although insulin increases net protein synthesis in bovine mammary tissue it is not known whether these effects are due to increased amino acid extraction or increased efficiency of protein synthesis due to changes in synthesis and degradation rates, or a combination of the two.

The effects of insulin on amino acid concentrations may represent increased amino acid removal, decreased protein breakdown, or a combination of both processes. Insulin stimulates muscle protein synthesis in growing rats when given as a single bolus injection but not during sustained insulin infusion unless branch chain amino acids, particularly leucine, are administered simultaneously [101]. Similarly insulin stimulates muscle protein synthesis in the neonatal pig, although the effect of insulin is greater in 7-day-old compared with 26-day-old pigs [102]. In growing rats, ruminants [103] and perhaps pigs [102], there is an age-related decline in the protein fractional synthesis rate in muscle so that in adult mature animals there is little effect of insulin on muscle protein synthesis.

The effects of insulin to rapidly restore postabsorptive protein synthesis in nonruminants have not been observed in ruminants. In lambs insulin acts to reduce protein breakdown in muscle tissue but only when nutrients are limiting [104]. In general the effects of insulin on muscle synthesis are primarily through an increased rate of synthesis in nonruminants and decreased rate of protein degradation in ruminants.

The effect of insulin to stimulate protein synthesis appears to be mediated through changes in translation initiation. In myoblast cell lines insulin acts to increase the activation of the eucaryotic initiation factor (eIF)-4E and the eIF-4E binding proteins eIF4A and eIF4G to increase mRNA and 40S ribosome association and transcription initiation [92].

Glucagon, in contrast to insulin appears to play no direct role in protein turnover in muscle but acts to increase hepatic amino acid extraction [22], to indirectly decrease the supply of amino acids to peripheral tissues. Concomitant increases in ureagenesis are observed in response to excess protein feeding and starvation and are mediated in part by increased expression of the ureagenic enzymes, in turn mediated by high glucagon relative to insulin concentrations [105].

7. SOMATOSTATIN, GROWTH HORMONE AND NUTRIENT METABOLISM

Somatostatin, a 14-amino-acid peptide derived from the 116-amino-acid preprosomatostatin protein acts to control the release of somatotropin from the pituitary and is also termed somatotropin (growth hormone) release inhibitory factor. Somatostatin produces a variety of effects including modulation of somatotropin, glucagon, insulin, and neurotransmitter release. Somatostatin indirectly impacts protein synthesis to decrease basal and nutrient-induced increases in growth hormone concentrations [22]. Immunisation against somatostatin indicates that it is a potent GH-governing factor, and when inhibited, baseline mean growth hormone levels increase, accompanied by a consistent response to growth hormone releasing factor [106].

The effects of somatostatin on glucose and amino acid metabolism are indirect [107] and are mediated through changes in other endocrine signals, primarily somatotropin. However, short-term somatostatin infusion increased glucose turnover during concomitant insulin infusion in dairy cattle, suggesting a role for somatostatin in modulating insulin sensitivity [64]. On the other hand, data from cattle immunised against somatostatin [108] indicate a lack of lean growth advantage, perhaps as a consequence of increased insulin concentrations. Therefore the effects of somatostatin immunisation may be distinct from those of somatotropin on growth and nutrient metabolism. To better understand the role of somatotropin in the regulation of adipose tissue metabolism and muscle lean body growth in domestic livestock the reader is directed to recent reviews [51,71].

8. CONCLUDING REMARKS

The multifaceted regulation of animal growth and performance by pancreatic hormones is impacted by a number of nutritional and physiological factors. Despite these complexities some common themes have emerged in our understanding of the role of insulin and glucagon in regulation of animal metabolism and performance, particularly with regard to the synthesis and disposal of glucose. The infinite complexity and integration of cellular and tissue events that result in changes in whole animal performance is staggering yet it is apparent that the endocrine pancreas plays a key role in this process. Continued efforts to reduce the multifaceted actions of insulin, glucagon, somatostatin to their basic components, particularly with regard to cellular signalling and regulation of gene expression, are necessary to further understand current growth and production phenomena and to seek methods to modify the efficiency of animal production.

REFERENCES

1. A. Trenkle, Fed. Proc., 40 (1981) 2536.
2. C.K. Reynolds, G.B. Huntington, T.H. Elsasser, H.F. Tyrell, and P.J. Reynolds, J. Dairy Sci., 71 (1989) 1803.
3. T.E.C. Weekes, P.J. Buttery, D.B. Lindsay and N.B. Haynes (eds.), Control and Manipulation of Animal Growth, Butterworths, London, 1986.
4. A. DeLong, L.P. Milligan, W.I. Grovum and A. Dobson (eds.), Control of Digestion and Metabolism in Ruminants, Prentice Hall, Englewood Cliffs, NJ, 1986.

5. L.E. Armentano, S.E. Mills, G. de Boer and J.W. Young, J. Dairy Sci., 67 (1984) 1445.
6. J.D. Sutton, I.C. Hart, S.V. Morant, E. Schuller and A.D. Simmonds., Brit. J. Nutr., 60 (1986) 265.
7. M.A. Lomax, Baird, G.D. Mallinson, C.B. Symonds, H.W., J. Biochem., 180 (1979) 281.
8. C.K. Reynolds, G.B. Huntington, T.H. Elsasser, H.F. Tyrell and P.J. Reynolds, J. Dairy Sci., 72 (1989) 1459.
9. U.A. Parman, Insulin, C.H. Gray and V.T.H. James (eds.), Hormones in Blood, Academic Press, London, 1979.
10. R.P. Brockman and E.N. Bergman, Amer. J. Physiol., 229 (1975) 1338.
11. H.J. Balks and K. Jungermann, Eur. I. Biochem., 141 (1984) 645.
12. R.P. Brockman, J.G. Manns and E.N. Berpman, Can. J. Physiol. Pharm., 54 (1976) 666.
13. S. Cosimi, P. Marchetti, R Giannarelli, P. Masiello, M. Bombara, M. Carmellini, F. Mosca, C. Arvia, R. Navalesi, Transplant Proc., 26 (1994) 3421.
14. J. Achmadi H. Ynagisawa, H. Sano, and Y. Terashima, Domest. Anim. Endo., 10 (1993) 279.
15. E. Evans, J.G. Buchanan-Smith, G.K. McLead, and J.B. Stone, J. Dairy Sci., 58 (1975) 672.
16. N. Janes, T.E.C. Weekes, and D.G. Armstrong, Brit. J. Nutr., (1985) 459.
17. G.B. Huntington, Reprod, Nutr. Dev., 30 (1990) 35.
18. R.P. Brockman, Biochem. Physiol., 74A (1983) 681.
19. J. T, Bosnan, Fed. Proc., 41 (1982) 91.
20. E. Debras, J. Grizard, E. Aina, S. Tesseraud, C. Champredon, and M. Arnal, Amer. J. Physiol., 256 (1989) E295.
21. R.P. Brockman, Can. J. Physiol. Pharmacol., 63 (1985)1460.
22. R.P. Brockman and B Laaveld, Can. J. Physiol. Pharmacol., 64 (1986) 1055.
23. R.P. Brockman, Brit. J. Nutr., 64 (1990) 95.
24. R.P. Brockman and C. Greer, Aust. J. Biol. Sci., 33 (1980) 457.
25. R.P. Brockman, E.N. Bergman, P.K. Joo and J.G. Manns, Amer. J. Physiol., 229 (1975) 1344.
26. T.R. Overton, J.K. Drakley, L.S. Emmert and J.H. Clark, J Dairy Sci., Suppl. 1 (1998) 295.
27. E.N. Bergman and J.E. Wolff, Amer. J. Physiol., 221 (1971) 586.
28. W.D. Steinhour, D.E. Bauman, A. Dobson and M.J. Dobson, (eds.), Aspects of Digestive Physiology in Ruminants, Comstock Publishing Associates, Ithaca, NY, 1988.
29. G.J. Barritt, G.L. Zander, M.F. Utter. R.W. Hanson and M.A. Mehiman (eds.), John Wiley and Sons, London, 1976.
30. K. Jungermann, Diabetes Metab. Rev., 3 (1987) 269.
31. W.G Guder and U. Schmidt, 1976, Hoppe-Seyler's Z. Physiol. Chem., 357 (1976) 1793.
32. H. Miethke, B. Wittig, A. Nath, S. Zierz, and K. Jungermann, Biol Chem. Hoppe-Seyler, 366 (1985) 493.
33. G.M Lawrence, M.A. Jepson, I.P Trayer, and D.G. Walker, Histochem. J., 18 (1986) 45.
34. N. Katz, H.F. Teutsch, and K. Jungermann, FEBS Lett., 76 (1977) 226.
35. D.G Tosh, G.M.M. Alberti, and L. Agius, Biochem. J., 256 (1988) 197.
36. Probst, P. Schartz, and K. Jungermann, Eur. J. Biochem., 126 (1982) 271.
37. S.S. Donkin and L.E. Armentano, Amer. J. Physiol. 266 (1994) R1229.
38. A, Faulkner and H.T. Pollock, Biochem. Biophys. Acta, 1052 (1990) 229.
39. P.M.J. Savan, M.K. Jeacock and D.A.L. Shepard, J. Agric. Sci., 106 (1986) 259.
40. M.C. Looney, R.L. Balswin and C.C. Calvert, J. Anim. Sci., 64 (1987) 283.
41. G.A. DeBoer, A. Trenkle, and J. W. Young, J. Dairy Sci., 69 (1986) 721.

42. S.J. Pilkis and T.H. Claus, Annu Rev. Nutr., 11 (1991) 465.
43. R.M. O'Brien and D.K. Granner, Diabetes Care, 13 (1990) 327.
44. F.D. Sistare and R.C. Haynes, J. Biol. Chem., 260 (1985) 12748.
45. G. Jones, S.K. Hothi, and M.A. Titheradge, Biochem J., 289 (1993) 821.
46. F.P. Lemaigre and G.G. Rousseau, Biochem J. 303 (1994)1.
47. F.J. Ballard, R.W. Hanson, and D.S. Kronfeld, Fed. Proc., 28 (1969) 218.
48. E. Bauman, C.J. Peel, W.D. Steinhour, P.J. Reynolds, H.F. Tyrrell, A.C.G. Brown, and G. Haaland, J. Nutr., 118 (1988) 1031.
49. N. Emmison, L. Agius and V. Zammit, Biochem. J., 274 (1991) 21.
50. J. R. Knapp, H.C. Freetly, B.L. Reis, C.C. Calvert, and R.L. Baldwin, J. Dairy Sci., 75 (1992) 1025.
51. T.D. Etherton, S.S. Donkin, D.E. Bauman, S.B. Smith, and D.R. Smith, Biology of Fat in Meat Animals: Current Advances. American Society of Animal Science. Champaign, IL, 1995.
52. R.W. Smith and A. Walsh, J. Agr. Sci. Camb., 98 (1982) 563.
53. R.B. Greenfield, S.S. Donkin, and M.J. Cecava, J. Dairy Sci., 81, Suppl 1 (1998) 320.
54. J.E. Pessin and G.I. Bell, Ann. Rev. Physiol., 54 (1992) 911.
55. E.J. Hajduch, M.C. Guerre-Millo, I.A. Hainault, C.M Guichard, M.M. Lavau, J. Cell. Biochem., 49 (1992) 251.
56. P.Y. Chiu, S. Chaudhuri, P.A. Harding, J.J. Kopchick, S.S. Donkin and T.D. Etherton, J. Anim. Sci., 72 (1994) 1196.
57. K.A. Magri, M. Adamo, D. Leroith, T.D. Etherton, Biochem. J., 266 (1990) 107.
58. S.S. Donkin, P.Y. Chiu, D. Yin, I. Louveau, B. Swencki, J. Vockroth, C.M. Evock-Clover, J.L. Peters, and T.D. Etherton, J. Nutr., 126 (1996) 2568.
59. H. Abe, M. Morimatsu, H. Nikami, T. Miyashige, M. Saito, J. Anim. Sci., 75 (1997) 182.
60. R.J. Boado, W.M. Pardridge, Biochem. Biophys. Res. Commun., 166 (1990) 174.
61. J.F. Hocquette and M. Balage, Proc Nutr. Soc., 55 (1996) 254.
62. T.D. Etherton and C.M. Evock, J. Anim. Sci., 62 (1986) 357.
63. R.G. Vernon, E. Finley E. Taylor; and D.J. Flint, Endocrinology, 116 (1985) 1195.
64. M.T. Rose, Y. Obara, F. Itoh, H. Hashimoto, Y. Takahashi, J. Dairy Res., 64 (1997) 341.
65. N. Janes, T.E.C. Weekes, and D. G. Armstrong, Brit. J. Nutr., (1985) 459.
66. Gottesman, L. Mandarino and J. Gerich, Amer. J. Physiol., 24 (1983) E632.
67. D. Baron, G. Brechtel, P. Wallace, and S.V. Edelman, Amer. J. Physiol., 255 (1988) E769.
68. J.H. Eisemann and G.B. Huntington, J. Anim. Sci., 72 (1994) 2919.
69. R.A. Jackson, Diabetes Care, 13 (1990) 9.
70. Burchell, Biochem. Soc. Trans., 22 (1994) 658.
71. F.Q. Zhao, D.R. Glimm, J.J Kennelly, Int. J. Biochem., 25 (1993) 1897.
72. B, Cherbuy, B. Darcy-Vrillon, L; Posho, P; Vaugelade, M.T., Morel MT, F. Bernard, A. Leturque, L. Penicaud, and P.H. Duee, Amer. J. Physiol., 272 (1997) G1530.
73. G.A. Leveille, D.R. Romsos, Y. Yeh, and E,K. O'Hea, Poult. Sci., 54 (1975) 1075.
74. S.B. Smith and D.R. Smith (eds.), The Biology of Fat in Meat Animals, American Society of Animal Science, Champaign, 1995.
75. T.D. Etherton and P.E. Walton, J. Anim. Sci., 63(Suppl. 2) (1986) 76.
76. D.E. Bauman Fed Proc., 35 (1976) 2308.
77. K.H. Kim and H.J.J Tae, J. Nutr., 124 (8 Suppl) (1994) 1273S.

78. F. Lopez-Casillas, K.H Kim, Eur. J. Biochem., 201 (1991) 119.
79. M.C. Barbers and T. Tavers, Gene, 154 (1995) 271.
80. El Khadir-Mounier, N. Le Fur, R.S. Powell, C. Diot, P. Langlois, J. Mallard, and M. Douaire, Biochem J., 314 (1996) 613.
81. M.C. Barber and M.T. Travers, Trans. Bichem. Soc., 24 (1996) 360S.
82. Wang and H.S. Sul, J. Biol. Chem., 270 (1995) 28716.
83. M. Harris, F.R. Dunshea, D.E. Bauman, R.D. Boyd, S.Y. Wang, P.A. Johnson, and S.D. Clarke, J Anim. Sci., 71 (1993) 3293.
84. J. Christophe, Biochim Biophys Acta., 1241 (1995) 45.
85. J.M. Miles and M.D. Jensen, J. Clin. Endocrinol. Metab., 77 (1993) 5A.
86. P.A. She, A.R, Hippen, G.L. Lindberg, D.C. Beitz, J.W. Young, R.W. Tucker, and L.F. Richardson, J. Dairy Sci., 80 (1997) 251.
87. Laarveld, D.A. Christensen, and R.P. Brockman, Endocrinology, 108 (1981) 2217.
88. M.O. Nielsen and K. Jakobsen, Comp. Physiol., 106 (1993) 359.
89. J. Hajduch, M.C. Guerre-Millo, I.A. Hainault, C.M. Guichard, and M.M. Lavau, J. Cell. Biochem., 49 (1992) 251.
90. M.F. White, Diabetologia, 40 (1997) S2.
91. P. Cohen, D.R. Alessi, and A.E. Cross, FEBS Lett., 410 (1997) 3.
92. C.G. Proud and R.M. Denton, Biochem. J., (1997) 329.
93. L.A. Wilson, S.E Mills, E. Finley, E. Kilgour, P.J. Buttery, and R.G. Vernon, J. Endocrinol., 151 (1996) 469.
94. M.D. Houslay, Eur J. Biochem., 195 (1991) 9.
95. R.M. Campbell and C.G. Scanes, Gen. Comp. Endocrinol., 26 (1987) 243.
96. R.T. Premont and R. Iyengar, Endocrinology, 125 (1989) 1151.
97. D.L. Russell-Jones and M. Umpleby, Eur. J. Endo., 135 (1996) 631.
98. T. Kuhara, S. Ikeda, A. Ohneda, Y. Sasaki, Amer. J. Physiol., 260 (1991) E21.
99. R. L.Prior and S.B. Smith, J. Nutr., 113 (1983) 1016.
100. J.M. Griinari, M.A. McGuire, D.A. Dwyer, D.E. Bauman, D.M. Barbano, W.A. House, J. Dairy Sci., 80 (1997) 2361.
101. P.J. Garlick, M.A McNurlan, T. Bark, C.H. Lang and M.C.J Gelato, J. Nutr., 128 (1998) 356S.
102. Wray-Cahen, P.R. Beckett, H.V. Nguyen, and T.A. Davis, Amer. J. Physiol., 273 (1997) E305.
103. G.E. Lobley, J. Nutr., 123 (1993) 337.
104. V.H. Oddy, D.B. Lindsay, P.J. Barker, and A.J. Northrop, Brit. J. Nutr., 58 (1987) 437.
105. M. Takiguchi, M. Mori, Biochem. J., 312 (1995) 649.
106. P. Dubreuil, G. Pelletier, D. Petitclerc, H. Lapierre, P. Gaudreau, and P. Brazeau, Endocrinology, 125 (1989) 1378.
107. J.A. Roe, A.S.H. Baba, J.M.M. Harper, and P.J. Buttery, Comp. Biochem. Physiol., 110A (1995) 107.
108. J.M. Dawson, J.B. Soar, P.J. Buttery, J. Craigon, M. Gill, and D.E. Beever, Animal Science : an International Journal of Fundamental and Applied Research. 64 (1997) 37.

Biology of the Pancreas in Growing Animals
S.G. Pierzynowski and R. Zabielski (Editors)
329

Feed protein and exocrine pancreatic secretion in monogastric animals

T. Żebrowska

The Kielanowski Institute of Animal Physiology and Nutrition, Polish Academy of Sciences, Instytucka 3, 05-110 Jabłonna, Poland

The entry of protein and its hydrolysis products into the duodenum affects pancreatic enzyme secretion. Amino acids and peptides are more effective in stimulating exocrine pancreatic secretion in dogs, but non-hydrolysed protein in rats. In growing pigs, increasing levels of protein in the diet stimulate the secretion of proteolytic enzymes but only slightly effect the pancreatic secretion of protein. The source of dietary protein influences pancreatic secretion; however feed protein is often accompanied by substances that can change the exocrine pancreatic secretion more than the protein itself.

1. INTRODUCTION

The pancreas plays a key role in maintaining the protein status of an animal because it produces a variety of proteolytic enzymes which hydrolyse feed protein within the intestine so that it can be absorbed and utilised by the body. The functions of the pancreas include the synthesis of proteolytic enzymes (which are important in the initiation of hydrolysis) and their secretion into the duodenum. Proteolytic enzymes secreted by the pancreas include trypsinogens, chymotrypsinogens, proelastases, collagenases and procarboxypeptidases. The majority of these proteolytic enzymes are secreted as inactive zymogens that are activated in the duodenum in a succession of steps: first enterokinase cleaves trypsin from trypsinogen, then trypsin acts on the zymogens, converting them to the active forms of the enzymes.

In animals, pancreatic proteolytic enzyme synthesis and secretion are modified by dietary protein content. The influence of dietary proteins on pancreatic enzyme activity can be assessed by measuring changes in pancreatic tissue enzyme contents in response to dietary composition, by estimating the activity of proteolytic enzymes in pancreatic tissue and juice or in digesta after ingestion of a meal.

2. EFFECT OF AMINO ACIDS AND PEPTIDES ON PANCREATIC ENZYME SECRETION

Studies conducted as early as in the '40s and '50s by Thomas and Crider [1] and Wang and Grossman [2] on dogs showed that protein and its products stimulate pancreatic exocrine activity. Peptides and L-amino acids present in the intestinal lumen were identified as substances stimulating secretion of protein and enzymes.

Meyer *et al.* [3] measured the pancreatic secretion of protein and bicarbonates in dogs receiving an infusion of individual amino acids or a mixture of them into the duodenum. They showed that phenylalanine and tryptophan were strong stimulators of pancreatic secretion, while alanine, leucine and valine increased the secretion of protein, but their effect was small and statistically insignificant. The reaction to phenylalanine infused at a concentration exceeding 8 mM depended on the load and length of the intestinal segment. On the basis of their results the authors concluded that receptors mediating the reaction to phenylalanine are distributed along the upper part of the intestine. Of the remaining 11 amino acids, tryptophan had only slightly less stimulatory effect than phenylalanine, while alanine, leucine and valine increased protein secretion only insignificantly and the remaining amino acids showed no stimulatory properties.

Although some individual amino acids were found to stimulate pancreatic secretion, the role of this mechanism in the context of protein consumption remains unknown. It is known that after feeding protein, most amino acids are in peptide form, not free form, in the small intestine. It was necessary to show which of the products of protein degradation - peptides or others - stimulate the secretion of pancreatic enzymes. In experiments on dogs [4] peptide solutions were infused into the duodenum. Of the studied peptides, only glycylphenylanine, phenylalanylglycine and glycyltryptophan exhibited significant stimulatory effects, indicating that polypeptides containing phenylalanine or tryptophan could stimulate pancreatic secretion. Further experiments were carried out on dogs to investigate whether protein or its degradation products could stimulate the pancreas to secrete protein and bicarbonate [5]. The perfusates administered into the intestine contained bovine serum albumin, bovine haemoglobin, casein, crude egg albumin and crude gelatine, as well as pepsin or pancreatic hydrolysates of these proteins. None of the proteins increased pancreatic secretion, but their hydrolysates did. The authors concluded that peptides comprising four or more amino acids and the products of enzymatic protein hydrolysis present in the intestinal lumen after protein consumption can stimulate pancreatic secretion. Both types of hydrolysates (peptic and pancreatic) stimulated secretion of a small volume of pancreatic juice with a low bicarbonate concentration but high protein content.

These results did not fully agree with the earlier results of Konturek *et al.* [6], who studied the effect of 16 amino acids individually administered into the intestine of dogs. These authors showed that although phenylalanine and tryptophan exhibited the greatest stimulatory effect on pancreatic secretion, the remaining amino acids, with the exception of asparagine, cysteine and threonine, also acted in a similar manner.

Experiments in which amino acids are infused into the duodenum do not reflect the conditions normally prevalent in the digestive tract. In normally fed animals, the amount of free amino acids in the digesta in the upper part of the digestive system is small, and their concentration much lower than in the cited experiments. Part of the amino acids freed by proteolytic enzymes are rapidly absorbed, while others are absorbed in the form of small peptides.

The amino acids that stimulate pancreatic secretion the most are the ones that are most rapidly freed by proteolytic enzymes in the intestine. They include phenylalanine, valine, leucine, methionine, lysine, arginine, tyrosine, alanine and probably tryptophan. It may be supposed that as the result of hydrolysis of considerable amounts of feed protein, the concentration of amino acids that can stimulate the pancreas may rise sufficiently high for them to effectively react with their receptors, but this in turn depends on a sufficient production of pancreatic proteases to free these amino acids.

The studies described above on pancreatic secretion were carried out on dogs. Other studies revealed differences among species in the reaction of the pancreas to protein and the products of its digestion. It was found, for example, that administering undigested protein into the duodenum does not increase pancreatic secretion in dogs [5]. In rats the infusion of casein into the duodenum increased the secretion of protein in pancreatic juice, but the infusion of free amino acids or totally hydrolysed casein did not stimulate secretion [7].

The effect of partial exclusion of pancreatic juice from the small intestine on the pancreatic response to intraduodenal infusion of casein, casein hydrolysate, and trypsin inhibitor was investigated in conscious rats with chronic pancreatic and biliary fistulas [8]. The casein hydrolysate increased secretion of pancreatic juice and protein, but this rise was much smaller than when non-hydrolysed casein was administered. The small rise after administration of free amino acids found in that study, as well as by other researchers [9], points to large differences among species in the reaction of the pancreas to protein and the products of its hydrolysis.

The reaction of the pancreas to intestinal perfusion of amino acids depends more on the perfused load of amino acids per unit of time than on their concentration in the perfusate. This observation suggests that mucosal amino acid and peptide receptors in the intestinal lumen need only small amounts of amino acids to be activated and that the length of the intestine exposed to digestion products is an important factor in the secretory response of the pancreas.

In animals, the activity of proteolytic enzymes, both in pancreatic tissue and in the juice it secretes into the duodenum, can be modified by the protein content of the diet. The type of protein in the diet also affects pancreatic secretion, and it takes the pancreas anything from a few hours to 7-8 days to adapt to a new diet, with adaptation to a high-protein diet occurring faster than to a high-carbohydrate diet [10].

The mechanism by which the pancreas adapts to a new diet is not yet fully understood. In animals, supplying a dietary component in greater amounts causes a rapid rise in the level of the relevant enzyme in the pancreas, although there is no direct contact between this component and the pancreas. Protein undergoes rapid hydrolysis, first in the stomach and then in the small intestine. A mixture of protein and its hydrolysis products in the stomach flows into the duodenum, which is why information sent to the pancreas may be generated by the products of hydrolysis. It is presently accepted that the products of protein hydrolysis act on the mucous lining of the intestine. This hypothesis is supported by the example of the lack of pancreatic stimulation in rats [11] and dogs [12] when amino acids are administered intravenously. Most studies have shown that products of hydrolysis exert their stimulatory effect in the intestinal lumen before they are absorbed, which points to the role of the mucous lining of the intestine. Most likely these mechanisms are different for each enzyme.

Among the regulatory peptides, cholecystokinin (CCK) is assumed to be the main intestinal factor involved in the adaptation of the pancreas to diet. It is known that CCK is freed in the intestine by protein or the products of its hydrolysis.

The role of digestion of dietary protein in the stomach on the secretion of pancreatic enzymes and release of CCK in rats was studied by Guan and Green [14]. Casein or bovine serum albumin were infused either into the stomach or into the duodenum and the effect of peptic predigestion on pancreatic secretion and on plasma CCK was determined. In duodenal infusion, casein was a stronger stimulator of CCK release (5.8+0.6 vs. 1.6+0.2 PM) and protein secretion (5592+736 vs. 750+461 mg/kg/min) than bovine serum albumin. Infusion of bovine serum albumin into the stomach increased pancreatic protein secretion and plasma CCK levels considerably, but casein had no effect.

3. EFFECT OF PROTEIN LEVEL IN THE DIET ON PANCREATIC SECRETION

Many studies have shown that diet composition can modulate pancreatic secretion. It was found that the activity of proteolytic enzymes in pancreatic tissue and juice is modified by the protein content, and the effect on particular enzymes is different and dependent on the amount of protein ingested. In rats [15] and pigs [16], trypsin and chymotrypsin activities increase as the protein content of the diet rises, with the activity of chymotrypsin showing a more sensitive response to changes in protein consumption. According to Giorgi et al. [17] the activity of carboxypeptidase A in the pancreas remained unchanged when the protein content of the diet was increased from 150 to 700 g/kg, while the activities of trypsin, chymotrypsin and elastase increased 1.4, 2.8 and 2.0-fold, respectively. The authors concluded that adaptation to dietary protein content is a characteristic trait of the serine protease family.

Corring and Saucier [18] showed that in pigs fed diets containing 0, 10, 30 or 40% protein, the activity of chymotrypsin in pancreatic juice clearly increased as the protein content of the diet rose, while changes in trypsin and amylase activities were less distinct.

A similar relationship was observed in the studies by Hee et al. [19]. When the dietary protein content was 15%, total secretion of chymotrypsin and trypsin increased approximately 2-fold higher than in the protein - free diet, while the pancreatic secretion of protein was non-significantly lower on a protein-free diet (Table 1). These studies confirmed earlier findings by Corring and Saucier [18], showing that the secretion of protein in pancreatic juice is less responsive to dietary changes in the protein content than the secretion of the proteolytic enzymes and amylase.

Table 1
Effect of protein level in the diet on the volume, protein and enzyme secretion in pancreatic juice of pigs in 24 h

	Diet	
	Control (15 % protein)	Protein-free
Volume (ml)	3990	3476
Protein (g)	15.1	13.1
Trypsin	243.4[a]	115.3[b]
Chymotrypsin	166.2[a]	73.8[b]
Amylase	340.4	180.6
Lipase	654	578

Enzyme secretions are expressed as U x 10^3
Hee et al. [19].

Li *et al.* [20] studied pancreatic secretion in pigs fed diets containing 12 or 24% protein in a cross-over design with initial body weights of 24 and 31 kg at the start of the experimental period. No differences were found in the daily amount of secreted protein in pancreatic juice, although the protein concentration was higher in pigs on the diet with the higher protein content. The level of protein in the diet did not affect the total trypsin, chymotrypsin, amylase or lipase activities, although their specific activities were higher on the high-protein diets. It was also shown that as body mass rose, so did the volume of pancreatic juice, and the total protein content and enzyme activity.

4. EFFECT OF SOURCE OF PROTEIN ON PANCREATIC SECRETION

The source of dietary protein also affects pancreatic proteolytic enzymes. Sook and Meyer [21] showed that in rats, whole-egg protein increased the synthesis and secretion of trypsin and chymotrypsin as compared with casein. These authors as well as Johnson *et al.* [22] postulated that proteins with a high biological value stimulate the secretion of pancreatic enzymes more than proteins with a low value.

In experiments on rats the effects of a low-protein diet with casein or soya bean protein isolate on the secretion of pancreatic juice and its protein content and trypsin and chymotrypsin activity were studied [23]. It was shown that the secretion of protein, trypsin and chymotrypsin were significantly higher on the casein diet than on the soya bean protein isolate. These results show that pancreatic exocrine activity under physiological conditions reacts to low levels of dietary protein content. Green and Nasset [24] showed in experiments on rats that a diet containing 24% soya bean protein stimulates the secretion of trypsin more than a diet with 24% casein. Berger and Scheeman [25] also showed that the secretion of carboxypeptidases A and B was higher when rats were given soya bean protein isolate than a casein diet. These results are in disagreement with those of Hara *et al.* [23], possibly due to differences in feeding conditions and dietary components. Pancreatic secretion also depends on factors other than protein, such as the rate of passage from the stomach of various dietary components, the secretion of gastric juices, the type and content of fat in the diet, and the presence of protease inhibitors.

The results of studies in pigs weaned early and fed diets containing skimmed-milk powder (SMP), soya-bean-protein concentrate (SPC), soya bean meal (SBM) or fish meal (FM) showed that 10 days after weaning, dietary protein content affected the weight of the pancreas and enzyme activity [26]. The SPC diet caused a rise in the weight of the pancreas, while the SMP and SPC diets were associated with a rise in the activity of trypsin and chymotrypsin. After 10 days these differences disappeared, although the amount of consumed feed continued to affect chymotrypsin activity.

Digestion and pancreatic enzyme activity in response to proteins of varying solubility in early-weaned pigs were studied by Peiniau *et al.* [27]. The proteins studied were: casein, soluble fish protein concentrate, soya bean meal and soya bean meal concentrate. The weight of the pancreas and its protein content in pigs slaughtered at the age of 56 days differed considerably and were significantly lower in animals that had been fed diets containing soluble fish protein concentrate than in the others. This may have been related to the poor stimulation of the pancreas to synthesise chymotrypsin and trypsin in the animals fed the soluble fish protein concentrate.

The total activity of enzymes was also reduced accordingly, but specific activity was not affected by the treatments (Table 2).

Table 2
Effect of source and solubility of protein on pancreas and pancreatic enzymes

	Diet			
	Casein	SFPC[1]	SBM[2]	SC[3]
Pancreas				
Fresh weight (g)	22.6^A	14.4^B	21.1^A	21.2^A
Protein (mg g^{-1})	194^a	174^b	187^a	219^a
Total activity (IV/pancreas)				
Trypsin	9340^a	6566^b	8628^a	9129^a
Chymotrypsin	56900^a	27300^b	36500^{ab}	44800^{ab}
Lipase	11916	6725	12768	13202
Amylase x 10^3	5663^a	2090^b	5431^a	6022^a

1 - soluble fish protein concentrate
2 – soya bean meal
3 – soya bean concentrate
A, B - P $\langle$ 0.01; a, b - P $\langle$ 0.05
Peiniau *et al.* [27].

In an experiment on growing pigs fed diets containing casein or rapeseed meal as protein sources, Valette *et al.* [28] showed that the daily amount of protein secreted in pancreatic juice did not differ significantly, but the activities of trypsin, chymotrypsin, and carboxypeptidase B in pancreatic juice were significantly different when pigs were fed diets containing rapeseed than when they received casein. The average daily activities of elastase and carboxypeptidase A were lower on the ration containing rapeseed meal (Table 3).

The results of these studies are in disagreement with those of Partridge *et al.* [29] and Żebrowska *et al.* [30], who did not find a significant effect of the type of protein on the activity of pancreatic proteases and peptidases.

This discrepancy can be explained by the fact that semi-synthetic diets were used by Valette *et al.* [29], while in the experiments of Żebrowska *et al.* [30] and Partridge *et al.* [29] a semi-synthetic diet with casein as the protein source was compared with a feed mix, based on cereal feeds and fish meal, used in practice for growing pigs. In short, these results lead to the conclusion that the type of protein in the diet modifies the synthesis and activity of proteolytic enzymes secreted in pancreatic juice.

There is limited information on the effect of cereal grains fed alone or supplemented with high protein feeds, including legume seeds, on exocrine pancreatic secretion in pigs. The effects of different protein supplements and different cereal grains on pancreatic secretions of pigs have been studied by Imbeah et al. [31], Żebrowska and Długołęcka [32], Buraczewska et al. [34] and Pohland et al. [34]. The latter authors used pigs with a weight ranging from 40 to 65 kg, fed a diet based on corn starch supplemented with soya bean meal or canola meal, containing 18.6 and 16.9% crude protein, and diets made only of wheat or barley containing 14.4 and 11.2% crude protein.

Table 3
Mean daily pancreatic juice volume, protein output and total enzyme activities in pigs adapted to casein or rapeseed meal diet (µmol substrate hydrolysed/min)

| | Diet | |
	Casein	Rapeseed
Volume (ml)	2383	1677*
Protein (g)	13.2	15.6
Trypsin	62.0	83.8
Chymotrypsin	453.0	647.4*
Elastase	27.6	24.6
Carboxypeptidase A	279.8	232.3*
Carboxypeptidase B	17.4	26.2

* Mean values were different from those for casein (P $<$ 0.05)
  Valette et al. [28].

They found no effect of diet on the volume of pancreatic juice, pH, or secretion of total and TCA-precipitable nitrogen, total activity of trypsin, chymotrypsin, α-amylase, and lipase. This was in contrast to the results reported by, Żebrowska and Długołęcka [32] who found that the volume of pancreatic juice secreted was greater when barley was fed rather than rye, wheat or triticale (Table 4). The protein content was also significantly higher with rye and barley than with the wheat and triticale diets, but total trypsin, chymotrypsin and amylase activities were similar for all diets. The greater volume of pancreatic juice secreted when the barley diet was fed could be related rather to the higher NDF content in the barley than in the wheat, triticale and rye diets, than to protein content. As shown by, Żebrowska and Low [35], noncellulose components of fibre may be involved in regulating the volume of pancreatic juice.

Table 4
Mean 12h weight of pancreatic juice, total protein content and enzyme activities in pigs fed cereal grain diet

| | Diet | | | |
	Rye	Wheat	Barley	Triticale
Juice, g	1875	1679	2085	1800
Protein, g	11.0	8.7	11.4	8.3
Trypsin, $\mu \times 10^{-3}$	134.4	107.4	122.1	125.1
Chymotrypsin, $\mu \times 10^{-3}$	44.0	39.6	35.5	50.5
Amylase, $\mu \times 10^{-3}$	344.0	244.3	327.0	249.8

Żebrowska and Długołęcka, [32].

Imbeah et al. [31] measured the rate of pancreatic secretion in pigs of about 47 kg live weight fed semi-synthetic diets containing soya bean meal or canola meal as the source of protein. There was no effect of the diet used on the rate of pancreatic juice secretion or contents of protein and activity of trypsin and chymotrypsin. The total activities of trypsin and chymotrypsin were in agreement with those found by Partridge et al. [29] and Żebrowska et al. [30]. In studies of Pohland et al. [34] there was also no difference in the activities of the enzymes that were measured in the pancreatic juice of pigs fed soybean or canola diets. In experiments by Buraczewska et al. [33], the influence of diets based on barley supplemented with pea, lupine or field bean on pancreatic secretion in pigs of about 35 kg was studied. The diets contained 10% total protein (5% from barley and 5% from pea and lupine or 10% from field bean). They showed that the mean volume of pancreatic juice was not affected by the diet. The average daily protein, trypsin, chymotrypsin, and amylase output was similar for barley, pea, and lupine diets but significantly lower for the field bean diet (Table 5). Changes, both in protein and in daily enzyme secretion, might have been elicited by differences in proteins, starches and type of dietary fibre of the diets or content of antinutritional factors of the field bean seeds.

The results of experiments by Partridge et al. [29], Żebrowska et al. [30], Imbeah et al. [31], and Pohland et al. [34] were quite variable but this variation could be of biological origin. As pointed out by Imbeah et al. [31], variation was observed in separate experiments in which different methods were used to collect pancreatic juice; diet compositions and live weight also differed. The high level of within-study variation observed in many studies and the relatively small numbers of observations in particular experiments may possibly mask dietary effects on pancreatic secretions.

Table 5
Mean daily output of pancreatic juice, protein and enzyme activities expressed per 1 kg DM intake of different diets

| | Diet | | | |
	Barley	Pea+barley	Lupin+barley	Field+starch
Volume, ml	3752	4142	3721	3918
Protein, g	12.9^a	10.6^a	12.7^{Ab}	8.8^{Bb}
Trypsin$^{1/}$	164^a	171^A	173^A	117^{Bb}
Chymotrypsin$^{1/}$	50^a	47^a	63^A	28^B
Amylase$^{1/}$	963^a	631^a	748^a	466^b
Lipase$^{1/}$	746^{ac}	1159^b	1139^{bc}	693^a

$1/ - U \times 10^{-3}$
A, b - $P \langle 0.01$; a, b, c - $P \langle 0.05$
Buraczewska et al. [33].

CONCLUSIONS

Exocrine pancreatic secretion is influenced by the level and source of protein. The response to protein is due to increased proteolytic enzyme synthesis and secretion.

However, determining to what degree feed protein affects this process is difficult, due to the presence of naturally occurring substances (e.g. inhibitors, fibre), that can change the magnitude of synthesis and secretion of proteolytic enzymes and the volume of pancreatic juice. The large variations in data reported in the cited papers may have resulted from variations in the applied experimental and analytical methods, or could be of biological origin and not an artifact.

REFERENCES

1. J.E. Thomas and J.O. Crider, Amer. J. Physiol., 134 (1941) 656.
2. C.C. Wang and M.I. Grossman, Amer. J. Physiol., 164 (1951) 527.
3. J.H. Meyer, G.A. Kelly, L.J. Spingola and R.S. Jones, Amer. J. Physiol., 231 3 (1976a) 669.
4. J.H. Meyer, G.A. Kelly and R.S. Jones, Amer. J. Physiol., 231 3 (1976b) 678.
5. J.H. Meyer and G.A. Kelly, Amer. J. Physiol., 231 3 (1976c) 682.
6. S.J. Konturek, T. Radecki, P. Thor and A. Dembiński, Proc. Soc. Exptl. Biol. Med., 143 (1973) 305.
7. B.O. Schneeman, I. Chang, L.B. Smith and R.L. Lyman, J. Nutr. 107, (197)7 281.

338

8. G.M. Green and Miyasaka K., Amer. J. Physiol., 245 (1983) G394-G398.
9. G.M. Green, Olds B.A., Matthews G., R.L. Lyman, Proc. Soc. Exptl. Biol. Med. 142 (1973) 1162.
10. T. Corring, C. Juste and E.F. Lhoste, Nutr. Res. Rev., 2 (1989) 161.
11. M. Lavau, R. Bazin and J. Herzog, J. Nutr., 104 (1974) 1432.
12. B.E. Stabile, M. Borzatta, R.S. Stubbs and H.T. Debas, Amer. J. Physiol. 246 (1984) G274.
13. M.V. Singer, Scand. J. Gastroenterol., 22 (suppl. 139), (1987) 1.
14. D. Guan and G.M. Green, Amer. J. Physiol. 271 (1) (1996) G42.
15. V. Keim, Ann. Nutr. Metab., 30 (1986) 113.
16. T. Corring, World Review of Nutrition and Dietetics 27, (1977) 132.
17. D. Giorgi, W. Renaud, J.P. Bernard and J.C. Dagorn, Biochemical and Biophysical Research Communications 127 (1985) 937.
18. T. Corring and R. Saucier, Biol. Anim. Bioch. Biophys., 12 (1972) 233.
19. J.Hee., W.C. Sauer and R. Mosenthin, J. Anim. Physiol. Anim. Nutr., 60 (1988) 241.
20. S. Li, W.C. Sauer, S.X. Huang and V. M. Gabert, J. Anim. Feed Sci., 6 (1997) 207.
21. J.T. Snook and J.H. Meyer, J. Nutr., 82 (1964) 409.
22. A. Johnson, R. Hurwitz and N. Kretchmer, J. Nutr., 107 (1977) 87.
23. H. Hara, A. Fujibayashi and S. Kiriyama, J. Nutr. Biochem., 3 (1992) 177.
24. G.M. Green and E.S. Nass, J. Nutr., 113, (1983) 2245.
25. J. Berger and B.O. Schneeman, J.Nutr., 116 (1986) 265.
26. C.A. Makkink, G.P. Negulescu, Q. Guixin and M.W.A. Verstegen, Brit. J. Nutr., 72 (1994) 353.
27. J. Peinian, A. Aumaitre, and Y. Lebreton, Livest. Prod. Sci., 45 (1996) 197.
28. P. Valette, H. Malouin, T. Corring, L. Savoie, A.M. Guengneau and S. Berot, Brit. J. Nutr, 67 2 (1992) 215.
29. I.G. Partridge, A.G. Low, I.E. Sambrook and T. Corring, Brit. J. Nutr., 48 (1982) 137.
30. T. Żebrowska, A.G. Low and H. Żebrowska, Brit. J. Nutr., 49 (1983) 401.
31. M. Imbeah, W.C. Sauer and R. Mosenthin, J. Anim. Sci., 66 (1988) 1409.
32. T. Żebrowska and Z. Długołęcka, In: Proc. 4th International Seminar on Digestive Physiology in the Pig, Jabłonna, Poland, (1988) 104.
33. L. Buraczewska, U. Pöhland, J. Gdala, W. Grala, G. Janowska and W.B. Souffrant, In: Digestive physiology in pigs. M.W.A. Verstegen, J. Huisman and L.A. den Hartog (eds.) Wageningen EAAP Publication No 54, (1991) 167.
34. U. Pöhland, W.B. Souffrant, W.C. Sauer, R. Mosenthin and C.F.M. de Lange, J. Sci. Food Agric., 62 (1993) 229.
35. T. Żebrowska and A.G. Low, J. Nutr., 117 (1987) 1212.

Biology of the Pancreas in Growing Animals
S.G. Pierzynowski and R. Zabielski (Editors)
© 1999 Elsevier Science B.V. All rights reserved.

The contribution of exocrine pancreatic secretions to fat digestion

V.M. Gabert[a] and M.S. Hedemann[b]

[a]Department of Animal Sciences, University of Illinois, Urbana, Illinois, USA

[b]Department of Animal Nutrition and Physiology, Danish Institute of Agricultural Sciences, DK-8830 Tjele, Denmark

Fat digestion occurs in the small intestine and absorption of fatty acids, as mono- and diacylglycerols, is nearly complete at the distal ileum. The whole process of fat digestion is dependent on the exocrine pancreas and without pancreatic secretions, fat digestion would be severely impaired.

There are three enzymes: lipase, carboxyl ester hydrolase and phospholipase A_2 and one cofactor: colipase, which act in concert to digest dietary fat. The exocrine pancreas of both the monogastric animal and the ruminant animal secretes these enzymes. The existence of carboxyl ester hydrolase in sows' milk remains to be demonstrated; the activity of this enzyme in pancreatic tissue increases very rapidly during the suckling period, and it is suggested that the pig may compensate for the missing enzyme in the milk by secreting more carboxyl ester hydrolase from the pancreas during the suckling period. Exocrine pancreatic secretion responds to changes in the level of fat in the diet and lipase secretion increases with an increase in the level of dietary fat. The exocrine pancreas also responds to changes in the fatty acid profile of dietary fat and these changes may have implications for fat digestion and digestive function. We observed significant effects of the type of fat on the total activities of chymotrypsin and carboxyl ester hydrolase, when the catheter method was used to collect pancreatic juice. Recently, additional research has been conducted in weanling pigs to further investigate the effect of dietary fat source on exocrine pancreatic secretions, and it has been found that the secretion of carboxyl ester hydrolase is increased by the inclusion of fish oil in the diet. We have applied the ileal analysis method to study the digestion of different sources of fat, which were also used in studies designed to investigate the nutritional regulation of exocrine pancreatic secretions. Different batches of the same sources of fat were used and both ileal and faecal digestibilities of fat and fatty acids were determined. The secretion and action of pancreatic lipolytic enzymes is not only dependent on the amount and type of dietary fat; the amount and type of protein, carbohydrates, minerals and antinutritional compounds may influence the digestion and absorption of fat as well.

Fat digestion is a complex process and involves many different factors. The amount and type of dietary fat is probably the most important factor affecting the secretion of lipolytic enzymes. When the content of dietary fat in the diet is increased an increased secretion of lipase follows. Lipase is the most thoroughly studied lipolytic enzyme and future studies will have to elucidate whether there is a parallel increase in the other lipolytic enzymes, i.e. carboxyl ester hydrolase and phospholipase A_2 and in the cofactor colipase, when there is an increase in dietary fat. In addition, the quantitative role of specific enzymes in the process of fat digestion needs to be investigated.

1. INTRODUCTION

The digestive tract of an animal enables it to digest and assimilate a wide variety of foodstuffs. The exocrine pancreas secretes polypeptide enzyme cofactors and inhibitors, mucins, bicarbonate, urea, sodium, potassium and chloride [1-3].The pancreas consists of 90-95% exocrine tissue and only 2-3% endocrine tissue [4]. It supplies enzymes needed for the digestion of lipids, carbohydrates and proteins [3].

The regulation of secretion and activities of the various enzymes has been extensively studied [5-7]. The activities are highly dependent on diet composition, age, feeding regimen and time of sampling in relation to time of feeding [6,8]. Adaptation of the exocrine pancreatic secretion is most likely necessary to optimise digestion. Exocrine pancreatic secretions adapt to the level of protein, fat and starch in the diet [9,10]. The secretion of lipolytic enzymes, proteolytic enzymes and amylase increases when the level of dietary fat, protein and starch increases, respectively, and the changes in secretion are nonparallel, i.e. the proportions of pancreatic enzymes change [11]. Pancreatic adaptation to a change in diet composition is usually complete within 5-7 d [6,12].

Fatty acids as a proportion of total fat and fat digestibility are the most important factors determining the nutritive value of fat [13]. For monogastric animals, the fatty acid pattern of the dietary lipids is reflected in the fatty acid profile of animal products arising from them [14]. Fat digestion occurs in the small intestine and absorption of fatty acids, as mono- and diacylglycerols is nearly complete at the distal ileum [15]. The whole process of fat digestion is dependent on the exocrine pancreas and without pancreatic secretions fat digestion would be severely impaired. The intent of this chapter is to provide a very detailed and integrated information on the contribution of the exocrine pancreas to the digestion of dietary fat. A number of topics are covered. Firstly, the enzymes responsible for fat digestion are examined. Secondly, changes in fat digestion during an animal's life cycle are discussed and thirdly, the relationship between dietary fat level and exocrine pancreatic secretions is described. A fourth topic is the effect of fat source, primarily the fatty acid composition of dietary fat, on the secretion of lipolytic enzymes from the exocrine pancreas. The stability of lipolytic enzymes in the digestive tract is discussed as well as quantitative approaches to studying fat digestion. Potential interactions between pancreatic secretions and other nutrients and compounds in the diet are also investigated and potential ways to improve fat digestion in animals are mentioned.

2. LIPOLYTIC ENZYMES

The secretions of the exocrine pancreas are responsible for digesting most dietary fat. Some fat digestion, especially in young animals occurs in the stomach as a result of gastric lipase but most of the dietary fat is digested in the small intestine [16]. Bicarbonate secretion neutralises hydrochloric acid from the stomach, thereby making the pH of the duodenal contents slightly alkaline and favourable for digestion [2]. In growing pigs, when a catheter is used to collect pancreatic juice from the pancreatic duct, bicarbonate secretion ranges from 406 to 679 mmol/d and the pH of pancreatic juice is approximately 8.5 [17]. The fact that dietary fats are not water-soluble and are primarily nonpolar compounds makes the emulsification of lipids necessary before they can be digested and absorbed. Bile salts and phospholipids secreted in bile are responsible for this [15,18].

There are three enzymes: lipase, carboxyl ester hydrolase and phospholipase A_2 and one cofactor: colipase, which act in concert to digest dietary fat [3,15]. The exocrine pancreas of both the monogastric animal and the ruminant animal secretes these enzymes. Carboxyl ester hydrolase is also sometimes referred to as milk lipase, because it is present in milk, bile salt stimulated lipase or carboxyl esterase [15]. It is a relatively non-specific lipase which cleaves ester linkages and it most likely makes a substantial contribution to fat digestion. This enzyme is also responsible for hydrolysing ester forms of vitamin A (retinol esters) and vitamin E (tocopherol esters). However, its quantitative contribution to fat digestion remains to be elucidated. Pancreatic lipase is the main lipolytic enzyme secreted by the pancreas and it cleaves triacylglycerols at positions one and three to form mono- and diacylglycerols. For lipase to be active, dietary fat, which is primarily in the form of triacylglycerols, needs to be emulsified. This results in the formation of micelles. In addition colipase is needed to allow attachment of the lipase to the micelle. Colipase is secreted as an inactive proenzyme known as procolipase, which is activated to colipase by the action of trypsin [3,15]. The secretion of lipase and colipase in pancreatic juice are highly correlated [19,20]. Phospholipase A_2 is secreted in pancreatic juice as inactive prophospholipase A_2 which is activated by trypsin. Phospholipase A_2 is responsible for hydrolysing phospholipids such as phosphatidylcholine (lecithin) [3,15].

The amount of lipolytic enzymes secreted in pancreatic juice is usually determined by conducting enzyme activity assays. However, other approaches, such as electrophoretic or chromatographic separation of the various enzymes can also be employed (21). Enzyme activity is often expressed in units (U), where one U is defined as the hydrolysis of 1 μmol of substrate in 1 min. Enzyme activity can be expressed in a number of different ways. The term specific activity refers to units per litre or units per milligram protein. The term total activity refers to units per unit time such as units per hour or per 8 or 24 h. Total enzyme activities are calculated as specific activity x volume of pancreatic juice secreted per unit time. If many samples need to be analysed, the analyses can be semi-automated to decrease costs and improve efficiency. We have successfully modified a method for measuring carboxyl ester hydrolase activity [22] so that it can be performed on a 96-microwell plate and the samples can be read by a microplate reader [23].

Reliable and reproducible methods for measuring enzyme activities in pancreatic juice are required for investigating the effect of dietary modifications and the effects of different secretagogues on exocrine pancreatic secretions. The choice of method depends on the resources and equipment available to the researcher as well as personal preference. We have compared the two most commonly used methods for measuring lipase activity in pancreatic juice [24]. In the first method (Method A), tributyrin was used as the substrate in the presence of bile salts and excess colipase, and lipase activity was determined by autotitration [25]. In the second method (Method B), a stabilised olive oil emulsion was used and lipase activity was determined spectrophotometrically [26]. We have also routinely measured the activity of colipase, an essential cofactor for lipase, with Method A by determining the amount of lipase activity dependent on the presence of colipase. The lipase assay was performed without adding colipase prior to titration [27].

In Method B, preliminary analysis indicated that the addition of colipase did not result in a higher activity of lipase [24]. It was very difficult to obtain duplicate results with a reasonably low level of variation. Most samples were analysed two or three times. Part of the problem was most likely due to incomplete removal of excess copper when the aqueous top layer was aspirated off the bottom layer of chloroform which contained copper salts of fatty acids released during hydrolysis of triacylglycerols by lipase [26]. If traces of the aqueous layer remain and are transferred to the second set of tubes (to which diethyldithiocarbamate is added to produce the colour reaction), the results will be greatly affected. This problem may be resolved if the chloroform layer is removed through the bottom of the tube following centrifugation to separate the layers. Another concern is the effectiveness of the olive oil emulsion; further investigation is needed on whether or not this contributes to the variation in the assay. It was also difficult to obtain a linear standard curve for stearic acid, which may also have been due to traces of copper interfering with the colour reaction, as previously discussed. The photometric method of assaying lipase activity needs to be improved and investigated further. The results of our comparative work [24] do not agree with those of another comparative study [26], in which there was a high correlation between lipase activity measured with the titrimetric and photometric method in duodenal aspirate, serum and pancreatin. We observed a poor relationship between the titrimetric and the photometric method for determining lipase activity ($R^2 = 0.42$). The titrimetric method [25] is much simpler, more straightforward and there is substantially less variation between duplicates.

3. FAT DIGESTION AND STAGE OF DEVELOPMENT

In vitro studies have shown that the concerted action of different lipolytic enzymes is a prerequisite for complete digestion of human milk triacylglycerol [28]. Gastric lipase and lipase-colipase in combination hydrolysed about two thirds of all ester bonds, and addition of bile salt-stimulated lipase resulted in hydrolysis of monoacylglycerols also [28]. Furthermore the hydrolysis of phosphorylcholine by phospholipase A_2 stimulates the activity of lipase by product activation [15].

Suckling pigs digest the nutrients in sows' milk very efficiently, and an apparent fat digestibility of 96% has been reported [29] in spite of a low level of the most important lipolytic enzyme, pancreatic lipase [16]. During the suckling period gastric lipase may play a major role in the hydrolysis of triacylglycerols [30]. In preterm infants it has been shown that the enzyme bile salt-stimulated lipase, which is found in human milk, is very important for the digestion of human milk triacylglycerols [31]. The existence of bile salt-stimulated lipase in sows' milk remains to be demonstrated. However, this enzyme is identical to carboxyl ester hydrolase [31] which is secreted from the exocrine pancreas. Studies have shown that the activity of this enzyme in pancreatic tissue increases very rapidly during the suckling period, and it has been suggested that the pig may compensate for the missing enzyme in the milk by secreting more carboxyl ester hydrolase from the pancreas during the suckling period [16].

The digestion of fat is to a very large extent dependent on pancreatic enzymes [15]. It has been shown that the activity of a number of digestive enzymes in pancreatic tissue declines upon weaning (Table 1, [6,32]) and in association with this decline a poor digestibility of nutrients has been observed in weanling pigs. The activity of lipase and its cofactor colipase as well as the activity of carboxyl ester hydrolase in pancreatic tissue reach a minimum on day 5 after weaning [Hedemann, unpublished results]. An increase in the activity of the lipolytic enzymes is observed approximately two weeks after weaning [16]. In agreement with this observation, it has been shown that the digestibility of fat declines to between 65 and 80% at weaning, and increases again during the following weeks [33]. The digestibility of fat is of special concern because it has been demonstrated that piglets have a high energy requirement that is not met because feed intake is not adequate; consequently body fat is mobilised to meet the deficit [34].

In the growing pig, pancreatic lipase is quantitatively the most important lipolytic enzyme, as it hydrolyses triacylglycerols which make up the major proportion of dietary fat.

Table 1
Activity of lipolytic enzymes in pancreatic tissue (U/g tissue) from day 3 to 56 in piglets which were weaned at day 28[1]

Age	Lipase		Colipase		Carboxyl ester hydrolase	
	Mean	SD[2]	Mean	SD	Mean	SD
3	727	315	569	228	35	0.31
7	2417	1025	1657	620	111	0.15
14	1959	1267	1267	739	72	0.17
21	2686	1291	1226	639	58	0.49
28	4994	4004	2108	2161	49	0.52
35	1133	763	502	298	7	1.04
42	1083	626	480	183	8	0.74
49	3407	2192	1143	706	15	1.53
56	3973	532	1450	242	11	0.50

[1]Adapted from reference 16.
[2]Standard deviation (n = 5).

However, carboxyl ester hydrolase and phospholipase A_2 also contribute substantially to fat digestion by hydrolysing a variety of other substrates such as cholesterol esters, ester forms of vitamin A and E and phospholipids.

Developmental studies on exocrine pancreatic function in ruminants have addressed three time periods. During the preweaning period, when the animals are consuming milk, they can be considered monogastric. The ingested milk bypasses the forestomachs and is digested as in monogastric animals. The second period is that of progressive weaning, and the third is the ruminant period, in which the animal has a fully functional rumen.

In preruminant calves, the activity of lipase in pancreatic tissue increased 1.6-fold between birth and day 70 and the activity of colipase decreased by 44% during the same period, whereas phospholipase A_2 activity did not change significantly during postnatal development [35]. In lambs, a similar development of lipase activity in pancreatic tissue was observed [36]. In both calves and lambs, a decrease in activity of enzymes in the pancreatic tissue was observed between birth and day two, indicating that secretion of enzymes was faster than synthesis during the first two days of life [35,36]. At weaning, the activity of lipase in pancreatic tissue in calves was observed to increase [35] despite the fact that lipid intake was much lower than in preruminants. The colipase content in the pancreas decreased further after weaning, resulting in a colipase:lipase ratio that was more than 62% lower in ruminants than in preruminants [35]. It was suggested that the changes in enzyme activities with age and upon weaning were related more to the increase in dry matter intake than to variation in amount of substrates.

In suckling goats, chronically catheterised for collection of pancreatic juice, it was found that the lipase activity was significantly lower in the group fed with milk replacer when compared to those fed goats' milk [37]. The milk replacer had a lower fat content than the goats' milk and this indicates that the pancreatic lipase adapted to the amount of fat in the diet. When the effect of age on exocrine pancreatic secretion was studied in goats it was seen that the basal (without feed stimulation) output of amylase and lipase activity increased during the fourth week of life [38]. After ingestion of milk, the lipase output was also increased [38].

The importance of pancreatic lipase differs in monogastric animals and ruminants. In monogastric animals there are only minor differences between the amount of fat ingested and the amount that reaches the duodenum. In the stomach, 10-30% of the triacylglycerols are hydrolysed by lingual or gastric lipase, and this is important especially in new-born animals and animals with pancreatic insufficiency. The young milk-fed ruminant can be compared with monogastric animals, as stated earlier. In an animal with a functional rumen the situation is far more complicated [39-41]. In the rumen the dietary fat is hydrolysed by the microflora and free unsaturated fatty acids are to a large part hydrogenated. Some of the fatty acids will be incorporated in the microbes, and furthermore a microbial de novo fatty acid synthesis takes place. This means that the lipid fraction that reaches the duodenum is very different from the ingested lipid, both in amount and composition, in the ruminant animal. Whether or not there is adaptation of the exocrine pancreatic secretion of lipase to an increase in the level of dietary fat in the ruminant animal remains to be investigated [40,41].

4. AMOUNT OF FAT AND PANCREATIC SECRETIONS

When the amount of dietary fat is increased, lipase secretion from the exocrine pancreas increases [6]. An increase in total lipase activity from 654 to 3950 U/24 h x 10^{-3} was reported when the level of dietary fat was increased from 2% (control diet) to 10% (tallow) [9]. In other studies, also with pigs, a 5% fat diet (control) and a 25% fat diet were used and lipase activity in pancreatic tissue increased by 83 0% and colipase activity increased by 37.5% [42]. Similar results were reported in rats [43]. A pre-translational regulatory mechanism appears to be responsible for increased lipase synthesis, regardless of the degree of saturation of dietary fat [44]. Enzyme adaptation to a change in diet is rapid and in pigs it is usually complete within 5 d [6,12]. However in dogs no adaptation of exocrine pancreatic secretion was observed after 8 d of feeding two different diets, one with a high fat content and the other containing a large amount of starch [45]. In the rabbit, it has been shown that pancreatic lipase activity increased when the amount of fat in the diet was increased from 2.7% to 12% [46]. At the same time the amount of colipase did not change in pancreatic tissue; consequently the colipase:lipase ratio decreased. In the same study it was observed that the fatty acid composition of triacylglycerols did not change the adaptive response of pancreatic lipase or colipase [46].

5. FATTY ACID COMPOSITION AND PANCREATIC SECRETIONS

Exocrine pancreatic secretion responds to changes in the level of fat in the diet and lipase secretion increases with an increase in the level of dietary fat. The exocrine pancreas also responds to changes in the fatty acid profile of dietary fat and these changes may have implications for fat digestion and digestive function. In the rat, the effect of the degree of saturation and (or) chain length of dietary fatty acids on lipase activity remains controversial. In some studies, unsaturated fat stimulated lipase secretion and long-chain fatty acids increased lipase content in pancreatic tissue more than medium-chain triacylglycerols [4]. However, in experiments with rats fed diets containing 45% fat, lipase and colipase activities were not affected by the degree of saturation or the chain length of fatty acids [47]. Inclusion of polyunsaturated fatty acids in the diet has been shown to increase lipase activity in pancreatic homogenate [43,44,48]. The question of whether the relative activities of enzymes in pancreatic homogenate taken from an animal that has been killed at one particular instant are similar to the relative activities in an hourly or pooled sample of pancreatic juice, from the same animal, remains to be investigated.

Secretin, ketones and fatty acid metabolites are proposed mediators of pancreatic adaptation to dietary fat [4]. Recent studies with rats suggest that the type of fat may act through a translational mechanism: moderate levels of saturated fat may reduce the efficiency of translation or decrease the synthesis of lipase through a pre-translational mechanism [44]. Whether or not the same mechanism exists in the pig remains to be determined. In pigs, there is a scarcity of information on the effect of fatty acid composition on pancreatic secretion of lipase as well as colipase, an essential cofactor for lipase activation. In addition, there is lack of information on the effect of the amount or source of dietary lipids on the activity of porcine carboxyl ester hydrolase, an enzyme that hydrolyses a variety of lipid substrates [3]. With the exception of two studies [17,49], the pig has not been used as a model to study the effect of the fatty acid composition of dietary fat on exocrine pancreatic secretion. It was found that pigs fed diets containing 21% sunflower oil had higher lipase activity in pancreatic homogenate than pigs fed diets with the same level of lard [49]. The quality of dietary fat has been shown to affect pancreatic secretion. The total activity of lipase in pancreatic juice increased when 15% peroxidized canola oil (heated to 180°C for 12 or 24 h) was fed to growing pigs [10].

Table 2
The secretion of lipolytic enzymes in pancreatic juice collected from growing pigs prepared for the collection of pancreatic juice with either the pouch method or the catheter method, and the apparent faecal digestibilities of fat when the pigs were fed diets supplemented with 15% fat[1]

Pouch method

Diet:	Fish oil diet	Rapeseed oil diet[2]	Coconut oil diet	SEM[3]
Total enzyme activities				
Lipase (U/24 h x 10^{-3})	6998.3	6928.3	4582.7	706.7
Colipase (U/24 h x 10^{-3})	755.0	528.7	287.0	303.3
Carboxyl ester hydrolase (U/24 h)	252.7	277.7	189.3	35.0
Apparent faecal digestibility of fat (%)	83.5	85.6	78.1	2.85

Catheter method

Diet:	Fish oil diet	Rapeseed oil diet[2]	Coconut oil diet	SEM[3]
Total enzyme activities				
Lipase (U/24 h x 10^{-3})	4771.0	4765.0	6432.0	989.4
Colipase (U/24 h x 10^{-3})	2041.0	2026.0	3149.0	828.8
Carboxyl ester hydrolase (U/24 h)	2964.7[a]	2090.3[b]	2293.0[b]	63.1
Apparent faecal digestibility of fat (%)	79.1	82.1	82.0	2.74

[1]Adapted from reference 17.
[2]The rapeseed oil was extracted from double-low rapeseed (low erucic acid, low glucosinolate) which is now grown in Denmark.
[3]Standard error of the mean (n = 3).

    We observed significant effects of the type of fat on the total activities of chymotrypsin and carboxyl ester hydrolase when the catheter method was used to collect pancreatic juice (Table 2) [17]. Similar results were observed in studies with rats fed high-fat diets (50%); chymotrypsin activity in pancreatic homogenate was increased when tristearin and arachid oil were fed [48]. Pigs fed a coconut oil diet had a higher total activity of chymotrypsin in pancreatic juice [17], in contrast to previous studies with rats or pigs fed diets containing either 17.4% safflower oil or 21% sunflower oil [44,49], where no such increase was observed. The higher (P < 0.05) total activities of carboxyl ester hydrolase in pancreatic juice from pigs fed the fish oil diet may have been due to an effect of the type of fat on the translational regulatory mechanism of carboxyl ester hydrolase synthesis [50]. Fish oil may have had a stimulatory effect, or rapeseed and coconut oil may have had an inhibitory effect. Our results suggest that the catheter method may be more sensitive than the pouch method in determining the effect of diet composition on exocrine pancreatic secretion [17]. This is the first time that both collection methods have been used under the same conditions. An approach similar to the one used in this study is needed to further compare the techniques and investigate the sensitivity of each. Regardless of collection method, pancreatic secretion responds to changes in the levels of fat, protein and starch [6,9,51]. However, future research must reveal whether both methods, under the same conditions, give similar results when different levels of dietary fat, starch and protein are fed. Trypsin and chymotrypsin in the duodenal pouch, activated by enterokinase secreted by the duodenal mucosa, may hydrolyse some of the enzymes in the pancreatic juice, explaining the lower activities of carboxyl ester hydrolase and colipase in pancreatic juice collected from pigs prepared with the pouch method [21]. The susceptibility of pancreatic enzymes to hydrolysis by proteases in the pancreatic juice and the occurrence of active enzymes in the duodenal pouch warrant further study.

Recently, additional research has been conducted in weanling pigs to further investigate the effect of dietary fat source on exocrine pancreatic secretions [52]. Since previous studies have shown that the dietary fat source influences the digestibility of fat in weaned pigs [33,53], it can not be ruled out that the fatty acid composition has an effect on the secretion of enzymes from the exocrine pancreas in newly weaned pigs. In the study, 10% coconut oil, lard or fish oil was included in the diet. For continuous collection of pancreatic juice, the pigs were surgically fitted with a pancreatic catheter and a T-shaped duodenal fistula. Pancreatic juice was collected continuously for 8 h. The volume of pancreatic juice secreted was clearly affected by the fat source. Piglets fed fish oil secreted 265 ml/8 h compared to piglets fed coconut oil or lard, who secreted 158 and 161 ml/8 h, respectively. The output of lipase over eight hours was significantly higher in piglets fed fish oil ($98.6 \text{ U} \times 10^3/8$ h) when compared to piglets fed coconut oil ($36.1 \text{ U} \times 10^3/8$ h) and lard ($12.7 \text{ U} \times 10^3/8$ h), whereas the output of colipase only differed between the piglets fed fish oil or lard ($32.2 \text{ U} \times 10^3/8$ h and $12.7 \text{ U} \times 10^3/8$ h, respectively). Carboxyl ester hydrolase was also clearly affected by the inclusion of fish oil in the diet. Piglets fed fish oil secreted 259 U/8 h of carboxyl ester hydrolase in the pancreatic juice whereas piglets fed coconut oil or lard secreted 138 U/8 h and 120 U/8 h, respectively. These results suggest that young pigs (7 - 8 wk old, 9 - 15 kg) are more sensitive to the fatty acid composition of the diets than growing pigs (35 – 45 kg) [17]. However, the output of carboxyl ester hydrolase was stimulated by diets containing fish oil irrespective of the age of the pig, and it is suggested that the secretion of this enzyme is increased by the long-chain polyunsaturated fatty acids in fish oil [17,52]. A specific effect of both the quality and quantity of dietary triacylglycerols on pancreatic lipase in pancreatic tissue of growing pigs has been observed [49]. The inducibility of pancreatic lipase was higher when the triacylglycerols were rich in unsaturated fatty acids than when they were rich in saturated fatty acids.

The activity or output of enzymes is regulated by the level of substrate for the given enzyme in the diet [4]. The results discussed here suggest that fatty acid composition not only regulates the activity of the lipolytic enzymes; a general stimulation of the exocrine pancreatic secretion (volume and composition) was observed when the piglets were fed the fish oil diet, compared to the lard diet [52]. Intestinal perfusion with fatty acids strongly stimulates pancreatic secretion [5] and it has been shown that they are potent releasers of hormones and peptides that regulate pancreatic secretion [54]. Studies have suggested that type and amount of fat together regulate the lipase activity at a translational or post-translational level [44]. In fact it has been shown that lipase, colipase and carboxyl ester hydrolase are regulated at the translational level by gastrointestinal hormones [50,55]. Studies in dogs demonstrated that those fed diets containing sunflower oil had a higher output of amylase and lipase than those fed olive oil [56]. It was shown by the same group that feeding these diets resulted in higher basal levels of peptide YY (PYY) and pancreatic polypeptide (PP), peptides that both inhibit pancreatic secretion, in the group fed olive oil [57]. The different effect of the diets containing sunflower oil and olive oil was attributed to the content of oleic acid (C18:1) in these diets [56,57]. Oleic acid has been shown to stimulate secretion of CCK, which stimulates pancreatic secretion [54], but at the same time it is the most potent stimulator of PYY and PP release [58,59]; i.e. it may modulate pancreatic secretion. In the study with weanling pigs [52], the lard diet had the highest content of oleic acid and further studies are needed to show whether a balance between stimulatory and inhibitory mechanisms explains the different exocrine pancreatic secretion observed in piglets fed fish oil diets and lard diets.

The relative potency of fatty acids with differing chain lengths to stimulate pancreatic secretion has been proposed to have the following order: C18:1 > C12:0 > C8:0; however, the order remains to be determined in detail [5]. It has been suggested that because long-chain fatty acids are absorbed at the lowest rate they expose the intestinal mucosa to the fatty acid stimulus over a longer time [60]. In the study with weanling pigs [52] the lard diet had the highest content of oleic acid (C18:1) but the piglets fed this diet had the lowest volume of pancreatic juice secreted. Feeding piglets the fish oil diet, containing the longest and most unsaturated fatty acids, resulted in the highest volume of pancreatic juice secretion [52]. These results suggest that the longer the fatty acids are, the higher is the stimulation of exocrine pancreatic secretion. Furthermore, as the long-chain fatty acids in fish oil are highly unsaturated, an effect of the degree of saturation cannot be ruled out. Further investigations are needed to elucidate the effect of chain length and degree of saturation of fatty acids and their possible interaction on exocrine pancreatic secretion.

It has been suggested that coconut oil is a good fat source for piglets due to its high content of medium-chain fatty acids, since these are absorbed at a faster rate from the intestinal lumen than long-chain fatty acids [53]. The weanling piglet study [52] did not show any stimulation of pancreatic secretion due to the inclusion of coconut oil in the diet, which may have been due to the short exposure of the intestinal mucosa to the aforementioned fatty acids. The results reported from the weanling pig study [52] suggest that the beneficial effect of coconut oil in diets for piglets observed in previous experiments [33,53] was the result of more rapid absorption of the fatty acids rather than a stimulation of the exocrine pancreas.

It has been suggested that the ratio between unsaturated and saturated fatty acids (U/S ratio) is of importance when determining the suitability of a diet with a given fatty acid composition for weaning pigs [61,62]. A fatty acid composition with a U/S ratio of 0.93 [61] or 5.71 [62] has variously been suggested to provide an ideal fatty acid profile [61]. These highly different ratios and the fact that in the previously discussed experiment [52], the fish oil diet had an U/S ratio of 1.72 and the lard diet had an U/S ratio of 1.14, imply that the U/S ratio should be used with caution.

The stimulation of pancreatic lipase secretion may be of limited value if colipase secretion is not stimulated at the same time. Colipase has been shown to adapt to dietary fat content in pigs [42], but it is more sensitive to protein intake [63]. In the weanling pig study [52], colipase responded to the type of fat in the diet; a higher colipase output was observed with the fish oil diet, but the lipase-colipase ratio was also increased, indicating that the secretion of lipase was stimulated more than that of colipase. The colipase activity determined in that study represents the relative colipase activity and is equal to the residual lipase activity described in other studies [42]. This may also help to explain the different lipase-colipase ratio reported in the literature [19,52]. When the relative colipase activity is measured, a risk of misinterpreting the adaptation of colipase to the diet arises [63]. As a consequence, no definite conclusions concerning the adaptation of colipase to the fatty acid composition of the diet can be drawn from the weanling pig study [52].

The use of fish oil in diets is accompanied by the risk that the feed will go rancid during storage, due to oxidation of the polyunsaturated fatty acids. It has been demonstrated that oxidised canola oil stimulates the secretion of lipase from the exocrine pancreas [10]. Oxidation could therefore be an explanation for the higher secretion observed in the fish oil fed piglets, but feeding with oxidised canola oil did not cause an increase in volume or in other enzyme activities [10] as the fish oil did [52]. In the study with fish oil for weanling pigs [52] care was taken to avoid fatty acid oxidation. The vitamin-mineral premix contained an antioxidant (butylated hydroxytoluene, 100 mg/kg feed), the feed was stored in a refrigerated room and only a few meals were weighed out at a time while the experiment was being conducted. The use of fish oil in practical pig feeding is limited due to its effects on meat quality [64], but these results indicate that further investigation into its use in diets for weanling pigs is warranted.

6. STABILITY OF LIPOLYTIC ENZYMES

For optimal digestion, lipolytic enzymes in the digestive tract must be stable and resist degradation by proteolytic enzymes for long enough to allow them to cleave their substrates. From a research and a diagnostic perspective, there should not be degradation of the lipolytic enzymes before the samples have been assayed for enzyme activity or the enzymes have been quantitatively measured. Samples of duodenal aspirate or ileal digesta contain active proteolytic enzymes and depending on which method is used to collect pancreatic juice it can also contain active proteolytic enzymes [20]. Information on the stability of lipolytic enzymes is scarce and much of the information there is has been derived from studies examining the effect of storage conditions on their activity.

The activity of digestive enzymes in digesta decreases during transit from the duodenum to the distal ileum [65]. This inactivation may be due to bacterial degradation, most prominent in the colon, acid denaturation, particularly of ingested enzymes, or digestion of the enzymes. In the healthy animal, digestion of enzymes by proteases is most important. Lipase activity decreases more than that of other enzymes; more than 95% of its activity disappears during small intestinal transit [65]. Delivery of lipase activity increased significantly after luminal protease inhibition [65]. Both trypsin and chymotrypsin are responsible for this degradation but chymotrypsin seems to be of greater importance [66]. Intraluminal nutrients increase the survival of enzyme activities in the proximal intestine [67], but after nutrient absorption chymotrypsin and bile acids regulate the survival of lipolytic activity in the ileum [67].

We investigated the stability of lipolytic enzymes by comparing the pouch method (PM) and the catheter method (CM) for collecting pancreatic juice from growing pigs [20] and by examining the effect of freezing and thawing on the activities of lipolytic enzymes [24]. The specific and total activities of carboxyl ester hydrolase (CEH) in pancreatic juice collected from CM pigs were much higher ($P < 0.001$) than for PM pigs. The specific activity of lipase was higher ($P < 0.001$) in pancreatic juice from PM pigs than from CM pigs. The specific and total activities of colipase in pancreatic juice from CM pigs were greater ($P < 0.01$) than in pancreatic juice collected from PM pigs. A plot of specific lipase activity in relation to colipase activity for PM pigs indicated that there was a weak but significant relationship between lipase and colipase activity [20]. Generally the colipase activity in pancreatic juice from PM pigs was relatively low, indicating that there was a substantial amount of degradation by active proteolytic enzymes in the duodenal pouch [20]. In contrast, a linear relationship ($P < 0.001$) was observed between lipase and colipase activity in CM pigs. It has been reported that 99% of lipase activity is inactivated during passage from the duodenum to the ileum [68]. In contrast, *in vitro* experiments in which lipase activity was measured over time in pancreatic juice which was being activated demonstrated that lipase was relatively resistant to inactivation until the proteases had been active for some time [15]. However, lipase is less resistant to inactivation than either trypsin or chymotrypsin [69]. Procolipase is activated to colipase relatively quickly, before trypsin and chymotrypsin activities plateau, and colipase is inactivated to a large extent during and following the activation of these two proteolytic enzymes [15].

Before analysis, refrigerated or frozen storage of samples is often required due to technical and logistical limitations, especially if a large number of samples are to be analysed. Changes in enzyme activities during storage could affect the results of an experiment and its interpretation (i.e., artefacts) and/or result in an incorrect diagnosis of pancreatic insufficiency [70]. Repeated freezing and thawing may be necessary if there is a small amount of sample and several analyses are to be performed. Very few studies have been conducted to examine the effect of storage conditions on enzyme activities in pancreatic juice. An additional concern is that thawing conditions are not specified in the literature and could affect enzyme activities. It was observed that storage of pancreatic juice for 3 wk at -20 or -80°C did not affect lipase activity [71], but at 4°C, enzyme activity declined significantly. Most studies involving storage have been carried out with samples of duodenal aspirate which definitely contains active proteolytic enzymes. In other studies it was variously reported that lipase activity steadily declined during storage at -20°C [72], that lipase activity in duodenal aspirate, stored at -20°C for 4 wk was quite stable [70] and that lipase activity did not decrease during storage at -15°C [27].

We have observed a reduction in the activities of trypsin, chymotrypsin and especially of lipase which is of practical significance because it indicates that repeated freezing and thawing of pancreatic juice leads to an underestimation of enzyme activities [24]. It would have been very useful to determine the impact of one freezing and thawing cycle on enzyme activities in fresh pancreatic juice, but unfortunately this was not possible in this study because the enzyme assays could not be carried out immediately after collection.

Several modifications have been made to prevent a decline in enzyme activities in duodenal aspirate during storage but none of these approaches has been applied to the storage of pure pancreatic juice. A decline in lipase activity was prevented by adding albumin or casein, which act as alternative substrates for chymotrypsin and trypsin, or a chymotrypsin inhibitor (turkey egg white) to duodenal aspirate prior to freezing [66,72,73]. The addition of Trasylol (aprotinin, a trypsin inhibitor), glycerol or glucose was used to reduce or prevent the inactivation of amylase, chymotrypsin, lipase and trypsin during frozen storage of duodenal aspirate [73,74]. However, whether or not the Trasylol was removed from the samples prior to carrying out the enzyme assays was not reported. Trasylol may interfere with the determination of trypsin activity and other proteolytic enzymes; further studies are required to see if this is so.

Depending on the concentration of enzymes (reflected by the magnitude of enzyme activity present), the effect of storage may vary [24]. Regardless of the results of our first lipase assay, the activity measured in the second assay was always considerably lower. After a second freezing and thawing cycle, lipase activity had decreased by 83% [24]. Lipase and other lipolytic enzymes are resistant to repeated freezing and thawing but are susceptible to hydrolysis by chymotrypsin [72]. In our samples, there was a very small amount of chymotrypsin activity present (< 1 U) and there was no trypsin activity. Proteolysis or inactivation of lipase in pancreatic juice does not occur until the proteolytic enzymes have been active for approximately 1 h [15]. Furthermore, as mentioned earlier, lipase is less resistant to inactivation than either trypsin or chymotrypsin [69]; this was confirmed in this study. Repeated freezing and thawing of pancreatic juice is not recommended due to the sensitivity of lipase to inactivation [24] by trypsin and chymotrypsin, which can be activated by thawing and freezing.

7. QUANTIFICATION OF FAT DIGESTION

In order to study the consequences of the secretion of pancreatic lipolytic enzymes on fat digestion, the events taking place in the small intestine must be studied. Fatty acids as a proportion of total fat and fat digestibility are the most important factors determining the nutritive value of fat [13]. The lipids used in diets for domesticated animals are extremely diverse in chemical structure, which may influence their digestibility and energy value. Fat digestion occurs in the small intestine and absorption of fatty acids, as mono- and diacylglycerols is nearly complete at the distal ileum [15]. However, the fatty acids which have not been absorbed in the small intestine will enter the caecum and large intestine where microbial hydrogenation of unsaturated fatty acids has been shown to be significant [13,75]. Therefore, the absorption of the individual fatty acids must be measured at the terminal ileum. In contrast, for total fat the faecal digestibility is similar to the ileal digestibility, because the net disappearance is very small [13]. Dietary fat from animal sources may have a lower digestibility and therefore energy value than dietary fat from vegetable sources due to a higher content of saturated fatty acids (16:0 and 18:0). Saturated fatty acids may have a lower ileal digestibility than unsaturated fatty acids (18:1, 18:2 and 18:3) [13,64,76]. Depending on the degree of saturation, fatty acids may have different rates of absorption. Whether or not a difference in ileal digestibility could be observed between saturated and unsaturated fatty acids using diets containing coconut oil, rapeseed oil or fish oil was investigated in our recent experimental work [77], discussed below.

In a recent study examining the effect of the type of dietary fat on the secretions of the exocrine pancreas in growing pigs, there was a significant effect of fat source on the secretion of carboxyl ester hydrolase [17]. Carboxyl ester hydrolase is a relatively non-specific enzyme which hydrolyses a variety of lipid substrates [3] and its contribution to fat digestion has not yet been quantified. However, the apparent faecal digestibilities of fat, protein and energy were not affected by the inclusion of fish oil, rapeseed oil or coconut oil in the diet (Table 2) [17]. Nevertheless, there may have been some differences between the fat sources which were masked by the modifying and equalising effects of the microflora in the hindgut [78]. The rapeseed oil used in the aforementioned study as well as in the recent study on ileal digestibilities [77] was extracted from double-low rapeseed (low erucic acid, low glucosinolate) which is now grown in Denmark.

In-vivo studies addressing the events occurring in the small intestine allow the assessment of the effects on fat digestion of factors which change or modify pancreatic secretions. One way in which this is done is by taking samples of duodenal aspirate via nasal intubation; this is the approach used in studies with human subjects [70,72].

We used the ileal analysis method to study the digestion of different sources of fat, which were also used in studies designed to investigate the nutritional regulation of exocrine pancreatic secretions (Table 2) [17], Different batches of the same sources of fat were used

Table 3
The apparent ileal digestibilities of fat and selected fatty acids in growing pigs fitted with a simple T-cannula in the distal ileum and fed the same diets, containing different batches of the respective fats, as those fed to pigs prepared for the collection of pancreatic juice with the pouch or the catheter method[1]

Diet:	Fish oil diet	Rapeseed diet[2]	Coconut oil diet	SEM[3]
Apparent ileal digestibilities (%):				
Fat	91.6	91.1	91.4	0.94
Linoleic acid (18:2)	85.4[b]	93.9[a]	82.6[b]	1.62
Linolenic acid (18:3, n-3)	96.2[a]	97.2[a]	85.2[b]	1.12
Timnodonic acid (20:5, n-3)	98.1	96.7	96.9	0.96
Cervonic acid (22:6, n-3)	96.8[a]	90.0[b]	94.4[a]	1.40
Apparent faecal digestibility of fat (%)	92.8[a]	93.4[a]	88.4[b]	1.61

[1]Adapted from reference 77.
[2]The rapeseed oil was extracted from double-low rapeseed (low erucic acid, low glucosinolate), which is now grown in Denmark.
[3]Standard error of the mean (n = 4).

and both ileal and faecal digestibilities of fat and fatty acids were determined (Table 3, [77]). Four barrows (initial weight 35 kg) were fitted with a simple T-cannula in the terminal ileum. Three wheat starch and fish meal-based diets were formulated to contain 15% of either fish oil, rapeseed oil or coconut oil. A basal diet which did not contain oil was also prepared. The diets were fed according to a 4 times 4 Latin square design. Each experimental period comprised 5 d adaptation to the diets, 3 d faecal collection and 2 d digesta collection. Recent research has shown that 24 h continuous collection of ileal digesta is not needed in order to obtain a representative sample; it is adequate to sample ileal digesta between two feeding periods [79]. In our current experiments, we collect ileal digesta continuously from 8:00 to 20:00 h on two consecutive days and pool the samples. The apparent ileal digestibility of fat in the basal diet (83.1%) was lower than that measured for the other diets which were supplemented with 15% fat (91.1 to 91.6%). The differences in the ileal digestibilities of fat were due to differences in the level of dietary fat. Ileal digesta from pigs fed the diets supplemented with fat most likely had a lower level of endogenous fat relative to dietary fat than ileal digesta from pigs fed the basal diet. Due to the lower level of fat in the basal diet, the amount of endogenous fat at the end of the small intestine, relative to dietary fat, would most likely be higher than for pigs fed the other diets. However, there were no differences in the ileal digestibilities of fat between the diets which were supplemented with 15% fat, indicating that the source of dietary fat did not affect fat digestion in the small intestine.

Neither was there any difference between the ileal and faecal digestibility of fat when absolute values were compared. These findings are in agreement with previous results (13), and suggest that there is essentially no net disappearance of long-chain fatty acids during the transit of digesta through the caecum-colon.

However, there were differences in the ileal digestibilities of individual fatty acids and in the digestibilities of different classes of fatty acids (Table 3). As with the ileal digestibilities of fat, the ileal digestibilities of individual fatty acids were relatively high (82.6 to 97.2%) indicating that most of the fat in the diets was digested and absorbed. In the diet containing coconut oil, the ileal digestibility of fatty acids (8:0 to 16:0) decreased with increasing chain length (from 100 to 86%). The ileal digestibility of C18:1, C18:2 and C18:3 in the rapeseed oil diet ranged from 94 to 97% and the ileal digestion of the unsaturated long-chain fatty acids C20:5(n-3) and C22:6(n-3) in fish oil was nearly complete (97-98%). However, observed digestibilities were largely affected by the concentration of individual fatty acids in ileal digesta relative to the levels occurring in the diets. The low and negative digestibilities for 18:0 were most likely due to the very low levels of 18:0 in the diets [77] which would make the endogenous secretion of C18 decrease the apparent digestibility [18,76]. The digestibility of stearic acid was much lower than that determined in diets supplemented with animal fat [13]. The highest ileal digestibilities for 18:1 and 18:3 (n-3), observed in pigs fed the fish oil and rapeseed oil diets, were due in part to the high levels of 18:1 and 18:3 (n-3) in these diets. The highest digestibility for 18:2 was observed in pigs fed the rapeseed oil diet, which had the highest level of 18:2 [77].

The faecal digestibilities of fat observed in the aforementioned study (Table 3) are similar to those reported previously [13,14] for pigs fed diets containing a similar level of animal fat or rapeseed oil. We determined faecal digestibilities in order to investigate how fat supplementation affects digestion and fermentation in the caecum and colon. There were no differences in the digestibilities of energy and protein and the digestibilities were high, suggesting that the supplemented fats did not greatly affect digestion.

The diets fed in the study to determine ileal and faecal digestibilities of fatty acids [77] and our previous study concerning the effect of dietary fat source on exocrine pancreatic secretion [17] were formulated to have exactly the same composition. The faecal digestibilities of energy, dry matter, protein and fat, determined in this study [77] were slightly higher than those

354

measured in growing pigs fitted with a pancreatic pouch re-entrant cannula or a catheter in the pancreatic duct. The animals in the two studies had a similar feeding regimen and a similar genetic background. This qualitative comparison, which has not been made before, suggests that surgical intervention may have an effect on digestion. However, before a definitive statement is made more research is warranted, including comparison within a single study, under the same conditions. Within the study, we did not observe any differences in digestibilities related to the method used for collection of pancreatic juice [17].

The higher faecal digestibilities of fat in the fish and rapeseed oil diets, compared to the basal diet [77], were most likely due to the higher level of fat in these diets, as previously discussed. The lower faecal digestibility of fat (88.4%) compared to the ileal digestibility of fat (91.4%) was most likely due to the hydrogenation of mono- and polyunsaturated fatty acids by the microflora in the caecum and colon.

Biohydrogenation of fatty acids has been shown to occur in the caecum and colon in the pig [13,75], i.e. the microflora in the hindgut can have a modifying and equalising effect on faecal fatty acid digestibilities [78]. Therefore, faecal fatty acid digestibilities are not reflective of ileal digestibilities. Compared to the ileal digestibilities of 18:0, the faecal digestibilities were highly negative, suggesting that additional 18:0 was synthesized by hydrogenation of mono- and polyunsaturated 18 carbon fatty acids [77]. For 18:1, 18:2 and 18:3 (n-3), faecal digestibilities were numerically higher than the ileal digestibilities [77], which was most likely a result of biohydrogenation of these fatty acids. There may also have been some degradation of fatty acids in the caecum and colon.

Hydrogenation also most likely occurred for the long-chain fatty acid 20:5 (n-3); faecal digestibilities [77] suggest that the digestion of this fatty acid was essentially complete. However, this was not the case for 22:6 (n-3) where faecal digestibilities were lower than ileal digestibilities, suggesting that there may have been a net appearance of 22:6 (n-3) in the caecum and large intestine.

The daily flow of fatty acids in ileal digesta is influenced by the fatty acid composition of dietary fat. In our previous work [77], pigs fed the coconut oil diet, as expected, had the highest daily intake of saturated fatty acids which most likely led to these animals having the highest ileal flow of saturated fatty acids. The high faecal flow, which may have been due, in part, to the high ileal flow was also a result of biohydrogenation of mono- and polyunsaturated fatty acids. However, for all diets, the amount of saturated fatty acids excreted in faeces was approximately twice as high as the amount flowing into the caecum-colon [77]. Although the disappearance of mono- and polyunsaturated fatty acids in the caecum and colon was high, it was exceeded by the increase in saturated fatty acids in faeces of pigs fed the basal, fish oil or rapeseed oil diets, which suggests that there were modifications in fatty acid chain length. The disappearance of mono- and polyunsaturated fatty acids in the caecum and colon of animals fed the coconut oil diet was 8.9 g/d less than the appearance of saturated fatty acids in the caecum and colon, indicating that synthesis of saturated fatty acids exceeded biohydrogenation.

The endogenous flow of fatty acids can be used to determine the true digestibilities of fatty acids [18,76]. Once apparent digestibilities are corrected for the endogenous contributions of fatty acids or endogenous losses, then a correct estimate of how much of a particular fatty acid was taken up by and disappeared from the digestive tract can be made. The regression method, in which the amount of digested fatty acids is regressed onto fatty acid intake, allows the endogenous contribution of fatty acids to be determined. This approach was used in studies with growing pigs [76]. The level of endogenous fat was estimated to be approximately 4.5 g/kg dry matter intake. However, for specific fatty acids the endogenous flows were usually very low. For example, the following endogenous flows were reported for palmitic, palmitoleic, stearic, oleic, linoleic and linolenic acids: 0.17, 0.03, 0.06, 0.12, 0.08 and 0.02 g/kg of dry matter intake, respectively [Jørgensen et al., 1993]. In this study a semipurified basal diet was used, containing casein, whey, cellulose (3%), ground barley straw (3%), potato starch, corn starch, cassava meal and sucrose [2%]. More research, with commonly used commercial-type diets, is required to identify the factors which affect the endogenous flow of fatty acids. They may originate from sloughed epithelial cells, bacteria and secretions from the digestive tract, for example bile [18].

8. INTERACTIONS AND LIPOLYTIC ENZYMES

Once the pancreatic enzymes enter the duodenum, their action is dependent on the gastrointestinal environment and their interaction with other nutrients and compounds. The secretion and action of pancreatic lipolytic enzymes is not only dependent on the amount and type of dietary fat; the amount and type of protein, carbohydrates, minerals and antinutritional compounds may influence the digestion and absorption of fat as well.

In vitro studies have shown that dietary fibre has an inhibitory effect on the activity of pancreatic enzymes [80]. This effect has been attributed to viscosity, pH and adsorption. However, studies with rats have shown a positive effect of pectin and wheat bran in the diet on the activity of pancreatic enzymes in small intestinal contents [81]. The effect of dietary fibre on activity of lipolytic enzymes may be very dependent on the type of fibre and hence a definite conclusion is difficult to reach.

In experiments with pigs, it has been shown that ileal digestibility of certain fatty acids is increased when the protein content of the diet is increased [13]. Conversely, the level of dietary fat has been shown to affect the digestion of protein. A significant increase in apparent ileal amino acid digestibility was observed as the level of canola oil in the diet was increased [82]. Similar results were observed with the apparent faecal digestibility of protein when growing pigs were fed diets containing 4, 8 and 16% rapeseed oil [14]. The observed results may have been due to a positive effect of fatty acids on amino acid absorption or a reduction in endogenous protein secretions caused by coating of feed particles with fat, and a consequent reduction of their abrasive effect [77,82]. We hypothesised that there may be differences in protein digestibility between the basal diet and the diets with added fat or an effect of differences in fatty acid composition on protein digestion [77]. Protein digestibility was not affected, but this does not mean that there were no differences in amino acid digestibility [77]. In weaned pigs, different fat sources have been shown to have different effects on nutrient digestibility [53], although the differences decrease with age [53]. Endogenous and undigested protein may contribute to the formation and stabilisation of micelles in the intestinal contents [83]. Removal of the free fatty acids from the triacylglycerol-lipase interface may reduce their inhibitory action on lipolysis [83].

Variation in the level of minerals (± 40% from the normal level) had no significant effect on the ileal digestibilities of fat and fatty acids. However, a significant reduction of the faecal digestibilities of a number of fatty acids was observed. The decreased digestibility of saturated fatty acids indicates that insoluble Ca-soaps are formed in the large intestine [13].

Since the absorption of fatty acids takes place in the small intestine, even large variations in the level of minerals will not affect the amount of fatty acids absorbed.

The existence of lipase inhibitors has been demonstrated in several seeds, e.g. soya bean and wheat [84]. Studies performed in rats have shown that the inclusion of wheat flour lipase inhibitor in the diet decreases serum triacylglycerol levels and increases faecal lipid excretion [84].

9. IMPROVING FAT DIGESTION

One of the goals of research on digestive physiology should be to identify ways of improving fat digestion for domesticated farm animals. Improving fat digestion may be especially important in the young animal. Attempts could be made to augment the role of the pancreas, perhaps by using feed enzymes. Another approach would be to develop specific strategies whereby certain types of fat are given at certain stages of development. The way in which fat is applied to feeds and blended into feeds may have an effect on fat digestion. More research is needed on the way in which fats are applied to feeds and the potential effect on fat digestion. Various ways of processing feeds, such as pelleting and extrusion, may also affect the digestion of fat.

10. CONCLUSIONS

In conclusion, the process of fat digestion is a complex process and involves many different factors. The amount and type of dietary fat is probably the most important factor affecting the secretion of lipolytic enzymes. When the content of dietary fat in the diet is increased an increased secretion of lipase follows. Lipase is the most thoroughly studied lipolytic enzyme and future studies will have to elucidate whether there is a parallel increase in all lipolytic enzymes, i.e. colipase, carboxyl ester hydrolase and phospholipase A_2, when there is an increase in dietary fat. In this respect, the type of fat included in the diet may play an important role. Considerable controversy exists on the significance of type of dietary fat and fatty acid composition on the secretion of lipolytic enzymes, but it seems that the species and age of the animal affect the results obtained. Future experiments are warranted to further elucidate this question and investigation of all lipolytic enzymes in such studies may provide better insight. In addition, very little is known about how the exocrine pancreas in the ruminant responds to the intake of dietary fat, and its fatty acid composition.

In the present review focus has been placed on the secretion of lipolytic enzymes from the exocrine pancreas, and it should be noted that bile secreted from the gallbladder also plays a very significant role in the hydrolysis and absorption of lipids. It is beyond the scope of this chapter to discuss this interaction and excellent reviews have been made on this topic (e.g. 15).

In order for fat digestion to occur, lipolytic enzymes must be active throughout most of the small intestine. Degradation of lipolytic enzymes occurs due to the action of proteolytic enzymes in the small intestine. Inactivation can be rapid; therefore the process of fat digestion must be complete in a relatively short time. More research is needed to identify factors which affect the stability of lipolytic enzymes in the digestive tract.

To know the effect of various factors on fat digestion, factors which affect the secretion of lipolytic enzymes need to be quantitatively evaluated by studying the events taking place in the small intestine. The ileal analysis method must be used to measure the uptake of fatty acids by the small intestine. Extensive biohydrogenation occurs in the caecum and large intestine and this confounds faecal (total tract) measurements of fatty acid digestibility. The ileal analysis method is an excellent approach, which allows factors such as other nutrients or compounds that affect fat digestion to be evaluated. These types of studies complement studies which investigate the nutritional regulation and adaptation of the exocrine pancreas. Future research is needed on factors which affect the action of lipolytic enzymes in the digestive tract, and the quantitative role of specific enzymes in the process of fat digestion.

REFERENCES

1. D.E. Kidder and M.J. Manners, Digestion in the pig, University of Bristol, Bristol, UK, 1978.
2. I. Schulz, Electrolyte and fluid secretion in the exocrine pancreas, In: L.R. Johnson (ed.), Physiology of the Gastrointestinal Tract, 2nd ed. Raven Press, New York. Pages (1987) 1147.
3. H. Rinderknecht, Pancreatic secretory enzymes, In: V.L.W. Go, E.P. DiMagno, J.D. Gardner, E. Lebenthal, H.A. Reber and G.A. Scheele (eds.), The Pancreas: Biology, Pathobiology, and Disease. Raven Press, New York. 219 (1993).
4. P.M. Brannon, Ann. Rev. Nutr. 10 (1985) 85.
5. T.E. Solomon, Control of exocrine pancreatic secretion, In: L.R. Johnson (ed.), Physiology of the Gastrointestinal Tract. 2nd ed. Raven Press, New York (1987) 1173.
6. T. Corring, C. Juste and E. Lhoste, Nutr. Res. Rev. 2 (1989) 161.
7. W.Y. Chey, Hormonal control of pancreatic enzyme secretion. In: V.L.W. Go, E.P. Dimagno, J.D. Gardner, E. Lebenthal, H.A. Reber and G.A. Scheele (eds.), The pancreas: biology, pathobiology, and disease, Raven Press, New York., 403 (1993).
8. J. Hee, W.C. Sauer and R. Mosenthin, J. Anim. Physiol. Anim. Nutr. 60 (1988) 249.
9. J. Hee, W.C. Sauer and R. Mosenthin, J. Anim. Physiol. Anim. Nutr. 60 (1988) 241.
10. L. Ozimek, R. Mosenthin and W.C. Sauer, Eur. J. Nutr. 34 (1995) 224.
11. J.S. Davidson, Control of the exocrine pancreas, In: J. S. Davidson (ed.), Gastrointestinal secretion, Wright, London, UK (1989) 102.
12. I.G. Partridge, A.G. Low and I.E. Sambrook, Brit. J. Nutr. 48 (1982) 137.
13. H. Jørgensen, K. Jakobsen and B.O. Eggum, Acta Agric. Scand. Sect. A Anim. Sci. 42 (1992) 177.
14. H. Jørgensen, S.K. Jensen and B.O. Eggum, Acta. Agric. Scand. Sect. A Anim. Sci. 46 (1996) 65.
15. B. Borgström, Luminal digestion of fats, In V.L.W. Go, E.P. Dimagno, J.D. Gardner, E. Lebenthal, H.A. Reber and G.A. Scheele (eds.), The Pancreas: Biology, Pathobiology, and Diesase, Raven Press, New York (1993) 475.
16. M.S. Jensen, S.K. Jensen and K. Jakobsen, J. Anim. Sci. 75 (1997) 437.
17. V.M. Gabert, M.S. Jensen, H. Jørgensen, R.M. Engberg, and S.K. Jensen, J. Nutr. 126 (1996) 2076.
18. H. Jørgensen, K. Jakobsen and B.O. Eggum, J. Anim. Feed Sci. 1 (1992) 139.

19. S.G. Pierzynowski, B.R. Weström, J. Svendsen, L. Svendsen and B.W. Karlsson, Int. J. Pancreatol. 18 (1995) 81.
20. M.S. Jensen, V.M. Gabert, H. Jørgensen and R.M. Engberg, Int. J. Pancreatol. 21 (1997) 173.
21. V.M. Gabert, M.S. Jensen, B.R. Weström and S.G. Pierzynowski, Int. J. Pancreatol. 22 (1997) 39.
22. C. Erlanson, Scand. J. Gastroenterol. 5 (1970) 333.
23. J. Lainé, M. Beattie and D. LeBel, Pancreas 8 (1993) 383.
24. V.M. Gabert and M.S. Jensen, Pancreas 15 (1997) 183.
25. C. Erlanson-Albertsson, A. Larsson and R. Duan, Pancreas 2 (1987) 531.
26. F.H. Schmidt, H. Stork and K. von Dahl, Lipase: photometric assay. In: H.U. Bergmeyer (ed.), Methods of Enzymatic Analysis. Volume 2. New York: Verlag Chemie Weinheim, Academic Press. (1974) 819.
27. B. Borgström and H. Hildebrand, Scand. J. Gastroenterol. 10 (1975) 585.
28. S. Bernbäck, L. Bläckberg and O. Hernell, J. Clin. Invest. 85 (1990) 1221.
29. P.D. Cranwell and P.J. Moughan, Biological limitations imposed by the digestive system to the growth performance of weaned pigs. In: J.L. Barnett and D.P. Hennessy (eds.), Manipulating pig production II. Victoria, Australia (1989) 140.
30. M.J. Newport and G.L. Howarth, Contribution of gastric lipolysis to the digestion of fat in the neonatal pig. In: A Just, H Jørgensen and JA Fernandez (eds) Proc. 3rd Int. Seminar on Digestive Physiology in the Pig. Copenhagen, Denmark. (1985) 143.
31. O. Hernell and L. Bläckberg, Acta Paediat. Suppl. 405 (1994) 65.
32. W.F. Owsley, D.E. Orr and L.F. Tribble, J. Anim. Sci. 63 (1986) 497.
33. K.R. Cera, D.C. Mahan and G.A. Reinhart, J. Anim. Sci. 66 (1988) 1430.
34. A. Chwalibog, K. Jakobsen and G. Thorbek, J. Anim. Physiol. Anim. Nutr. 72 (1994) 80.
35. I. Le Huerou-Luron, P. Guilloteau, C. Wicker-Planquart, J.-A. Chayvialle, J. Burton, Mouats, R. Toullec and A. Puigserver, J. Nutr. 122 (1992) 1434.
36. P. Guilloteau, T. Corring, P. Garnot, P. Martin, R. Toullec and G. Durand, J. Dairy Sci. 66 (1983) 2373.
37. J.A. Naranjo, M. Manas, A. Valverde, M.D. Yago and E. Martinez-Victoria, Arch. Physiol. Biochem. 105 (1997) 190.
38. J.A. Naranjo, E. Martinez-Victoria, A. Valverde, M.D. Yago and M. Manas, Arch. Physiol. Biochem. 105 (1997) 144.
39. W.J. Croom, Jr., L.S. Bull and I.L. Taylor, J. Nutr. 122 (1992) 191.
40. D.L. Harmon, J. Anim. Sci. 70 (1992) 1290.
41. D.L. Harmon, J. Dairy Sci. 76 (1993) 2102.
42. J. Mourot and T. Corring, Ann. Biol. Anim. Bioch. Biophys. 19 (1979) 119.
43. J.E. Sabb, P.M. Godfrey and P.M. Brannon, J. Nutr. 116 (1986) 892.
44. J. Ricketts and P.M. Brannon, J. Nutr. 124 (1994) 1166.
45. M. Manas, M.D. Yago, J.L. Quiles, J.R. Huertas and E. Martinez-Victoria, Arch. Physiol. Biochem. 104 (1996) 819.
46. P. Borel, M. Armand, M. Senft, M. Andre, H. Lafont and D. Lairon, Gastroenterology 100 (1991) 1582.
47. B. Saraux, A. Girard-Globa, M. Ouagued and D. Vacher, Amer. J. Physiol. 243 (1982) G10.

48. M. Deschodt-Lanckman, P. Robberecht, J. Camus and J. Christophe, Biochemie 53 (1971) 789.
49. C. Simoes-Nunes, Reprod. Nutr. Develop. 26 (1986) 1273.
50. Y. Huang and D.Y. Hui, J. Biol. Chem. 266 (1991) 6720.
51. C.A. Makkink and M.W.A. Verstegen,. J. Anim. Physiol. Anim. Nutr. 64 (1990) 190.
52. M.S. Hedemann, A.R. Pedersen and R.M. Engberg, Brit. J. Nutr. (1999) (submitted).
53. K.R. Cera, D.C. Mahan, and G.A. Reinhart, J. Anim. Sci. 67 (1989) 2040.
54. O. Olsen, O.B. Schaffalitzky de Muckadell and P. Cantor, Scand. J. Gastroenterol. 24 (1989) 74.
55. R.-D. Duan and C. Erlanson-Albertsson, Amer. J. Physiol. 262 (1992) G779.
56. M.C. Ballesta, M. Manas, F.J. Matiax, E. Martinez-Victoria and I. Seiquer, Brit. J. Nutr. 64 (1990) 487.
57. M.D. Yago, E. Martinez-Victoria, M. Manas, M.A. Martinez and J. Mataix, Nutr. Biochem. 8 (1997) 502.
58. G.W. Aponte, A.S. Fink, J.H. Meyer, K. Takemoto and I.L. Taylor, Amer. J. Physiol. 249 (1985) G745.
59. A.S. Fink, I.L. Taylor, M. Luxemburg and J.H. Meyer, Metabolism 30 (1983) 1063.
60. J.-R. Malagelada, E.P. DiMagno, W.H.J. Summerskill and V.L.W. Go, J. Clin. Invest. 58 (1976) 493.
61. D.F. Li, R.C. Thaler, J.L. Nelssen, D.L. Harmon, G.L. Allee and T.L. Weeden, J. Anim. Sci. 68 (1990) 3694.
62. J. Powles, J. Wiseman, D.J.A. Cole and B. Hardy, Anim. Prod. 58 (1994) 411.
63. M. Ouagued, B. Saraux, A. Girard-Globa and G. Bourdel, J. Nutr. 110 (1980) 2302.
64. M. Øverland, Z. Mroz and F. Sundstøl, J. Anim. Sci. 72 (1994) 2022.
65. P. Layer, J.B.M.J. Jansen, L. Cherian, C.M.H.W. Lamers and H. Goebell, Gastroenterology 98 (1990) 1311.
66. R. Thiruvengadam and E.P. DiMagno, Amer. J. Physiol. 255 (1988) G476.
67. G. Holtmann, D.G. Kelly, B. Sternby and E.P. DiMagno, Amer. J. Physiol. 273 (1997) G553.
68. P. Layer, V.L.W. Go and E.P. DiMagno, Amer. J. Physiol. 251(1986) G475.
69. D. Pelot and M.I. Grossman, Amer. J. Physiol. 202 (1962) 285.
70. E.P. Legg and A.M. Spencer, Clin. Chim. Acta. 65 (1975) 175.
71. C.A. Makkink, L.A.J. van der Westerlaken, L.A. den Hartog, M.J. van Baak and J. Huisman, J. Anim. Physiol. Anim. Nutr. 63 (1990) 267.
72. D.G. Kelly, B. Sternby and E.P. DiMagno, Gastroenterol. 100 (1991) 189.
73. G. Lake-Bakaar, S. McKavanagh, C.E. Rubio, O. Epstein and J.A. Summerfield, Gut 21 (1980) 402.
74. D.P.R. Muller and G.K. Ghale, Ann. Clin. Biochem. 19 (1982) 89.
75. W.E. Can. J. Anim. Sci. 48 (1968) 315.
76. H. Jørgensen, K. Jakobsen and B.O. Eggum, Acta Agric. Scand. Sect. A Anim. Sci. 43 (1993) 101.
77. H. Jørgensen, V.M. Gabert, M.S. Hedemann and S.K. Jensen, J. Nutr. (1999) (submitted).
78. W.C. Sauer and L. Ozimek, A Review. Livest. Prod. Sci. 15 (1986) 367.
79. H. Jørgensen, J.E. Lindberg and C. Anderson, J. Sci. Food Agric. 74 (1997) 244.
80. G. Isaksson, I. Lundquist and I. Ihse, Gastroenterology 82 (1982) 918.

81. B.O. Schneeman, Pancreatic and digestion function. In: Vahouny GV and Kritchevsky (eds), Dietary Fiber in Health and Disease, New York, Plenum., (1982) 73.
82. S. Li and W.C. Sauer, J. Anim. Sci. 72 (1994) 1737.
83. N.F. LaRusso, Amer. J. Physiol. 247 (1984) G199.
84. H. Tani, H. Ohishi and K. Watanabe, J. Nutr. Sci. Vitaminol. 41 (1995) 699.

Biology of the Pancreas in Growing Animals
S.G. Pierzynowski and R. Zabielski (Editors)
© 1999 Elsevier Science B.V. All rights reserved.

Carbohydrates and exocrine pancreatic secretions in pigs

S. Jakob[a], R. Mosenthin[a] and W.C. Sauer[b]

[a]Institute of Animal Nutrition (450), Hohenheim University, D-70599 Stuttgart, Germany

[b]University of Alberta, Department of Agricultural, Food and Nutritional Science,
Edmonton, Alberta, T6G 2P5, Canada

The response of the pancreas to nutritional and dietary factors and the divers mechanisms controlling the exocrine pancreas are of particular interest. In this review, the effect of dietary carbohydrates, including different fibre sources on quantitative and qualitative aspects of pancreatic secretion will be addressed. The importance of describing dietary fibre (DF) in as much chemical and physical detail as possible needs to be emphasised, since the lack of information makes comparison of most published studies on the effect of DF on pancreatic secretion extremely difficult. Starch is hydrolysed in the intestinal lumen by pancreatic α-amylase into maltose, triose and α-dextrins. Pancreatic adaptation of piglets to dietary starch starts immediately after weaning. Studies carried out with growing pigs and rats have shown that the production of pancreatic α-amylase is very sensitive to changes in the dietary starch a content increasing starch content (in a diet) evoking increased α-amylase activity. The effect of NSP on the exocrine pancreas remains unclear, as some authors have reported stimulatory effects while others authors have obtained equivocal results. For example, an increase in the volume of secretion of pancreatic juice and total nitrogen was reported when the crude fibre content of the diet originated from native sources (wheat bran) rather than pure cellulose. This supports the idea that the type of diet and source of DF are important, i.e. diets made up of natural rather than purified components stimulate the exocrine pancreas. Methodological sources of variation must be taken into consideration when comparing results obtained with different surgical techniques to collecting pancreatic juice. For example, the pouch technique showed a higher secretion of volume but a lower α-amylase activity when compared with the catheter method.

1. INTRODUCTION

An understanding of digestive processes and physiological mechanisms is essential for developing optimal feeding strategies for pigs. This may be a key factor in the prevention of nutritional diseases and moreover, it is crucial for the application of feeding strategies which will also conserve the environment. In this context, the role of the pancreas as a major source of enzyme production is of specific interest. The development of pancreatic fistulation techniques [1,2,3,4,5,6,7,8] allows for long term *in vivo* studies in several species including the pig. The response of the pancreas to nutritional and dietary factors and the different mechanisms controlling the secretions of the exocrine pancreas are of particular interest. In this review, the effect of dietary carbohydrates, including different fibre sources on quantitative and qualitative aspects of pancreatic secretion will be addressed.

2. DEFINITION AND CLASSIFICATION OF DIETARY FIBRE

It is still a matter of controversy how to define dietary fibre (DF) and several definitions have been suggested. The terms crude fibre (CF), neutral-detergent fibre (NDF), acid-detergent fibre (ADF) and non-starch polysaccharides (NSP) have been used interchangeably. Trowell *et al.* [9] defined the term DF as "the sum of the polysaccharides and lignin which are not digested by the endogenous secretions of the gastrointestinal tract". This definition covers both chemical and physiological aspects of DF, but from an analytical point of view it is too imprecise to be used as the basis for devising routine methods for fibre estimation. A common and widely accepted chemical definition of DF is "the sum of all non-starch polysaccharides and lignin". However, this basic and reductionist approach does not take into account many other dietary components, including starch resistant to amylase (resistant starch, RS), several non-digestible oligosaccharides (NDO) and some protein and lipid fractions [10] which, in the large intestine, behave similarly to some sources of NSP and might be included within the definition by those taking a holistic view. An overview over the classification of carbohydrates present in feedstuffs including feed additives is presented in Table 1.

Finally, another approach to defining DF is to divide it into a soluble and insoluble fraction. This differentiation is made on the basis of its physiochemical properties and nutritional effects. Soluble fibre may evoke viscous conditions in the stomach and the small intestine, thus affecting digestion and absorption, whereas the insoluble fibre fractions usually exert their effects in the large intestine (bulking effect). Consequently, many analytical procedures have been developed to differentiate between soluble and insoluble fibre fractions. However, as pointed out by Graham and Åman [12], this distinction is often designed to fit into an analytical procedure rather than to correspond to actual physiological conditions since the fibre complex is continuously modified during gastrointestinal transport.

The importance of describing DF in as much chemical and physical detail as possible needs to be emphasised since the lack of information makes comparison of most published studies on the effect of DF on pancreatic secretions extremely difficult.

3. THE RESPONSE OF THE EXOCRINE PANCREAS TO DIETARY STARCH

Starch is the principal dietary carbohydrate. Apart from RS, starch is hydrolysed in the intestinal lumen by pancreatic α-amylase into maltose, triose and α-dextrins [13]. The remaining dissacharides are hydrolysed into monomeric sugars by intestinal enzymes such as maltase, lactase and saccharase.

Pancreatic adaptation of piglets to dietary starch starts immediately after weaning. Young pigs weaned at 35 d of age showed a sharp increase in α-amylase activity 7 d after the diet

Table 1
Classification of carbohydrates

Category	Monomeric residues	Source
Non-starch polysaccharides (NSP)		
Cell Wall NSP		
Cellulose	Glucose	Most feedstuffs
Mixed linked β-glucans	Glucose	Barley, oats, rye
Arabinoxylans	Xylose, arabinose	Rye, wheat, barley
Arabinogalactans	Galactose, arabinose	Cereal by-products
Xyloglucans	Glucose, xylose	Cereal flour
Rhamnogalacturans	Uronic acid, rhamnose	Hulls of peas
Galactans	Galactose	Soya bean meal, sugar beet pulp
Non-cell wall NSP		
Fructans	Fructose	Rye
Mannans	Mannose	Coconut cake, palm cake
Pectins	Uronic acids, rhamnose	Sugar beet pulp
Galactomannans	Galactose, mannose	Guar gum
Non-digestible oligosaccharides (NDO)		
α-Galacto-oligosaccharides	Galactose, glucose, fructose	Soya bean meal, peas, rapeseed meal
Fructo-oligosaccharides	Fructose	Cereals, feed additives
Transgalacto-oligosaccharides	Galactose, glucose	Feed additives, whey and other milk products
Resistant starch (RS)		
Physically inaccessible starch	Glucose	Peas, faba beans
Native starch	Glucose	Potatoes
Retrograded starch	Glucose	Heat-treated starch products

Bach Knudsen [11]

was changed from milk to a diet with high starch content [3]. These results were confirmed by Flores *et al.* [14] who found an increased specific activity of α-amylase after substitution of fat with starch in 7 to 10-wk - old piglets. The process of adaptation to changes in the level of dietary starch takes 5 to 7 d in growing pigs [13].

There is convincing evidence that the pancreas adapts to the level of starch in the diet. Studies with growing pigs [15] and rats [16] showed that the production of pancreatic α-amylase is very sensitive to changes in the dietary starch content. Corring and Chayvialle [17] observed a 2.3, fold increase in specific α-amylase activity in growing pigs after a 3 - fold increase of starch in the diet. Studies by Ozimek *et al.* [15] showed a 50% decrease in total α-amylase production when 15% corn starch was replaced by 15% fat in a corn starch-based diet including 15% crude protein. Mosenthin and Sauer [18] included 7.5% pectin in a diet for growing pigs at the expense of corn starch. There was a decrease (P<0.05) in the total activity of α-amylase. As pointed out by Corring [13], the total secretion of α-amylase in both treatments exceeded by far the amounts theoretically required for intestinal hydrolysis of starch under optimal conditions. Therefore, the physiological importance of the observed decrease remains unclear.

Hansen [19] pointed out that maldigestion in humans is likely to occur only if the pancreatic enzyme secretion drops below 10% of the normal output. A possible explanation could be the carbohydrate, related feedback mechanism reported by Jain *et al.* [20] in humans. These authors infused carbohydrates (a solution of rice starch and glucose) at different rates (0; 12.5; 25; 50; 100 mg/min) into the ileum of human subjects. As the amount of unabsorbed carbohydrates in the ileum increased, the ratio of α-amylase to trypsin secretion increased (P<0.005) as well. It was suggested that the increase in α-amylase secretion following infusion of carbohydrates into the ileum is regulated via a feedback mechanism at the ileal rather than the duodenal level, because at the same time there was a decline in the rate of passage of dietary carbohydrate from the stomach to the duodenum.

It may be assumed that these changes in the volume of pancreatic secretion and activity of enzymes are dependent on the level of glucose in the blood. Glucose administered via the jugular vein of pigs evoked a significant decrease in the secretion of pancreatic juice, protein and, in addition, a decrease in the total activities of α-amylase, chymotrypsin and lipase [21]. However, Rudick and Janowitz [22] observed a higher α-amylase output after elevation of the blood glucose level in humans, whereas Karlsson *et al.* [23] could not show any effect on the exocrine pancreas of pigs after intravenous 2-deoxy-D-glucose infusion, although the plasma levels of glucagon and insulin were elevated (P<0.01). Pierzynowski and Barej [24] suggested that insulin enhances the stimulatory action of the vagus nerve on the pancreatic secretion of sheep and a very good correlation between changes in the plasma insulin concentration and the secretion of pancreatic enzymes was observed in cows [25]. The picture of the response of the exocrine and endocrine pancreas to infused glucose remains unclear.

Moreover, it seems that the duration of glucose infusions has an influence on the pancreatic response, as short term infusions decrease and long term infusion stimulate the enzymatic secretion [26]. A feedback mechanism most likely controls pancreatic secretion and the blood glucose level, but further investigation focusing on the regulation of the exocrine and endocrine pancreas are warranted.

4. THE RESPONSE OF THE EXOCRINE PANCREAS TO DIETARY NSP AND DIETARY FIBRE

The exocrine pancreas of pigs adapts its secretion not only to the type and level of starch in the diet, but also the type and level of NSP in the diet.

In studies reported by Mosenthin and Sauer [18] four barrows (initial BW 70 kg), fitted with permanent pancreatic cannulas according to the "pouch method" [7], were fed two corn starch-based diets, containing 16% crude protein from soya bean meal, with or with out 7.5% pectin included at the expense of corn starch. The pigs were fed twice daily, and pancreatic juice was collected continuously at 1- h intervals for a total of 24 h. The inclusion of pectin at the expense of corn starch had no effect (P>0.05) on the rate of secretion of pancreatic juice and specific activities of trypsin, chymotrypsin, α-amylase or lipase. In addition, total activities of trypsin, chymotrypsin and lipase were not affected by the variations in diet. However, there was a reduction (P<0.05) in the total activity of α-amylase when corn starch was replaced by pectin. To our knowledge, no reports have yet been published yet on the effect of pectin or other gel-forming polysaccharides on pancreatic secretions in pigs. On the other hand, several studies have been conducted with rats. It is difficult to draw conclusions from these studies because the results obtained more equivocal, which main part be attributed to the different techniques used to measure pancreatic secretions. According to Forman and Scheeman [16] and Calvert et al. [27] there is only a little evidence that pectin might affect the exocrine pancreas, either (by affecting the secretion) via hormonal pathways (cholecystokinin and secretin) or via a negative feedback mechanism, as described in detail by Owyang [28] and Miyasaka and Funakoshi [29]. However, it must be remembered that these studies were carried out on slaughtered animals, which may lead to distortion when there results are compared with the results of studies chronically fistulated animals.

Several studies have been carried out that focus on the effect of different sources of NSP on exocrine pancreatic secretions. As pointed out by Mosenthin and Sauer [30], differences in the source of fibre could, in part, explain differences both in ileal amino acid digestibilities between feedstuffs and among different samples of the same feedstuff, as described by Sauer and Ozimek [31]. These differences may be attributed to changes in the rate of secretion of protein and digestive enzymes in the pancreatic juice following consumption of feedstuffs rich in fibre.

Mosenthin and Sauer [30] determined the effect of source of fibre on the rate of secretion of protein, trypsin, chymotrypsin, α-amylase and lipase. Six barrows (initial BW 50 kg) were fitted with a permanent pancreatic re-entrant cannula according to Hee et al. [7]. The animals were fed three different corn starch-based diets: a basal diet containing 49.9% corn starch and two experimental diets in which 10% corn starch was replaced by 10% Alphafloc (cellulose), or 10% straw meal, respectively. The inclusion of Alphafloc had no effect (P>0.05) on the secretion of pancreatic juice, nitrogen and the specific as well as total activities of trypsin, chymotrypsin, α-amylase and lipase. In addition, the secretion of pancreatic juice and of nitrogen was not (P>0.05) affected by the inclusion of straw, but there was a decrease (P<0.05) in the specific activities of chymotrypsin and α-amylase. However, most likely because of the higher volume of secretion of pancreatic juice (although not significant, P<0.10) in pigs fed the straw-containing diet, there were no differences (P<0.05) between the total enzyme activities.

The results of Mosenthin and Sauer [30] and Mosenthin et al. [32] who reported no effect of level and source of fibre on the total activities of enzymes secreted in pancreatic juice, are in agreement with those of Żebrowska et al. [6] and Fevrier et al. [33]. The results of a study by Żebrowska and Low [34] revealed that substitution of 50% of the wheat in a wheat-based diet (88.7% wheat) by 50% wheat bran or by 50% wheat flour, respectively, did not affect the volume of secretion. However, a level of 20% NSP in the diet based onwheat and wheat bran induced a 78% higher secretion (P<0.01) of pancreatic juice compared to the diet based on wheat and wheat flour, containing 5% NSP. Despite the higher secretion of volume, total enzyme activities were not significantly affected by the differences in diet.

However, these results are in contrast to these obtained by Langlois et al. [35] in growing pigs fitted with a pancreatic duct cannula. The control group was fed a cereal-based diet without wheat bran whereas the experimental group received a diet containing 40% wheat bran included at the expense of wheat. Wheat bran induced an increase (P<0.05) in the volume (+115%) and protein content (+36%) of pancreatic juice during a 24-hour period. Moreover, in contrast to the findings of Żebrowska and Low [34], total enzyme activities were enhanced (P<0.05) when wheat bran was included in the diet. This study confirms observations made by Jakob et al. [36] in piglets. Three 8-wk-old, piglets with a BW of 12.4 kg at surgery were fitted with a chronic pancreatic duct catheter and a re-entrant duodenal fistula according to Pierzynowski et al. [8]. After a post-operative recovery period of 7 d the pigs were fed two diets according to the following experimental design: all pigs received a commercial weaner diet as a control diet for a period of 7 d, followed by a period in which the same diet supplemented with 2% potato fibre was fed. Thereafter, the control diet without potato fibre was fed for another 7 d. The chemical composition of potato fibre is presented in Table 2. The volume of pancreatic juice, the protein secretion and the total and specific trypsin, lipase and α-amylase activities increased (P<0.05) after adaptation to the diet supplemented with potato fibre. After re-adaptation to the control diet without potato fibre supplementation, no decrease to the initial levels was observed in the parameters measured.

In previous growth trials by Pierzynowski [26], potato fibre supplementation to a diet for growing pigs was observed to have positive effects on production traits. This improvement in performance may be related to the increased secretion of pancreatic enzymes (due to potato fibre supplementation) which, in turn, may have a positive effect on nutrient digestibility, resulting in a better nutrient supply to the pig. A possible explanation is given by Botermans and Pierzynowski [37] who showed that better performance of piglets compared to litter mates is related to a higher protein content and trypsin activity in the pancreatic juice.

The stimulatory effects of DF on the secretion of pancreatic enzymes observed by Langlois et al. [35] and Jakob et al. [36] are in contrast to the results obtained by Żebrowska and Low [34], Mosenthin and Sauer [18] and Mosenthin et al. [32]. Langlois et al. [35] reported a

Table 2
Chemical composition of Potato Fibre (%)

Crude fibre	Cellulose	Lignin	Pectin + hemicellulose	Starch	Protein	Fat
70%	23%	2%	45%	10%	7%	0.3%

stimulatory effect of DF after replacement of starch by DF, whereas Mosenthin *et al.* [32] obtained a decrease in α-amylase activity after the replacement of starch by DF. One explanation for this can be derived from the studies by of Żebrowska and Low [34] who suggested that the volume of secretion of pancreatic juice as well as the protein secretion (apparently) are more closely related to the content of NSP in the diet than to the crude fibre content. This emphasises the importance of a precise definition of DF when comparing the results of different studies .

This necessity for a clear definition of DF can also be seen in the studies by of Partridge *et al.* [5] and Żebrowska and Low [34]. These authors showed that semi-synthetic diets based on either starch and casein or wheat flour and casein induced a distinctly lower (P<0.05) pancreatic juice secretion compared to cereal-based diets. Enzyme activities were not affected by the source of fibre. Especially the results reported by Żebrowska and Low [34] support the idea that the type of diet and source of DF are important, i.e. diets made up of natural rather than purified components stimulate secretions from by of the exocrine pancreas. There was an increase (P<0.01) in the volume of secretion of pancreatic juice and total nitrogen when the crude fibre content of the diet originated from natural sources (wheat bran) rather than pure cellulose. The volume of secretion and protein output reported in the literature in response to different diets in growing pigs are summarised in Table 3.

Part of the variation between studies regarding the effect of DF on exocrine pancreatic secretions may be attributed to different techniques regarding used to collect pancreatic juice. Whereas Żebrowska *et al.* [6], Żebrowska and Low [34], Mosenthin and Sauer [30] and Mosenthin and Sauer [18] used the "pouch method" [38] to collect pancreatic juice, the animals in the studies of Langlois *et al.* [35] and Jakob *et al.* [36] were fitted with a pancreatic duct cannula as described by Corring *et al.* [4], Pierzynowski *et al.* [8] and Zabielski *et al.* [39]. After replacement of 50% wheat by wheat bran in a cereal- based diet Langlois *et al.* [35] an increase in total protein secretion despite a decrease in protein concentration. Gabert *et al.* [40] reported considerable differences in the volume of secretion and enzyme activities in a comparative study obtained with different surgical methods for collecting pancreatic juice. Jensen *et al.* [41] found, considerable differences in the volume of pancreatic juice secreted and in the chemical and enzyme composition of the pancreatic juice when the "pouch method" and the "catheter method" more compared. For example, the concentration of protein in pancreatic juice from pigs prepared with the "pouch method" was higher (P<0.001) than in pigs fitted with a pancreatic duct catheter. In addition, specific and total α-amylase activities were increased (P<0.01) in pigs fitted with a fistula according to the "catheter" method. Moreover, the volume of secretion was enhanced (P<0.05) in pigs prepared with the pancreatic duct catheter. In conclusion, the method for collection of pancreatic juice must be taken into consideration when comparing results (Table 3).

In addition, when comparing results from different studies, the effect of breed on pancreatic secretion must be considered. Fevrier *et al.* [33] did not observe any differences in enzyme activities in pancreatic juice when different breeds (Large white and Mei Shan) were given different level of wheat bran (0%, 20%, 51.8%) in the diet on enzyme activities in pancreatic juice. On the other hand, Freire *et al.* [42] reported differences when different levels of wheat bran (0% or 15%) were fed to different breeds of pigs. Total activities of pancreatic lipase, trypsin and α-amylase were 2.0, 1.5 and 5.0 – fold higher in Alentejano compared to Large White piglets. Both groups were weaned at the age of 21 d, respectively. It should be

Table 3
Influence of type of diet on daily volume of secretion of pancreatic juice and protein output
secretion in pigs

Reference	Feed intake (kg/d)	Volume (l)	Protein (g)	Body weight (kg)	Surgical procedure
Żebrowska et al.	1.5 barley / soya bean meal	2.2	12.1	40	pouch
[6]	1.5 starch /casein	1.2	10.9	40	pouch
	1.5 starch / soya bean meal	3.8	14.4	35 – 50	pouch
Żebrowska and Low [34]	1.4 wheat	4.1	17.9	34*	pouch
	1.4.wheat / wheat bran	4.6	19.0	34*	pouch
	1.4 wheat / wheat flour	2.6	15.8	34*	pouch
	1.4 wheat flour / cellulose	1.8	13.0	34*	pouch
Langlois et al. [35]	1.6 no wheat bran	1.7	14.6	38	catheter
	1.6 40% wheat bran	3.6	19.7	38	catheter
Mosenthin and Sauer [30]	1.8 starch	3.7	26.9	60	pouch
	1.8 cellulose	3.2	22.8	59	pouch
	1.8 straw meal	4.6	28.5	69	pouch
Mosenthin and Sauer [18]	1.8 0% pectin	3.8	25.5	70	pouch
	1.8 7.5% pectin	4.7	27.0	70	pouch
Jakob et al. [36]	0.5 0% potato fibre	1.2	11.7	12.4*	catheter
	0.5 2% potato fibre	1.9	20.2	12.4*	catheter

* Body weight at surgery

mentioned that in the studies of Freire et al. [42] and Jakob et al. [36] piglets (12 kg) were used, whereas in the other studies animals weighing between 35 and 70 kg were used. As reviewed by Makkink and Verstegen [43], it is evident that pancreatic secretion (volume, protein and enzyme activities) increases with age and, moreover, dietary changes may interact with development of the exocrine pancreas. Thus, the effect of age on pancreatic secretion must also be considered when comparing the results of different studies.

5. CONCLUSIONS

The results of studies that relate to the effect of different sources and levels of dietary carbohydrate on exocrine pancreatic secretions in pigs show considerable variation. According to Partridge et al. [5] this variation is of biological origin rather than an artefact. The nutritional implications of these studies, however, may be minor as long as the quantity of pancreatic enzymes secreted is sufficient for digestion. Corring [13] claims that under physiological conditions the quantity of pancreatic enzymes secreted is sufficient for digestion of approximately ten times the amount of food usually consumed. Moreover, as pointed out by Imbeah et al. [44], comparison of results from different studies relating to pancreatic secretion in pigs is difficult, because these comparisons are confounded by differences in feed intake, feeding regimen, diet composition, body weight and the method used to collect pancreatic juice.

The effect of dietary fibre and its mode of action in piglets still remains open unclear. Further studies are warranted to clarify possible physiological implications in the nutrition of piglets. However, comparison of results between different research groups require standardisation of the methods used to collect pancreatic juice and to determine pancreatic enzyme activities. Furthermore, a clear description and definition of DF is necessary in order to obtain conclusive results.

REFERENCES

1. W.M. Wass, Amer. J. Vet. Res., 26 (1965) 1106.
2. J.C. Pekas, Thompson A.M. and V.W. Hays, J. Anim. Sci., 25 (1966) 113.
3. A. Aumaitre, World Rev. Anim. Prod., 8 (1972) 54.
4. T. Corring, A. Aumaitre and A. Rerat, Ann. Biol. Anim. Biochim. Biophys., 12 (1972) 109.
5. I.G. Partridge, A.G. Low, I.E. Sambrook and T. Corring, Brit. J. Nutr., 48 (1982) 137.
6. T. Żebrowska, A.G. Low and H. Żebrowska, Brit. J. Nutr., 49 (1983) 401.
7. J.H. Hee, W.C. Sauer, R. Berzins and L. Ozimek, Can. J. Anim. Sci., 65 (1985) 451.
8. S.G. Pierzynowski, B.R. Weström, B.W. Karlsson, J. Svendsen and B. Nilsson, Can. J. Anim. Sci., 68 (1988) 953.
9. H. Trowell, D.A. Southgate, T.M. Wolever, A.R. Leeds, M.A.Gassull and D.J. Jenkins, Lancet, 1 (1976) 967.
10. H.N. Englyst, H. Trowell, D.A. Southgate and J.H. Cummings, Amer. J. Clin. Nutr., 46 (1987) 873.
11. K.E. Bach Knudsen, R.Hartemink, (ed) in International Symposium "Non-digestible oilgosaccharides: Healthy food for the Colon?", Wageningen, The Netherlands (1997).
12. H. Graham and P. Åman, Anim. Feed Sci. Technol., 32 (1991) 143.
13. T. Corring, Reprod. Nutr. Dev., 20 (1980) 1217.

14. C.A. Flores, P.M. Brannon, S.A. Bustamante, J. Bezerra, K.T. Butler, T. Goda and O. Koldovsky, J. Pediatr. Gastroenterol. Nutr., 7 (1988) 914.
15. L. Ozimek, W.C. Sauer and G. Ozimek, 3rd International Seminar on Digestive Physiology in the Pig, Copenhagen, Denmark (1985).
16. L.P. Forman and B.O. Scheeman, J. Nutr., 110 (1980) 1992.
17. T. Corring and J.A. Chayvialle, Reprod. Nutr. Dev., 27 (1987) 967.
18. R. Mosenthin and W.C. Sauer, Z. Ernährungswiss., 32 (1993) 152.
19. W.E. Hansen, Int. J. Pancreatol., 1 (1986) 341.
20. N.K. Jain, M. Boivin, A.R. Zinsmeister and E.P. DiMagno, Pancreas, 6 (1991) 495.
21. C. Simoes Nunes and T. Corring, Reprod. Nutr. Dev., 21 (1981) 705.
22. J. Rudick and H.D. Janowitz, Gastroenterology, 58 (1970) 130.
23. S. Karlsson, S.G. Pierzynowski, B.R.Weström, M.J. Thaela, B.Ahren and B.W. Karlsson, Pancreas, 11 (1995) 271.
24. S.G. Pierzynowski and W. Barej, Q. J. Exp. Physiol., 69 (1984) 35.
25. S.G. Pierzynowski, W. Barej, R. Mikołajczyk and R. Zabielski, J. Anim. Physiol. Anim. Nutr., 60 (1988) 234.
26. S.G. Pierzynowski, Personal comminication, (1999) Dept. Anim. Physiol., Lund Univ., Sweden.
27. R. Calvert, B.O. Schneemann, S. Satchithanandam, M.M. Cassidy and G.V. Vahouny, Amer. J. Clin. Nutr., 41 (1985) 1249.
28. C. Owyang, J. Nutr., 124 (1994) 1321S.
29. K. Miyasaka and A. Funakoshi, Pancreas, 16 (1998) 277.
30. R. Mosenthin and W.C. Sauer, J. Anim. Physiol. Anim. Nutr., 65 (1991) 45.
31. W.C. Sauer and L. Ozimek, Livest. Prod. Sci., 15 (1986) 367.
32. R. Mosenthin, W.C. Sauer and F. Ahrens, J Nutr, 124 (1994) 1222.
33. C. Fevrier, D. Bourdon and A. Aumaitre , J. Anim. Physiol. Anim. Nutr., 68 (1992) 60.
34. T. Żebrowska and A.G. Low, J. Nutr., 117 (1987) 1212.
35. A. Langlois, T. Corring and C. Fevrier, Reprod. Nutr. Dev., 27 (1987) 929.
36. S. Jakob, S.G. Pierzynowski, B. Weström, R. Mosenthin, M.J. Thaela, S. Karlsson and B.W. Karlsson, J. Anim. Physiol. Anim. Nutr., submitted (1999)
37. J.A.M. Botermans and S.G. Pierzynowski, J. Anim. Sci., in press (1999)
38. J. Hee, W.C. Sauer and R. Mosenthin, J. Anim. Physiol. Anim. Nutr., 60 (1988) 241.
39. R. Zabielski, V. Leśniewska and P. Guilloteau, Reprod. Nutr. Dev., 37 (1997) 385.
40. V.M. Gabert, M.S. Jensen, H. Jørgensen, R.M. Engberg and S.K. Jensen, J. Nutr., 126 (1996) 2076.
41. M.S. Jensen, V.M. Gabert, H. Jørgensen and R.M. Engberg, Int. J. Pancreatol., 21 (1997) 173.
42. J.P.B. Freire, J. Peiniau, L.F. Cunha, J.A.A. Almeida and A. Aumaitre, Ann. Zootech., 45 (1996) 357.
43. C.A. Makkink and M.W.A. Verstegen, J. Anim. Physiol. Anim. Nutr., 64 (1990) 190.
44. M. Imbeah, W.C. Sauer and R. Mosenthin, J. Anim. Sci., 66 (1988) 1409.

Biology of the Pancreas in Growing Animals
S.G. Pierzynowski and R. Zabielski (Editors)
© 1999 Elsevier Science B.V. All rights reserved.

Anti-nutritional factors and exocrine pancreatic secretion in pigs

W.C. Sauer[a] and R. Mosenthin[b]

[a] University of Alberta, Department of Agricultural, Food and Nutritional Science,
Edmonton, Alberta, Canada T6G 2P5

[b] Hohenheim University, Institute of Animal Nutrition (450),
D-70593 Stuttgart, Germany

The effect of protease inhibitors, tannins and lectins on exocrine pancreatic secretion in the pig is reviewed. Two surgical approaches to the collection of total pancreatic juice are discussed, and the importance of basing interpretations of experimental results on total rather than specific enzyme activities is stressed.

1. INTRODUCTION

Of the anti-nutritional factors, protease inhibitors, tannins and lectins have received most attention in research. These are present in variable amounts in most legumes [1]. Comprehensive reviews on anti-nutritional factors have been provided by Birk [2] on protease inhibitors, by Marquardt [3] and Jansman [4] on tannins, and by Pusztai [5] on lectins. These anti-nutritional factors have in common that they exert detrimental effects on the digestive and/or absorptive processes.

The objective of this review is to assess the effect of protease inhibitors, tannins and lectins on pancreatic exocrine secretion in the pig. Where necessary, reference has been made to studies with chicks and rats. Furthermore, for reasons discussed in this review, results from studies with pigs surgically modified to allow total collection of pancreatic juice have been given particular attention. Two basic approaches have been used to collect exocrine pancreatic secretions in pigs: (1) direct cannulation of the pancreatic duct [6] and (2) collection of pancreatic juice from a duodenal pouch [7]. Sometimes the techniques have been used with modifications [8, 9]. The advantages and disadvantages of these techniques have been discussed by Makkink and Verstegen [10] and by Gabert [11].

2. EFFECT OF PROTEASE INHIBITORS ON EXOCRINE PANCREATIC SECRETION

Although protease inhibitors are found in most legumes, those present in soya bean have received most attention, especially in studies with rats and chicks. Feeding raw soya bean or soya bean trypsin inhibitors will elicit adverse nutritional, biological and physiological responses in rats [12] and chicks [13]. As shown in studies with rats and chicks, soya bean trypsin inhibitors inactivate trypsin, inducing the intestinal mucosa to release cholecystokinin, a hormone which stimulates the acinar cells of the pancreas to produce more trypsin as well as other digestive enzymes such as chymotrypsin, elastase and α-amylase. Rats and chicks fed raw soya bean or soya bean trypsin inhibitors respond by hypersecretion of pancreatic enzymes and hypertrophy of the pancreas. Trypsin, which contains 8.1% cystine, accounts for half of the cysteine secreted in the pancreatic juice of rats fed raw soya bean [14]. Hypersecretion of pancreatic enzymes results in a higher demand for cysteine by the pancreas, which may create a deficiency of the sulphur–containing amino acids [15]. A negative feedback mechanism in chicks and rats was proposed by Green and Lyman [16].

A comprehensive scheme explaining the experimental evidence relating to the effect of soya bean protease inhibitors on the nutritive value of protein, including the metabolic pathways of methionine, valine, and threonine (in relation to the formation of cysteine and its incorporation into trypsin) has been provided by Liener and Kakade [12]. Schingoethe et al. [17] suggested that there is a direct relationship between the size of the pancreas (in relation to body weight) and the sensitivity of response to soya bean trypsin inhibitors or raw soya bean. It was suggested that species with a pancreas weight exceeding 0.3 % of body weight (which includes rats and chicks) are more prone to pancreatic hypertrophy than species in which the ratio of the pancreas to body weight is less than 0.3 % (Table 1).

Table 1
Relationship between size of the pancreas of various species of animals and the response of the pancreas to raw soya bean or trypsin inhibitors

Species	Size of pancreas (% of body weight)	Pancreatic hypertrophy
Mouse	0.6 – 0.8	+
Rat	0.5 – 0.6	+
Chick	0.4 – 0.6	+
Guinea pig	0.29	± [a]
Dog	0.21 – 0.24	-
Pig	0.10 – 0.12	-
Human being	0.09 – 0.12	(-) [b]
Calf	0.06 – 0.08	-

[a] Observed in young guinea pigs but not in adults
[b] Predicted response
Liener and Kakade [12].

Only a few studies, in which total pancreatic juice was collected, have been carried out to determine whether the feedback mechanism is also present in pigs. Li *et al.* [18] recently measured the pancreatic secretory response to diets with low and high levels of soya bean trypsin inhibitors in growing pigs. Six pigs, prepared for total collection of pancreatic juice with the pouch method [7], were fed two corn starch-based diets formulated to contain 20 % crude protein from either Nutrisoy (food grade defatted soy flour) or autoclaved Nutrisoy. The trypsin inhibitor activities in Nutrisoy and autoclaved Nutrisoy were 38.1 and 9.3 respectively. The trypsin inhibitor activities in Nutrisoy and autoclaved Nutrisoy in the diets were 13.4 and 3.0 g per kg, respectively. The results of these studies are presented in Table 2.

Table 2
Effect of diet on the secretion volume, nitrogen and protein content, and enzyme activities of pancreatic juice in growing pigs

Diets		Nutrisoy	Autoclaved Nutrisoy	SE [a]
Volume	ml (24 h) $^{-1}$	3803.6^D	2633.1^E	104.38
Nitrogen	g litre $^{-1}$	1.3^e	2.0^d	0.08
	g (24 h) $^{-1}$	5.0	5.2	0.16
Protein	g litre $^{-1}$	6.2^e	10.3^d	0.58
	g (24 h) $^{-1}$	22.8^e	25.7^d	1.26
Enzyme activities:				
Amylase	Specific [b]	107.4^E	159.5^D	0.61
	Total [c]	414.3	420.8	18.68
Lipase	Specific [b]	32.7	36.3	2.07
	Total [c]	108.1	95.6	9.22
Chymotrypsin	Specific [b]	42.1^E	60.3^D	1.38
	Total [c]	139.0	154.0	6.96
Trypsin	Specific [b]	46.0^e	73.5^d	6.62
	Total [c]	168.5	178.9	10.60

[a] Standard error of the mean (n=10)
[b] U litre $^{-1}$ x 10 $^{-3}$
[c] U (24 h) $^{-1}$ x 10 $^{-3}$
[d, e] Means in the same row with different superscript letters differ (P<0.05)
[D, E] Means in the same row with different superscript letters differ (P<0.01).

The incorporation of Nutrisoy compared with autoclaved Nutrisoy in the corn starch-based diet increased (P<0.05) the total volume of pancreatic juice secretion. There was a decrease (P<0.05) in the concentration of nitrogen (Kjeldahl method) but not total secretion. There was a slight but significant (P<0.05) increase in the total secretion of protein (Lowry method). The inclusion of Nutrisoy decreased the specific activities of α-amylase (P<0.01), chymotrypsin (P<0.01) and trypsin (P<0.05) but not of lipase. However, there was no effect (P>0.05) on the total activities of the enzymes assayed. The results obtained by Li et al. [18] are in general agreement with those reported by Żebrowska et al. [19] in studies in which pigs were fed raw or normal soya bean meal. In these studies, the pigs were prepared for total collection of pancreatic juice according to the procedure described by Żebrowska et al. [8]. They reported an increase (P<0.01) in the volume of secretion of pancreatic juice when raw compared to normal soya bean meal was fed but found no differences (P>0.01) in the total activities of trypsin, chymotrypsin, carboxypeptidases A and B and amylase. The results obtained by Li et al. [18] and Żebrowska et al. [19] are not in agreement with those reported by Schumann et al. [20], in studies with pigs prepared with the pancreatic duct cannulation technique and fed untoasted (solvent-extracted) or toasted soya bean meal. In addition to an increase (P<0.01) in the volume of secretion of pancreatic juice there was a doubling (P<0.01) of protein secretion. The authors also claimed that soya bean trypsin inhibitors increased the secretion of pancreatic enzymes, including chymotrypsin and trypsin. However, it should be noted that this conclusion was based on the interpretation of specific rather than total enzyme activities.

The previous studies show that it is important to obtain a total collection of pancreatic juice, so that total enzyme activities can be determined. The slaughter technique in which enzyme activities are measured in digesta collected from the small intestine (or when digesta are collected via a cannula) provides specific activities. Results expressed in total rather than specific activities are a true reflection of the effect of soya bean trypsin inhibitors (or other dietary treatment) on exocrine pancreatic secretion. Differences in specific activities may simply reflect the dilution of the pancreatic juice, as previously discussed by Hee et al. [21, 22].

Makkink and Verstegen [10] suggested that studies on the effect of diet composition (or for that matter of soya bean trypsin inhibitors) on pancreatic enzyme secretion should be combined with digestibility studies in order to obtain a more complete understanding of the digestive processes. Further studies by Li et al. [23] suggest that the detrimental effect of feeding soya bean trypsin inhibitors (exemplified by feeding Nutrisoy and autoclaved Nutrisoy diets) in pigs is simply due to the formation of complexes between the soya bean trypsin inhibitors and trypsin (and chymotrypsin), which will result in an overall decrease in the efficiency of protein digestion in the small intestine (Table 3).

As shown by Blow et al. [24] and Sweet et al. [25], the enzyme-inhibitor complex is very strong, due to the close complementary fit of these two interacting molecules. The binding force is further reinforced by a large number of non-covalent hydrophobic and hydrogen bonds. Based on the very low ileal amino acid digestibilities in the Nutrisoy diet (Table 3), only small amounts of free trypsin (and chymotrypsin) may have been available for digestion.

The faecal digestibilities of the amino acids are not presented but were higher (P<0.05) than the respective ileal digestibilities for both diets. However, the differences in digestibilities of amino acids between the diets were much less pronounced than those observed between the ileal digestibilities, due to the modifying action of the microflora in the large intestine, as discussed by Sauer and Ozimek [26].

Table 3
Effect of diet on ileal digestibilities (%) of nutrients and energy in growing pigs

Items	Ileal digestibilities Nutrisoy	Autoclaved Nutrisoy	SE [a]
Dry matter	64.3 [c]	73.9 [b]	1.11
Organic matter	67.0 [c]	76.2 [b]	0.95
Crude protein	37.4 [c]	77.1 [b]	2.69
Energy	66.0 [c]	77.9 [b]	1.12
Amino acids			
Indispensable			
Arginine	45.4 [c]	90.0 [b]	2.34
Histidine	43.9 [c]	82.5 [b]	2.88
Isoleucine	40.4 [c]	86.3 [b]	2.81
Leucine	37.1 [c]	86.3 [b]	2.43
Lysine	40.8 [c]	79.6 [b]	3.09
Methionine [d]	58.9 [c]	85.9 [b]	3.87
Phenylalanine	39.1 [c]	87.8 [b]	1.98
Threonine	36.5 [c]	73.3 [b]	3.96
Valine	38.2 [c]	83.6 [b]	2.46
Dispensable			
Alanine	43.4 [c]	81.1 [b]	2.78
Aspartic acid	42.4 [c]	72.6 [b]	1.92
Cysteine	35.5 [c]	67.7 [b]	4.43
Glutamic acid	48.6 [c]	83.7 [b]	1.60
Glycine	29.4 [c]	70.2 [b]	4.18
Serine	36.8 [c]	80.6 [b]	2.16
Tyrosine	34.1 [c]	84.9 [b]	3.06

[a] Standard error of the mean (n = 6)
[b, c] Means with different superscript letters differ (P<0.01)
[d] Digestibility after correction for dietary supplementation of methionine.

One study, in which total collections were obtained, was performed to determine the effect of trypsin inhibitors in peas on exocrine pancreatic secretion [27]. Five barrows, with an average initial body weight of 18.1 kg, prepared with the pouch technique, were fed one of two diets according to a cross-over design. The diets were formulated to contain 15 % crude protein from peas (cv. Ascona or cv. Radley). The trypsin inhibitor activities were 1.12 and 4.60 in cv. Ascona and cv. Radley, respectively. In the diets containing cv. Ascona and cv. Radley, the corresponding values were 0.76 and 3.24, respectively. The trypsin inhibitor activity values for the peas are within the range of values reported by Leterme *et al.* [28] for spring cultivars. As expected, the values for cv. Radley were higher than for cv. Ascona. As shown in Table 4, the trypsin inhibitor activity in the diet had no effect on either the specific or the total activities of the enzymes assayed, including α-amylase and lipase for which the results were not presented.

Table 4
Effect of diet on volume of pancreatic juice and flows of nitrogen, protein and enzymes, in pigs

Diets		AP [a]	RP [a]	SE [b]
Volume	ml 24 h $^{-1}$	2029	2221	250
Nitrogen	g litre $^{-1}$	0.60	0.59	0.01
	g 24 h $^{-1}$	1.20	1.29	0.13
Protein	g litre $^{-1}$	2.12	1.84	0.11
	g 24 h $^{-1}$	4.30	4.09	0.34
Enzyme activities:				
Chymotrypsin	Specific [c]	14.2	13.1	0.6
	Total 24 h [d]	28.8	29.1	2.6
Trypsin	Specific [c]	24.6	22.8	1.5
	Total 24 h [d]	49.9	50.6	5.5

[a] AP, cv. Ascona peas as protein source; RP, cv. Radley peas as protein source
[b] Standard error of the mean (n=15 except for 24 h means where n = 5)
[c] Units litre $^{-1}$ x 10 $^{-3}$
[d] Units 24 h $^{-1}$ x 10 $^{-3}$
Gabert *et al.* [27]

3. EFFECT OF TANNINS ON EXOCRINE PANCREATIC SECRETION

Marquardt *et al.* [29] identified condensed tannins as the predominant anti-nutritional factor in faba beans, especially in dark- (also referred to as coloured) flowering varieties.

Tannins bind to proteins by the interaction of their reactive hydroxyl groups with the carbonyl groups of the proteins. Hydrogen bonds and hydrophobic interactions appear to be the principal linkages involved [30].

Since digestive enzymes are proteins, they can also form complexes with tannins which has been shown for trypsin, chymotrypsin and α-amylase in many *in vitro* experiments [31]. *In vivo* studies with pigs have also shown that tannins bind to enzymes and inhibit their activities in the small intestine [32, 33]. Studies by Grala *et al.* [34] with pigs showed that condensed tannins in faba beans can decrease apparent ileal amino acid digestibilities and nitrogen retention.

It was suggested that dietary tannins increase the pancreatic secretion of enzymes in a manner similar to that of protease inhibitors from legume seeds [35]. This suggestion was based on the observation that in some cases tannins increase the activity of lipase in digesta. Furthermore, this observation was based on the assumption that total pancreatic enzyme secretion is increased by tannins and that the relative affinity of tannins for trypsin and α-amylase is higher than for lipase [4].

Table 5
Effect of diet on volume of pancreatic juice and flows of nitrogen, protein and enzymes in pigs

Diets		SBM [a]	SF [a]	SE [b]
Volume	ml 24 h $^{-1}$	854	714	89
Nitrogen	g litre $^{-1}$	1.64	1.77	0.06
	g 24 h $^{-1}$	1.40	1.26	0.15
Protein	g litre $^{-1}$	5.51	5.68	0.23
	g 24 h $^{-1}$	4.71	4.06	0.35
Enzyme activities				
Chymotrypsin	Specific [c]	36.8	37.3	1.9
	Total 24 h	31.4	26.6	3.2
Trypsin	Specific [b]	41.2 [e]	53.7 [d]	3.6
	Total 24 h	35.2	38.3	4.2

[a] SBM, soya bean meal; SF, 50 % crude protein from soya bean meal and 50 % from faba beans
[b] Standard error of the mean (n=12 except for 24 h means where n = 4)
[c] Units litre $^{-1}$ x 10 $^{-3}$
[d, e] Means in the same row followed by different superscripts letters differ (P<0.05)

Gabert *et al.* [27] investigated the effect of a diet containing faba beans on exocrine pancreatic secretion in young pigs, using the pouch technique. Eight barrows, with an average initial body weight of 8.5 kg, were fed one of two corn starch-based diets formulated to contain 20 % crude protein, according to a completely randomised design. In one diet, soya bean meal was the sole protein source; in the other diet, soya bean meal and faba beans (cv Fibro; dark-flowering) each supplied 50 % of the dietary crude protein. The soya bean meal and faba beans contained 0.08 and 0.50 % tannins, respectively (expressed as % catechin equivalents). The respective diets contained 0.04 and 0.21 % tannins. The effect of the diets on the volume of pancreatic juice secreted and concentrations and flows of nitrogen, protein and enzymes are presented in Table 5.

There was no effect (P>0.05) of diet on the volume of secretion of pancreatic juice, nitrogen and protein concentrations and the specific and total activities of α-amylase, lipase and chymotrypsin. The activities of α-amylase and lipase are not presented in Table 5. The specific trypsin activity was higher (P<0.05) in pancreatic juice from pigs fed the soya bean meal – faba bean diet than from pigs fed the soya bean meal diet. However, there were no differences (P>0.05) in total activities of trypsin between the two diets. As previously discussed, differences in specific activities are of little nutritional significance, as total enzyme activities reflect the quantity of enzymes that can participate in digestion.

These results are in general agreement with those reported by Jansman *et al.* [32]. When growing pigs, prepared with the pouch technique, were fed diets containing faba bean hulls with either a low or high content of condensed tannins there was no effect (P>0.05) on the volume of secretion of pancreatic juice and total activities of trypsin and chymotrypsin.

4. EFFECT OF LECTINS ON EXOCRINE PANCREATIC SECRETION

Most dietary lectins are resistant to hydrolysis in the digestive tract. They bind to membrane receptors of epithelial cells of the small intestine and interfere with the digestion and absorption of nutrients [5]. There is very little information on the effect of lectins on exocrine pancreatic secretion. Lectins from soya beans and beans (*Phaseolus vulgaris*) induce an increase in the size of the pancreas in rats (36, 37). As discussed by Grant *et al.* [38], this enlargement (hyperplasia and hypertrophy) is different to the changes induced by trypsin inhibitors.

5. CONCLUSIONS

There is a scarcity of information on the effect of anti-nutritional factors on exocrine pancreatic secretion. The major problem in research relating to the effect of different diets or anti-nutritional factors on exocrine pancreatic secretion is that interpretations are often based on results pertaining to specific rather than total enzyme activities. It is important to obtain a total collection of pancreatic juice so that total enzyme activities can be determined. The latter can only be achieved with the use of surgically–modified animals, unfortunately. Based on the limited information available it seems that protease inhibitors and condensed tannins have no effect on total enzyme activities.

REFERENCES

1. I.E. Liener, Recent Advances of Research in Antinutritional Factors in Legume Seeds, J. Huisman, T.F.B. van der Poel and I.E. Liener (eds.), Pudoc, Wageningen, The Netherlands, (1989) 6.
2. Y. Birk, Recent Advances of Research in Antinutritional Factors in Legume Seeds, J. Huisman, T.F.B. van der Poel and I.E. Liener (eds.), Pudoc, Wageningen, The Netherlands (1989) 83.
3. R.R. Marquardt, Recent Advances of Research in Antinutritional Factors in Legume Seeds, J. Huisman, T.F.B. van der Poel and I.E. Liener (eds.), Pudoc, Wageningen, The Netherlands (1989) 141.
4. A.J.M. Jansman, Nutr. Res. Rev., 6 (1993) 209.
5. A. Pusztai, Recent Advances of Research in Antinutritional Factors in Legume Seeds. J. Huisman, T.F.B. van der Poel and I.E. Liener (eds.), Pudoc, Wageningen, The Netherlands, (1989) 17.
6. T. Corring, A. Aumaitre and A. Rerat, Ann. Biol. Anim. Biochim. Biophys., 12 (1972) 109.
7. J. Hee, W.C. Sauer, R. Berzins and L. Ozimek, Can. J. Anim. Sci., 65 (1985) 451.
8. T. Żebrowska, A.G. Low and H. Żebrowska, Brit. J. Nutr., 29 (1983) 401.
9. S.G. Pierzynowski, B.R. Weström, B.W. Karlsson, J. Svendsen and B. Nilsson, Can. J. Anim. Sci., 68 (1988) 953.
10. C.A. Makkink and M.W.A. Verstegen, J. Anim. Physiol. Anim. Nutr., 64 (1990) 190.
11. V.M. Gabert, Ph.D. Thesis. University of Alberta, Edmonton, Canada, (1997).
12. I.E. Liener and M.L. Kakade, In Toxic Constituents of Plant Foodstuffs, Liener; I.E. (ed.), 2nd Edition, Academic Press, Inc., New York, USA, (1980) 7.
13. J.T. Yen, A.H. Jensen, T. Hymowitz and D.H. Baker; Poultry Sci., 52 (1973) 1875.
14. R.H. Barnes, G. Fiala and E.J. Kwong, J. Nutr., 85 (1965 a) 127.
15. R.H. Barnes, E.J. Kwong and G. Fiala, J. Nutr., 85 (1965 b) 123.
16. G.M. Green and R.L. Lyman; Proc. Society Exp. Biol. Med., 140 (1972) 6.
17. D.J. Schingoethe, A.D.L. Gorrill, J.W. Thomas and M.G. Yang, Can. J. Physiol. Pharmacology 48 (1970) 43.
18. S. Li, W.C. Sauer, S. Huang and R. T. Hardin, J. Sci. Food Agric., 76 (1998) 347.
19. T. Żebrowska, T.D. Tanksley Jr. and D.A. Knabe, In: Digestive Physiology in the Pig. A. Just, H. Jørgensen and J.A. Fernandez (eds.), National Institute of Animal Science. Copenhagen, Denmark, (1985) 149.
20. B. Schumann, W.B. Souffrant, R. Matkowitz and G. Gebhardt, Wiss. Z. Karl-Marx-Universität Leipzig; Math.-Naturwiss. R., 32 (1983) 570.
21. J. Hee, W.C. Sauer and R. Mosenthin, J. Anim. Physiol. Anim. Nutr., 60 (1988 a) 241.
22. J. Hee, W.C. Sauer and R. Mosenthin, J. Anim. Physiol. Anim. Nutr., 60 (1988 b) 249.
23. W.C. Sauer and W.R. Caine, J. Sci. Food Agric., 76 (1998 b) 357.
24. D.M. Blow, J. Janin and R.M. Sweet, Nature (London) 249 (1974) 54.
25. R.M. Sweet, H.T. Wright, J. Janin, C.H. Chochia and D.M. Blow; Biochemistry, 13 (1974) 4212.
26. W.C. Sauer and L. Ozimek, Livest. Prod. Sci., 15 (1986), 367.
27. V.M. Gabert, W.C. Sauer, S. Li, M.Z. Fan and M. Rademacher, J. Sci. of Food and Agric., 70 (1996) 247.

28. P. Leterme, T. Monmart and A. Théwis, Anim. Feed Sci. Technol., 37 (1992) 309.
29. R.R. Marquardt, A.T. Ward, L.D. Campbell and P.E. Cansfield, J. Nutr., 107 (1977) 1313.
30. W.E. Artz, P.D. Bishop, A.K. Dunker, E.G. Schanus and B.G. Swanson, J. Agric. Food Chem., 35 (1987) 417.
31. D.W. Griffiths, J. Sci. Food Agric., 30 (1979) 458.
32. A.J.M. Jansman, H. Enting, M.W.A. Verstegen and J. Huisman, Brit. J. Nutr., 71 (1994) 627.
33. P. Van Leeuwen, A.J.M. Jansman, J. Wiebenga, J.F.J.G. Koninks and J.M.V.M. Mouwan, Brit. J. Nutr., 73 (1995) 31.
34. W. Grala, A.J.M. Jansman, P. Van Leeuwen, J. Huisman, G.J.M. Van Kempen and M.W.A. Verstegen, J. Anim. Feed Sci., 2 (1993) 169.
35. D.W. Griffiths and G. Moseley, J. Sci. Food Agric., 31 (1980) 255.
36. J.T.A. de Oliveira, A. Pusztai and G. Grant; Nutrition Research., 8 (1988) 943.
37. G. Grant, J.T.A. de Oliveira, P.M. Dorward, M.G. Annand, M. Waldron and A. Pusztai, Nutrition Reports Intern., 36 (1987) 763.
38. G. Grant, W.B. Watt, J.C. Stewart and A. Pusztai, Medical Sci. Res., 15 (1987) 1197.

Biology of the Pancreas in Growing Animals
S.G. Pierzynowski and R. Zabielski (Editors)
© 1999 Elsevier Science B.V. All rights reserved.

381

Growth and digestion in pancreatic duct ligated pigs. Effect of enzyme supplementation

P.C. Gregory[a], R.Tabeling[b] and J. Kamphues[b]

[a]Department of Pharmacology Research, Solvay Pharmaceuticals GmbH,
Hans-Böckler-Allee 20, D-30173 Hannover, Germany

[b]Department of Animal Nutrition, Hannover School of Veterinary Medicine,
Hannover, Germany

The importance of pancreatic enzymes for the growth and performance of pigs was investigated by comparing control pigs with pigs made pancreatic exocrine insufficient (P.I.), by ligation of the pancreatic duct, before and after enzyme supplementation. The studies were made in German Landrace and Göttingen minipigs chronically fitted with duodenal, jejunal and/or ileal T-fistulae, or ileo-caecal re-entrant fistulae. Pancreatic duct ligation caused: complete pancreatic exocrine insufficiency, with retention of low, level "intestinal lipase" activity; complete cessation of growth; a lowering of duodenal pH by 2-3 units but of ileal pH by only 0.5 units; a severe reduction in total (T) and pre-caecal (P-C) digestibility and absorption of fat (T from 95.5 to 31.5, P-C from 95.2 to 43.0%) and protein (T from 89.9 to 56.9, P-C from 79.1 to 27.3%) of a 30% fat, 15% protein diet; T of starch was >98% in all groups but P-C was reduced to 87.7 and 61.9% with a 25% and 54% starch diet respectively; a huge increase in the microbial content of the small and large intestine and compensatory increase in hindgut fermentation of undigested protein and carbohydrates; a net hindgut production of fat. Enzyme supplementation (Creon® 10,000 Minimicrospheres™, Solvay Pharmaceuticals GmbH, 8-24 capsules/meal) dose-dependently, partially/completely reversed most of these changes except hindgut production of fat. This last effect may be relevant to the clinical situation in some P.I. patients in whom normalization of faecal fat excretion has proved very difficult.

1. PANCREATIC EXOCRINE INSUFFICIENCY

1.1. Introduction
Pancreatic exocrine insufficiency (P.I.) is a severe problem in human patients suffering for example, from cystic fibrosis or chronic pancreatitis. The symptoms of P.I., maldigestion/malabsorption especially of fat and protein, diarrhoea, loss in weight and increased susceptibility to infection are seen most dramatically in cystic fibrosis, since about 90% of these patients are pancreatic insufficient at birth. Great advances in treatment of cystic fibrosis have been made, especially concerning antibiotic and enzyme treatment, and life expectancy has been increased to around 30 at the present time. Most clinical literature (based

upon faecal estimates of digestibility) suggests that adequate enzyme supplementation normalizes protein digestion [1], but that although fat digestion is also greatly improved, it is not *normalized* in a proportion of patients [e.g. 2,3]. On the other hand, despite enzyme supplementation it is generally difficult for the patients to achieve a normal rate of growth, and many patients are still below the accepted growth/weight levels for their age [4]. The nutritional status of the patients has been shown to have a great impact on their life expectancy [5], and nowadays, in contrast to previous advice, patients are encouraged to consume a high energy diet incorporating a high fat and high protein content [4]. Therefore, to improve therapy it has been necessary to develop an animal model of P.I., and for this purpose the pig is arguably one of the best, having pancreatic enzymes and a G.I. system similar to those in man [6].

The influence of P.I. on weight gain was investigated in growing German Landrace (pigs), aged approx. 12 to 22 weeks. In contrast, in order to reduce anticipated problems with re-entrant fistulae and of health in growing animals, all digestibility studies were performed in mature ($\geq$ 1 year) minipigs (full-grown at 30-35 kg). This allows comparative studies to be made over long periods (1-3 years) under reasonably steady-state conditions (stable body weight).

1.2. Methods

The following studies were performed in either German Landrace (male and female), or Göttingen minipigs (Ellegaard; female), 20-30 kg at surgery. All pigs were sedated with Tilest® (Tiletamin/Zolazepam; im), intubated, and anaesthetised with a mixture of halothane, nitrous oxide and oxygen. Following a mid-line laparotomy the pancreatic duct was carefully isolated and ligated (P.I.; pancreatic insufficient); while no ligation was performed in the control pigs. The pigs were variously fitted with titanium T-fistulae in duodenum, jejunum, and/or ileum, or with an ileo-caecal, re-entrant titanium fistula. All fistulae were exteriorized on the right flank of the animals. The pigs were prophylactically treated with antibiotic (Tardomyocel®, Benzylpenicillin, Dihydrostreptomycin) and with an analgetic (Tramal®, Tramadol). At least 4 weeks were allowed between surgery and the first studies, to ensure that the pigs had fully recovered. The pancreatic enzyme status (control or P.I.) was confirmed by measurement of faecal chymotrypsin activity (Boehringer Mannheim) and by measurement of lipase, trypsin, chymotrypsin and amylase activity from chyme samples withdrawn from the various intestinal fistulae. Results were discarded from any pancreatic duct ligated pig found to have more than a negligible faecal or intestinal enzyme activity and/or found on post mortem examination to have an intact pancreatic duct.

In digestibility studies, pigs were fed 2 meals per day (250 g/meal in 500ml H_2O, of a finely milled high-fat diet, or 315 g/meal of a high-starch diet; see Table 1), at 08.00 and 20.00h, plus Cr_2O_3 (Aldrich; 0.625 g/meal) as a marker. At least 7 days adaptation were allowed with each change of diet or enzyme supplementation (0, 8, 16 or 24 capsules [caps] Creon® 10,000 Minimicrospheres™; each capsule contained 11,200 amylase, 14,000 lipase, 665 protease Fédération Internationale Pharmaceutique (FIP) units) before any measurements were made. Thereafter, all faeces were collected for 5 days, and ileal chyme was collected on ice for 12h on 3 successive days. All samples were stored at –20°C until analysis. The frozen samples as well as the original diet were freeze-dried and a Weender analysis was performed [7] for dry matter (DM), crude ash, crude protein, crude fat and crude fibre. In brief, DM was estimated by weight after freeze-drying followed by 8h at 103°C; crude ash was estimated after 6h in a

Table 1
Composition of diets used in digestibility experiments (g per kg fresh diet)

High-fat diet

Values analysed		Values calculated from Manufacturer's data (Ssniff)		
Dry matter (DM)	936.3	Trace elements		
Raw ash	39.0	Calcium		
Raw protein	148.7	Phosphorus		
Raw fat	301.1	Sodium		
Raw fibre	38.8	Magnesium		
Starch	249.2	Vitamins:		
Sugar	21.8	Vitamin A	(I.U.)	12240
N-free extract (NFE)	408.7	Vitamin D3	(I.U.)	870
Organic matter	897.3	Vitamin E	(mg)	334
		Vitamin B1	(mg)	13.6
		Vitamin B2	(mg)	20.4
		Vitamin B6	(mg)	6.8
		Vitamin B12	(µg)	40.8
		Biotin	(µg)	163
		Pantothenic acid	(mg)	27.2
		Folic acid	(mg)	2.72
		Nicotinic acid	(mg)	81.6
		Vitamin K	(mg)	1.4
		Choline	(mg)	1088

High-starch diet

Values analysed		Values calculated from Manufacturer's data (Ssniff)		
Dry matter	907.1	Trace elements		
Raw ash	27.9	Calcium		5.4
Raw protein	116.5	Phosphorus		4.1
Raw fat	81.7	Sodium		1.1
Raw fibre	26.3	Magnesium		1.3
Starch	543.8	Vitamins:		
Sugar	16.3	Vitamin A	(I.U.)	9720
N-free extract (NFE)	654.7	Vitamin D3	(I.U.)	690
Organic matter	879.2	Vitamin E	(mg)	265
		Vitamin B1	(mg)	10.8
		Vitamin B2	(mg)	16.2
		Vitamin B6	(mg)	5.4
		Vitamin B12	(µg)	32.4
		Biotin	(µg)	129
		Pantothenic acid	(mg)	21.6
		Folic acid	(mg)	2.2
		Nicotinic acid	(mg)	64.8
		Vitamin K	(mg)	1.1
		Choline	(mg)	864

The high-fat diet comprised Ssniff's standard minipig diet supplemented with soya oil (Roth) and soyamin (Lukas Meyer). The high-starch diet comprised the Ssniff diet supplemented with maize starch. Pigs were fed daily 2 x 250 g/meal of the high-fat diet, or 2 x 315 g/meal of the high-starch diet - mixed with 500 ml water. All digestibility studies were performed within a time-span of 10 months in 1-2 year old, ileo-caecal re-entrant fistulated minipigs. The controls weighed 31.8 ± 3.3, and the P.I. minipigs 30.1 ± 2.7 kg over the course of these studies.

muffle furnace; crude protein was determined by Kjeldahl analysis (raw protein = nitrogen x 6.25); crude fat was determined gravimetrically after boiling for 30 min in conc. HCl, followed by a 6h extraction with petrol ether; raw fibre was determined after boiling for 30 min in 5% H_2SO_4 followed by boiling for 30 min in 5% NaOH, and ashing the sediment in a muffle furnace. Starch was analysed polarimetrically after acid hydrolysis, sugar was estimated gravimetrically. Cr_2O_3 was oxidized to chromate and chromium content calculated via extinction at 365 nm (spectrophotometer; [8]).

Lipopolysaccharide (LPS), a cell wall constituent of gram negative bacteria was used as an indicator of the counts of these bacteria within the chyme [9], and was measured in frozen faecal or ileal samples by the Limulus-Test [®]. Short chain fatty acid (SCFA) content of fresh faecal samples was determined by gas chromatography. Bacterial counts were made from samples of fresh faeces (obtained from rectum) obtained under sterile conditions in Dormicum® (Midazolamin) plus Ketavet® (Ketamin) anaesthetised minipigs.

Digestibility values for each food component were estimated according to the formula:

$$\text{digestibility of a nutrient (\%)} = \frac{\text{g/day in feed - g/day in faeces (or ileum)}}{\text{g/day in feed}} \times 100$$

Pre-caecal digestibility values were corrected for 100% recovery of Cr_2O_3.

Means and standard deviations were calculated using Excel 5.0, and statistical procedures were performed using the SAS® Software programme. Treatment effects were tested by analysis of variance. Independent samples were checked with the t-test for independent observations (controls vs PI-0), dependent samples with the t-test for dependent observations (PI-0 vs PI-8, PI-16, PI-24). Significant differences of the means, $P<0.05$, are indicated in the respective tables by different superscripts (a,b,c,d).

2. INFLUENCE OF PANCREATIC DUCT LIGATION ON PIG GROWTH

In normal healthy adult humans it has been demonstrated that the pancreas produces a large excess of pancreatic exocrine secretion, such that it has been suggested that up to 80-90% of the normal secretory capacity can be lost before any symptoms of pancreatic exocrine insufficiency are seen [10]. Such a large overproduction of enzymes would seem to be very wasteful, and if it exists it can only be an indication of the vital importance of a sufficient enzyme secretion for the growth and development of the animal. This can perhaps be demonstrated most simply and dramatically by artificially inducing total pancreatic exocrine insufficiency, e.g. by ligation of the pancreatic duct, and then comparing the rate of growth of pair-fed pancreatic insufficient pigs with that of control pigs.

Only a few such studies have previously been reported, and these have given surprisingly different results; i.e. although all studies reported reductions in rate of weight gain after duct ligation, these varied from as little as 25% over 12 weeks ([11]; Large White male castrates starting weight 40 kg) of 50% over 3 weeks which could be reversed by enzyme supplementation ([12]; Yorkshire, starting weight 14 kg) to as much as 100% over 6 weeks (studies cited in [13], starting weight 10 kg; [14], starting weight 10-14 kg). In our limited studies on this point with German Landrace (both sexes), we observed that appetite was retained but weight gain ceased completely for at least 10 weeks, with no signs of any recovery, following pancreatic duct ligation (Figure 1)

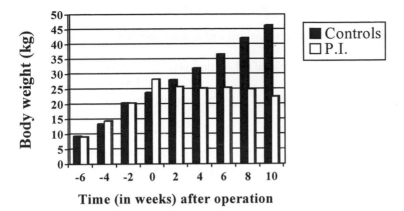

Figure 1. Influence of pancreatic duct ligation on weight gain in German Landrace.

The reasons for such disparate findings are presently unclear. A variety of factors could be involved, e.g. different races, different ages, possible failure in some cases to completely eliminate pancreatic exocrine secretion (overall some 10- 20% of pigs have two pancreatic ducts), but one critical factor is likely to be the diet chosen and the efficiency with which the pancreatic insufficient pig is able to digest this diet.

3. INFLUENCE OF PANCREATIC DUCT LIGATION ON INTESTINAL LUMINAL CONTENTS

3.1. Intestinal enzyme activity

Ligation of the pancreatic duct directly or indirectly produced a variety of dramatic changes to the intestinal luminal environment. Most importantly trypsin, chymotrypsin and amylase activities in duodenum, jejunum and ileum were undetectable, but interestingly, low chymotrypsin-like activity was often observed in the faeces (i.e. mean value of 0.3 ± 0.7, when measured at least 1 week after duct ligation, compared to control values of 12.8 ± 5.6 U/g), presumably derived from bacterial sources. In contrast to the above enzymes, a low baseline level of lipase activity was retained in the intestinal lumen of the P.I. pig (Table 2); similar findings have also been reported elsewhere [15]. Since ileal and jejunal lipase activity were similar this is unlikely to represent gastric lipase activity. It seems most likely that this activity corresponds to an intestinal lipase [16], or alternatively to an exogenously secreted bacterial lipase. It has been reported that the pig is able to increase gastric and pancreatic lipase activity according to dietary needs [17], however there was no indication that the pancreatic insufficient pig is able to increase the levels of this "intestinal lipase" to accommodate for the loss of its pancreatic lipase. Thus, in pancreatic duct ligated minipigs fed a 30% fat diet there was no change in the level of this "intestinal lipase" activity over periods of up to 3 months. No animals were prepared with gastric fistulae, and so it is not clear whether or not the pig can increase its gastric lipase activity in circumstances of pancreatic insufficiency.

Table 2
Influence of pancreatic duct ligation on intestinal pH and enzyme activities

Pig group	Duod. pH	Duod. pH	Jejunal pH	Ileal pH	Jejunal Lipase	Ileal
	Preprandial	Postprandial (¼ - 4h)	Preprandial	Postprandial (0 – 12h)	(0 – 6h)	Lipase (0 – 6h)
Control	6.97 ± 1.13^a	6.81 ± 1.22^a	6.40 ± 0.64^a	7.74 ± 0.05^a	759 ± 691^a	242 ± 334^a
P.I. 0 cap	4.33 ± 0.91^b	4.79 ± 0.93^b	5.96 ± 0.55^b	7.33 ± 0.16^b	4.7 ± 8.6^b	5.1 ± 6.0^b

All values are mean ± S.D; duodenal pHs are from German Landrace, all other values are from Göttingen minipigs; ileal pH from complete 12h collection of chyme, all other values from spot samples; lipase activities in F.I.P. units/ml.

3.2. Intestinal pH

Another result of pancreatic duct ligation was a fall in intestinal pH due to the loss of pancreatic bicarbonate secretion (Table 2). This is an important point in respect of enzyme supplementation for human pancreatic insufficiency, since nowadays most enzyme products are enteric coated to prevent gastric acid inactivation of lipase, (in most products enzymes are released at pH ≥ 5.5) and an acid intestinal content could cause delayed release of enzymes. Our studies showed that both pre- and postprandial proximal duodenal pH (approx 30 cm from the pylorus) in German Landrace fell by some 2.0-2.7 units after pancreatic duct ligation (Table 2). Since pH rises steeply along the duodenum, this is roughly comparable with the situation in pancreatic insufficient cystic fibrosis patients, in whom the pre-and post-prandial pH of mid to distal duodenum is some 1.0-1.5 units lower than in controls [18].

In contrast to the duodenum, we observed that the preprandial jejunal pH (1m from the pylorus) in the minipig was at most only 0.5 units lower than control (Table 2), while postprandial pH was unaffected (6.03 ± 0.54, and 5.95 ± 0.58 for control and P.I. respectively). It seems likely therefore that biliary secretion has a major buffering effect on the intestinal contents in the pig (indeed, in one P.I. pig, later found to have an obstructed bile duct, and whose results have not been included, the pre- and post-prandial jejunal pH was 2-3 units lower than in controls). It is not clear how important biliary secretion is in the human in this respect, but in any event in pancreatic insufficient humans jejunal pH (pre- and post-prandial) seems to be at most only some 0.5-1.0 units lower than in controls [18].

In the ileum, spot sampling failed to show any difference in pH between P.I. and control minipigs. However, when the complete ileal chyme was collected (re-entrant cannulated pigs), it became evident that ileal pH was significantly lower in untreated P.I. pigs, especially in the first 4h collection, i.e. from the undigested remains of the previous meal. But the pH was still somewhat lower even when the contents from the whole 12h were compared (see Table 2).

The few human ileal data published [18] do not seem to differ significantly from these findings in the P.I. pig.

3.3. Intestinal flora

Only preliminary studies have so far been performed concerning changes in intestinal bacterial colonisation following induction of pancreatic insufficiency. Owing to the difficulty in anaerobically obtaining a sample of ileal chyme, the level of gram negative bacteria was indirectly assessed by measuring the level of lipopolysaccharide (LPS) present. Our studies showed that in minipigs fed 500 g/day of a fat diet there was approximately a 40-fold increase in the amount of LPS passing through the ileum /day in P.I. pigs compared to control pigs (Table 3), i.e. there was bacterial overgrowth of the small intestine in these minipigs.

Table 3
Influence of pancreatic duct ligation on intestinal flora

Animal Group	Ileal chyme	Faecal content	E. coli	Gram –ve. Anaerobes
	(μg LPS/g)	(μg LPS/g DM)	(cfu/g faeces)	(cfu/g faeces)
Control (fat diet)	29 ± 12^a	85 ± 25^a	$8.8 .10^7$	$9.0.10^7$
P.I. (fat diet)	634 ± 254^b	2700 ± 797^b	$9.8. 10^8$	$3.5.10^8$
P.I. (starch diet)	105 ± 31^c	2240 ± 798^b	Not measured	Not measured

LPS = lipopolysaccharide; DM = dry matter; cfu = colony forming units.

This bacterial overgrowth is presumably a result of the massive increase in the levels of unabsorbed nutrients passing through the intestines. If the amount of faeces produced/day is considered, there was a 45-fold increase in viable E.coli and 15-fold increase in viable gram negative anaerobic bacteria in P.I. compared to control minipigs.

It is probable that the dietary content itself influenced these results, since a high fat content [19], especially of oil [20], as well as a reduction in protein content of the diet [21] can inhibit growth of gram positive bacteria, and this could have led to an exaggerated increase in gram negative bacteria. In any event, P.I. pigs fed a starch diet showed a much smaller increase in ileal gram negative bacteria (i.e. LPS content), but a similar large increase in faecal LPS (Table 3). An increase in small intestinal content of gram positive as well as gram negative bacteria has been observed in dogs following ligature of the pancreatic duct [22,23], and has sporadically been reported in humans with pancreatic insufficiency.

Since pancreatic juice has antibiotic properties [24], this microbial overgrowth in pancreatic insufficiency may not only derive from the rich source of nutrients available to them due to the poor digestibility of the diet in the absence of pancreatic enzymes.

4. INFLUENCE OF PANCREATIC DUCT LIGATION ON PRE-CAECAL AND TOTAL DIGESTION/ABSORPTION

In comparison to humans with pancreatic insufficiency the minipigs showed far fewer outward signs of disturbed digestion. Even when fed a diet containing 30% fat they did not develop diarrhoea; the only observation was that the faeces (which are like pellets in control minipigs) became softer and more formless. Greater changes were seen only in the first week on the new diet, when the pigs produced foul-smelling, watery faeces. But these changes were transient, and within a few days the smell disappeared and the faeces became more solid again – presumably as a result of altered hindgut metabolism of the undigested feedstuffs.

4.1. Total digestion/absorption (faecal output)

Pancreatic duct ligation strongly reduced total digestibility/absorption of the diet as shown by the very large increase in dry matter (DM) and especially of fat excreted, as well as by a considerable increase in faecal protein output (Table 4). In contrast, there was no increased loss of carbohydrates. Overall, digestibility of fat was reduced from 95.5 ± 0.9 to 31.5 ± 8.1% and protein from 89.9 ± 3.3 to 56.9 ± 2.6%, while digestibility of starch was 99% in controls and P.I. pigs. These data are in good agreement with clinical data collected from untreated human patients with pancreatic insufficiency [1], and from dogs with induced P.I. [25].

Table 4
Influence of pancreatic duct ligation on faecal output (g/24h)

Pig group	Dry matter	Fat	Protein	NFE	Starch
Control	58.8 ± 15.3[a]	6.9 ± 1.3[a]	7.3 ± 2.4[a]	23.1 ± 7.0	1.2 ± 0.4[ab]
P.I. 0 caps	175.4 ± 15.7[b]	103.1 ± 12.2[b]	32.0 ± 1.9[b]	14.5 ± 4.0	1.1 ± 0.3[a]
P.I. 8 caps	147.9 ± 16.9[c]	72.7 ± 18.8[c]	23.4 ± 1.9[c]	26.6 ± 3.9	1.8 ± 0.3[ab]
P.I. 16 caps	128.4 ± 16.8[d]	58.6 ± 10.8[c]	20.0 ± 3.2[cd]	25.1 ± 1.3	2.0 ± 0.1[b]
P.I. 24 caps	106.4 ± 19.4[d]	47.4 ± 10.2[c]	14.6 ± 2.7[d]	21.9 ± 5.2	1.9 ± 0.2[b]

All values are mean ± SD; sugar excretion was zero in all pig groups

Table 5
Relative ratios of faecal SCFA (in %)

Pig group	Acetate	Propionate	Iso-butyrate	n-butyrate	Iso-valerate	n-valerate
Control	69.6 ± 6.2[a]	16.1 ± 3.8[a]	1.5 ± 0.3[a]	7.9 ± 1.4	2.9 ± 0.5[a]	2.0 ± 0.3[a]
P.I. 0 caps	41.6 ± 2.5[b]	33.4 ± 2.4[b]	3.2 ± 0.5[b]	9.3 ± 0.6	6.1 ± 0.6[b]	6.6 ± 0.6[b]

All values are mean ± S.D. from fresh faecal samples.

However, although no increases were observed in faecal values of starch or sugar, differences were seen in faecal SCFA values. Clear-cut changes were seen in the relative ratios of the SCFA (Table 5), such that following duct ligation there was a large fall in acetate counteracted by a doubling in propionate, iso-butyrate and iso-valerate, and a trebling of n-valerate content. Similar changes have been observed in human pancreatic insufficiency [26]; the changes in C_4 and C_5 have previously been reported to be a consequence of increased hindgut metabolism of protein [27]. In addition, there was a moderate increase in overall SCFA content, from a mean of 121 to 138 mmol/l, which however, when combined with the increase in amount of faeces produced, i.e. from 85 ± 21 to 352 ± 51 g/day, represented an approximate 7-fold increase in daily excretion rate of SCFA in the pancreatic insufficient minipig, and when one considers that SCFA are well absorbed from the hindgut [27] this gives some indication of the great increase in hindgut fermentation that must have occurred.

4.2. Pre-caecal digestion/absorption (ileal outflow)

When analysed at the level of the ileum, pancreatic duct ligation had even more widespread effects, causing strong increases in the ileal flow of undigested fat, protein and dry matter, as well as a moderate increase in the flow of undigested starch and nitrogen-free extract compared to that of control pigs (Table 6); no comparable published data are available from pig, human or dog studies concerning pre-caecal digestibility in pancreatic exocrine insufficiency.

In conjunction with this increase in ileal flow after duct ligation, there was also a substantial increase in the dry matter content of the ileal chyme, from 14.4 ± 0.8 to $21.3 \pm 0.9\%$, but without change in the viscosity. This led to periodic problems of blockage of the ileo-caecal re-entrant fistula in the P.I. minipigs, but since enzyme supplementation rapidly normalized dry matter content it is unlikely to make much contribution to distal ileal obstruction syndrome in cystic fibrosis unless these patients are insufficiently supplemented.

Table 6
Influence of pancreatic duct ligation on ileal outflow (g/24h)

Pig Group	Dry matter	Fat	Protein	N-free extract	Starch	Sugar
Control	104 ± 7	7.3 ± 0.5	15.1 ± 2.3	51.3 ± 3.4	3.8 ± 0.3	2.5 ± 0.2
P.I. 0 caps	269 ± 1	85.8 ± 13.6	54.0 ± 5.8	88.7 ± 12.3	15.3 ± 7.8	2.4 ± 0.9
P.I. 8 caps	190 ± 1	45.5 ± 5.5	35.6 ± 3.2	72.5 ± 1.2	6.0 ± 1.6	1.3 ± 0.2
P.I. 16 caps	162 ± 14	32.9 ± 13.9	28.6 ± 1.8	64.1 ± 0.9	5.3 ± 0.2	1.2 ± 0.2
P.I. 24 caps	153 ± 13	25.2 ± 8.5	27.2 ± 5.3	65.8 ± 6.3	4.6 ± 0.8	1.6 ± 0.5

All values are mean $\pm$ SD, corrected for 100% recovery of Cr_2O_3 in ileo-caecal re-entrant fistulated minipigs

These results indicate that as far as pre-caecal digestibility is concerned, the most severe effects of pancreatic insufficiency were on protein digestibility, which was reduced from 79.1 ± 3.2 to $27.3 \pm 7.8\%$, and on fat digestibility, which fell from 95.2 ± 0.4 to $43.0 \pm 9.0\%$.

On the other hand, digestibility of starch (87.7 ± 6.3% as compared to 97.4 ± 0.2% in the controls) was remarkably well maintained in the absence of any pancreatic secretion, and digestibility of nitrogen-free extract only fell to 56.6 ± 6.0 from 75.5 ± 1.6%. This surprising result raises the question of whether pancreatic amylase is after all essential for efficient carbohydrate digestion. However, pig diets would normally have a higher starch content than that (25%) used in this experiment, and so a further study was performed in which the pancreatic duct ligated pigs were fed another diet much richer in starch (54% starch). With this diet total digestibility of starch was again complete (99.3 ± 0.1%), but this time the pre-caecal digestibility was only 61.9 ± 5.5%, and an ileal flow of 130.1 ± 18.6 g/day of undigested starch was seen. Clearly therefore, although the pancreatic insufficient pig can digest starch more efficiently than protein or fat, pancreatic amylase is nevertheless necessary if the pig is to achieve a normal pre-caecal digestibility of starch. Due to the extensive hindgut fermentation poor carbohydrate digestibility cannot be detected from analysis of faeces alone. Only relatively recently, using breath tests as an indirect measure of pre-caecal digestion and absorption, has it been shown that contrary to previous belief there is carbohydrate maldigestion/malabsorption also in humans with pancreatic exocrine insufficiency [1].

4.3. Hindgut fermentation

Comparison of the faecal output with ileal outflow gives information concerning the digestive events taking place in the hindgut, and demonstrated two major points (Figure 2). Firstly, the pig is able to partially compensate for poor pre-caecal digestibility by an increased capacity for hindgut fermentation. Undigested starch reaching the hindgut is completely fermented, but undigested protein (estimated from nitrogen excretion) is apparently only partially fermented.

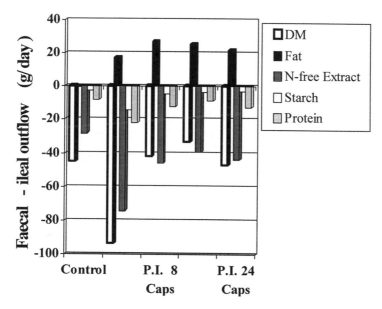

Figure 2. Hindgut fermentation in control and P.I. minipigs ± enzyme supplements.

The latter is probably an oversimplification, since faecal protein is mainly of bacterial origin rather than undigested dietary protein [28,29], and the supranormal nitrogen excretion is therefore more likely to be an indication of the increased microbial excretion observed rather than a failure to ferment all undigested dietary protein.

Secondly, in agreement with the generally accepted view in humans [e.g. 29,30] the daily faecal excretion of fat was almost identical with to the ileal outflow of fat in the control pigs. Unexpectedly however, there was an increase of about 20 g/day in the amount of fat excreted in the faeces compared to ileal outflow in the pancreatic duct ligated pig. This finding is not completely novel, since hindgut addition of fat, albeit of lesser amounts, has been sporadically reported also in control pigs [e.g. 31,32] . The source of this "extra hindgut fat" in the P.I. pigs is presently under investigation, but it would seem unlikely to derive from secretion of fat into the hindgut and more likely to reflect the fat content of sloughed intestinal cells and/or bacterial cells i.e. to follow either a faster turnover of hindgut epithelial cells in the face of the increased workload and SCFA energy supply [33] and/or from the huge increase in microbial population observed. In this context it is noteworthy that administration of antibiotics in the diet has been observed to enhance total digestibility of fat in control pigs [34], and it might be interesting to investigate the influence of antibiotics on fat digestibility in the P.I. pigs.

5. INFLUENCE OF ENZYME SUPPLEMENTATION IN PANCREATIC DUCT LIGATED MINIPIGS

Most if not all of the changes observed and discussed here following pancreatic duct ligation were reversible. Thus, when the pigs were given enzyme supplementation with Creon® 10,000 Minimicrospheres there was a dose-dependent improvement in total (Table 4) and more importantly in pre-caecal (Table 6) digestion/absorption of fat and protein, together with normalization of pre-caecal starch digestion). The small intestinal bacterial overgrowth (as judged by LPS values) seen in untreated pancreatic insufficient minipigs was completely reversed following enzyme supplementation (ileal LPS of 30.5 ± 31.7 µg/g after 24 capsules Creon®). In contrast the increased microbial content of the faeces was only moderately reduced (1980 ± 1093 µg/g LPS after 24 capsules Creon®), presumably because there was still a richer than normal nutrient supply for the hindgut flora. This is a point that may well have clinical significance. Somewhat unexpectedly there was also a partial restoration of normal ileal pH after enzyme supplementation (e.g. mean 12h ileal chyme pH of 7.55 ± 0.23 after 16 caps/meal). Therefore it is likely that the lack of pancreatic bicarbonate secretion was not solely responsible for the lowered ileal pH. Either the improved digestion and greater absorption of dietary content e.g. fatty acids, and/or the reduction in intestinal bacterial colonisation and concomitant lower intestinal fermentation were responsible. In contrast to all these findings, enzyme supplementation with up to 24 capsules Creon® 10,000 Minimicrospheres per meal did not reverse the hindgut production of fat (Figure 2) observed in the pancreatic duct ligated minipig, and this finding above all remains to be clarified. In particular it raises the question of whether a similar production of hindgut fat might occur in human patients with pancreatic insufficiency, and whether this might have some significance in patients in which it has proven difficult or impossible to completely normalize faecal fat excretion, even with high levels of enzyme supplementation. Likewise, it would be interesting to investigate whether the difficulty to normalize fat excretion in dogs with artificially induced pancreatic insufficiency, even after supplementing lipase at 100% of its normal postprandial secretion with a new, highly potent acid-stable bacterial lipase [35], is in any way related to hindgut production of fat.

6. CONCLUSIONS

Ligation of the pancreatic duct clearly and simply demonstrates just how important the pancreatic exocrine secretion is for digestion/absorption, for maintaining a healthy intestinal environment and ultimately for the growth and performance of the pig. In the event of pancreatic insufficiency huge changes take place in the intestinal flora, and considerable compensation of poor pre-caecal digestion results via increased hindgut fermentation, with large changes in daily excretion of protein, carbohydrate and fat compared to ileal outflow. This renders impossible an accurate estimation of the status of pancreatic insufficiency or its therapy purely by analysis of faecal samples (as usually is performed clinically). Hindgut fermentation however, although rescuing dietary energy that would otherwise be lost to the animal, is nevertheless a much less efficient process than small intestinal digestion. Thus for starch, fermentation to SCFAs represents a loss of about 40% metabolizable energy, while fermentation of protein represents not only a loss of amino acids to the animal, but moreover results in increased uptake of nitrogen as ammonia [36], which is hepatotoxic. These points should not be overlooked in diseases such as chronic pancreatitis and especially in cystic fibrosis and it emphasises how important it is that enzyme supplementation is able to *normalize pre-caecal digestibility*. It was shown that the pig has a surprisingly high capacity for pre-caecal digestion of starch in the absence of pancreatic amylase, but that dependence upon pancreatic proteases and lipase is far higher. It was further demonstrated that although improvements in pre-caecal digestion/absorption of protein and fat were achieved following enzyme supplementation it was difficult to bring about *normalization* of either, for reasons that still need to be clarified. Finally, the pancreatic duct ligated minipig looks to be a good model for studying problems related to pancreatic exocrine insufficiency in humans and its therapy with enzyme supplementation.

REFERENCES

1. E.P. DiMagno, Gastroenterology, 104 (1993) 1255.
2. P.T. Regan, J-R. Malagelada, E.P. DiMagno, S.L. Glanzman and V.L.W. Go, New Engl. J. Med. 297 (1977) 854.
3. M.J. Bruno, E.A.J. Rauws, F.J. Hoek, and G.N.J. Tytgat, Dig. Dis. Sci. 39 (1994) 988.
4. R.W. Shepherd, G. Cleghorn, L.C. Ward, C.R. Wall and T.L.Holt, Nutr. Res. Rev. 4 (1991) 51.
5. R. Kraemer, A. Rudeberg, B. Hadorn and E. Rossi, Acta Pediatr. Scand. 67, (1978) 33.
6. P.J. Moughan, P.D. Cranwell, A.J. Darragh and A.M. Rowan, Proceedings the VIth International Symposium on Digestive Physiology in Pigs, eds W-B Souffrant and H. Hagemeister; Dummerstorf, EAAP publication 80, Vol 2 (1994) 389.
7. C. Naumann and R. Bassler, Die chemische Untersuchung von Futtermitteln. 3. Aufl. VDLUFA-Verlag, Darmstadt, (1993).
8. H. Petry and W. Rapp, Z. Tierphysiol., 27 (1979) 181.

9. J. Kamphues, Tierärztl. Hochschule Hannover, Habil. - Schr. (1987).

10. E.P. DiMagno, V.L.W. Go and W.H.J. Summerskill., N. Engl. J. Med., 288 (1973) 813.

11. T. Corring and D. Bourdon, J. Nutr., 107 (1977) 1216.

12. H. Saloniemi, T.V. Kalima and T. Rahko, Acta Vet. Scand., 30 (1989) 367.

13. A.R. Imondi, R.P. Stradley and R. Wolgemuth, Proc. Soc. Exp. Biol. Med., 141, (1972) 367.

14. P. Pitkaranta, L. Kivisaari, S. Nordling, A. Saari, and T. Schröder, Scand. J. Gastroenterol., 24 (1989) 987.

15. J. Abello, X. Pascaud, C. Simoes-Nunes, J.C. Cuber, J.L. Junien, and C. Rozé, Pancreas 4 (1989) 556.

16. G. Serrero, R. Négrel and G. Ailhaud, Biochem and Biophys. Res. Commun. 65 (1975) 89.

17. M. Armand, P. Borel, P.H. Rolland, M. Senft, H. Lafont, and D. Lairon, Nutrition Research 12 (1992) 489.

18. P.C. Gregory, J. Pediatric Gastroenterol. Nutr., 23 (1996) 513.

19. J. Czerkawski and J. Clapperton, In: J. Wiseman (ed), Fats in animal nutrition, Butterworths, London, (1984) 249.

20. M. Götting, Tierärztl. Hochschule Hannover, Diss. 1989.

21. J. Inborr and K. Suomi, J. Agric. Sci. Fin. 60 (1988) 673.

22. K.W. Simpson, D.B. Morton, S.H. Sorensen, L. McLean, J.E. Riley and R.M. Batt, Res. Vet. 47 (1989) 338.

23. E. Westermarck, V. Myllys and M. Aho, Pancreas 8 (1993) 559.

24. S.G. Pierzynowski, P. Sharma, J. Sobczyk, S. Gaswacki, W. Barej and B. Weström, Pancreas 8 (1993) 546.

25. A. Suzuki, A. Mizumoto, A. Metzger, R. Rerknimitr, M.G. Sarr and E.P. DiMagno, Gastroenterology. 110, Suppl. (1996) A434.

26. T. Nakamura, K. Tabeke, A. Terada, K. Kudoh, N. Yamada, Y. Arai and H. Kikuchi, Acta Gastro-Entcrol. Belg. 56 (1993) 326.

27. H. Ruppin, S. Barmeir, H. Soergel, C.M. Wood CM and M.G. Schmitt, Gastroenterology 78 (1980) 1500.

28. A.M. Stephens and J.H. Cummings, JH. J. Med. Microbiol. 13 (1980) 45.

29. O.M. Wrong, C.J. Edmonds and V.S. Chadwick, In: " The large intestine: its role in mammalian nutrition and homeostasis". MTP Press, Lancaster, England, (1981) 123.

30. H.S. Wiggins, K.E. Howell, T.D. Kellock and J. Stalder, Gut 10 (1969) 400.

31. I.E. Sambrook, Brit. J. Nutr. 42 (1979) 279.

32. N.A. Nierick, I.J. Vervaeke, J.A. Decuypere, and H.K. Henderickx, J. Anim. Physiol. Anim. Nutr. 63 (1990) 220.

33. T. Sakata, Brit. J. Nutr. 58 (1987) 95.

34. V.C. Mason and A. Just, Z. Tierphysiol. Tierernährg. u. Futtermittelkde. (1976), 301.

35. A. Suzuki, A. Mizumoto, A. Metzger, R. Rerknimitr, M.G. Sarr and E.P. DiMagno, Gastroenterology 110 Suppl, (1996) A433.

36. W. Drochner and H. Meyer, Fortschr. Tierphysiol. Tierernährg., Beih. Verlag Parey, Berlin, Hamburg, 22 (1991) 18-14

Biology of the Pancreas in Growing Animals
S.G. Pierzynowski and R. Zabielski (Editors)
© 1999 Elsevier Science B.V. All rights reserved.

The exocrine pancreas in pig growth and performance

J.A.M. Botermans[a], J. Svendsen[a], L.S. Svendsen[a] and S.G. Pierzynowski[bc]

[a] Department of Agricultural Biosystems and Technology,
Swedish University of Agricultural Sciences, P.O. Box 59, 230 53 Alnarp, Sweden

[b] Department of Animal Physiology, University of Lund, Helgonavägen 3B,
223 62 Lund, Sweden

[c] Gramineer Int. AB, Ideon, 223 70 Lund, Sweden

The relationship between exocrine pancreatic secretion and pig performance is discussed with respect to the different production phases of the pig, its ingestive behaviour and growth capacity. In suckling pigs, exocrine pancreatic secretion is low; however, it plays an indispensable role in the digestion and absorption of milk components. Weaning induces a gradual and significant increase in pancreatic secretion. During the first few days after weaning the secretion may still be insufficient to cope with the rapid influx of difficult-to-digest feed. This may not only greatly affect production but also the occurrence of gastrointestinal tract disorders. It has been shown that during the growing period, different feeding techniques result in different feed intake patterns, which alter exocrine pancreatic secretion. There is a positive relationship between exocrine secretion and daily weight gain in catheterised growers. Exocrine secretion might limit performance in growing pigs, whereas in finishing pigs the tendency towards fat deposition may be more limiting for performance than pancreatic secretion.

1. INTRODUCTION

The ultimate aim of the pig industry is the production of high quality meat for human consumption. This production should be efficient in terms of economy, and sustainable. In addition, it has to take into consideration the physiological and behavioural needs of the pig.

A high feed conversion efficiency is important for farm economy and for a sustainable pig production. This means that the overall performance has to be on a high level, turning feed into meat in an optimal manner. For this, pigs with a high health status and a high genetic capacity for growth are needed, as well as feed with a high nutritive value and an optimal environment. If one of these four factors is limiting, performance will never reach a high level, no matter how optimal the other factors may be.

The feed intake level is the engine in performance; a pig with a low daily feed intake will never reach a high daily weight gain. However, ingestion of feed alone is not enough: the feed has to be digested/absorbed and metabolised for the deposition of protein and other body components. In this, the pancreas plays a key role.

The exocrine pancreas in the pig, as in other mammals, produces pancreatic juice which contains enzymes, nonenzymatic proteins, and salts. The enzymes, which are able to digest proteins, carbohydrates, lipids, and nucleic acids, are produced in the acinar cells of the exocrine pancreas [1,2]. Electrolytes capable of neutralising the acidic stomach contents and establishing the proper pH for enzymatic action are produced mainly in the intra-acinar and ductal cells [3]. The islet cells of the endocrine pancreas produce the hormones (e.g., insulin, glucagon) that regulate the utilisation of the absorbed digestion products [4,5,6,7]. Thus the pancreas, as the largest secretory gland associated with the digestive system, is directly involved in the digestion, absorption and utilisation of nutrients and thereby in carbohydrate, fat and protein metabolism.

The exocrine pancreatic secretion adjusts to the composition of the feed, and the quantity and quality of fat, protein and carbohydrates present in the diet will modulate exocrine secretion [8].

The poorer the nutritive value of the feed, the harder it is to digest and the greater the secretion has to be to break it down. For example, fibre has a stimulating effect on exocrine secretion, while secretion is low in the presence of sows' milk [9].

Table 1
Body weight (BW), main nutrient source, daily feed intake in dry matter, daily weight gain (DWG), DWG as percentage of BW, and exocrine pancreatic protein secretion per kg BW (catheterised pigs) during different stages of pig development, in commercial pig production

Pig category	BW (kg)	Nutrient source	Daily feed intake in dry matter (kg/day)	DWG (g/day)	DWG as % of BW	Exocrine protein output per kg BW (mg/kg/24h)
Piglet (1 d)	1	milk	0.2	150	11	17[a]
Piglet (28 d)	7	milk	0.3	350	5	24[a]
Weaner	15	feed	1.0	500	3	400[b]
Grower	40	feed	2.2	850	2	550[b]
Finisher	80	feed	3.0	950	1	375[b]
Adult sow	250	feed	2.4	200	0.1	?
Sow in lactation	250	feed	10	0	0	?

[a] Pierzynowski et al. (1995)
[b] Botermans, unpublished.

The exocrine secretion also adjusts to the biological needs of the animal, changing during the pig's development (Table 1). While the exocrine pancreas does not appear to be mainly responsible for digestion of milk during the suckling period, it plays a crucial role in the digestion and absorption of nutrients in pigs after weaning (5-10 kg liveweight at weaning until 20 kg liveweight) and during the growing period (20-60 kg liveweight). No information is available about exocrine pancreatic secretion in sows, but the fact that 90% of the pancreas in adult humans can be damaged without an impaired digestion [10] shows that exocrine secretion may be less important in full-grown adults than in growing individuals.

Many investigators have studied the regulation and development of the pancreas during the lifetime of the pig, and the effect of different nutrients on exocrine secretion. However, almost no data are available relating exocrine pancreatic secretion to pig performance. From a practical point of view, the question arises of whether secretion only reflects an adaptation of the animal to the feed or whether a high exocrine secretion is advantageous for performance. This question might have different answers, depending on which of the following factors limits pig performance: feed intake, digestion and absorption, or (protein) deposition. If feed intake is the limiting factor, an increase in exocrine secretion alone will not improve performance. If protein deposition is the limiting factor, an improvement in digestion and absorption will not help. However, when digestion and absorption of nutrients are the limiting factors (both the quality and quantity of metabolic products), alteration of the exocrine secretion may improve the availability of metabolites for pig growth. The limiting factor for performance might depend on where in the production phase (developmental stage) the pig is, the type of feed used, and the genetic background of the pig. For this reason it seems important to discuss exocrine pancreatic secretion in relation to the production phase of the pig, its ingestive behaviour and growth capacity.

The questions we want to address in this chapter are related to whether a high exocrine pancreatic secretion determines optimal growth, at a specific feed intake level and feed quality.

2. INGESTIVE BEHAVIOUR AND GROWTH DURING SUCKLING AND THE INVOLVEMENT OF THE EXOCRINE PANCREAS

2.1. Suckling pigs

In the pig, nursing takes place 20-30 times per 24-h period during the first days after farrowing [11,12]. In intensive housing systems the number of nursings per 24-h period remains rather constant at about 24 for 3 to 6 weeks [13], and then decreases rapidly [14]. During the first week after birth, relatively many nursings are initiated by the sow and terminated by the piglets, while later in lactation relatively many nursings are initiated by the piglets and terminated by the sow [14]. During suckling, milk is available to the piglet for only about 20 sec [15]. Milk is available only as long as oxytocin causes contraction of the myoepithelial cells in the udder [16]. Therefore, during the first weeks after farrowing the sow basically regulates the ingestive behaviour and feed intake of the piglets, permitting many small meals spread out over the whole 24-h period. The interactive processes between mother and offspring, however, are also very important for milk yield and successful suckling [17,18].

2.2. Digestion of milk and pancreatic function

The newborn pig is dependent upon the acquisition of colostrum and milk from the dam for development and growth, and for passive protection against pathogens. Sows' milk has a high biological/nutritive value and newborn pigs may easily double their body weight during the first 7 days of life. Thus the sow's capacity for milk production may be a limiting factor for pig growth and development.

Before intestinal closure at 18-36 hours after birth [19,20,21,22], large amounts of macromolecules are unselectively transported to the blood. This process is vital for an adequate construction of the immune defence system, and for intestinal maturation processes. It is enhanced by sow colostrum, probably due to its high content of proteins and protease inhibitors [22,23]. During the remainder of the suckling period, the digestive system is mainly adapted to the digestion of milk. Lingual and pancreatic amylase secretion is low while luminal and mucosal lactase in the small intestine are involved in the digestion and absorption of lactose. Proteins are digested by pepsin and chymosin in the stomach; thereafter in the intestine pancreatic chymotrypsin is also involved, while pancreatic trypsin plays a minor but important role [24]. Lack of trypsin in pancreatic juice in suckling pigs is correlated to a complete lack of gain (Pierzynowski, unpublished). Sixty percent of all milk fat is digested by lingual and gastric lipase and pancreatic lipase is not as important as later in life, when fat in solid feed can generally not be digested by lingual and gastric lipase. Pancreatic Cholesterol Ester Lipase (CEL) plays a major role in fat digestion during the suckling period, and the activity of this enzyme decreases in importance after weaning [25, 26]. CEL allows the digestion of acylglycerols, fat soluble vitamins and cholesteryl esters [27].

Although enzymes have been detected in pancreas homogenates from young pigs, albeit differing somewhat both qualitatively and quantitatively [24,28] from those in growing animals, the exocrine pancreas function remains low during suckling [26,29,30,31,32]. There may be several explanations for this. Because of its ingestive behaviour, the piglet is exposed to a steady flow of digesta into the duodenum, resulting in constant stimulation of the exocrine pancreas. The immaturity of the GI tract hormone receptors and the entero-pancreatic reflexes [33,34] may also play a role. In addition, observations in chronically catheterised pigs have shown that the intra-duodenal administration of enterostatin inhibits pancreatic juice secretion. Thus lipid digestion, described above for the neonate, and the relatively high levels of colipase from which enterostatin is formed, might be associated with direct regulation of exocrine secretion [35]. Intracellular degradative processes may also be of importance, since milk digestive products, e.g., glucomacropeptide, administered intravenously [36], have been observed to reduce gastrin-stimulated gastric juice secretion, and casomorphines administered intraduodenally [37] can stimulate somatostatin secretion, which will inhibit pancreatic secretion. In addition, the presence of milk hormones in the small intestine, e.g., insulin, somatostatin, and bombesin [38,39] could be involved in the regulation of the exocrine pancreas, either from the luminal side or after absorption into the circulation. However, such effects have not yet been demonstrated experimentally. Probably the most important factor in the refractoriness of the exocrine pancreas to milk stimulation is the fact that sows' milk is 98-99% digestible [40]. While the qualitative content of the pancreatic juice rather than the quantitative enzyme content may be of importance for the requirements of milk digestion, it is likely that there is no requirement for a high pancreatic secretion at this stage. Milk compounds probably 'trim' pancreatic secretion to the level strictly required for milk digestion.

3. INGESTIVE BEHAVIOUR AND GROWTH AFTER WEANING AND THE INVOLVEMENT OF EXOCRINE PANCREATIC FUNCTION

3.1. No regulation by the sow any longer

At weaning (3-5 weeks of age in commercial production), there is an abrupt change in nutrient source from a diet consisting predominantly of milk to one usually consisting of solid feed. As a result the pigs have to change their ingestive behaviour, from eating many small, warm liquid meals (about 25-50 ml sows' milk per suckling) to eating larger quantities of dry, cool, solid feed given once or twice a day or with *ad libitum* access. The eating behaviour changes from massaging and sucking to rooting and chewing [41]. Before weaning, nutrient intake is predominantly regulated by the sow. After weaning, the pig has to regulate its own feed intake, resulting in fewer and frequently larger meals, which may lead to overconsumption. Three to six days after weaning, pigs spend 40-60 minutes daily in eating and drinking [42].

3.2. Solid feed and exocrine pancreatic function

Even before weaning, solid feed nutrients in the gastrointestinal tract can stimulate exocrine pancreatic secretion; however, as long as sow's milk is present in the diet, this stimulation is 'trimmed' by milk factors [31]. The sow's milk has to be completely replaced by solid feed before the exocrine pancreatic secretion shows an increase [26].

After weaning, exocrine secretion increases gradually in catheterised pigs [43], resulting in a significant increase in secretion after 3-5 days as compared to 1 day before weaning. Studies of pig pancreas homogenates and luminal contents show that around weaning the enzyme content of the pancreatic tissue also increases greatly and its composition changes [24]. Using chronically catheterised pigs it has been shown that the trypsin:protein and amylase:protein ratios increased in pancreatic juice after weaning, whereas the lipase and colipase:protein ratios remained more or less constant during the period studied. The CEL:protein ratios showed a tendency to decrease after weaning [26].

The hormonal consequences of the stress of weaning may also play a role in pancreatic maturation. Corticosteroids might be one of the mediators of pancreatic development in early weaning [44]. Injection of dexamethasone or hydrocortisone 21-acetate 2 to 6 days before weaning enhances digestive enzyme activity, in particular pancreatic amylase activity, in weanling pigs [45, 46]. This increase in exocrine secretion as a result of higher cortisol levels reduces postweaning mortality [45].

During the first 2-3 days after weaning, exocrine secretion appears to be insufficient for the necessary digestion and absorption of nutrients, especially if the pigs overeat. This may facilitate the rapid multiplication of pathogenic *Escherichia coli* [47], which is frequently associated with the occurrence of diarrhoea during the postweaning period. Lack of antibacterial substances in pancreatic secretions may also play a role [48]. Reducing the feed intake of piglets during day 3 to day 8 after weaning reduces this explosive bacterial growth, resulting in less diarrhoea [47].

It can be concluded that exocrine secretion might be a limiting factor during the first days after weaning and that feed intake and exocrine secretion are poorly regulated during this period, resulting in a risk of metabolic disturbances and diarrhoea.

4. INGESTIVE BEHAVIOUR AND PERFORMANCE IN GROWING AND FINISHING PIGS AND THE SIGNIFICANCE OF THE EXOCRINE PANCREAS

4.1. Feed consumption and pig performance

The amount of feed consumed in relation to the pig's production phase greatly influences performance. At the start of the growing period (growing period: 20-60 kg liveweight), high feed consumption leads to a high daily weight gain [49,50] and good feed conversion efficiency [49,51]. However, at the end of the finishing period (finishing period: 60-110 kg liveweight), high feed consumption not only can lead to a high daily weight gain but also to high fat deposition, resulting in a low carcass lean meat percentage and poor feed conversion efficiency [52, 53], especially in castrated males [51]. Thus, a high daily feed intake during the growing period has a positive effect on performance, while during the finishing period it may have adverse effects. Therefore, a restricted feed intake is often recommended during the finishing period, depending on the breed and sex of the animals [54,55,50].

The daily feed intake can differ depending on the feeding system. For example, the daily feed intake in pigs fed by a wet/dry feeder is significantly higher in comparison to pigs fed by a dry feeder, where there is *ad libitum* access to crumbles [49]. Even within feeding systems there are differences in daily feed intake between individual pigs, depending on the social status of the pig and the feeding system. An increased variation in daily feed intake has been observed with a decreasing number of feeding places. Low-ranking pigs in a system with a high level of competition for feed eat less than low-ranking pigs in a system with a lower level of competition [56].

Besides differences in the amount of feed consumed, differences in feed intake patterns exist, depending on the feeding system and social status of the pigs. Trough feeding in pens of 16 pigs results in an individual feed intake pattern which is closely related to feeding time, while feeding 16 pigs with 4 dry feeders results in a more spread individual feed intake pattern (Figure 1). With a high level of competition for feed (e.g. 1 feeding place per 16 pigs), low-ranking pigs are forced to eat during the night, while the high-ranking pigs are resting (Botermans, unpublished)

Digestion/absorption of the nutrients can also be a limiting factor for high performance. When the nutritive value of the feed is limited [57] and/or when the digestive system is not adapted to the feed, weight gain is reduced. When the nutritive value of the feed is low, pigs will compensate by increasing their feed intake. However, this adaptation of feed intake is limited to a certain level, since a high percentage of undigested compounds in the distal part of the intestines may lower the rate of stomach emptying, resulting in a lower daily feed intake because of constant stimulation of the satiety centre in the hypothalamus [58,59]. This problem may be partly avoided by using feeds with high digestibility and net energy level, and breeds with a high digestive capacity (selection for growth rate rather than for feed conversion efficiency or lean growth) [60]. Limitations in the digestive capacity of the pig may depend on several factors, including saliva production, stomach, gallbladder, pancreas, and intestinal function.

Deposition of proteins or other body constituents may also be a limiting factor in pig production and pigs with a high genetic capacity for meat deposition are desirable, if deposition is the limiting factor. High levels of metabolites such as glucose [61,62], volatile fatty acids [61], amino acids [63] urea [64] etc. in the blood down-regulate voluntary feed intake.

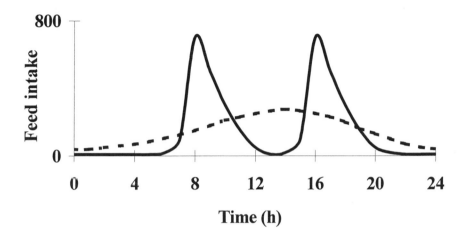

Figure 1.   Individual feed intake patterns for 16 pigs fed *ad libitum* with a trough (———) or four dry feeders (- - - -) (unpublished).

4.2. Ingestive behaviour and exocrine pancreatic secretion

Feeding stimulates exocrine pancreatic secretion. However, the amount of feed consumed does not seem to affect the amount of pancreatic secretion [65]. The fact that the pig is eating appears to be enough to elevate pancreatic secretion, indicating that the cephalic phase of secretion plays an important role. Therefore, feeding many small meals results in a higher exocrine secretion than does feeding the same amount of feed in only two large meals per day (Figure 2). Thus, exocrine pancreatic secretion may be altered by manipulating the ingestive behaviour of the pig [66].

No difference in exocrine pancreatic secretion could be detected in pigs fed the same amount of feed and the same number of meals during the day or night, respectively (Botermans, unpublished). Exposing pigs to social stress by grouping did not appear to affect secretion either. However, treatment with ACTH significantly enhanced preprandial exocrine pancreatic secretion by 70%, while a neuroleptic drug reduced exocrine preprandial secretion by 80% (Botermans, unpublished).

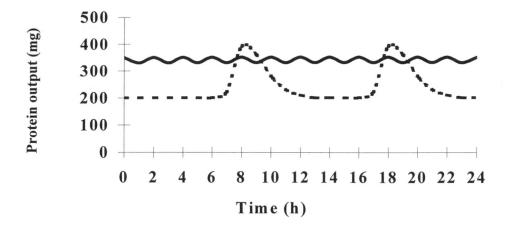

Figure 2. Exocrine pancreatic protein output on feeding two large meals a day (- - - -) as compared to many small meals spread over the entire 24-h period (———), at the same daily feed intake (empirical model based on Botermans, unpublished)

4.3. Exocrine pancreatic secretion and performance in growing animals

The importance of exocrine pancreatic secretion for pig development has been reported by Saloniemi *et al.* [67], who induced exocrine pancreatic insufficiency by ligation of the main pancreatic duct and resection of the other parts of the head of the pancreas. They observed that the ligated pigs (age 40-47 days, 13.6 kg) had a daily weight gain of 240 g, ligated pigs with enzyme supplementation had a daily weight gain of 454 g, and sham-operated pigs had a daily weight gain of 483 g.

In a second experiment done by Soloniemi *et al.* [67], healthy pigs without surgical manipulation (33 days, 9.6 kg) receiving a feed supplementation of 10 g pancreatic enzyme preparation per animal per day for 14 days had a daily weight gain of 360 g (S.E. 45 g, n=6), while pigs not receiving these enzymes gained 332 g (S.E. 17 g, n=6).

In one of our own experiments the second experiment (Botermans, unpublished) one pig developed pancreatitis, but did not show any clinical signs of illness. The volume of exocrine secretion in this pig was reduced by 72%, protein output was reduced by 86 %, trypsin activity by 90% and amylase activity by 99%. Daily feed consumption was comparable to that of the other pigs which had the same body weight at the start of the experiment. However, the pig did not gain any weight during the two-week experimental period, while the other pigs had an average experimental DWG of 305 g.

Differences in exocrine pancreatic secretion exist between pigs depending on their performance. In one study (Pierzynowski, pers. obs), pigs weighing 20 kg at 8 weeks of age had a higher secretion per kg body weight than did pigs weighing 13 kg at 8 weeks (Figure 3). In the heavier pigs, interprandial secretion was higher and secretion was less stimulated by feeding than in the lighter pigs; in heavy pigs postprandial protein output was seven percent of the total output, while in lighter pigs it was 20 percent (Figure 3).

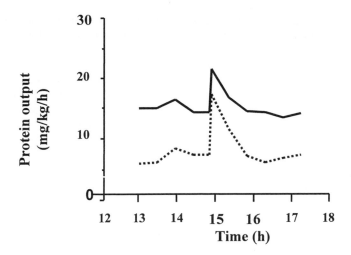

Figure 3. Exocrine pancreatic protein output in catheterised pigs weighing 20 kg at 8 weeks of age (——) (n=3) or weighing 13 kg at 8 weeks of age (----) (n=3), feeding at 15:00 hours (Pierzynowski, unpublished).

The difference in secretion between heavy and light pigs was clearest in the interprandial periods, which can be explained by how pigs respond to CCK and secretin stimulation during these interprandial periods. In an experiment using anaesthetised pigs, in which the response exocrine pancreas to CCK-8 (125 mmol/kg BW, bolus injection) plus secretin was tested, it

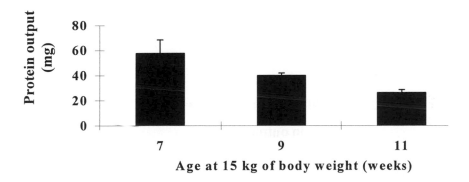

Figure 4. Exocrine pancreatic protein output during 10 min. in sedated pigs, using CCK and secretin stimulation, according to the age of the pigs when they reached 15 kg BW (total n=9) (Pierzynowski, unpublished).

was found that pigs weighing 15 kg at 7 weeks of age responded much more strongly to these hormones than did pigs weighing 15 kg at 11 weeks (Figure 4). Thus pigs showing better performance also had a greater response to key hormones.

In studies with catheterised pigs it is always difficult to know whether there is a causal relationship between exocrine pancreatic secretion and performance or whether pigs with high performance and high exocrine secretion are less affected by surgery, compared to pigs with low performance and low exocrine secretion. In other words: how good are catheterised pigs as a model to study pancreatic secretion in healthy pigs in a commercial herd?

In an investigation using 10 pigs, a positive correlation between exocrine secretion and performance (compared at the same daily feed intake) was observed in catheterised pigs (16-32 kg liveweight) [65]. The question is whether performance would have improved more if the exocrine secretion had been increased. The answer depends very much on whether secretion is the limiting factor for performance (Figure 5) or whether other factors in digestion/absorption or metabolism (deposition) are limiting. Exaggerated exocrine secretion, especially if not appropriate to the amount of feed consumed, may result in pancreatic endogenous losses [68] due to a high production of enzymes, although ileal endogenous losses appear to be of greater importance than pancreatic endogenous losses [69].

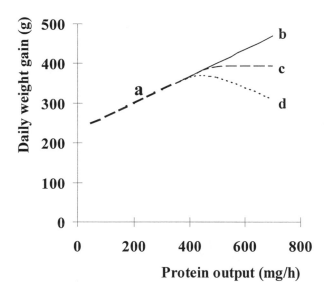

Figure 5. Theoretical relationship between exocrine pancreatic protein output and daily weight gain (DWG) with standardised feed intake a) own observations (n=10) b) where exocrine pancreatic secretion is the limiting factor (theoretical), c) where exocrine pancreatic secretion is not the limiting factor (theoretical), d) where exocrine pancreatic secretion results in endogenous losses of protein (theoretical).

5. FUTURE AREAS OF RESEARCH

The relationship between exocrine pancreatic secretion and performance needs further elucidation. The function of the pancreas in balancing digestion/absorption on the one side and metabolism on the other also needs investigation. It is known that different amounts of individual enzymes and different ratios between types of enzymes, (e.g. endopeptidase (trypsin, chymotrypsin, elastase) to exopeptidase ratios, and colipase to lipase ratios), result in different metabolic products, which in turn will affect performance. This indicates that exocrine pancreatic secretion (different enzyme profiles) not only affects digestion quantitatively but also qualitatively. It has recently been shown that protein can be absorbed both in amino acid form and as short peptides [70,71,72], and it may be hypothesised that the composition of the pancreatic endo- and exopeptidases may directly affect the composition of available peptides for absorption. Thus the quality of digestion can affect the quality of absorption, and this might affect the quality of deposition.

6. CONCLUSIONS

Performance is affected by many factors and exocrine pancreatic secretion may only be limiting in certain pig categories/stages of pig production. During the suckling stage, pancreatic secretion plays a minor role, while directly after weaning an impaired exocrine pancreatic secretion may result in disturbances in the performance and health of the pigs. In growing pigs, exocrine secretion may also be limiting for performance. In finishing pigs, the tendency to deposit fat might be the limiting factor, not the digestion capacity, and exocrine pancreatic secretion may be of minor importance. However, if the quality of the digestion can be changed by changes in exocrine pancreatic secretion, fat- and protein deposition may be altered. No information is available on exocrine secretion in the adult pig; however, data from humans indicate that it plays a minor role in fully grown adults.

Research on the relationship between exocrine pancreatic secretion and performance is very limited. There is a need to elucidate the role of the pancreas (both endocrine and exocrine) in balancing digestion/absorption and metabolism, and how this affects pig performance.

REFERENCES

1. J. R. Malagelada, Physiology of the Gastrointestinal Tract, L. R. Johnson (ed.), Raven, New York (1981) 172.
2. C.S. Pitchumoni, G. Sheele, L.C. Lee and E. Lebenthal, The Exocrine Pancreas: Biology, Pathobiology and Diseases J.D Gardner, F.P. Brooks *et al.* (ed.), Raven, New York (1986) 387.
3. I. Schulz, Ann. NY Acasd. Sci., 341 (1980) 191.
4. G. Sitbon and P. Mialhe, Horm. Metab. Res., 10 (1978) 12.
5. K. Christensen and A. Just, Comp. Biochem. Physiol., 91A (1988) 279.

6. T. Motyl, B. Dębski, W. Kukulska, P. Ostaszewski and P. Krupa, J. Anim. Physiol. Anim. Nutr., 55 (1986) 110.
7. K. Malmlöf, J. Örberg, S. Helberg, Z. Cortova, S. Björkgren, J. Anim. Physiol. Anim. Nutr., 63 (1990) 180.
8. T. Corring, Rev. Nutr. Diet., 27 (1977) 132.
9. S.G. Pierzynowski, B.R. Weström, J. Svendsen and B.W. Karlsson, J. Pediatr. Gastroenterol Nutr., 10 (1990) 206.
10. P. Layer and G. Hdtman, Int. L. Pancreatol, 15 (1994).
11. M.J. Bryant, P. Rowlinson and H.A.M. van der Steen, Anim. Prod., 36 (1983) 445.
12. A-Ch. Olsson and J. Svendsen, Observations at farrowing and mother-offspring interactions in different housing systems, Report 65, Swedish Univ. of Agric. Sci., Dept. of Farm Buildings, Lund, Sweden, 1989.
13. G.M. Cronin and J.A. Smith, Appl. Anim. Behav. Sci., 33 (1992) 175.
14. K. Bøe , Appl. Anim. Behav. Sci., 35 (1993) 327.
15. D. Fraser, Appl. Anim. Ethol., 6 (1980) 247.
16. F. Ellendorff, M.L. Forsling and D.A. Poulain, J. Physiol., 333 (1982) 577.
17. B. Algers, Vocal and tactile communication during suckling in pigs. Aspects on functions and effects of continuous noise, Thesis, Univ. of Agric. Sci., Skara, 1989.
18. H. Castén, Suckling behaviour, milk consumption and hormone release in the sow relative to nest building and early milk ejections, Ph.D. thesis, College of Vet. Med., Helsinki, Finland, 1993.
19. F.W.R Brambell (ed.), The Transmission of Passive Immunity from Mother to Young, Elsevier/North Holland Biomedical Press, Amsterdam, 1970.
20. J.P. Kraehenbuhl, C. Bron and B. Sordat. Current Topics in Pathology (ed.), E. Grundman), Springer-Verlag, Berlin (1979) 105.
21. W.A. Walker, Ciba Foundation Symposium on Development of Mammalian Absorptive Processes, Excerpta medica, Amsterdam (1979) 751.
22. B.R. Weström, J. Svendsen and B.W. Karlsson, Biol. Neonate, 42 (1982) 185.
23. B.R. Weström, J. Svendsen, B.G. Ohlsson, C. Tagesson and B.W. Karlsson, Biol. Neonate, 46 (1984) 20.
24. T. Corring, A. Aumaitre and G. Durand, Nutr. Metab., 22 (1978) 231.
25. M.S. Jensen, S.K. Jensen and K. Jakobsen, J. Anim. Sci., 75 (1997) 437.
26. S.G. Pierzynowski, B.R. Weström, C. Erlansson-Albertsson, B. Ahrén, J. Svendsen and B.W. Karlsson, J. Pediatr. Gastroenterol. Nutr., 16 (1993) 287.
27. O. Hernell and L. Bläckberg, Acta Pætdiatr. Suppl., 405 (1994) 65.
28. B.R. Weström, B. Ohlsson and B.W. Karlsson, Pancreas, 2 (1987) 589.
29. S.G. Pierzynowski, B.R. Weström, B.W. Karlsson, J. Svendsen and B. Nilsson, Can. J. Anim. Sci., 68 (1988) 953.
30. S.G. Pierzynowski, B. R. Weström, B.W. Karlsson and J. Svendsen, Development of the exocrine pancreas function: Regulatory mechanisms in pigs during early postnatal period, Proceedings of the 4th International Seminar at the Kielanowski Institute of Animal Physiology and Nutrition, S. Buraczewska et al (eds.), Jabłonna, Poland, 1988, 44.
31. S.G. Pierzynowski, Int. J. Pancreat,, 18 (no. 2) (1995) 81.

32. B.R. Weström, S.G. Pierzynowski, B.W. Karlsson and J. Svendsen, Digestion Physiology in the Pig, Proceedings of the 4th International Seminar at the Kielanowski Institute of Animal Physiology and Nutrition, S. Buraczewska *et al.* (eds), Jabłonna, Poland, 1988, 36.
33. A. Chang and J.D. Jamieson, J. Cell Biol., 103 (1986) 2353.
34. L. Larose and J. Morisset, Gastroenterology, 73 (1977) 530.
35. C. Erlanson-Albertsson, B.W. Weström, S.G. Pierzynowski, S. Karlsson and B. Ahrén, Pancreas, 6 (1991) 619.
36. L.S. Vasilevskaya, Y. Stan, M.P. Chernikov and G.K. Shlygin, Vopr Pitan, 4 (1977) 21.
37. V. Schusdziarra, R. Schick, A. de la Fuente, H.V. Brantl and E.F. Pfeiffer, Endocrinology, 112 (1983) 1948.
38. O. Koldovsky and V. Thornburg, J. Ped. Gastroenterol. Nutr., 6 (1987) 172.
39. B.R. Weström, R. Ekman, L. Svendsen, J. Svendsen and B.W. Karlsson, J. Ped. Gastroenterol Nutr., 6 (1987), 440.
40. D.E. Kidder and M.J. Manners, Digestion in the Pig, Scientechnica, Bristol, 1978.
41. M. Schmidt, Ugeskrift for Jordbrug 127, 13 (1982) 253.
42. D. Rantzer, J. Svendsen and B. Weström, Swed. J. Agric. Res., 25 (1995) 61.
43. D. Rantzer, P. Kiela, M-J. Thaela, J. Svendsen, B. Ahrén, S. Karlsson and S.G. Pierzynowski, J. Anim. Sci., 75 (1997) 1324.
44. P.C. Lee and E. Lebenthal, J. Nutr., 113 (1983) 1381.
45. R.P. Chapple, J.A. Cuaron and R.A. Easter, J. Anim. Sci., 67 (1989) 2985.
46. S. Gómez, M.L. Angeles and J.A. Cuarón, J. Anim. Sci., 75 (1997) 993.
47. D. Rantzer, J. Svendsen and B. Weström, Acta Agric. Scand. A. Animal Sci., 46 (1996) 219.
48. S.G. Pierzynowski, P. Sharma, J. Sobczyk, S. Garwacki and W. Barej, Int. J. Pancreatol., 12 (1992) 121.
49. J.A.M. Botermans, J. Svendsen and B. Weström, Livestock Environment Symp. V, ASAE, St. Joseph, Michigan (1997) 591.
50. S. Thomke, A. Madsen, H. P. Mortensen, F. Sundst.l, O. Vangen, T. Alaviuhkola and K. Andersson, Acta. Agric. Scand. Sect. A, Anim. Sci., 45 (1955) 45.
51. S. Thomke, T. Alaviuhkola, A. Madsen, F. Sundst, l, H. P. Mortensen, O. Vangen and K. Andersson, Acta Agric. Scand. Sect. A, Anim. Sci., 45 (1995) 54.
52. K.A. Leymaster and H.J. Mersmann, J. Anim. Sci., 69 (1991) 2837.
53. E. Kanis, Anim. Prod., 46 (1988) 111.
54. L.A. den Hartog and C.M.C. van der Peet-Schwering, Pig News and Information, 16 (1995) 51.
55. K. Andersson. Konsulentavdelningens rapporter 67, Uppsala, Sweden, 1985.
56. L. Berg, S. Pierzynowski, J. Botermans and J. Svendsen, 15th IPVS Congress, Birmingham, England, 1998.
57. J. Håkansson, M-A. Cidh and N. Lundeheim, Fakta 3., Swedish Univ. of Agric. Sci., Uppsala, Sweden, 1997.
58. P. Tybirk, Ugeskrift for Jordbrug, 35 (1987) 1063.
59. H. Spiekers. Schweine-Zucht und Schweine-mast, 39 Heft 10 (1991) 335.
60. P. Tybirk, A Model of Food Intake Regulation in the Growing Pig, In: The Voluntary Intake of Pigs, J. M. Forbes, M.A. Varley and T.L.J. Lawrence (eds.), (1989) 105.

61. J.M. Forbes, Voluntary Food Intake and Diet Selection in Farm Animals, CAB international, Oxon, U.K. 1995.
62. P.C. Gregory, M. Mcfadyen and D.V. Rayner, Quarterly J. of Exp. Phys., 72 (1987) 525.
63. Y. Henry, Livest. Prod. Sci., 12 (1985) 339.
64. H.Y. Chen, A.J. Lewis and P.S. Miller, Nebraska Swine Report (1997) 18.
65. J.A.M. Botermans and S. G. Pierzynowski, J. Anim. Sci., accepted.
66. J. Hee, W.C. Sauer and R. Mosenthin, J, Anim. Physiol. Anim. Nutr., 60 (1988) 249.
67. H. Saloniemi, T.V. Kalima and T. Rahko, Acta Vet. Scand., 30 (1989) 367.
68. T. Corring, Annls. Biol. Anim. Biochim. Biophys., 15 (1975) 115.
69. C.A. Makkink, Of Piglets, Dietary Proteins, and Pancreatic Proteases, Ph.D thesis, Dep. of Anim. Nutr., Agric. Univ. Wageningen, The Netherlands, 1993.
70. W.R. Caine, Ileal Recovery of Endogenous Amino Acids in Pigs, Ph.D. thesis, Dep. of Anim. Nutr., Agric. Univ. Wageningen, The Netherlands, 1997.
71. A.H. Danzig, J-A. Hoskins, L.B. Tabas, S. Bright, R.L. Shepard, I.L. Jenkins, D.C. Duckworth, J.R. Sportsman, D. Mackensen, P.R. Rosteck Jr. and P.L. Skatrud, Science, 264 (1994) 430.
72. H. Daniel, M. Boll and U. Wenzel, VIth International Symp. on Digestive Physiology in Pigs, EAAP 80 (1981) 1.

Biology of the Pancreas in Growing Animals
S.G. Pierzynowski and R. Zabielski (Editors)

Exocrine pancreatic functions of carnivores

R.K. Buddington[a] and A.J. Lepine[b]

[a] Department of Biological Sciences, Mississippi State University,
Mississippi State, Mississippi, 39762

[b] Research and Development, The Iams Company, Lewisburg, OH, 45338

Although basic mechanisms of exocrine pancreatic functions are shared among mammals, the wide diversity of evolutionary diets is associated with differences among species for the composition of the exocrine secretions and the responses to changes in diet composition. Differences between species are less pronounced during suckling and begin to increase at weaning. This contribution reviews exocrine pancreatic secretion in carnivores with the emphases on patterns of secretion, responses to diet composition, ontogenetic development, and common pathologies.

1. INTRODUCTION

The exocrine pancreas has been extensively investigated in omnivores, such as the rat, and much less is known about carnivores, which consume a diet that places different functional demands on the digestive system. Although basic pancreatic functions are similar among mammals, there is increasing evidence that the composition of the exocrine secretions, patterns of development, and adaptive responses of omnivores differ markedly from those of carnivores and even humans [1,2]. This severely limits the ability to extrapolate results from rats, pigs and other omnivores to carnivorous species.

Most of what is known about pancreatic functions of carnivores is based on pathological conditions of dogs and cats (see reviews by Williams [3] and Williams and Guilford [4]), or the use of the dog as a model for the human because of several similarities [5]. As a result, the modulation of pancreatic secretions in response to diet composition is poorly understood for the dog, with virtually nothing known for the cat. Even less is known about age-related changes in exocrine pancreatic secretions of dogs, cats, and other carnivorous mammals. The exception is the mink for which there are reports of postnatal changes in the activities of pancreatic digestive enzymes.

The objective of this contribution is to familiarise readers with what is known about the exocrine pancreas of carnivores. It expands on a previous description of the pancreas of dogs and cats [6]. The first sections describe structural and functional features of the pancreas in carnivores, based on what is known for dogs, cats, and mink. Subsequent sections present information about methods used to study pancreatic functions of carnivores, adaptation of exocrine secretions in response to changes in diet composition, ontogenetic development of pancreatic exocrine secretions, and pathological conditions associated with the exocrine pancreas. The majority of references are restricted to carnivores, but information for omnivores is included when relevant and/or not available for carnivores.

2. THE PANCREAS OF CARNIVORES

The anatomical arrangement of the cat and dog pancreas has been reviewed by Williams [3]. Unlike many other mammals, dogs have two pancreatic ducts [7], and in some individuals even more ducts can be found (personal observations). The cranial, and actually smaller, main pancreatic duct empties into the intestine through the major duodenal papilla, which it shares with the bile duct. The greater part of the pancreatic secretions are drained by the larger accessory pancreatic duct and enter the intestine through the minor duodenal papilla, which is distal to the major duodenal papilla pancreatic duct. In cats, the main pancreatic duct is larger and in some individuals the only duct.

Histologically, the acinar cells represent more than 80% of the exocrine pancreas. These cells synthesise and secrete over 20 proteins, including the enzymes that are responsible for hydrolysing the macronutrient components of food (proteins, fats, carbohydrates, nucleic acids). Also present in the secretions is a protein(s) considered to be an antibacterial factor. The remainder of the exocrine pancreas is mainly ductal tissue that secretes water with ions and varying concentrations of bicarbonate.

2.1. Composition of exocrine pancreatic secretions

Several recent reviews describe the composition and regulation of pancreatic secretions in mammals [8-13]. Readers are referred to these reviews for detailed descriptions of the various enzymes [8], the structure-function relations of the pancreatic acinar cells responsible for enzyme synthesis [9,10], *in vitro* synthesis of enzymes and requirements [11], and the signals and signal transduction pathways that trigger exocrine pancreatic secretion [12-14]. In addition to the large volume of water added to the intestine, pancreatic juice contains three functional groups of solutes. These include digestive enzymes, electrolytes, and the antibacterial factor.

The exocrine pancreatic secretion of the dog contains proteins in excess of 20 mg/ml. This is markedly higher than the 4 mg protein/ml measured in the exocrine secretions of pigs and other omnivores and herbivores [15]. Reports for other species indicate that over 20 proteins are present in the pancreatic juice. When the concentrations of protein and large volumes of secretion measured for omnivores are considered together, the rate of protein synthesis and secretion by the pancreas on a per gram basis exceeds that of any other tissue in the body [16]. Rates of synthesis and secretion may be even greater in carnivorous mammals, because of the need to rapidly digest a more nutrient-dense diet as it transits the relatively short intestines (only 4 to 5 times the body length; [17]) in a short period of time (e.g., only 4 hours in adult mink [18]). In mink the nitrogen content of the chyme in the first part of the small intestine 1.5 hours after a meal is 20% higher than of the food itself [19]. This is consistent with a very high rate of exocrine pancreatic secretion.

There are multiple forms (isozymes) of the digestive enzymes synthesised by the exocrine pancreas, with some of the isozymes having different substrate specificities [20]. The major proteases include endopeptidases and exopeptidases, whose function is to reduce proteins into small peptides, with the release of some free amino acids. The principal endopeptidase of the cat and dog is trypsin, with lower activities for chymotrypsin and elastase. The different types of endoproteases cleave proteins at different sites, releasing a diversity of oligopeptides, which are further reduced in size by exopeptidases that remove amino acid residues from the carboxyl and amino terminal ends of proteins and peptides. The dominant forms in dogs and cats are carboxypeptidases A and B. The proteases are secreted as inactive proenzymes (zymogens) to prevent activation and autodigestion prior to secretion. In addition to an inherent resistance to the various pancreatic hydrolases, protease inhibitors are present in the pancreatic tissues. The proteases are activated only after entering the intestine, by enterokinase, which is produced by the intestinal mucosa and activates trypsin. The activated trypsin then activates additional trypsin as well as chymotrypsin and the other proteases.

Other enzymes present in the pancreatic juice of carnivores include phospholipases for digestion of phosphoglycerides, lipase and its necessary cofactor colipase for degrading long-chain triglycerides, amylase for digestion of complex carbohydrates, and ribonucleases and deoxyribonucleases for degradation of nucleic acids.

Although digestive enzyme activities are better understood for dogs, a large fraction of the information about fluid and electrolyte secretion by the ductal tissue is from studies of the cat pancreas. The pancreatic juice contains bicarbonate to neutralise gastric acid and other electrolytes. Whereas the concentrations of Na^+ and K^+ in pancreatic juice are relatively stable and parallel plasma levels, bicarbonate concentrations vary widely [21] and are reciprocally related to Cl^- concentrations due to exchange mechanisms. The amount of digesta entering the small intestine is an important determinant of bicarbonate secretion and fluid production.

The pancreatic juice of dogs has been shown to have antibacterial properties [22-24] (and personal observations), and similar antibacterial activity has been reported in the pancreatic juice of other mammals (e.g., pigs; personal observations), but not of rats. Although the antibacterial properties of feline pancreatic secretions have not been assessed, the high densities of bacteria that are normally present in the proximal small intestine of many cats [25] may be indicative of low antibacterial activity. In other species, secretion of the antibacterial factor is affected by changes in quantitative input, but is not responsive to the composition of the diet. The active component has been identified as a protein with a molecular weight estimated to be less than 4,000 daltons. The protein is resistant to pancreatic proteases, but is pH-sensitive, and loses its activity when the pH is less than 7.0. The protein is relatively heat stable, as activity is retained and can even be increased on exposure to 65° for 15 min. The protein is inactivated when exposed to 100° C.

The antibacterial factor present in dog pancreatic secretions is reported to have a broad spectrum of activity. Bactericidal activity has been demonstrated for E coli, Shigella, Salmonella, and Klebsiella, whereas the secretions are considered to be bacteriostatic for coagulase positive and negative staphylococci and Pseudomonas, and for Candida albicans. The antibacterial factor does not adversely affect all bacterial groups. Interestingly, many groups considered to be symbiotic, such as Bacteroides and Streptococcus faecalis are not affected, and our preliminary studies indicate that lactic acid bacteria and other groups considered to be beneficial may not be affected. Additional studies are needed to better characterise the responses of the various groups of bacteria present in the gastrointestinal tract and environment to the antibacterial factor. Although it is generally thought that the antibacterial factor is important for preventing bacterial invasion of the pancreatic ducts, leading to pancreatitis, it is possible that the apparent selective action against specific, but not all, bacterial groups may help to "manage" the gastrointestinal bacterial populations. This speculation is corroborated by the common occurrence of small intestinal bacterial overgrowth in dogs with exocrine pancreatic insufficiency (EPI; see later section).

Carnivores differ from omnivores in the proportions of the different digestive enzymes. This is exemplified by the nearly 200-fold higher activity of amylase relative to trypsin in pigs, corresponding to the much higher levels of carbohydrate in the diet. The corresponding ratio for adult mink is less than 1.0, matching the low carbohydrate to protein content of the diet. Although comparable data are not available for dogs and cats, limited values from the literature and our own measurements indicate that the ratios for cats and dogs are lower than those for pigs and more comparable to those for mink.

3. ASSESSING EXOCRINE PANCREATIC FUNCTIONS

Exocrine pancreatic functions are usually assessed indirectly by assaying for the activities of enzymes in peripheral blood or in faecal samples. Although a variety of methods are available to clinicians [reviewed by Williams and Guilford 4], they have limited diagnostic value, on the whole allowing a clinician to determine whether a condition exists, but not the severity of the pathology. For example, faecal samples are easy to collect, but probably do not provide accurate estimates of enzyme activities and secretory patterns, due to autodigestion and bacterial degradation of secreted enzymes. Furthermore, trypsin activity represents 0 - 77% of faecal protease activity [26] even though it is the dominant secreted protease. Measurement of trypsin activity in blood samples (serum trypsin-like immunoreactivity) tends to be preferred by many clinicians and has proven to be dependable for diagnosing EPI. An *in vivo* approach sometimes used involves feeding N-benzoyl-L-tyrosyl-p-aminobenzoic acid (Bentiromide) and measuring plasma or urine concentrations of p-aminobenzoic acid that are absorbed after hydrolysis of the Bentiromide. Although the indirect measures are of diagnostic use, as of now they have only limited applications for establishing the patterns of secretion during development and in response to changes in diet composition.

Direct measures of pancreatic secretions include the use of pancreatic tissue (acute), usually obtained at necropsy, and repeated collection of pancreatic secretions from a single individual (chronic studies). By collecting the entire pancreas and assaying for activity, investigators are able to determine the total secretory capacity of an animal. Although enzyme activities associated with pancreatic tissue correspond to those measured in secretions [27], it is not possible to determine the actual rate of secretion. Furthermore, data from tissue studies are restricted to a single time point and thereby do not contribute to an understanding of diurnal rhythms, meal-induced patterns of synthesis and secretion, and changes over extended periods of time (hours to days or weeks). Chronic collection of pancreatic secretions requires surgical approaches that allow either sampling of the contents of the duodenum at the level of the duodenal papilla or collection of pancreatic secretions by means of a catheter inserted into the duct [reviewed by Zabielski *et al.* 7]. The second approach has proven to be very informative as it is possible to measure the volume and composition of the secretions over prolonged periods of time without contamination and activation of proteases by intestinal secretions. Furthermore, by placing a reentrant catheter into the duodenum after aliquots of pancreatic secretion have been collected and the volume recorded, the remainder can be introduced into the intestine, permitting normal digestive function. To date, chronic investigations of pancreatic juice have been largely restricted to the dog, [32] with only a few similar studies in cats.

Although chronic methods have proven to be very useful to investigators studying the development, adaptation, and regulation of exocrine pancreatic secretion, such approaches are not practical for clinical diagnosis. There is a need to define the relationship between serum faecal enzyme activities and activities in actual pancreatic secretions. This could be done by developing correlative relationships based on chronic and simultaneous measurements of activities in blood, faecal samples and pancreatic juice. These findings would be useful in assessing the magnitude of pancreatic dysfunction in clinical settings.

4. REGULATION AND ADAPTATION OF PANCREATIC SECRETIONS

4.1 Neural and endocrine regulation

Exocrine pancreatic secretion in dogs, cats, and other mammals is regulated by hormonal and nervous signals [28-32]. The presence and composition of nutrients in the small intestine provide critical signals triggering pancreatic secretion. In a similar manner, the presence of food in the duodenum induces postprandial intestinal hyperaemia in dogs, with rates of perfusion highest when high-fat diets are fed, lowest for high-carbohydrate diets, and intermediate for high-protein diets [33]. Several factors and regulatory pathways are implicated in causing the hyperaemia [34], and it is likely that some of these may also influence exocrine pancreatic functions in carnivores.

The pancreas of dogs and cats are well innervated by branches of the vagus and splanchnic nerves [31]. The cholinergic influences associated with the parasympathetic inputs stimulate the acinar and ductal cells, whereas sympathetic inputs are vasoactive, hence affecting the perfusion of the pancreas. Infusion of nutrients into the duodenum triggers parasympathetic inputs that increase the rate of secretion.

Secretin is the best known humoral regulator of pancreatic secretion and is released in response to luminal contents. Secretin causes an increase in the diameter of the canine pancreatic duct and reduces the tonicity of the pancreatic duct sphincter, thereby reducing resistance to flow and increasing secretion [35]. Another key hormone produced by canine mucosa is cholecystokinin (CCK) [36], which triggers secretion of proteins and bicarbonate, and potentiates the responses to secretin [37]. Hormonal regulation of pancreatic functions is made more complex by the involvement of other hormones [32]. For example, parathyroid hormones influence feline exocrine pancreatic secretions indirectly via serum calcium concentrations [38]. Parathyroid dysfunction that results in higher serum calcium lowers pancreatic secretion by altering responses to secretagogues. Another interesting interaction in the dog involves the dependency of normal CCK secretion and gall bladder responses on the digestion of dietary fat by pancreatic lipase [39].

4.2 Responses to diet

Ever since Pavlov's experiments more than 100 years ago with dogs it has been known that both the rate of secretion and the composition of the pancreatic juice are responsive to changes in diet composition. Since then the omnivorous rat has been the principal model used for studying dietary modulation of pancreatic enzyme secretion. More recently, investigators have increasingly been using the pig as a model. Studies with rats have shown that the magnitude of adaptation is greater for proteases and carbohydrases than for lipase, which is only slightly responsive to the amount of fat in the diet [27,40].

There are scattered reports dating as far back as Pavlov's studies, of a correlation between the composition of the diet and the secretion of pancreatic enzymes by carnivores. Analysis of pancreatic juice collected directly from cannulas placed in the duodenum of dogs fed diets high in protein, fat, or carbohydrate has shown that dogs have a capacity to modulate the enzyme composition to match changes in concentrations of substrates [41]. Dogs, unlike rats, can up and down-regulate lipase secretion [42]. The response to diet appears to be somewhat nonspecific, as lipase secretion is higher when dogs are fed a high-protein diet, though the increase is not as great as when a high-fat diet is fed.

The dietary influences are not as obvious when pancreatic enzyme activity is measured indirectly using faeces or serum samples [43] and protease values for some dogs are unchanged even after 6-fold increases in dietary protein. Although faecal protease activity and serum trypsin-like immunoreactivity tend to increase when dogs are fed diets high in protein, differences between dogs and even for samples collected from the same individual can obscure diet effects [43-45]. Still, trypsin-like immunoreactivity is considered by some to be a suitable indicator for studying adaptation to different levels of dietary protein.

The feedstuffs used to formulate diets are an important determinant of adaptive responses. Meat-based diets are more effective at stimulating trypsin secretion than diets prepared with cereal grains [44]. The fat source also influences rates of secretion and adaptive responses in a nonspecific manner. Dogs fed diets with sunflower oil, which is high in polyunsaturated fatty acids, secreted more amylase and lipase, but less chymotrypsin, than dogs fed an identical diet, but with the sunflower oil replaced by olive oil, which is mainly monounsaturated [46]. The differences between the two groups were not apparent when secretions were studied in the basal state. Fatty acid composition has little influence on the pancreatic secretions of the pig, highlighting another difference between omnivorous and carnivorous species that can be traced to the evolutionary diets.

Dogs and cats differ with respect to nutrient requirements and metabolic characteristics [47], and their respective abilities to adaptively modulate the volume and composition of pancreatic secretions. Cats are obligate carnivores and their evolutionary diet contains very little carbohydrate. Accordingly, cats are unable to digest or tolerate high dietary loads of carbohydrate [47, 48], have little ability to up-regulate amylase secretion [48], and the majority of dietary carbohydrate is degraded (fermented) in the colon [50]. Mink, another strict carnivore, similarly has no capacity to adapt secretion of amylase and proteases to match changes in dietary levels of carbohydrate and protein. However, mink can modulate lipase activity [51]. Despite the cat's inability to modulate amylase secretion, chymotrypsin activity will increase when dietary protein is increased. However, feeding a diet low in protein does not lead to a reduction in protease secretion. Dogs are considered to be more omnivorous, and when fed diets with varying proportions of carbohydrate, protein, and lipid there are adaptive changes in the secretion of amylase, proteases, and lipase. Pancreatic secretions of dogs are also responsive to dietary fibre, and even more so than those of rats [52] and pigs [53]. Inclusion of fibre in the diet of dogs increases the volume of pancreatic secretion. Even though the activity of most enzymes per ml does not change, because of the greater volume of secretion there is an increase in total activity secreted. The exception is the decline in lipase, which may partly explain the higher faecal fat content of dogs fed diets containing insoluble fibres.

There are also species differences for the responses to enzyme inhibitors present in feedstuffs. This is particularly true for the trypsin inhibitors present in leguminous plants, such as peas and soya beans, which are often used to lower the cost of sources of protein in animal feeds. Adult dogs fed diets containing up to 15% raw soya bean did not have altered pancreatic growth or secretion of digestive enzymes [54,55]. This contrasts sharply with the pronounced pancreatic hypertrophy reported in young rats and chickens fed diets with trypsin inhibitors. There are also differences between species for the sensitivity of proteases to the inhibitors. For example, trypsin from mink is up to 3,000 times more sensitive to inhibitors extracted from peas than trypsin isolated from pigs and rats [56]. Adding amylase inhibitors to the diet of dogs results in an increase of amylase relative to proteases in the pancreatic secretion and an enhanced response to CCK [5]. These responses have been attributed to the presence of undigested food in the ileum. If the carbohydrate, or any other feedstuff, can be digested, its presence in the ileum will increase enzyme secretion whereas dietary components that can not be absorbed do not elicit a response.

The patterns, mechanisms, and time course of adaptation for the pancreatic digestive enzymes have not been adequately defined for dogs and cats. This is partly related to recent concerns and limitations surrounding the use of dogs and other carnivores as experimental animals as well as the use of different methods to collect secretions and measure enzyme activities. In omnivorous mammals dietary adaptation begins as early as 2-4 hours after a change in diet, is evident after 24 h, with full adaptation requiring 5-7 days [57,58]. Regulation of enzyme activity is by pretranscriptional mechanisms. These findings are consistent with the shifts in proportions of isozymes and the time course of adaptive responses.

The responses of fluid and HCO_3^- secretion to hormonal stimulation are better developed in cats and dogs compared to rats. This may be related to how the evolutionary diet of carnivores requires them to eat large, sporadic, meals that require larger volumes of fluid and high concentrations of HCO_3^- to neutralise gastric acid. In contrast, omnivores tend to eat smaller meals on a frequent basis, need a more constant secretion of fluid and HCO_3^-, and have a reduced secretory response to hormonal stimulation.

There are several other considerations about pancreatic functions that have yet to be explored in carnivores. Fermentation of feedstuffs in the caecum and colon of rats is known to influence pancreatic secretion [59]. Infusing fatty acids into the colon of dogs up-regulates sodium-dependent glucose transport by the proximal intestine, with glucagon-like peptide 1 acting as a signal [60]. Therefore, it can be speculated that the composition of digesta in the distal small intestine, colon, and caecum of dogs and cats could affect pancreatic functions. It is also possible that pancreatic secretions of carnivores influence mucosal absorptive functions, as reported for pigs [61].

5. DEVELOPMENT OF EXOCRINE PANCREATIC SECRETIONS IN CARNIVORES

Digestive system structure and functions change during ontogenetic development [62]. The gastrointestinal tract and associated organs appear during gestation, and subsequent growth and differentiation prepare neonatal mammals so that they are born with a functional digestive system capable of processing and absorbing milk. The pancreas first appears during gestation as a diverticulum from the proximal intestine and this origin is retained by the ducts that carry the digestive secretions to the duodenum. Growth of the pancreas and differentiation of the acinar and ductal cells during gestation prepare mammals for birth, when pancreatic digestive secretions are essential for processing dietary inputs. Mammals differ as to the state of digestive system development at birth and postnatal patterns of change, with the species variation related to length of gestation and evolutionary diets.

The best known age-related changes in digestive functions are those that occur at weaning, when mammals switch from drinking milk to eating the adult diet. Weaning is a critical period of development for puppies and other mammals, and problems of digestion and nutrition are common [63]. A successful transition from milk to the adult diet is dependent on numerous changes in the proportions of digestive enzymes secreted by the intestine and those associated with the brush border of the enterocytes. Although weaning-associated changes are well understood for omnivores, particularly those of agricultural importance, there is little known about age-related changes in the digestive functions of carnivores. This is somewhat surprising when one considers that commercial diets for dogs and cats have been available for nearly 140 years [64]. Only recently have data been available for age-related changes in digestive enzyme activity in intestinal contents of developing dogs and cats [6, 65]. A more comprehensive set of data is available for the digestive enzymes associated with the intact pancreas of developing mink [66].

Trypsin is the dominant endoprotease of adult dogs and cats, with activities about 50-fold higher than those of chymotrypsin [6]. Trypsin activity increases during the first 3 weeks after dogs are born and remains relatively stable thereafter. There is a slight and transient decline at 6 weeks that coincides with when experimental dogs are weaned. Cats differ from dogs in that protease activity is very low at birth, and can not be detected in some individuals. Furthermore, the postnatal increase for trypsin is more gradual compared to dogs, with highest activities measured in the intestinal contents of adult cats.

Lipase activity of dogs increases 4-fold between birth and 3 weeks, with peak activity detected at 9 weeks of age. In the cat, lipase activity was not consistently detected during the first 24 h after birth, but by 3 weeks activities had reached levels that remained stable thereafter. It is likely that a portion of the detected lipase activity in the intestinal contents of developing dogs and cats originated from lingual or gastric secretions and from lipases present in milk [67]. These alternative sources of lipase activity may be of critical importance to neonatal cats to compensate for low levels of pancreatic lipase.

Amylase activity of the intestinal contents is low during suckling for both dogs and cats, corresponding with the virtual absence of substrates in milk. In dogs, amylase activity increases up to 10-fold between 4 and 8 weeks of age [65], which coincides with when puppies begin to eat solid food. Although amylase can be detected in the intestinal contents of cats, activities are lower than those of dogs and the magnitude of the postnatal increase is much lower.

Mink are born at an earlier stage of development than dogs and cats and are considered to be altricial. Corresponding with this, the postnatal pancreatic development is delayed relative to that of the more precocial dogs and cats. For example, protease and lipase activities in intact pancreas do not reach their peaks until the kits are more than 3 months old [66]. Mink are more similar to cats than dogs in that protease and lipase activities are maximal in adults, not in younger animals. Amylase activity is surprisingly high in mink kits for the first 4 weeks after birth after which there is a gradually decrease to the low values characteristic of adults.

The different patterns of pancreatic development appear to be related to the phylogeny and evolutionary diets of dogs, cats, and mink. Dogs are omnivores, and although adult mink are strict carnivores they are members of the marten family (*Mustelidae*), which includes several representatives that are omnivores (e.g. the badger and the skunk). It is possible that the presence in mink of relatively high amylase activities and a paradoxical well-developed ability to transport fructose and glucose [6] represents the retention of an ancestral omnivorous trait. In contrast, cats are members of the *Felidae* which are exclusively carnivores and have either lost or not acquired the ability to process or tolerate high dietary loads of digestible carbohydrate or adapt to changes in the levels of dietary carbohydrate [47-49,68].

From a comparative perspective, dogs, cats, and mink share several similarities with the pancreatic enzyme activities of pigs and other mammals [15]. All of these species are characterised by low activities of amylase, lipase, and the various proteases during suckling, with increases in these activities and a heightened responsiveness to hormonal stimulation. The magnitude of differences between species begins to increase at the time of weaning when mammals switch to the adult diet.

During pregnancy and lactation the secretion of digestive enzymes by the dog pancreas is higher in both the resting and stimulated states [69]. This would enhance digestive capacities when dietary inputs are increased to meet higher metabolic requirements. Similarly, the capacity of the entire length of mouse small intestine to absorb nutrients increases during pregnancy and lactation. Although there is an increase in the volume and bicarbonate content of the dog pancreatic secretion during pregnancy [69], information is lacking for carnivores about age-related changes.

Data are also lacking for age-related changes in pancreatic antibacterial activity of dogs and cats. In pigs there is an increase at the time of weaning [24]. This may allow young pigs to compensate for the loss of antibacterial factors present in milk while at the same time there are increases in the numbers of food-borne bacteria, many of which are potential pathogens.

The very few data that are available for exocrine pancreatic secretion of senescent individuals preclude any generalities about flow rates, composition, and responses to changes in diet composition.

6. COMMON PATHOLOGIES OF EXOCRINE PANCREATIC SECRETION

The most common pancreatic problem facing veterinarians is exocrine pancreatic insufficiency (EPI). The incidence is thought to be greater in dogs than cats, but this might be related more to difficulties in diagnosing the disease in cats than to species differences [70]. EPI is generally associated with atrophy of the pancreatic acinar cells, but in some cases can be attributed to pancreatitis. The risk factors most commonly mentioned include a high-fat diet, age, breed (large breeds, particularly German Shepherds, are at greater risk), and pregnancy [71-73]. The low activities of digestive enzymes are associated with malabsorption of the diet [74] and weight loss [72]. Long-term management of EPI is usually addressed by a combination of reducing the fat content of the diet and providing exogenous pancreatic enzymes [75]. Enzyme supplements are considered effective at increasing digestibility and improving weight recovery and body condition [76-77]. Enteric coating of enzyme tablets does not improve efficacy because of low bicarbonate secretion and impaired dissolution of the coating [72]. The use of low-fat diets is controversial. Although low-fat diets are generally accepted as an appropriate therapeutic approach [76,77], their effectiveness has been questioned by some investigators [78]. Another common manifestation of EPI is bacterial overgrowth of the small intestine (SIBO). The provision of enzyme supplements and modification of diet composition do not reduce the bacterial densities, and they are usually treated by broad spectrum antibiotics. More recently fermentable fibres have been explored as a means to alleviate SIBO due to EPI [79].

Pancreatitis is another common problem for dogs [80], and is often accompanied by biliary disease [81]. The pathogenesis and epidemiology of pancreatitis remain uncertain, but hypersecretion does not appear to be a cause [82]. Elemental diets are often prescribed for pancreatitis to reduce pancreatic stimulation and allow recovery. However, these are not always effective [81]. The pancreas is capable of recovering from damage and can regenerate tissue [83]. Full recovery is possible after short-term blockage of the pancreatic ducts (2-5 days), but long-term blockage (>10 days) can lead to permanent damage.

7. CONCLUSIONS AND PERSPECTIVES

The use of dogs, cats and various omnivores in biomedical research has shown that the cellular and mechanistic bases of exocrine pancreatic functions are shared by mammals. However, these same studies have revealed species-specific patterns of basal secretion, adaptation, and development that are set by genetic determinants that reflect the evolutionary diets of species. As a consequence, data from rats, pigs and other omnivores are of limited value when trying to understand adaptation and development of exocrine pancreatic functions in carnivores.

A better understanding of the patterns and mechanisms of pancreatic functions of carnivores during development into senescence and in health and disease, and their relations with diet composition will facilitate efforts to formulate more effective diets. Although adult dogs have the capacity to adapt pancreatic enzyme secretion to match changes in diet composition, there is a need to understand when these abilities are acquired during development, the range of adaptation, the regulatory signals and mechanisms, and whether these capacities are present in the more carnivorous cats and mink. A better understanding of exocrine pancreatic functions in carnivores will also assist in the advancement of therapeutic approaches for treating diseases and dysfunction of exocrine pancreatic secretion in companion animals and carnivorous species of agricultural importance.

REFERENCES

1. E. Janle-Swain, H.D. Jackson, O.F. Roesel, Insulin and amylase in the postnatal canine pancreas. Proc. Soc. Exp. Bio. Med. 164 (1980) 303.
2. C. Stock-Damge, P. Bouchet, A. Dentinger, M. Aprahamian, J.F. Grenier, Amer. J. Clin. Nutr. 38 (1983) 843.

3. D.A. Williams, The Pancreas, In: Strombeck´s Small Animal Gastroenterology, Guilford, W.G., S.A. Center, D.R. Strombeck, D.A. Williams and D.J. Mejer (eds), 3rd. edition. Philadelphia: W.P. Saunders Company 381 (1996).
4. D.A. Williams and W.G. Guilford, Procedures for the evaluation of pancreatic and gastrointestinal tract diseases. In: Strombeck´s Small Animal Gastroenterology, Guilford, W.G., S.A. Center, D.R. Strombeck, D.A. Williams and D.J. Mejer (eds), 3rd. edition. Philadelphia: W.P. Saunders Company (1996) 77.
5. D. Koike, Z. Yamadera and E.P. DiMagno, Gastroenterology 108 (1995) 1221.
6. J. Elnif and R.K. Buddington, Adaptation and development of the exocrine pancreas in dogs and cats. In: Recent Advances in Canine and Feline Nutrition, Reinhart, G.A. and D.P Carey (eds.), Vol. 2, Orange Frazier Press, Wilmington, OH, (1998) 217.
7. R. Zabielski, V. Leśniewska, and P. Guilloteau, Reprod. Nutr. Dev. 37 (1997) 385.
8. M.E. Lowe, The structure and function of pancreatic enzymes, In: Physiology of the Gastrointestinal tract Johnson, L.R. ed), 3rd edition, Raven Press, New York, (1994) 1531.
9. F.S. Gorelick and J.D. Jamieson, The pancreatic acinar cell: Structure-function relationships, In: Physiology of the Gastrointestinal Tract, Johnson, L.R. (ed), 3rd edition, Raven Press, New York, (1994) 1353.
10. G. Scheele and R. Jacoby, J. Biol. Chem. 258 (1983) 2005.
11. H. Rinderknecht, I.G. Renner, A.P. Douglas and N.F, Adham, Gastroenterology 75 (1978) 1083.
12. R.T. Jensen, Receptors on pancreatic acinar cells, In: Physiology of the Gastrointestinal Tract, Johnson, L.R. (ed.), 3rd edition, Raven Press, New York, 1346 (1994) 1346.
13. D.I Yule and J.A. Williams, Stimulus-secretion coupling in the pancreatic acinus, In: Physiology of the Gastrointestinal Tract, Johnson, L.R. (ed), 3rd edition, Raven Press, New York, (1994) 1447.
14. T.E. Solomon, Control of exocrine pancreas secretion, In: Physiology of the Gastrointestinal Tract, Johnson, L.R. (ed), 3rd edition, Raven Press, New York (1994) 1499.
15. S.G. Pierzynowski , B.R. Weström, J. Svendsen, L. Svendsen, and B.W. Karlsson, Int. J. Pancreatol. 18 (1995) 81.
16. Rasmussen T., H. Harling, L. Thim, S. Pierzynowski, B. Westrom, and J. Holst. Amer. J. Physiol. 264 (1993) G22.
17. C.E. Stevens and I.A. Hume, Comparative Physiology of the Vertebrate Digestive System, 2nd edition, New York, Cambridge University Press (1996) 400.
18. N.E. Hansen, Z. Tierphysiol. Tierernährg. u. Futtermittelkde. 40 (1978) 285.
19. R. Scymeczko and A. Skrede, Acta Agric, Scand 40 (1990) 189.
20. I. Huerou-Luron, E. Lhoste, C. Wicker-Planquart, N. Dakka, R. Toullec, T. Corring, P. Guilloteau and A. Puigserver, Proc. Nutr. Soc. 52 (1993) 301-313.
21. B.E. Argent and R.M. Case, Pancreatic ducts: Cellular mechanism and control of bicarbonate secretion, In: Physiology of the Gastrointestinal Tract, Johnson, L.R. (ed.), 3rd edition, Raven Press, New York, (1994) 1473.
22. E. Rubenstein, Z. Mark, J. Haspel, G. Ben-Ari, Z. Dreznik, D. Mirelman, and A. Tadmor, Gastroenterology 88 (1985) 927.
23. S.G. Pierzynowski, P. Sharma, J. Sobczyk, S. Garwacki, W. Barej, and B. Weström, Pancreas 8 (1993) 546.

24. S.G. Pierzynowski, P. Sharma, J. Sobczyk, S. Garwacki, and W. Barej, Intern. J. Pancreatol.12 (1992) 121.
25. K. Johnston and R.M. Batt, Vet. Rec. 132 (1993) 362.
26. D.A. Williams, S.D. Reed and L. Perry. J. Amer. Vet. Med. Assoc. 197 (1990) 210.
27. M.I. Grossman, H. Greengard and A.C. Ivy, Amer. J. Physiol. 138 (1942) 676.
28. R. Zabielski, P. Podgurniak, S. Pierzynowski and W. Barej, Exp. Physiol. 75 (1990) 401.
29. A. Grossman, Comp. Biochem. Physiol 78B (1984) 1.
30. M.V. Singer, T.E. Solomon, J. Wood and M.L. Grossman, Amer. J. Physiol. 238 (1980) G23.
31. M. Singh and P.D. Webster, Gastroenterology 74 (1978) 294.
32. S.J. Konturek, J. Tasler, W. Obtulowicz, D.H. Coy and A.V. Schally, J. Clin. Invest. 58 (1976) 1.
33. H. Siregar and C.C. Chou, Amer. J. Physiol. 242 (1982) G27.
34. R.H. Gallivan and C.C. Chou, Amer. J. Physiol. 249 (1985) G301.
35. E.P. DiMagno, J.C. Hendricks, R.R. Dozois and V.L.W. Go, Dig. Dis. Sci. 26 (1981) 1.
36. V.K. Eysselein, G.A. Eberlein, W.H. Hesse, M.V. Singer, H. Goebell and J.R. Reeve Jr., J. Biol. Chem. 262 (1987) 214.
37. W.Y. Chey, K.Y. Lee, T.-M. Chang, Y.-F. Chen and L. Millikan, Amer. J. Physiol. 246 (1984) G248.
38. P. Layer, J. Hotz, H.P. Schmitz-Moormann and H. Goebell, Gastroenterology 82 (1981) 309.
39. S. Watanabe, K.Y. Lee, T.-M. Chang, L. Berger-Ornstein and W.Y. Chey, Amer. J. Physiol. 254 (1988) G837-G842.
40. P. Desnuelle, J.P. Reboud and A. Ben Abdeljill, Influence of the composition of the diet on the enzyme content of rat pancreas, In: The Exocrine Pancreas Normal and Abnormal Functions, (Reuck, A.V.S. and M.P. Cameron, (eds), Ciba Foundation, London, (1962) 90.
41. H.R. Behrman and M.R. Kare, J. Physiol. 205 (1969) 667.
42. C. Stock-Damgé, P. Bouchet, A. Dentinger, M. Aprahamian, and J.F. Grenier, Amer. J. Clin. Nutr. 38 (1983) 843-848.
43. P.J. Canfieldand A.J. Fairburn, Res. Vet. Sci. 34 (1983) 24.
44. A.M. Merritt, C.F. Burrows, L. Cowgill, and W. Street, J. Amer. Vet. Med. Assoc. 174 (1979) 51.
45. T. Carro, and D.A. Williams, Amer. J. Vet. Res. 50 (1989) 2105.
46. M.C. Ballesta, M. Mañas, F.J. Mataix, E. Martínez-Victoria and I. Seiquer, Brit. J. Nutr. 64 (1990) 487.
47. Legrand-Defretin, V. Keynote Lecture 2, Differences between cats and dogs: a nutritional view, Proc. Nutr. Soc. 53 (1994) 15.
48. J.G. Morris, J. Trudell, and T. Pencovic, Brit. J. Nutr. 37 (1977) 365.
49. E. Kienzle, J. Anim. Physiol. a. Anim. Nutr. 69 (1993) 92.
50. E. Kienzle, J. Anim. Physiol. a. Anim. Nutr. 69 (1993) 102.
51. C. Simoes-Nunes, G. Charlet-Léry and J. Rougeot, Adaptation of the exocrine pancreas secretion to diet composition in mink, Proc. III. Congr. Anim. Fur Prod. 16 (1984) 1.
52. C. Stock-Damage, M. Aprahamian, F. Raul, W. Humbert and P. Bouchet, J. Nutr. 114 (1994) 1076.
53. T. Żebrowska and A.G. Low, J. Nutr. 117 (1987) 1212.

54. J.R. Patten, E.A. Richards and J. Wheeler, Life Sci. 10 (1971) 145.
55. Patten J.R. and E.A. Richards,The effect of raw soybean on the pancreas of adult dogs. Proc. Soc. Exp. Biol. Med. 137 (1971) 59.
56. J. Elnif, N.E. Hansen, K. Mortensen, and H. Sørensen, Properties of mink trypsinogen/trypsin and chymotrypsinogen/chymotrypsin compared with corresponding properties of these enzymes from other animals. Proc. IV Int. Congr. Fur Anim. Prod. (1988) 308.
57. J.C. Dagorn and R.G. Lahaie, Biochim. Biophys, Acta 654 (1981) 111.
58. R.G. Lahaie and J.C. Dagorn, Biochim. Biophys. Acta 654 (1981) 119.
59. E.F. Lhoste, I. Catala, M. Fiszlewicz, A.M. Gueugneau, F. Popot, P. Vaissade, T. Corring, and O. Szylit, Brit. J. Nutr. 75 (1996) 422.
60. S.P. Massimino, M.I. McBurney, C.J. Field, A.B.R. Thomson, M. Keelan, M.G. Hayek, and G.D. Sunvold, J. Nutr. 128 (1998) 1786.
61. D.D.P. Lundin, S. Lundin, H. Olsson, B.W. Karlsson, B.R. Weström, and S.G. Pierzynowski. Pharm. Res. 12 (1995) 1478.
62. I.R. Sanderson and Walker, W.A. (eds), Development of the Gastrointestinal Tract, B.C. Decker Inc., Hamilton, Ontario, Canada, (1999).
63. H.F. Hintz, Vet. Tech. 9 (1988) 372.
64. L.P. Case, D.P. Carey and D.A. Hirakawa (eds), Canine and Feline Nutrition, Mosby, St. Louis, MO, (1995).
65. V.E. Kienzle, J. Anim. Physiol. a. Anim. Nutr. 60 (1988) 276-288.
66. J. Elnif, N.E. Hansen, K. Mortensen, and K. Sørensen, Production of digestive enzymes in mink kits, Proc. IV Int. Congr. Fur Anim. Prod. (1988) 320.
67. S.J. DeNigris, M. Hamosh, D.K. Kasbekar, T.C. Lee, and P. Hamosh, Biochem. Biophys. Acta 959 (1988) 38.
68. R.K. Buddington, J.W. Chen and J.M. Diamond, Amer. J. Physiol. 261 (1991) R293.
69. V. Rosenburg, J. Rudick, M. Robbiou, D.A. Dreiling, Ann. Surg. 181 (1975) 47.
70. M. Räihä and E. Westermarck, Acta Vet. Scand. 30 (1989) 447.
71. G. Pidgeon, and D.R. Strombeck, Amer. J. Vet. Res. 43 (1982) 461.
72. D.A. Williams, S.D. Reed, and L. Perry. J. Amer. Vet. Med. Assoc. 197 (1990) 210.
73. T.H.B. Haig, Surg. Gynecol. Obst. 131 (1970) 914.
74. R.M. Batt, J. Sm. Ani. Prac. 33 (1992) 161.
75. J.W. Simpson, I.E. Maskell, J. Quigg, and P.J. Markwell, J. Sm. Ani. Prac. 35 (1994) 133.
76. G. Pidgeon, J. Amer. Vet. Med. Assoc, 181 (1982) 232.
77. E. Westermarck, V. Myllys and M. Aho, Pancreas 8 (1993) 559.
78. E. Westermarck, J.T. Junttila and M.E. Wiberg, Amer. J. Vet. Res. 56 (1995) 600.
79. M.D.Willard, R.B. Simpson, E.K. Delles, N.D. Cohen, T.W. Fossum, D. Kolp and G. Reinhart, Amer. J. Vet. Res. 55 (1994) 654.
80. A.K. Cook, E.B. Breitschwerdt, J.F. Levine, S.E. Bunch, and L.O. Linn, Risk factors associated with acute pancreatitis in dogs: 101 cases (1985-1990), J. Am. Vet. Med. Assoc. 203 (1993) 673.
81. M.D.Kerstaein and R.M. Tonkens, Surg. Gynecol. Obst. 143 (1976) 253.
82. T. Kimura, G.D. Zuidema and J.L. Surg. 88 (1980) 661.
83. T.T. White and D.F. Magee, Surg. Gynecol. Obstet. 114 (1962) 463.

Biology of the Pancreas in Growing Animals
S.G. Pierzynowski and R. Zabielski (Editors)
© 1999 Elsevier Science B.V. All rights reserved.

Characteristics of pancreatic exocrine secretion in herbivores

E. Harada and T. Takeuchi

Department of Veterinary Physiology, Faculty of Agriculture,
Tottori University, Tottori 680-0945, Japan

The characteristics of pancreatic exocrine secretion in herbivores were compared with those in other species. The pig, rat, chicken and duck showed a high amylase to protein ratio in pancreatic juice. The rabbit and sheep secreted amylase-low juice; especially the sheep showed high trypsin and chymotrypsin to protein ratios, just like the mink. The pancreas of sheep showed a high responsiveness to secretin and CCK as well as to vagal stimulation. These characteristics of pancreatic exocrine secretion may correlate closely with food intake behaviour.

SCFAs, which are the major end products of microbial fermentation in the rumen of ruminants, stimulate pancreatic exocrine secretion directly. However, there are differences among species in the response induced by SCFAs: the pancreas of sheep, guinea pigs and voles responds to these fatty acids, but that of rats, rabbits, cats and fowl does not. These findings are compatible with the view that pancreatic enzyme secretion is induced by SCFAs only in those species in which SCFAs can be produced and utilized as a major energy source. Although it has been reported that the secretory process induced by SCFAs in ovine pancreatic acinar cells resembles that of ACh and may be mediated by intracellular Ca ions, the precise cellular mechanisms underlying the species specificity of the response of the exocrine pancreas to SCFAs have yet to be determined. A possible role for SCFAs in pancreatic exocrine secretion, as a potent stimulator and/or modulator, was proposed in the herbivores.

1. INTRODUCTION

A large number of investigations have been carried out in different species to elucidate the morphological and physiological characteristics of gastrointestinal tracts. It is very interesting to compare these characteristics in various species with different eating behaviours. Digestive enzyme components in the pancreas are drastically changed by food composition and are adapted to making the digestive system more effective. The predominant factor regulating pancreatic exocrine secretion may differ among species and may be related to specific eating behaviour [1]. In the ruminant, short-chain fatty acids (SCFAs), which are major end products of microbial fermentation in the rumen, are potent stimulators of pancreatic endocrine [2,3] and exocrine secretion [4]. In this chapter, the characteristics of exocrine pancreatic secretion in herbivores, a comparison of the pancreatic secretory response to SCFAs in several species, the mechanisms by which SCFAs influence secretion and the physiological significance of SCFAs will be described, primarily with reference to our own studies.

424

2. COMPARISON OF THE EXOCRINE PANCREAS IN VARIOUS ANIMALS

2.1. Digestive enzyme component in pancreatic juice
Adaptation of the pancreatic enzymes to dietary composition has been well documented in many species. In rats, pancreatic amylase and protease are increased within a few days of the introduction of a carbohydrate and protein diet, and the level of lipase is elevated by a high fat diet [5]. Furthermore, pancreatic enzyme alterations are observed on treatment with adrenaline, glucagon and thyroxin [6], on application of different stressful stimuli [7] and during cold acclimation [8].

Regarding digestive enzyme components, Harada *et al.* [1] analysed amylase, trypsin and chymotrypsin activities in pancreatic juice collected under anaesthesia in several species. As shown in Figure 1, the pigs, rats (omnivores), chickens and ducks (aves) showed a higher amylase to protein ratio than the other animals, and a lower trypsin to protein ratio, with the exception of pigs. The herbivores (rabbits and sheep) showed a lower amylase to protein and higher trypsin and chymotrypsin to protein ratios. The characteristic of a low amylase and high protease content in the pancreatic juice of sheep resembled that seen in mink (carnivore). A large proportion of the total protein of bovine pancreatic juice is composed of proteolytic enzymes or their respective zymogens. The proteolytic components which have been identified account for 72 % of the total protein of bovine pancreatic juice, whereas only 2 % of the protein has amylolytic activity [9]. Thus, it was concluded that the high level of proteolytic enzyme activities in ruminants may allow the digestion of microbial protein produced by fermentation in the rumen.

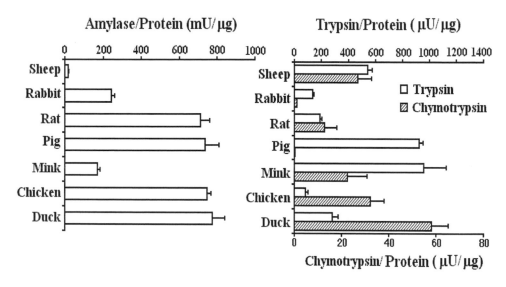

Figure 1. Comparison of the ratios of amylase, trypsin and chymotrypsin to protein in the pancreatic juice evoked by CCK injection in several species. Drawing made from data in Harada *et al.* [1] with permission.

2.2. Pancreatic secretory response

The major part of the pancreatic exocrine secretion during digestion depends on the release of secretin and CCK from the upper small intestine [10]. However, the degree of secretion induced by these peptides varies greatly from species to species. Although the cephalic, gastric and intestinal phases all contribute to the total response of the exocrine pancreas to feeding [12], the predominant factor regulating pancreatic exocrine secretion may differ from species to species and be related to specific feeding behaviour [1].

Pancreatic exocrine secretory responses induced by vagal stimulation, intravenous injection of CCK and intraduodenal infusion of synthetic trypsin inhibitor were compared in various mammalian and avian species under anaesthesia [1]. Trypsin inhibitor is known to induce endogenous CCK release from the intestine by direct and/or indirect actions. The secretory response of juice flow and protein output evoked by each stimulation is shown in Figure 2.

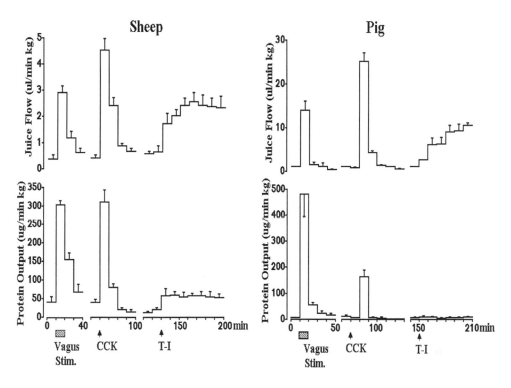

Figure 2. Time course of pancreatic secretory response of juice flow and protein output evoked by vagal stimulation (15 Hz, 5 mA, 5 ms), intravenous injection of CCK (2 U/kg) and intraduodenal infusion of synthetic trypsin inhibitor (T-I: 200 mg/kg) in sheep and pigs. Each figure is drawn on a different scale.

Although the response to vagal stimulation and CCK administration in sheep was much weaker than in pigs, it was fairly good, and both juice flow and protein output were stimulated by the infusion of trypsin inhibitor (Figure 2). These responses to vagal

426

stimulation, CCK injection and trypsin inhibitor infusion are compared with those of other species in Figure 3.

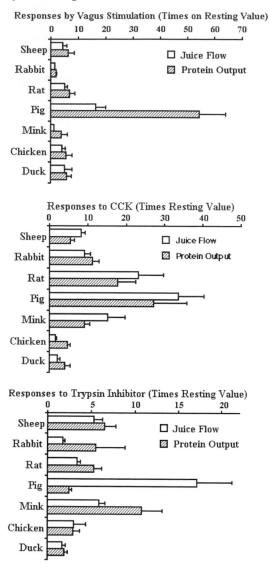

Figure 3. Comparison of pancreatic response to vagal stimulation (15 Hz, 5 mA, 5 ms), CCK injection (2 U/kg) and intraduodenal infusion of synthetic trypsin inhibitor (200 mg/kg) in several species. The magnitude of the response was calculated from the mean value of pancreatic juice flow or protein output for 20 min during and after stimulation compared to the basal value before stimulation. The response to trypsin inhibitor was calculated from the mean value for 60 min after the infusion.

The pancreas of pigs and rats (omnivores) which secreted amylase-rich juice was controlled vagally or hormonally. The pancreas of the mink (carnivore), which secreted protease-rich juice, was controlled predominantly by luminal stimulation. The pancreas of the rabbit and sheep (herbivores) secreted amylase-low juice and showed a high responsiveness to CCK. The chicken and duck (aves) secreted amylase- and chymotrypsin-rich juice, which was weakly controlled by the vagus and by hormones. Moreover, species differences in the basal level of pancreatic juice flow were also observed. The basal levels in rats, rabbits and aves were much higher than those in pigs and mink. These observations indicate that the basal level of pancreatic juice flow and the predominant factor in the pancreatic secretory response of each animal may correlate closely with food intake behaviour; carnivores eat intermittently while herbivores and aves eat more or less continuously.

Gastrointestinal peptides, particularly secretin, may be important in the regulation of lectrolyte secretion from the pancreas and of bile formation in dogs [13], in cats [14] and in man [15]. However, in herbivores, at least the non-ruminant type, bile formation may be relatively insensitive to gastrointestinal peptides [16]. Shaw and Heath [17] demonstrated that the control of bile formation in rabbits and guinea pigs differs from that in other species, and it is possible that these differences are related to the temporal pattern of their eating habits. Most herbivores eat more or less continuously, and thus bile and pancreatic juice may be expected to enter the duodenum at frequent intervals throughout the day [18]. In sheep, secretin is the major peptide that regulates pancreatic exocrine secretion and hepatic bile production [11]. Thus, the vagal nerve seems to dominate the regulatory mechanisms and secretin is suggested to be a key regulatory peptide in ruminants, whereas the relative importance of CCK and related peptides is minor [10, 11, 19-21].

3. PANCREATIC SECRETORY RESPONSES TO SCFAs

3.1. The secretory response in ruminants

The predominant factor regulating pancreatic exocrine secretion may differ from species to species and be related to specific eating behaviour [1]. Ruminants derive most of their energy from SCFAs, mainly acetate (AA), propionate (PA), and butyrate (BA). These fatty acids are major end products of microbial fermentation in the rumen and are absorbed into the portal circulation. SCFAs, with the exception of AA, are potent stimulators of insulin release in ruminants [2, 22], but not in monogastric animals [23]. Since plasma insulin levels increase rapidly after administration of physiological doses of BA and are not accompanied by an appreciable elevation of plasma glucose levels, Mann *et al.* [3] suggested that BA could have a direct action on the sheep pancreas.

In vitro studies have demonstrated that PA and BA act directly on the insulin secretory mechanism [25,26,36]. Manns *et al.* [2,3] showed that BA stimulates the secretion of insulin in sheep via its direct action on the pancreas, the process being independent of either hyperglycaemia or hyperketonaemia. Moreover, Horino *et al.* [23] demonstrated that all the lower fatty acids stimulate the secretion of insulin in sheep, valerate being the most effective in this respect. Acetate, acetoacetate and ß-hydroxybutyrate were without any effect on the secretion of insulin.

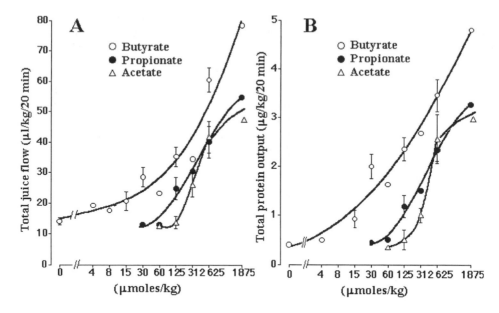

Figure 4. Relationship between dose of SCFAs and: pancreatic juice (A) and protein output (B) in anaesthetised sheep. Individual values were summed up over a 20-min period in response to each SCFA. Reproduced with permission from Harada and Kato [4].

Moreover, Basset [24] showed that intravenous administration of PA and BA causes striking increases in the plasma glucagon concentration of sheep.

Although some of the SCFAs are clearly potent stimulators of both glucagon and insulin release under appropriate conditions in ruminants, it had not been shown whether these fatty acids modified the secretory response of the exocrine pancreas. Harada and Kato [4] studied the secretory response of the exocrine pancreas to SCFA in sheep (Figure 4). BA, PA and AA dose dependently (15-1875 μmoles/kg) stimulated pancreatic juice flow and protein and amylase output under anaesthesia. The response to BA (625 μmoles/kg) wascomparable with thatobtained with 2 U/kg CCK pancreozymine (Boots), and was significantly greater than that observed with PA or AA. It was known that BA and PA are potent stimulators of insulin and glucagon release, whereas AA has little effect in sheep [2, 22, 24]. However, it was shown that the exocrine pancreas responded not only to BA and PA, but also to AA [4]. Detectable responses were obtained with 15 μmol/kg BA, 125 μmol/kg PA, and 312.5 μmol/kg AA. These secretory responses to SCFAs were confirmed in sheep [27], goats [28, 29] and cows [30]. Thus, in the ruminant, it is clear that SCFAs are potent stimulators not only of pancreatic endocrine [2] but also exocrine secretion [4].

3.2. Specific responses in herbivores

It is known that there are species differences in the secretory response induced by SCFAs, not only in the endocrine pancreas, but also in the exocrine pancreas. SCFAs are the major end products of microbial fermentation in the rumen and large intestine and are absorbed into the portal circulation. SCFAs, with the exception of AA, are potent stimulators of insulin [2, 22] and glucagon [24] release in ruminants, but not in monogastric animals [23]). Infusion of PA into rats, rabbits or pigs had no effect on the plasma insulin, whereas both PA and BA provoked a rise in plasma insulin in the sheep, goat and cow. Thus it was concluded that PA and BA are stimulators of insulin secretion in the sheep and cow but not in non-ruminant species [23].

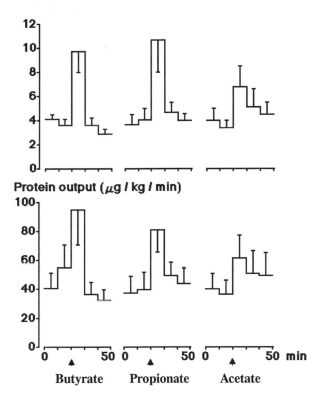

Figure 5. Secretory response of exocrine pancreas induced by SCFAs in guinea pigs. Butyrate, propionate and acetate were administered intravenously (625 µmoles /kg). Data from Harada [31].

The secretory response of the exocrine pancreas to SCFAs was examined under anaesthesia in monogastric species [31]. As shown in Figure 5, intravenous administration of BA, PA and AA (625 µmoles/kg) stimulated pancreatic juice flow and protein output in guinea pigs. The secretory response to BA and PA was higher than that to AA and was much less effective than that of sheep reported previously [4]. However, infusion of these SCFAs into rabbits, cats, rats, ducks and fowl had no effect on the exocrine pancreas. Thus it seems possible that in some species, SCFAs regulate pancreatic exocrine secretion as well as having nutritional value.

The Japanese field vole, *Microtus montebelli*, belonging to the Muridae family, lives mainly on grass in the field and has a large, well developed oesophageal sac which can digest plant cellulose [32]. Voles are natural grass eaters with a digestive system capable of gastric and caecal digestion of fibre. Kudo *et al.* [33,34] have shown that aerobic and anaerobic bacteria are present in the vole's oesophageal sac, where fermentation takes place to produce SCFAs. Consumption of PA and BA in the oesophageal membrane of voles was higher than that found in mice, and the pattern of metabolism of SCFAs in the vole liver is similar to that in domestic ruminants [35]. These results suggest that digestion and metabolism in the oesophageal sac of voles may be similar to that in ruminants. Moreover, Figure 6 shows that the plasma glucose concentration in the Japanese field vole is half of that in mice, similar to that seen in ruminants [28]. From these observations, it seems possible that pancreatic exocrine secretion in Japanese field voles may be regulated by SCFAs. Harada [28] has studied the digestive enzyme secretory response induced by SCFAs in Japanese field voles, mice and goats, using isolated pancreatic lobule preparations. As shown in Figure 7, there was a dose-dependent amylase release in response to SCFAs in goats. Some response was obtained in the voles with AA and PA, but in mice there was no response to SCFAs. The dose of AA and PA that induced a half-maximal response in voles was almost the same as the dose used for goats [28]. Further, it should be noted that the ratio of amylase to protein in the pancreas of voles is one to two, whereas trypsin levels are four times higher than in mice (Figure 6). Consequently, these results support the view that the secretory function of the exocrine pancreas in voles closely resembles that in domestic ruminants.

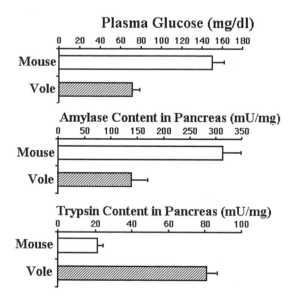

Figure 6. Comparison of the plasma glucose concentration, and the amylase and trypsin content in the pancreas of mice and Japanese voles. Drawing made from data in Harada [28].

4. MECHANISM BEHIND THE EFFECT OF SCFAs ON THE EXOCRINE PANCREAS IN HERBIVORES

As mentioned above, short-chain fatty acids are the major end products of microbial fermentation in the alimentary canal of some herbivores and stimulate pancreatic endocrine and exocrine secretion. Recently, Mineo *et al.* [37] revealed that a single carboxylic group and a definite number of hydrocarbon chains in SCFAs are necessary to induce insulin and glucagon secretion in sheep *in vivo*. However, no published data are available concerning the precise mechanism whereby SCFAs influence endocrine secretion.

On the other hand, there are some reports related to the cellular mechanisms that may be involved in stimulation of exocrine secretion by SCFAs. Ovine pancreatic exocrine secretion is evoked by vagal stimulation [1]. Harada and Kato [4] examined whether the secretory response to BA was mediated by the parasympathetic nervous system in sheep. The secretory response to BA was not affected by pre-treatment with atropine and hexamethonium, although the response to vagal stimulation was completely abolished, indicating that the effect of BA is not mediated by the parasympathetic nervous system. Magee [38] and Taylor [39] examined the effect of intra-ruminal and -duodenal infusion of SCFAs on the pancreatic exocrine secretion of sheep, and suggested that the indirect action was due to duodenal acidification of the SCFAs. However, in preparations of isolated lobules of sheep [4], goats and Japanese field voles [28], amylase release increased in response to SCFAs in a concentration-dependent manner. It was therefore concluded that SCFAs act directly on the pancreatic acinar cells to stimulate enzyme secretion, and not indirectly through vagalstimulation or via gut peptides.

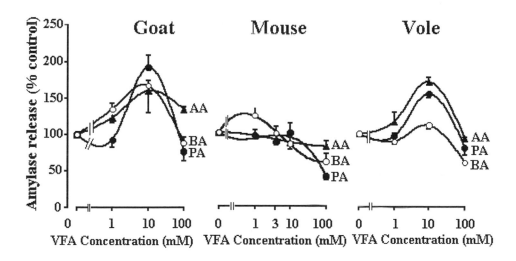

Figure 7. Concentration dependence of SCFA (VFA)-induced amylase release from isolated lobule preparations in the goat, the vole and the mouse. Individual values represent the response to acetate (AA), propionate (PA) and butyrate (BA). Reproduced with permission from Harada [28].

Katoh and Tsuda [27] investigated the action of ACh and SCFAs on acinar cells of the exocrine pancreas of sheep by measuring amylase release, ^{45}Ca efflux from superfused segments and the membrane potential in the acinar cells. They concluded that the cellular secretory process evoked by SCFAs was qualitatively similar to that evoked by ACh, and that Ca ions might be an important mediator for these secretagogues in the acinar cells of the pancreas in sheep. SCFAs are known to be involved in various physiological functions, including cell proliferation, Na+ transport, and colonic motility [40,41]. The administration of BA changes the fluidity of the membrane in colon cancer cells [41]. Vasorelaxant actions of SCFAs might be related to an increase in artery cAMP levels (42). The action appears to be mediated by the stimulation of adenylate cyclase rather than by an inhibition of phosphodiesterase [43, 44]. Changes in ionic Ca and cAMP have been linked as coupling factors between cell excitation and hormonal release [45]. Moreover, a mono-carboxylic group in the structure of SCFAs is essential for stimulation of pancreatic exocrine [29] and endocrine [37] secretion in ruminants. It was proposed that a specific receptor, which could recognise the chemical structure of SCFAs, may exist on the surface of the pancreas in ruminants. Recently, we observed that in isolated perifused pancreatic acini of the guinea pig the presence of PA (100 μM) in the solution significantly enhanced the amylase release induced by Ca ionophores (Figure 8). This result reveals that a dose of PA too low to evoke amylase release may modulate the pancreatic secretory responses induced by other secretagogues. The possible mechanisms of signal transduction in pancreatic exocrine secretion induced by SCFAs are summarised in Figure 9. Following are the presumed possibilities: [1] an increase in intracellular Ca ion concentration, [2] changes in IP3 and

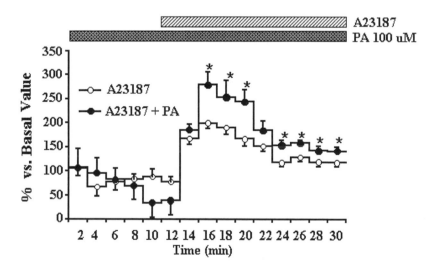

Figure 8. Effect of propionate on Ca ionophore-induced amylase release in pancreatic acini of the guinea pig. The response to a combination of Ca ionophore A23187 (5 μM) and propionate (PA; 100 μM) was compared to the value obtained with A23187 alone. Each value represents the mean (%) against the basal value before stimulation.

DAG, [3] changes in cyclic nucleotides, [4] the presence of a specific receptor, [5] changes in the fluidity of the cell membrane, [6] PK-C-related changes, [7] changes in ion channels. Thus, further investigations are required to reveal whether the response of the exocrine pancreas to SCFAs is mediated by changes in cyclic nucleotides or IP3 via specific receptors, or related to PK-C, in herbivores.

4. PHYSIOLOGICAL SIGNIFICANCE OF EXOCRINE SECRETION INDUCED BY SCFAs

In spite of the fact that the secretion of insulin [2,23,36] and glucagon [24] in ruminants, and amylase in some herbivores [4,28,31] can be altered by certain SCFAs, the physiological significance of the effect of SCFAs on the exocrine pancreas has remained in doubt, as well as that on endocrine secretion. This is because the peripheral concentration of SCFAs is very low, due to conversion to other substrates or clearance by the rumen epithelium and liver [46].

PA and BA are rapidly cleared from portal blood by the liver, and their concentrations in peripheral circulation remain extremely low, even in fed sheep [46]. Horino et al. [23] assumed that any species should eventually evolve an insulin secretory response mechanism to that nutrient or type of nutrient which represents the major metabolic or energy substrate for that particular organism. In these terms, the SCFAs, which represent the major source of energy for ruminants, should provoke insulin release primarily to aid in the conversion of SCFAs to two storage forms, namely, glycogen and fat.

The question was raised whether the insulinogenic effectiveness of SCFAs in ruminants was a constitutional characteristic present at birth or developed only after the animal ceased to be monogastric and had developed a functioning forestomach. The results obtained with the monogastric newborn lamb clearly indicate that the capacity to respond to SCFAs is a constitutional characteristic, present at birth, and support the concept that the evolution of an insulin secretory response mechanism in various species has been determined, at least in part, by the nature of the metabolites constituting the major nutritional mix for the species [23].

In regard to pancreatic exocrine secretion, Harada and Kato [4] demonstrated that the injection of 15 µmol/kg of BA into the jugular vein caused a 2.5-fold increase in protein output and 1.5-fold increase in juice flow. The threshold concentration of PA and AA was about one order of magnitude higher than that of BA; PA (125 µmol/kg) and AA (312.5 µmol/kg) caused a doubling of the protein output and juice flow. The higher threshold for AA compared with other SCFAs correlated with the relatively high concentration of AA in peripheral blood, as AA is not completely removed by the liver [23]. Thye et al. [47] determined that concentrations of AA, PA and BA in the carotid artery increased markedly during the first 90 min of feeding in lactating ewes. Peak concentrations were attained at 3 hours: about 3.4 mM, 140 µM, and 65 µM, respectively. These concentrations were roughly similar to the doses of SCFA that elicited detectable secretory activity in this study. Thus, it is concluded that SCFA is a potent stimulator of pancreatic exocrine secretion.

Recently, Harada et al. (1999) investigated the action of one of the major SCFAs, PA, on amylase release induced by several secretagogues, using isolated pancreatic acini from several different animals (unpublished data). Carbachol-induced amylase release from the pancreatic acini was enhanced by addition of PA to the perifused solution in the guinea pig,

434

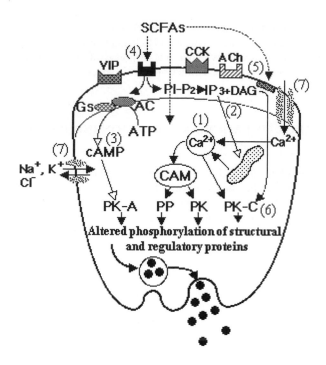

Figure 9. Possible mechanism of signal transduction in pancreatic exocrine secretion induced by SCFAs: (1) increases in intracellular Ca ion levels, (2) changes in IP3 and DAG, (3) changes in cyclic nucleotides, (4) the presence of a specific receptor, (5) changes in the fluidity of the cell membrane, (6) PK-C-related changes and (7) changes in ion channels.

but not in the mouse. Whether the mechanism of this enhancement involves the mobilisation of intracellular Ca ions or cAMP is now being analysed. Thus, the enhancing action of SCFAs on cholinergic control of pancreatic exocrine secretion may be physiologically relevant, and a characteristic phenomenon in some herbivores.

As described above, there is a species difference in the pancreatic exocrine secretion evoked by SCFAs. It may be that pancreatic enzyme secretion is induced by SCFAs only in those species in which SCFAs are produced and utilised as a major energy source. These findings support the view that the pancreatic response evoked by SCFAs may be useful as an index of the degree of production and utilisation of these fatty acids in each species. Furthermore, *Microtus montebelli* species might serve as a unique model for investigating nutritional and metabolic diseases in ruminants.

In conclusion, SCFAs are potent stimulators of pancreatic exocrine secretion at high concentrations and/or modulators at low concentrations, suggesting the presence of a specific regulatory system in the pancreas of the ruminant, guinea pig, and vole.

435

REFERENCES

1. E. Harada, K. Nakagawa and S. Kato, Comp. Biochem. Physiol., 73A (1982) 447.
2. J.G. Manns and J.M. Boda, Amer. J. Physiol., 212 (1967) 747.
3. J.G. Manns, J.M. Boda and R.F. Willes, Amer. J. Physiol., 212 (1967) 756.
4. E. Harada and S. Kato, Amer. J. Physiol., 244 (1983) G284.
5. J.C. Dagorn and D. Giogi, J. Morisset and J.E. Solomon (eds.), Gastrointestinal Hormone and Growth Factors, CRC Press, Boston, 1994, pp.89.
6. E. Harada and S. Kato, Jpn. J. Vet. Sci., 44 (1982) 589.
7. E. Harada, Comp. Biochem. Physiol., 98A (1991) 333.
8. E. Harada and T. Kanno, J. Physiol. Lond., 260 (1976) 629.
9. P. Keller, E. Cohen and H. Neurath, J. Biol. Chem., 233 (1958) 344.
10. J. Croom Jr, L.S. Bull and I.L. Taylor, J. Nutr., 122 (1992) 191.
11. E. Harada, M. Niiyama and B. Syuto, Comp. Biochem. Physiol., 85A (1986) 729.
12. J.E. Thomas, R.F. Pitts (ed.), The External Secretion of Pancreas, Charles C. Thomas, Springfield, 1950, pp.1.
13. R.S. Jones and W.C. Meyers, Ann. Rev. Physiol., 41 (1979) 67.
14. T. Scratcherd, W. Taylor (ed.), The Biliary System, Blackwells, Oxford, 1965, pp.515.
15. S.T. Konturek, A. Dabrowski, B. Adamczyk and J. Kulpa, Am. J. Dig. Dis., 14 (1969) 900.
16. H.M. Shaw and T.J. Heath, Aust. J. Biol. Sci., 25 (1972) 147.
17. H.M. Shaw and T.J. Heath, Q. J. Exp. Physiol., 59 (1974) 93.
18. H.N. Jordan and R.W. Phillips, Amer. J. Physiol., 234 (1978) E162.
19. R. Zabielski, S. Kato, S.G. Pierzynowski, H. Mineo, P. Podgurniak and W. Barej, Exp. Physiol., 77 (1992) 807.
20. R. Zabielski, T. Onaga, H. Mineo and S. Kato, Biomed. Sci., 13 (1992) 243.
21. R. Zabielski, T. Onaga, H. Mineo and S. Kato, Exp. Physiol., 78 (1993) 675.
22. J.P. Bell, L.A. Salamonse, G.W. Holland, E.A. Espiner, D.W. Beaven and D.S. Hart, J. Endocrinol., 48 (1970) 511.
23. M. Horino, L.J. Machlin, F. Hertelendy and D.M. Kipnis, Endocrinol., 83 (1968) 118.
24. J.M. Basset, Aust. J. Biol. Sci., 25 (1972) 1277.
25. H.N. Jordan and R.W. Phillips, Amer. J. Physiol., 234 (1978) E162.
26. Y. Sasaki, T.E.C. Weekes and J.B. Bruce, J. Endocrinol., 72 (1977) 415.
27. K. Katoh and T. Tsuda, J. Physiol. Lond., 356 (1984) 479.
28. E. Harada, Comp. Biochem. Physiol., 81A (1985) 539.
29. K. Katoh and T. Yajima, Pfluers Arch., 413 (1989) 256.
30. S. Kato, N. Asakawa, H. Mineo and J. Ushijima, Jpn. J. Vet. Sci., 51 (1989) 1123.
31. E. Harada, Vth World Conference on Animal Production, 2 (1983) 529.
32. F.B. Golley, J. Mammal., 41 (1960) 89.
33. H. Kudo, Y. Oki and H. Minato, Bull. Nippon Vet. Zootech. Coll., 28 (1979) 13.
34. H. Kudo and Y. Oki, Jap. J. Vet. Sci., 43 (1981) 299.
35. Y. Obara and N. Goto, Jap. J. Zootech. Sci., 51 (1980) 393.
36. F. Hertelendy, J.J. Machlin, Y. Takahashi and D.M. Kipnis, J. Endocrinol., 41(1968) 605.
37. H. Mineo, Y. Hashizume, Y. Hanaki, K. Murata, H. Maeda, T. Onaga, S. Kato and N. Yanaihara, Amer. J. Physiol., 267 (1994) E234.
38. D.F. Magee, J. Physiol. Lond., 158 (1961) 132.
39. R.B. Taylor, Res. Vet. Sci., 3 (1962) 63.

436

40. W. von Engelhardt, K. Ronau, G. Rechkemmer and T. Sakata, Anim. Feed Sci. Tech., 23 (1989) 43.
41. M.D. Dibner, K.A. Ireland, L.A. Koerner and D.L. Dexter, Cancer Res., 45 (1985) 4998.
42. C.W. Nutting, S. Islam and J.T. Daugirdas, Amer. J. Physiol., 261 (1991) H561.
43. J.R. Sheppard and K.N. Prasad, Life Sci., 12 (1973) 431.
44. K.N. Prasad and P.K. Sinha, In Vitro, 12 (1976) 125.
45. R.P. Rubin, Calcium and the secretory Process, N.Y. Plenum, 1974.
46. E.N. Bergman and J.E. Wolff, Amer. J. Physiol., 221 (1971) 586.
47. F.W. Thye, R.G. Warner and P.D. Miller, J. Nutr., 100 (1970) 565.

Biology of the Pancreas in Growing Animals
S.G. Pierzynowski and R. Zabielski (Editors)
1999 Elsevier Science B.V.

Characteristics of pancreatic function in fish

Å. Krogdahl and A. Sundby

The Norwegian School of Veterinary Science,
Department of Biochemistry, Physiology and Nutrition,
P. O. Box 8146 Dep., N-0033 Oslo, Norway

Great variation exists between fish species regarding the anatomy and physiology of the digestive organs. Present knowledge on the fish pancreas is only fragmentary and further work is needed. In most species of fish the pancreas is not a distinct organ, but spread as a *pancreas diffusum* between or on the walls of internal organs and vessels. Endocrine pancreatic tissue is found in the vicinity of exocrine pancreatic tissue or localised in specialised "Brockmann bodies". Pancreatic digestive enzymes in fish seem to have characteristics similar to those of the corresponding enzymes in other farm animals. One exception is the efficiency of nutrient hydrolysis by enzymes in cold water species, which in many cases is an order of magnitude higher than in mammals and birds. Carboxylester lipase is responsible for triglyceride hydrolysis. Endocrine, paracrine and neural mechanisms are involved in the regulation of enzyme secretion from the fish pancreas. Cholecystokinin plays a major role. Products of nutrient hydrolysis are more potent stimulators of enzyme secretion than the intact nutrients, at least in salmonids. Enzyme secretion also appears to be regulated according to the feeding level and diet composition. The ability to adapt amylase secretion to dietary carbohydrate level seems to be restricted to herbivorous and omnivorous species.

The major hormones produced in fish pancreatic islets are insulin, somatostatin-22-28 (SST-22-28), somatostatin-14 (SST-14), glucagon, glucagon-like-peptide (GLP) and pancreatic polypeptide (PP). Insulin seems to have a positive effect on growth. Insulin and glucagon/GLP have opposing metabolic effects. Insulin stimulates anabolism and accumulation of macromolecules, and has an inhibitory effect on regulatory enzymes catalysing lipolysis, glycogenolysis, and gluconeogenesis. The same enzymes are stimulated by glucagon and GLP. Basic amino acids stimulate insulin, glucagon and GLP secretion. In fish, the basic amino acids stimulate insulin directly, while in mammals, the stimulatory effect on insulin is mediated by the glucagon family peptides. Glucagon and GLP are strong insulin secretagogues in mammals, while in fish, glucagon and GLP have no effect on insulin secretion under most physiological conditions. Basic amino acids are stronger insulin secretagogues in fish than glucose. Somatostatins exert metabolic effects in fish indirectly through a reduction of insulin and glucagon levels, and directly by enhancing glycogenolysis and lipolysis. Pancreatic polypeptide from fish has been found to stimulate appetite in mammals. Whether it also has this effect in fish remains to be learned.

1. INTRODUCTION

Fish cultivation has ancient traditions, 3 – 4000 years, in China and Southeast Asia. In the Mediterranean area, fish ponds date back a thousand years or more as well. Reproduction under farming conditions, a prerequisite for efficient cultivation, was not successful until the 18th century. Since then fish cultivation has expanded rapidly all over the world, in particular during the last century, both regarding volume and number of species. The number of fish species presently under cultivation is not known, but it is certainly greater than the number of cultivated terrestrial animals. Among the cultivated fish species the anatomical and physiological diversity is also greater than that observed in the cultivated birds and mammals. The recent increase in economic importance of fish cultivation is closely related to increasing knowledge of fish physiology, nutrition and breeding. However, research into nutrition and breeding in fish has only gained strength during the last few decades. Progress in the accumulation of knowledge is slow due to the many species that need to be covered, from herbivorous fish in warm fresh water to carnivores in cold sea water. Knowledge of digestive physiology and nutrition is necessary for the development of efficient diets that can support the growth and health of the fish. Our knowledge of the fish pancreas is still limited and highly fragmentary compared to that of other domestic animals. Salmonids, being of high economic value to many countries in Europe and America, have gained more scientific attention than most other species.

The present chapter reviews results from recent investigations undertaken to understand the function of the fish pancreas, with the main emphasis on digestive enzymes, regulation of enzyme production and secretion, as well as on pancreatic hormones and their function. It should be kept in mind while reading this review, that our information is based on studies of a limited number of species. General statements regarding fish may therefore, in the future, be found to have many exceptions. As knowledge regarding salmonids is greater than that of other species, our presentation reflects this situation.

The pancreas as a source of bicarbonate for neutralisation of chyme in fish, has gained very little attention by the scientific community and will not be discussed in the present review.

2. THE EXOCRINE PANCREAS

2.1. Anatomy and morphology

2.1.1. Anatomy of the mature fish

The anatomy of the gastrointestinal tract and associated organs varies greatly between different species of fish. This variation is partly related to the variation in diet between carnivores, omnivores and herbivores [1]. Some species feed on dead, others on living material, some feed solely on microorganisms, others on larger plants and animals, and some just eat what they can get. However, even species that have a similar dietary selection may show great variation in intestinal anatomy. Even within species we find variation between developmental stages. The dietary selection of fish larvae differs from that of adults, being less complex during the larval period. Most fish species start out as carnivores.

In the majority of bony fish species (*Osteichytes*) pancreatic tissue takes the form of a *pancreas diffusum.* Pancreatic tissue may surround the intestine and pyloric caeca. The pyloric caeca are blind diverticula found in the pyloric region in some fish species, and greatly expand the absorptive surface area of the intestine. They are found in numbers ranging from a few to more than a thousand. Pancreatic tissue may also be located in the submucosa of the intestine or in the liver, on the gall bladder and along the major abdominal veins. In fish with a *pancreas diffusum* the tissue is often difficult to identify macroscopically. Figure 1 illustrates pancreatic tissue in Atlantic salmon (*Salmo salar* L.), located between the pyloric caeca, and in sea bream (*Sparus aurata*), located in the liver

A. ATLANTIC SALMON   B.   SEA BREAM

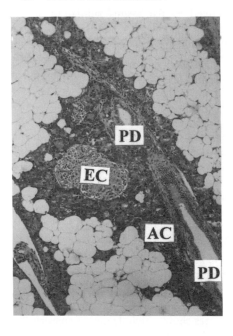   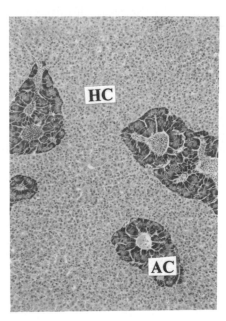

Figure 1. Exocrine pancreas of Atlantic salmon (*Salmo salar* L) (A) and sea bream (*Sparus aurata*) (B). Note in A: acinar cells (AC), endocrine cells (EC), fat cells (FC) and pancreatic duct (PD). Note in B: acinar cells (AC) and hepatocytes (HC). Photo: Trygve Poppe.

(hepatopancreas). The European eel (*Anguilla anguilla*) and catfish (*Parasilurus asotus*) are among the exceptional species, with compact pancreatic organs as in higher vertebrates. The tissue of the exocrine pancreas is, in all species, tubuloalveolar and the zymogen granules show supranuclear localisation. In Figure 1A both exocrine and endocrine pancreatic tissues are illustrated, but these tissues are not always found in close proximity. Rainbow trout

(*Oncorhynkus mykiss*) is one example, in which most of the endocrine pancreatic tissue is gathered in Brockmann bodies (See chapter 3).

The fish pancreas is supplied by nerve fibres from the pancreatic nerve. Both adrenergic and cholinergic fibres have been reported [2].

Collection of secreta from the pancreatic acini appears to differ between fish species. In the flounder (*Paralichthys olivaceus*), secreta seems to be collected from all the pancreatic tissue into one major duct, to be emptied in the vicinity of one of the few pyloric caeca [3]. The studies of Einarsson and Davies [4] indicate that in Atlantic salmon, pancreatic secreta is emptied into pyloric caeca and the anterior intestine through a large number of smaller ducts.

2.2. Enzymes in acinar cells and pancreatic juice

The variety of pancreatic digestive enzymes secreted by fish seems similar to that of mammals [5-10]; trypsin, chymotrypsin, elastase, carboxypeptidase A and B, carboxylester lipase, phospholipase A_2, ribonuclease, amylase. However, most of the enzymes from the various fish species are not well characterised regarding kinetics, temperature and pH-optima, amino acid sequence, secondary structure, immunological cross-reactivity with mammalian enzymes etc.

2.2.1. Proteinases

The endopeptidases trypsin, chymotrypsin and elastase are the best described pancreatic enzymes in fish [11-18]. Their specificity resembles, qualitatively, that found for pancreatic serine proteinases in other animals, although the degree of overlap between chymotrypsins and elastases may differ [19]. For the enzymes that have been investigated, pH optima are in the range 7 - 10 [20-22]. As in other animals, there are two or more isozymes for each enzyme [18,19,23-25]. The isozymes may possess different kinetic properties and show variation in substrate affinities, isoelectric point, pH optima and temperature stability [18,26].

Salmon isotrypsins, both anionic and cationic, have molecular weights of about 25 kDa [19]. Trypsins from Atlantic cod (*Gadus morhua*) also have molecular weights close to those of mammalian trypsins [24]. However, trypsins from capelin (*Mallotus villosus*) [27] and anchovy (*Engraulis enchrasicholus*) [28] are somewhat larger, 27 - 31 kDa. Trypsins from Atlantic cod have recently been subject to investigation of gene nucleotide structure, amino acid sequence and molecular structure [19]. The enzymes show a high degree of conservation in comparison with mammalian enzymes. About 90 % homology exists between trypsin from the Atlantic cod and the rat. However, immunological cross-reactions are weak.

Chymotrypsins from Atlantic cod and Atlantic salmon have also been described regarding gene nucleotide structure, amino acid sequence and molecular structure [20], confirming the conservation of the structure through evolution and the close relationship with trypsins. Work on chymotrypsins from common carp (*Cyprinus carpio*) and rabbitfish (*Siganus canaliculatus*) [7,18,22,29] emphasises that the main characteristics vary little between species.

Pancreatic elastase has been reported to exist in a large number of species [13,14,16,30-32], and elastase isoforms have been identified in dogfish (*Scyliorhinus canicula*) [25]. The two isoforms show different kinetic parameters, but are similar regarding pH and temperature optima. Their molecular weights are 26.5 kDa, close to the weight found for elastases in catfish (*Parasilurus asotus*) [30], Atlantic cod [33] and common carp [29]. The elastase from rainbow trout seems to consist of only one single polypeptide chain and to have an extremely high isoelectric point (pI>11) [32].

A non-serine pancreatic proteinase, which is a metalloproteinase with elastolytic activity, has also been reported in several fish species [30,34]. Both elastases solubilize cross-linked elastin.

Very little information exists regarding carboxypeptidase A and B in fish. In the study by Overnell [6] on enzymes from Atlantic cod, these enzymes showed pH optima of 8 - 10 and dependency upon zinc. Carboxypeptidase B purified from common carp, has a molecular weight of about 34.5 kDa [7]. This is close to the size of the corresponding porcine enzyme. However, the difference in amino acid composition seems to be greater than that between fish and porcine trypsins [7,29].

Pancreatic proteinases in fish species living under cold water conditions have higher catalytic efficiencies than the corresponding enzymes in mammals [16,24,27,35,36]. The main difference appears to be in K_m which is lower in cold water species of fish than in mammals [15]. For some species a higher K_{cat} also adds to this difference in enzyme efficiency. Modifications in amino acid sequence close to the active site of the enzymes are most likely the structural basis for the difference in efficiency. The difference is considered to be an evolutionary adaptation to compensate for the effect of temperature on enzyme activity [29,37].

2.2.2. Carboxylester lipase and phospholipase A$_2$

Carboxylester lipase seems to be the most important pancreatic lipase in fish [8,38-40]. The colipase-dependent triacylglycerol lipase found in mammals seems absent. Therefore, carboxylester lipase is considered to be responsible for triglyceride hydrolysis as well as hydrolysis of wax, cholesterol and vitamin esters. Carboxylester lipase has been purified from Atlantic cod and Atlantic salmon [40,41] showing characteristics similar to those of mammalian carboxylester lipases. The enzyme is dependent on bile salt for hydrolysis of water-insoluble substrates, whereas soluble substrates may be hydrolysed in the absence of bile salt. Lipase from Atlantic salmon has a molecular weight in the range of 56 - 60 kDa, comprising 257 amino acids [41]. A comparison with human, rat and bovine carboxylester lipase reveals 57 - 59 % homology [40]. Studies of substrate specificity show greater affinity for fatty acids in the 1,3-position of triglycerides than in the 2-position, with a pH optimum in the range 8 - 9. According to the work of Lie and Lambertsen [42] on homogenates of Atlantic cod pancreatic tissue, it appears that fish lipases hydrolyse triglycerides faster than wax esters, and that the enzymes hydrolyse ester bonds with polyunsaturated fatty acids at higher rates than bonds with saturated fatty acids. Ester bonds with myristic and palmitic acid seemed resistant to hydrolysis. Moreover, rapid release of glycerol from the reaction mixture indicates that Atlantic cod lipase, at least, is able to hydrolyse bonds in all positions of the triglyceride [42].

Phospholipase A$_2$ has been purified from red sea bream (*Pagrus major*) [10] in two isoforms [43]. Their molecular weights were estimated to be about 14 kDa, and the enzymes were dependent on both calcium and bile salt. Optimum activity appeared in the pH range 8 - 10. Choline- and glycerophospholipids seem to be hydrolysed more efficiently than ethanolamine and inositol phospholipids. However, the specific activities and substrate specificities were affected differently by calcium and bile salt concentrations [43].

2.2.3. Amylase

Amylase activities of pancreatic tissues and intestinal contents vary greatly between species of fish and are in general higher in herbivorous and omnivorous than in carnivorous fish [21,22,44-51]. In some carnivorous fish, amylase levels are very low. In our work with Atlantic salmon, we have made efforts to measure amylase activities in intestinal contents and pancreatic tissue [51]. The values found have been close to the detection limit, indicating that, in Atlantic salmon, amylase secretion is very low.

No information has been found in the literature on molecular characteristics of fish amylases.

2.3. Regulation of the exocrine pancreas

2.3.1. Regulatory mechanisms

Endocrine, paracrine and neural mechanisms are all involved [2] in the regulation of secretion from the exocrine pancreas in fish. Cholecystokinin (CCK) seems to play an important regulatory role through both endocrine and paracrine pathways. CCK-like immunoreactive peptides have been detected in endocrine cells of the mid intestine and the pyloric caeca of several fish species [52-56]. Moreover, there are indications that CCK may be a key substance in a neuro-endocrine regulation of the exocrine pancreas as well, at least in some species [57]. One should, however, keep in mind that both CCK and gastrin possess the same highly antigenic C-terminal pentapeptide, making it difficult to differentiate between them with the immunological methods most often used in these studies. On the other hand, porcine CCK injected intraperitoneally has been found to stimulate a dose-dependent release of enzymes from pancreatic/pyloric tissue, as well as contraction of the gall bladder in Atlantic salmon [58]. Porcine CCK also released trypsin and chymotrypsin from an *in vitro* preparation of Atlantic salmon pancreas [58]. In a similar experiment with killifish (*Fundulus heteroclitus*), CCK-octapeptide triggered secretion of pancreatic lipase [59].

2.3.2. Factors affecting enzyme secretion

Several studies have been concerned with factors that trigger regulatory mechanisms in fish, revealing important species differences. A series of experiments have been performed on rainbow trout, investigating the effects of infusion of nutrients and nutrient hydrolysates on enzyme secretion from the pancreas. The results showed that the products of hydrolysis are much more potent stimulators than the intact nutrients [60]. Amino acid mixtures caused increased enzyme secretion, whereas intact protein with a similar amino acid composition was ineffective. Hence, rainbow trout has been described as having a stimulatory response similar to that of the dog [60]. Single amino acids, such as phenylalanine and tryptophan, also stimulated enzyme secretion, whereas soya bean trypsin inhibitors were unable to trigger enzyme secretion under the prevailing experimental conditions. Sea bass (*Dicentrarcus labrax*) larvae have shown a similar response to amino acid mixtures and intact protein [61,62].

Under normal feeding conditions, adding increasing levels of soya bean trypsin inhibitors to fishmeal-based diets for Atlantic salmon has been found to stimulate trypsin secretion, and to decrease enzyme concentration in pancreatic tissue [63]. Atlantic salmon appeared to be able to compensate for the action of the trypsin inhibitors by increasing the enzyme secretion, but only to a certain degree. At higher levels of inhibitor, decreased trypsin activity of the chyme as well as decreased digestibilities of protein and fat were observed. Rainbow trout seem to react in a similar manner to Atlantic salmon when fed with soya bean trypsin inhibitors [64,65].

Studies with rainbow trout indicate that fish regulate their pancreatic enzyme stores according to diet composition. Proteolytic activity of pancreatic tissue, measured 24 hours after the last meal, increased with increasing levels of dietary protein [66].

In several fish species, intestinal amylase activity correlates positively with dietary carbohydrate level and feeding intensity [50,67]. The ability to adapt amylase secretion to match carbohydrate level in the diet and feed intake seems restricted to herbivorous and omnivorous fish. In rainbow trout, increasing the dietary starch level actually reduced the amylase activity in the chyme [68]. This reduction was, however, considered to be due to adsorption to the starch molecules.

According to results of experiments with Atlantic salmon [69] starvation causes accumulation of digestive enzymes in pancreatic tissue, whereas feeding causes emptying. These experiments also showed that feeding triggers secretion when food arrives in the intestine, about 4 - 14 hours after feeding, whereas resynthesis takes place during the ensuing hours.

2.4. Development of the exocrine pancreas in fish larvae

The development of gastrointestinal function in fish larvae has gained much attention in the great efforts made to find suitable nutrient sources and a suitable dietary composition for larval feed. Dietary composition is of crucial importance for survival, development and end-product quality. For many marine fish species live feed is still mandatory in the early larval stages for successful cultivation. Studies on turbot (*Scophthalmus maximus*) [70] and sea bass [71] showed a fully differentiated cytology in the exocrine pancreas from day one after hatching. Development after hatching appeared mainly to involve growth in tissue size, an increase in the number of zymogen granules and an elevation in enzyme concentration. However, a secretory response upon feed intake may be lacking during the first few days, and differences may exist in the onset of response for the different pancreatic enzymes, as demonstrated for sea bass [72]. Sea bass larvae showed an increase in amylase content in response to increasing dietary carbohydrate level from day 18 after hatching, whereas a corresponding response in proteinase content to changes in protein level was not apparent until after 35 days. Thus, even though structurally the pancreas seems fully developed, the regulatory system may not be functional, or is not turned on until later in the maturation of the larvae. This is in accordance with results of studies of the development of pancreatic enzyme activity in several species [61,62,70,71,73-76]. In some species amylase activity has been shown to decrease after an initial increase [72,77,78], which has been suggested to indicate that the early changes in digestive enzymes reflect different nutrient requirements at different stages of life [72,77].

3. THE ENDOCRINE PANCREAS IN FISH

In some teleost species, the pancreatic endocrine islet cells are found together with exocrine pancreas in small units in scattered locations around the gallbladder and in the adipose tissue between the pyloric caeca. In other species the endocrine pancreas may be almost completely separated from the exocrine pancreas and localised in whitish or pinkish oval or round structures called Brockmann bodies, adjacent to the gall bladder. The Brockmann bodies consist of many small islets of endocrine cells and several large islets, "principal islets". A principal islet is a large accumulation of endocrine tissue, surrounded by a thin layer of exocrine cells. The Brockmann bodies were first described by Heinrich Brockmann (1846) in sculpin (*Cottus scorpius)* and Atlantic cod. Later these structures were found in coho salmon (*Oncorhynchus kisutch*), halibut (*Hippoglossus hippoglossus*), tuna (*Thunnus germo),* anglerfish (*Lophius americanus*), sea bream, tilapia (*Orechronus nilotica*) and others.

Immunohistological studies have identified a concentration of insulin-producing B-cells in the central part of the islets. Close to the B-cells are D2-cells that produce somatostatin-14 (SST-14). Somatostatin-25 (SST-25) is produced in DI cells, located more to the periphery of the islets. [79,80,81]. The A-cells produce glucagon and glucagon-like peptide (GLP) and are located next to the SST-25 producing cells. The close topographic association between the different somatostatin immunoreactive cells and insulin and glucagon immunoreactive cells might indicate the existence of specific paracrine regulation of each endocrine cell type [82]. Pancreatic peptide (PP) and neuropeptide Y (NPY)-positive cells are also located in the periphery of the islets.

The comparative quantity of the major islet hormones in Brockmann bodies from coho salmon may be indicated by the amounts obtained after purification. This was in μg/mg: 1.2 for insulin, 1.0 for SST-25, 0.35 for GLP, 0.16 for glucagon, 0.08 for SST-14 and 0.004 for PP [83,84,85,86].

3.1. Insulin

3.1.1. Gene and peptide structure

The chum salmon (*Oncorhynchus keta)* insulin gene consists of 3 exons and 2 introns with a total of ca 1560 base pairs. Chain B and 6 amino acids of the C-peptide are coded for in exon 2, while the remainder of the C-peptide and the A-chain are coded for in exon 3 [87]. By southern blotting and PCR the presence of 2 insulin genes has been shown in the chum salmon [88].

Northern blots of Brockmann body RNA from anglerfish, hagfish (*Myxine glutinosa*) and chum salmon indicate a single mRNA transcript of 840, 1050 and 760 nucleotides [89,90,91], respectively. This transcript is translated into a single precursor molecule and processed into a single-chain proinsulin peptide consisting of B-chain-C-peptide-A-chain. In mammals it has been shown that the BCA chain is converted to insulin, where the B-chain and A-chain are joined by S-S bridges, by the serine proteinases prohormone convertase PC2 and PC3 [92].

Insulin has been purified and sequenced from many fish species. Sequence comparison shows that the insulin peptide is very well conserved through evolution. Human insulin has retained 72% amino acid identity with salmon insulin. In spite of this, salmon or other fish insulin can not be measured with a mammalian radioimmunoassay (RIA), because the cross-reactivity of salmon and other fish insulin with a mammalian system is too small. A homologous insulin RIA has been available for measuring cod insulin since the mid-seventies [93], and for measuring insulin in salmonids [84] and others, since the beginning of the eighties.

3.1.2. Factors affecting insulin production

For a long time it was believed that carnivorous fish e.g. salmonids were lacking in insulin, as the plasma glucose profile following a glucose load was quite similar to that found in human diabetic patients. However, after developing the homologous RIA a different picture evolved. Whereas the plasma level of insulin in humans is normally below 1 ng/ml and up to 3.2 ng/ml after a glucose load, the level in fish plasma is higher: about 5-10 ng/ml (range 0-50 ng/ml).

In mammals, glucose is the most important insulin secretagogue, while in fish, the amino acids: arginine, leucine, lysine, serine and threonine are more insulinotropic than glucose. The potency of these amino acids, however, varies among fish species.

In mammals, arginine stimulates insulin secretion through glucagon, while in fish, the insulinotropic effect of glucagon is very weak or nonexistent [94,95]. By giving arginine along with anti-glucagon and anti-GLP it was shown that arginine stimulates insulin secretion directly [96]. The negative effect of somatostatin on plasma insulin levels found in mammals has also been reported in fish. Injection of both SST-25 and SST-14 into juvenile coho salmon reduced plasma insulin levels [97]. The effect of glucose on plasma insulin levels is higher after oral than after intramuscular administration. This might be due to orally-induced secretion of secretin and GIP, which both stimulate insulin secretion [98].

Plasma insulin levels in salmonids vary during the life cycle; elevated levels are found in connection with critical energy-consuming periods, like smoltification and spawning. High plasma insulin levels are favourable for the accumulation of lipid and glycogen. These stores will subsequently be important in handling the critical energy-consuming periods [99,100,101]. As in mammals, it has been shown in rainbow trout (*Oncorhynchus mykiss),* that physical activity reduces plasma insulin levels [102].

The secretion of insulin from secretory granules is stimulated by nutrients and modulated by hormones and neurotransmitters. An elevation in plasma insulin has been measured as little as ½ hr after feeding in rainbow trout [103]. Maximum levels were reached 2 hours after feeding, both in rainbow trout and brown trout (*Salmo trutta*), [103,104]. Fish can handle a period of feed restriction and starvation much better than most mammals. This may be due to lower body temperature and a lower metabolism. Salmonids themselves may starve voluntarily for long periods before spawning. The size of the fish and the stage in their life cycle may influence the effect of starvation on plasma insulin levels. Thus, no changes in plasma insulin levels were found in large (about 8 kg) rainbow trout following 2 - 6 weeks of starvation, while a significant reduction in plasma insulin levels was recorded in small (about 2 kg) rainbow trout of the same age [105].

3.1.3. Effects of insulin

Insulin is primarily involved in the regulation of metabolic energy in connection with the nutritional state of the animal. Insulin is considered to be more important as a growth factor in non-mammalian than in mammalian vertebrates. A significant positive correlation between plasma insulin level and body weight has been demonstrated in rainbow trout, Atlantic and coho salmon, and juvenile sea bass [106, 107]. Similar results have been observed in the Atlantic cod [108,109]. Juvenile Chinook salmon (*Oncorhynchus tshawytscha*) reared on high and low rations with high and low fat content, showed significant correlation between plasma insulin and growth rate [110].

Most studies indicate anabolic effects of insulin on protein metabolism. Insulin has been found to increase ^{14}C-leucine entry into hepatocytes, to increase incorporation of ^{14}C-leucine into proteins and to increase protein secretion from isolated coho salmon liver cells [111]. Ablett et al. [112] reported significant increases in muscle protein in rainbow trout following bovine insulin injection every other day for about 2 months. A direct stimulatory effect of mammalian and salmon insulin on skeletal growth was shown by studying (^{35}S) sulphate and thymidine incorporation into the branchial cartilage of the European eel and several salmon species [113,114,115]. In mammals, it is reported that proinsulin is more potent than insulin in promoting growth [116]. In healthy humans, proinsulin makes up about 3-5% of the insulin levels, rising to 15-35% in familial diabetes [117]. Since proinsulin has not yet been isolated in salmonids, and since there are few mammalian insulin anti-sera which can distinguish between hormone and prohormone, we may be measuring proinsulin together with insulin in salmonids. The effects of proinsulin and insulin on skeletal growth in salmonids have been compared. Mammalian proinsulin and salmon and mammalian insulin were incubated with branchial cartilage from salmonid gills. Incorporation of (^{35}S) sulphate indicated that both insulin and proinsulin possess a growth-stimulating capacity. Insulin exerted effects at physiological concentrations, proinsulin only at supra-physiological levels [118].

In rainbow trout, bovine insulin injections caused a dose-related increase in lipids in skeletal muscle [112], and in juvenile Chinook salmon a significant correlation between plasma insulin levels and body fat has been reported [110].

The plasma triacylglycerol level appears to be regulated by insulin. The plasma fatty acid concentration tends to decrease following insulin administration as a result of increased esterification into triacylglycerols. Lipase activity was elevated in coho salmon following immunoneutralisation of insulin by a specific anti-insulin serum. Thus insulin inhibits lipase and thereby inhibits the degradation of triacylglycerol [119]. While studying lipase activation in rainbow trout liver, Harmon et al [120] found that increased lipolysis was correlated with increased phosphorylation of lipase. Insulin administration would depress phosphorylation and inhibit lipolysis. *De novo* synthesis of fatty acids from ^{14}C acetate in cultured trout liver cells was stimulated by insulin [121]. However, no effect of insulin was found on two regulatory enzymes of hepatic lipid synthesis in catfish [122].

In fish, as in mammals, insulin stimulates the uptake of glucose and amino acids from the blood into muscle cells and hepatocytes. In addition to activation of glucose uptake, insulin was found to depress the rate of gluconeogenesis in a dose-dependent manner in rainbow trout [123]. These authors also reported an insulin-dependent activation of pyruvate kinase activity in rainbow trout liver and thus activation of glycolysis. Here, insulin seems to exert its effect directly on pyruvate kinase activation, in contrast to the situation in the rat, where insulin acts indirectly on pyruvate kinase by antagonising the effects of glucagon. Ablett *et al.* [112] found an increased oxidative clearance of glucose in rainbow trout following insulin injection. However, this increased oxidative rate could not be observed by other investigators [123].

The effect of insulin injection on hepatic and muscle glycogen metabolism in fish is also controversial. Anti-insulin injection is reported to decrease liver glycogen [124], while insulin injection has been reported to have variable effects [125]. A reduction in liver glycogen after insulin injection might be due to an insulin-induced hypoglycaemia which will stimulate glycogen phosphorylase, and thus glycogen hydrolysis, through an allosteric control.

The message transduction of insulin in fish seems to be similar to that in mammals, including binding to a membrane receptor and a subsequent autophosphorylation of tyrosine residues on the receptor. However, the total specific binding and number of receptors per unit weight of piscine white skeletal muscle were lower than the corresponding values for mammalian skeletal muscle. When different fish species were compared regarding the insulin receptor along with tyrosine kinase activity, omnivorous fish such as carp had much higher values than the carnivorous salmonids [127]. Thus, the fish that naturally have more carbohydrate in the diet seem to have a more efficient apparatus for carbohydrate metabolism. There are indications that the insulin receptor concentration in liver and muscle is higher in large Atlantic salmon than in small, and that large fish also have higher plasma insulin levels. (Eliassen, Sundby, Plisetskaya, Gutierrez, unpublished). Long-term feeding of Atlantic salmon with a 30 % carbohydrate diet did not induce any changes in insulin receptor levels (Krogdahl, Sundby, Gutierrez, Eliassen, unpublished).

Recently, four cDNAs encoding the salmon insulin receptor in the branchial cartilage were cloned and sequenced. The cartilage insulin receptor mRNA yield was 56% of that obtained from the liver. This indicates that the branchial cartilage must also be a major insulin target, and thus also strengthens the possible effect of growth through increasing (^{35}S) sulphate incorporation in this tissue [128].

Destruction of pancreatic B-cells in juvenile coho salmon by streptozotocin was followed by a reduced plasma insulin concentration and reduced IGF-I mRNA expression, indicating an effect of insulin on IGF-I production [129].

3.2. IGF-I

In fish, as in mammals, the liver remains the major site of IGF-I production and the major supplier of systemic IGF-I [130]. Recently IGF-I mRNA expression and IGF-I immunoreactivity were demonstrated in the teleost pancreas. However, whether IGF-I from the pancreas is produced only for autocrine or paracrine use or also for systemic supply is still under debate [128]. The co-existence of IGF-I and the classic islet hormones insulin, glucagon, somatostatin and pancreatic polypeptide was studied using immunoreactivity. In one fish species, IGF-I was found only in insulin-immunoreactive cells, in another only in somatostatin-reactive cells, and in a third, in glucagon-, somatostatin- and PP-immunoreactive cells. Thus IGF-I had a varying localisation. In mammals, as in two of the fish species, insulin and IGF-I displayed a distinct cellular distribution, while in the third fish species, insulin and IGF-I were coexistent [131,132].

3.3. Glucagon and glucagon-like peptide

3.3.1. Proglucagon gene and peptides

A hyperglycaemic factor was discovered in tuna and anglerfish in 1952 [133], whereas isolation of proglucagon was first reported in 1973 from a study of Brockmann bodies in anglerfish [134]. The primary structure was determined from the cDNA sequence in 1983 [135]. Fish possess one or two closely-related proglucagon genes [134].

All islet A-cells in rainbow trout and coho salmon were found to be immunoreactive toward both anti-salmon glucagon and anti-salmon GLP [80]. Further studies also suggest that in fish, as in mammals, all glucagon family peptides are derived from a common proglucagon precursor [136].

The mammalian proglucagon gene contains 6 exons separated by 5 introns, coding for glicentin-related polypeptide, glicentin, glucagon (amino acid residue 33-66 in the prohormone), oxyntomodulin (amino acid residue 33-70) and two glucagon-like peptides (amino acid residues 72-108 and 126-159). Glucagon and oxyntomodulin are coded for by exon 3, GLP-1 and GLP-2 by exons 4 and 5, respectively.

In fish, the translational products of the pancreatic proglucagon gene are glucagon (amino acid 52-80), oxyntomodulin (amino acid 52-88), [87] and GLP-1 (amino acid 89-122). The pancreatic proglucagon cDNA in fish contains a stop codon immediately following GLP-1, while this is not the case for proglucagon in the intestine, where GLP-2 is produced as well. So far, there have been no reports of any production of a glicentin-like peptide in either the pancreas or gut in fish. In the rat, glucagon is processed by the liver into a mini-glucagon (Glucagon 19-29) with its own biological activity. As 15 out of 20 species of fish possess two basic residues in position 17 and 18, similar to the cleavage position in the rat, it is possible that similar processing take place in some fish species [136].

The glucagon sequence in various species of fish shows strong conservation, with 12 of the 29 amino acids being common to all fish. The similarity of salmon glucagon and mammalian glucagon is considered adequate for determining glucagon levels in salmonid plasma using a mammalian glucagon radioimmunoassay [137].

Glucagon release is stimulated by basic amino acids, adrenaline and KCl, and reduced by glucose.

The first native piscine GLP was isolated from the channel catfish (*Ictalurus punctatus*) endocrine pancreas by Andrews and Ronner [138]. The sequence corresponded to mammalian GLP, except that 6 amino acid residues were missing from the N-terminus. Between mammalian species, the primary structure of GLP is strongly conserved. In fish, however, the amino acid sequence is poorly conserved, with only 3 of the 31 residues in common [139].

Arginine is an important secretagogue for GLP-1 in the coho salmon 136].

3.3.2. Physiological action of glucagon

In mammals, glucagon is a major insulin secretagogue, while in fish glucagon administration does not have any effect on insulin secretion, as demonstrated in the European eel (*Anguilla anguilla* L.) and in the coho salmon [94,95]. However, in fish as in mammals, the major physiological effect of glucagon is its insulin-opposing effect, leading to an increased plasma glucose level through stimulation of glycogenolysis and gluconeogenesis. In addition, lipolysis is stimulated by fish glucagon, both in the liver and the adipose tissue [120]. A number of regulatory enzymes have been shown to be affected by fish glucagon, often through reversible phosphorylation. Studies in fish have shown that glucagon activates adenylyl cyclase [140] which will activate kinases necessary for phosphorylation. Glycogen phosphorylase is activated by fish glucagon through an increase in the total enzyme content as well as the proportion of the active phosphorylated form [141,142]. Glucagon has also been found to activate lipase by increased phosphorylation, giving increased lipolysis in isolated trout hepatocytes [120].

The rate of gluconeogenesis from lactate and amino acids is increased by fish glucagon. A glucagon-dependent increase in enzymes in this pathway has been documented for aspartate aminotransferase [143], alanine aminotransferase [144] and malic enzyme [145] in various species. Fish glucagon has an indirect effect on the gluconeogenetic pathway via glucagon-induced inhibition of enzymes in the «reversed pathways» such as glycolysis and glucose oxidation. This includes the regulatory enzymes pyruvate kinase [145], phosphofruktokinase [146] and glucose 6-phosphate dehydrogenase [147]. Fish glucagon also inhibits glycogen synthase [148] and hydroxyacyl-CoA dehydrogenase in the fatty acid oxidation pathway [145]. In addition, glucagon activates hepatic amino acid uptake and ammonia excretion in teleosts [143].

Mini-glucagon (Glucagon 19-29) showed no metabolic activity when tested in anglerfish [149]. This mini-glucagon is reported to exert its metabolic activity in the rat by inhibiting the liver Ca^{2+}-pump [150]. It is speculated that the lack of activity of mini-glucagon in fish might be due to a lack of calcium-dependent mechanisms in non-mammalian vertebrates.

Glucagon action in fish involves binding to cell membrane receptors. The properties of glucagon binding to hepatocytes in several teleosts is reported to be similar to that in mammals [151]. The further processes mainly involve activation of adenylyl cyclase and protein kinase A. However, alternative pathways cannot be excluded.

3.3.3. Physiological action of glucagon-like peptide

The physiological effects of GLPs in fish are very different from the effects of the same peptides in mammals. GLP has a predominantly endocrine role in mammals, being insulinotropic, while GLP in fish has a predominantly metabolic role, activating hepatic glycogenolysis, gluconeogenesis and lipolysis. In mammals, GLP-1 responds to glucose, activating insulin synthesis and secretion through cAMP-coupled receptors on the islet B-cells, and simultaneously suppressing glucagon secretion. Thus GLP-1 in mammals opposes glucagon action and because of its insulinotropic effect it appears to be an anabolic hormone [152]. In contrast, the metabolic actions of GLP in fish are mostly identical to or similar to those of glucagon. In fact, when comparing their relative efficiency, GLP-1 is more efficient than glucagon in activating glycogenolysis in fish [128]. In additional, in salmonids the GLP-1 concentration in plasma and in the Brockmann bodies is always higher than that of glucagon. In contrast, in the Atlantic cod, the measured plasma concentration of GLP is always lower than that of glucagon [108,109]. The reason for these discrepancies between species is unknown.

In mammals, GLP-1 neither binds to liver receptors nor is it degraded in the liver, while in salmonids the liver is the main target and also the primary degradation site for GLP. However, fish GLP-1$_{(1-31)}$ and truncated mammalian GLP-1$_{(7-36)}$ and GLP-1$_{(7-37)}$ are interchangeable, since salmon GLP-1 is insulinotropic in mammals and mammalian GLP-1 has glycogenolytic action in fish hepatocytes [153]. The fish GLP-1 is produced in the pancreas while the mammalian GLP-1 and GLP-2 are both produced in the gut. In fish, GLP-2 is produced in the intestine. In contrast to GLP-1, neither mammalian GLP-2 nor fish GLP-2 affects glycogenesis or glycogenolysis in isolated hepatocytes [154].

The binding sites for GLP-1 on hepatocytes isolated from the American eel (*Anguilla rostrata*) and brown bullhead (*Myxocephalus scorpius*) are different from those for glucagon [151].

Although GLP is metabolically more potent than glucagon in equimolar concentrations, cAMP production is stimulated much less by GLP [154]. Therefore, the intracellular message transduction for GLP does not seem to involve cAMP to any large degree, but may involve inositol trisphosphate (IP3), Ca^{2+} and other messengers [136].

3.3.4. Effect of feeding and fasting on glucagon /GLP levels

In spite of the insulin-opposing effects of fish glucagon and GLP on fish metabolism, most experiments show a parallel rather than an opposing variation in these hormones, in relation to feeding and fasting. In humans, plasma glucagon levels increase 48 hours after food deprivation, while in most studies in fish, both plasma glucagon and GLP levels, like the plasma insulin levels, are reduced in fasting and increased after feeding [106,109,155,156]. However, in several of these studies, the ratio of glucagon-family peptides to insulin tends to increase following food deprivation. Thus, the regulation of metabolism might be more affected by changes in the ratio between glucagon-family peptides and insulin than by the individual concentrations of these hormones. The decrease in plasma insulin, glucagon and GLP concentration during a fasting period may reflect a general regulatory mechanism used by fish to meet food deprivation, of slowing down the rate of metabolism. Thyroxin levels are also reduced in fasted rainbow trout [157].

3.4. Somatostatin (SST)

3.4.1. Gene structure and expression

The mammalian pancreas produces somatostatin consisting of 14 amino acids (SST-14). Somatostatin-14 from anglerfish islets has the same amino acid sequence as that found in mammals. In teleosts such as anglerfish (*Lopius Americanus*), catfish (*Ictalurus punctatus*), sea bream, European eel, salmon and trout, a larger N-terminally extended somatostatin, with 22-28 amino acids (SST- 22-28) is produced in addition to the SST-14.

Fish seem to have two somatostatin genes, gene I and gene II, which are located on different parts of the genome and which are expressed in different pancreatic cells. In the anglerfish, gene I and gene II mRNA have been cloned and sequenced, coding for a 121 and a 125 amino acid preprosomatostatin with about 45% amino acid sequence identity. The preprosomatostatin from the different cell types is exposed to different sets of processing enzymes. Somatostatin-14 will be produced from preprosomatostatin-I in cells adjacent to insulin producing cells, while SST-22-28 is produced from preprosomatostatin II in cells adjacent to glucagon/GLP producing cells [80,158]. Somatostatin-25 is quantitatively the major SST in the coho salmon pancreas [86].

3.4.2. Factors affecting the secretion and physiological action of somatostatin

Glucose is an important secretagogue for both SST-25 and SST-14 in fish. Elevated SST-25 levels were measured in Chinook salmon 30 minutes after glucose injection [159]. A dose-dependent stimulation of SST-14 by glucose has been reported in perfused anglerfish islet cells [160], and glucose evokes a biphasic release of SST-14 in Brockmann bodies from perfused European eel and catfish [161,162]. In the latter study it was shown that arginine had only a minor effect on SST-14 release. Both lipid and fatty acid infusion were found to stimulate SST-25 secretion in rainbow trout [163]. In this study rainbow trout was exposed to 2-min infusion of a triacylglycerol-rich lipid emulsion, and the effect of palmitic and oleic acid was studied in isolated Brockmann bodies. Three hrs after the lipid infusion a 2 – 5-fold increase was measured in plasma fatty acid levels and a 2-fold increase in plasma concentration of SST-25. Both palmitic and oleic acid were found to evoke an increased SST-25 secretion. A similar increase in fatty acids in rainbow trout was observed after fasting and after lipid infusion [164]. When studying the binding of SST-14 to the liver membrane in fed and fasted rainbow trout, two classes of binding sites, high-affinity and low-affinity sites, were found. The fasted fish, when compared with fed fish, had an increased number of high-affinity binding sites and elevated plasma SST-14 levels [165]. Studies of SST-25 and SST-14 release from Brockmann bodies in rainbow trout following insulin, glucagon and SST-14 administration showed effects to be dependent on the glucose level. At a high glucose level (10 mM), insulin would inhibit while glucagon would stimulate both SST-25 and SST-14 secretion. At normal and low glucose levels, insulin was found to stimulate SST-25 secretion, while insulin would stimulate SST-14 only at a low glucose level. SST-14 administration was also found to stimulate SST-25 secretion [166].

Recent work from the laboratory of M. Sheridan [167,168] suggests that SSTs in salmonids influence metabolism indirectly by reducing the pancreatic insulin and glucagon secretion, and directly by enhancing glycogenolysis and lipolysis in vitro.

In the coho salmon, it has been shown that SST-25 injection is followed by decreased plasma insulin, glucagon and GLP levels and a decreased liver glycogen content. In addition, SST-25 injection was followed by an elevated plasma glucose level. Injection of SST-25 anti-serum had the opposite effects, with increased plasma insulin levels and increased liver glycogen content [169].

Eilertson and Sheridan [168] report that SST-14 and SST-25 directly stimulate the mobilisation of triacylglycerol from the liver and adipose tissue by stimulating lipase activity, and fatty acid and glycerol release. The authors therefore suggest that SST-14 and SST-25 are important modulators of lipid metabolism in fish.

Following an intraperitoneal glucose injection into rainbow trout, elevated levels of plasma glucose and fatty acid were observed after 60 min [170]. In perfused catfish Brockmann bodies it was found that glucose evoked more response in SST-producing cells than in insulin-producing cells [171]. It is therefore possible that the glucose-induced somatostatin production and secretion suppresses insulin secretion. Hence, somatostatin might indirectly be responsible for delayed hyperglycaemia and directly responsible for the elevated fatty acid levels.

Somatostatin (SST) was originally named somatotropin-release inhibiting factor, SRIF, for its ability to inhibit the release of growth hormone from cultured rat pituitary cells [172]. The name changed as the hormone was found to affect many aspects of pituitary, pancreatic and gastrointestinal functions. Like the mammalian SST-14, fish SST-14 was found to inhibit growth hormone release. In contrast, neither catfish SST-22 nor coho salmon SST-25 showed any effect on growth hormone release from goldfish (*Carassius auratus*) pituitary fragments [173,174]. Somatostatin-14 and SST-25 also have differential effects on carbohydrate and lipid metabolism in rainbow trout [175]. Both hormones were found to increase plasma glucose, fatty acid levels and hepatic lipase activity. Both hormones also reduced plasma glucagon and GLP levels, SST-14 more so than SST-25. However, while SST-25 injection was followed by reduced plasma insulin levels and a reduced liver glycogen content, SST-14 injection affected neither plasma insulin nor liver glycogen levels. It caused a reduction in glucose-6-phosphate dehydrogenase activity, however, and thus decreased glucose metabolism through the pentose phosphate shunt.

The list of inhibitory effects of somatostatin in mammals that are unknown in fish is still long and includes effects on gastric and pancreatic enzymes, gastrointestinal motility, nutrient absorption and blood flow.

3.5. Pancreatic Polypeptide

The pancreatic polypeptides isolated from several fish species are more similar to mammalian neuropeptide Y (NPY) than to mammalian pancreatic polypeptide (PP). These peptides belong to the PP family, with 36 amino acids and similar structures. NPY in mammals is localised in the nervous system and its primary structure begins and ends with tyrosine (Y), while PP is expressed in the mammalian pancreas [176]. The sea bass pancreas was found to process PP and peptide Y (PYY) in islet cells that also produced glucagon [82]. Polypeptide YY also belongs to the PP family, having a similar structure and 36 amino acids. In mammals, PYY is found in the intestine. The first and last amino acid residue is tyrosine (Y). In the coho salmon, PP immunoreactive cells are localised to the periphery of the Brockmann bodies, close to the A cells [79].

Injection of pancreatic NPY-like peptide into dogfish (*Scyliorhinus canicula*) was followed by increased blood pressure [177]. When testing fish PP in mammalian systems, the peptide was found to have NPY-like effects, stimulating appetite, increasing blood pressure and decreasing heart rate [178].

In studies on fasted and fed Chinook and coho salmon, the preoptic area of the hypothalamus showed significantly higher NPY- like gene expression in the fasted than in the fed salmonids [179]. Since the fish PP has NPY-like effects, it might be asked whether fasting also will stimulate pancreatic PP expression in salmonids.

REFERENCES

1. C.E Stevens, Comparative physiology of vertebrate digestive system, Cambridge University Press, Cambridge, 1988.
2. A. Jönsson, in S. Nilsson and S. Holmgren (eds.), Comparative physiology and evolution of autonomic nervous system, Harwood Academic Publisher, Langhorn, 1994.
3. T. Kurokawa and T. Suzuki, J. Fish Biol., 46 (1995) 292.
4. S. Einarsson and P.S. Davies, J. Fish Biol., 50 (1997) 1120.
5. B.G. Kapoor, H. Smith and I.A. Verighina, Adv. Marine Biol., 13 (1975) 109.
6. J. Overnell, Comp. Biochem. Physiol., 46B (1973) 519.
7. T. Cohen, A. Gertler and Y. Birk, Comp. Biochem. Physiol., 69B (1981) 639.
8. D.R. Gjellesvik, A.J. Raae and B.T. Walther, Aquaculture, 79 (1989) 177.
9. I. Chakrabarti, M.A. Gani, K.K. Chaki, R. Sur and K.K. Misra, Comp. Biochem. Physiol., 112A (1995) 167.

10. N. Iijima, S. Chosa, K. Uematsu, T. Goto, T. Hoshita and M. Kayama, Fish Physiol. Biochem., 16 (1997) 487.
11. A. Gildberg and K. Overbo, Comp. Biochem. Physiol., 97B (1990) 775.
12. M.M. Kristjansson and H.H. Nielsen, Comp. Biochem. Physiol., 101B (1992) 247.
13. G.I. Berglund, A.O. Smalås, L.K. Hansen, A. Hordvik and N.P. Willassen, Acta Cryst., 51 (1995) 393.
14. G.I. Berglund, A.O. Smalås, A. Hordvik and N.P. Willassen, Acta Cryst., 51 (1995) 925.
15. H. Outzen, G.I. Berglund, A.O. Smalås and N.P. Willassen, Comp. Biochem. Physiol., 115B (1996) 33.
16. G.I. Berglund, A.O. Smalås, H. Outzen and N.P. Willassen, Mol. Marine Biol. Biotechnol., 7 (1998) 105.
17. F.J. Alarcon, J. Diaz, F.J. Moyano and E. Abellan, Fish Phys. Biochem., 19 (1998) 257.
18. W.P. Fong, E.Y.M. Chan and K.K. Lao, Biochem. Molec. Biol. Int., 45 (1998) 410.
19. R. Male, J.B. Lorens, A.O. Smalås and K.R. Torrissen, Eur. J. Biochem., 232 (1995) 677.
20. B. Asgeirsson and J.B. Bjarnason, Comp. Biochem. Physiol., 99B (1991) 327.
21. R. Munilla-Moran and J.R. Stark, Comp. Biochem. Physiol., 95B (1990) 625.
22. U. Sabapathy and L.H. Teo, J. Fish Biol., 42 (1993) 595.
23. K.R. Torrissen, Comp. Biochem. Physiol., 77B (1984) 669.
24. B. Asgeirsson, J.W. Fox and G.H. Thorgaard, Eur. J. Biochem., 180 (1989) 85.
25. A. Smine and Y.L. Gal, Mol. Marine Biol. Biotechnol., 4 (1995) 295.
26. K.R. Torrissen, G.M. Pringle, R. Moss and D.F. Houlihan, Fish Physiol. Biochem., 19 (1998) 247.
27. K. Hjelmeland and J. Raa, Comp. Biochem. Physiol., 71B (1982) 557.
28. A. Martinez, R.L. Olsen and J.L. Serra, Comp. Biochem. Physiol., 82B (1985) 607.
29. T. Cohen, A. Gertler and Y. Birk, Comp. Biochem. Physiol., 69B (1981) 647.
30. R. Yoshinaka, M. Sato, H. Tanaka and S. Ikeda, Comp. Bioch. Physiol., 80B (1985) 223.
31. R. Yoshinaka, M. Sato, H. Tanaka and M. Ikeda, Comp. Biochem. Physiol., 80B (1985) 227.
32. M. Bassompierre, H.H. Nielsen and T. Borresen, Comp. Biochem. Physiol., 106B (1993) 331.
33. B. Asgeirsson and J.B. Bjarnason, Biochim. Biophys. Acta, 1164 (1993) 91.
34. R. Yoshinaka, M. Sato, K. Tsuchiya and M. Ikeda, Comp. Biochem. Physiol. 83B (1986) 45.
35. Å. Krogdahl and H. Holm, Comp. Biochem. Physiol., 74B (1983) 403.
36. L.D. Taran and I.N. Smovdyr, Biokhimiya, 57 (1992) 55.
37. G.N. Somero, J. Exp. Zool., 194 (1975) 175.
38. D.R. Tocher and J.R. Sargent, Comp. Biochem. Physiol., 77B (1984) 561.
39. B.A. Rasco and H.O. Hultin, Comp. Biochem. Physiol., 89B (1988) 671.
40. D.R. Gjellesvik, J.B. Lorens and R. Male, Eur. J. Biochem., 226 (1994) 603.
41. D.R. Gjellesvik, A. Lombardo and B.T. Walther, Biochim. Biophys. Acta, 1124 (1992) 123.
42. Ø. Lie and G. Lambertsen, Comp. Biochem. Physiol., 80B (1985) 447.
43. H. Ono and N. Iijima, Fish Physiol. Biochem., 18 (1998) 135.
44. R. Hofer and C. Sturmbauer, Aquaculture, 48 (1985) 277.
45. H. Plantikow, Zool. J. Physiol., 89 (1985) 417.

46. S.V. Phadate and L.N. Srikar, Proc. Ind. Acad. Sci. Amin. Sci., 99 (1990) 387.
47. V.I. Ponomarev, Voprosy Ikhtiologii, 31 (1991) 292.
48. D.G. Yardley and S.E. Wild, Fish. Physiol. Biochem., 9 (1991) 31.
49. A.M. Ugolev and V.V. Kuzmina, Comp. Biochem. Physiol., 107A (1994) 187.
50. V.V. Kuzmina, I.L. Golovanova and G.I. Izvekova, Comp. Biochem. Physiol., 113B (1996) 255.
51. Å. Krogdahl, S. Nordrum, M. Sorensen and L. Brudeseth, Aquaculture Nutr., 5 (1999), In press.
52. M. Langer, S. van Noorden, J.M. Polak and A.G.E. Pearse, Cell Tiss. Res., 199 (1979) 493.
53. J. Noaillac-Depeyre and E. Hollande, Cell Tiss. Res., 216 (1981) 193.
54. J.H.W.M. Rombout and J.J. Taverne-Thile, Cell Tiss. Res., 227 (1982) 57.
55. S. Holmgren, C. Vaillant and R. Dimaline, Cell Tiss. Res., 223 (1982) 141.
56. S.R. Vigna, B.L. Fisher, J.L.M. Morgan and G.L. Rosenquist, Comp. Biochem. Physiol., 82C (1985) 143.
57. J. Jensen and Holmgren S., in S. Nilsson and S. Holmgren (eds.), Comparative physiology and evolution of autonomic nervous system, Harwood Academic Publisher, Langhorn, 1994.
58. S. Einarsson, P.S. Davies and C. Talbot, Comp. Biochem. Physiol., 117C (1997) 63.
59. R.E. Honkanen, J.W. Crim and J.S. Patton, Comp. Biochem. Physiol., 89A (1988) 655.
60. H. Plantikow, Fischerei. Forschung. Rostock, 29 (1991) 34.
61. C.L. Cahu and J.L. Zambonino Infante, Fish Biochem. Physiol., 14 (1995) 209.
62. C.L. Cahu and J.L. Zambonino Infante, Fish Physiol. Biochem., 14 (1995) 431.
63. J.J. Olli, K. Hjelmeland and Å. Krogdahl, Comp. Biochem. Physiol., 109A (1994) 23.
64. K. Dąbrowski, P. Poczyczyński, G. Köck and B. Berger, Aquaculture, 77 (1989) 29.
65. Å. Krogdahl, T. Berg Lea and J.J. Olli, Comp. Biochem. Physiol., 107A (1994) 215.
66. H. Plantikow, Wiss. Z. Wilhelm-Pieck-Universität Rostock, 31 (1982) 45.
67. C.B. Cowey and Walton M.J., in J.E. Halver (ed.), Fish Nutrition, Academic Press, San Diego, 1989.
68. L. Spannhof and H. Plantikow, Aquaculture, 10 (1983) 95.
69. S. Einarsson, P.S. Davies and C. Talbot, Fish Physiol. Biochem., 15 (1996) 439.
70. H. Segner, V. Storch, M. Reinecke and W. Kloas, Marine Biol., 119 (1994) 471.
71. J.P. Diaz, R. Connnes, P. Divanach and G. Barnabe, Annls. Sci. Nat. (Ser Zool.), 10 (1989) 87.
72. A. Péres, Fish Biochem. Physiol., 15 (1996) 237.
73. M. Lauff and R. Hofer, Aquaculture, 37 (1984) 335.
74. S.I. Kawai and S. Ikeda, Bull. Jap. Soc. Sci. Fisheries, 39 (1973) 877.
75. S.I. Kawai and S. Ikeda, Bull. Jap. Soc. Sci. Fisheries, 39 (1973) 819.
76. S. Ozkizilcik, F.L.E. Chu and R.P. Allen, Comp. Biochem. Physiol., 113B (1996) 631.
77. R.K. Buddington, J. Fish Biol., 26 (1985) 715.
78. C.L. Cahu and J.L. Zambonino Infante, Comp. Biochem. Physiol., 109A (1994) 213.
79. W. Yi-Qiang, E.M. Plisetskaya, D.G. Baskin and A. Gorbman, Zool. Sci., 3 (1986) 123.
80. M. Nozaki, K. Miyata,Y. Oota, A. Gorbman and E.M. Plisetskaya, Cell Tissue Res., 253 (1988) 371.

81. M.E. Abad, A. Garcia Ayala, M.T. Lozano and B. Agulleiro, Gen. Comp. Endocrinol., 86 (1992) 445.
82. M.T. Lozano A. Garcia Ayala, M.E. Abad and B. Agulleiro, Gen. Comp. Endocrinol., 81 (1991) 198.
83. E.M. Plisetskaya, H.G. Pollock, J.R. Kimmel and A. Gorbman, Amer. Zool., 25 (1985) 82A.
84. E.M. Plisetskaya, H.G. Pollock, J.B. Rouse, J.W. Hamilton, J.R. Kimmel and A. Gorbman, Peptides, 11 (1985) 105.
85. E.M. Plisetskaya, H.G. Pollock, J.B. Rouse, J.W. Hamilton, J.R. Kimmel and A. Gorbman, Reg. Pept., 14 (1986) 57.
86. E.M. Plisetskaya, H.G. Pollock, J.B. Rouse, J.W. Hamilton, J.R. Kimmel and A. Gorbman, Gen. Comp. Endocrinol., 63 (1986) 252.
87. S.J. Duguay and T.P. Mommsen, in: Fish Physiology, Molecular Biology of Fishes. C. Hew and N. Sherwood (eds), Acad. Press, New York, 1994.
88. V. Kavsan, A. Koval, O. Petrenko, C.T.Jr. Roberts and D. Leiroith, Biochem. Biophys. Res. Commun., 191 (1993) 1373.
89. P. Hobart, L. Shen, R. Crawford, R. Pictet and W.J. Rutter, Science, 210 (1980) 1360.
90. S.J. Chan, S.O. Edmin, S.C.M. Kwok, J. M. Kramer, S. Falkmer and D.F. Steiner, J. Biol. Chem., 256 (1981) 7595.
91. A.V. Sorokin, O.I. Petrenko, V. Kavsan, Y.I. Kozlov, V.B. Dababov and M.L. Zlochevskij, Gene, 20 (1982) 367.
92. N. Itoh, in Molecular Biology of the Islets of Lagerhans, H. Okamoto (eds.) Cambridge Univ. Press, New York, 1990.
93. L.F. Smith, Diabetes, 21 (1972) 457.
94. B.W. Ince and A. Thorpe, Gen. Comp. Endocrinol., 33 (1977) 453.
95. E.M. Plisetskaya, C. Ottolenghi, M. Sheridan, T. P. Mommsen and A. Gorbman, Gen. Comp. Endocrinol., 73 (1989) 205.
96. E.M. Plisetskaya, L.I. Buchelli-Narvaez, R.W. Hardy and W.W. Dickhoff, Gen. Comp. Endocrinol., 98A (1991) 165
97. E.M. Plisetskaya, J. Exp. Zool., 4 (1990) 53.
98. C. Pereira, A. Olsen, A. Sundby and K. Nilssen, in C. Pereira, Dr. Theses, NTNU, Trondheim, Norway, 1997.
99. W.W. Dickhoff, L. Yan, E.M. Plisetskaya, C.V. Sullivan, P. Swanson, A. Hara and M.G. Bernard, Fish. Physiol. Biochem., 7 (1989) 147.
100. E.M. Plisetskaya, E.M. Donaldson and H.M. Dye, J. Fish Biol., 30 (1987) 21.
101. E.M. Plisetskaya, P. Swanson, M.G. Bernard and W.W. Dickhoff, Aquaculture, 72 (1988) 51.
102. E. Virtanen, L. Forsman and A. Sundby, Comp. Physiol. Biochem., 9 (1990) 223.
103. A. Sundby, Eliassen, A.K. Blom and T. Åsgård, Fish Physiol. Biochem., 9 (1991) 253.
104. I. Navarro, M.N. Carneiro, M. Parrizas, J.L. Maestro, J. Planas and J. Gutierrez, Comp. Biochem. Physiol., 104A (1993) 389.
105. A. Sundby and T. Refstie, Proc. 15th Conf. Eur. Comp. Endocrinol., (1990) 145.
106. A. Sundby, K. Eliassen, T. Refstie and E.M. Plisetskaya, Fish Physiol. Biochem., 9 (1991) 23.
107. J. Perez, S. Zanuy and M. Carrillo, Fish Physiol. Biochem., 5 (1988) 191.

456

108. G-I. Hemre, Ø. Lie, G. Lambertsen and A. Sundby, Comp. Biochem. Physiol., 97A (1990) 41.
109. G-I. Hemre, Ø. Lie and A. Sundby, Fish. Physiol. Biochem., 10 (1993) 455.
110. J.T. Silverstein, J. Breininger, D.G. Baskin, and E.M. Plisetskaya, Gen. Comp. Endocrinol., 110 (1998) 157.
111. E.M. Plisetskaya, S. Brattacharya, W.W. Dickhoff and A. Gorbman, Comp. Biochem. Physiol., 78A (1984) 773.
112. R.F. Ablett, R.O. Sinnhuber, R.M. Holmes and D.P. Selvonchick, Gen. Comp. Endocrinol., 43 (1981) 211.
113. E.C. Urbinati, M.D. Willis and E.M. Plisetskaya, Amer. Zool., 34 (1994) 42A.
114. C. Duan and T. Hirano, J. Endocrinol., 133 (1992) 211.
115. C. Duan, T. Noso, S Moriyama, H. Kawauchi and T. Hirano, J. Endocrinol., 133 (1992) 221.
116. M.E. Roder, J. Eriksson, S.G. Hartling, L. Groop and C. Binder, Acta Diabetol., 30 (1993) 32.
117. G.L. King and C.R. Kahn, Nature, 292 (1981) 644.
118. E.M. Plisetskaya, Comp. Biochem. Physiol., 121 (1998) 3.
119. E.M. Plisetskaya, M.A. Sheridan and T.P. Mommsen, J. Exp. Zool., 249 (1989) 158.
120. J.S. Harmon, L.M. Rieniets and M.A. Sheridan, Amer. J. Physiol., 256 (1993) 255.
121. H. Segner, J.B. Blair, G. Wirtz, MR. Miller, In Vitro Cellular and Developmental Biology-Animal, 30A (1994) 306.
122. A.W. Warmann and N.R. Bottino (1978), Comp. Biochem. Physiol., 59B (1978) 153.
123. T.D. Petersen, P.W. Hochachka and R.K. Suarez, J. Exp. Zool., 243 (1987) 173.
124. T.P. Mommsen and E.M. Plisetskaya, Rev. Aquat. Sci., 4 (1991) 225.
125. E.M. Plisetskaya, H.G. Pollock and J.R. Kimmel, Can. J. Physiol. Pharmacol. 6th. Int. Symp. on Gastrointestinal Hormones., (1986) 29.
126. A. Sundby, in Recent Advances in Aquaculture. J.F. Muir and R.J. Roberts (eds.), Blackwell Scientific Publications, 1993.
127. M. Parrizas, M. Planas, E.M. Plisetskaya and J. Gutierrez, Amer. J. Physiol., 266 (1994) 1944.
128. S.J. Chan, E.M. Plisetskaya, E.C. Urbinati,Y. Jin and D.F. Steiner, Proc. Natl. Acad. Sci. USA, 94 (1997) 12446.
129. E.M. Plisetskaya and C.M. Duan, Amer. J. Physiol., 36 (1994) R1408.
130. C.M. Duan, S.J. Duguay, P. Swanson, W.W. Dickhoff and E.M. Plisetskaya, in: Peptides in Comparative Endocrinology. K. G. Dakvey, R. E. Peter and S.S. Tobe (eds), Natl. Res. Council, Ottawa, Canada, 1994.
131. M. Reinecke, C. Maake, S Falmer and V.R. Sara, Reg. Pept., 48 (1993) 65.
132. M. Reinecke, A. Schmid, R. Ermatinger and D. Loffing-Cueni, Endocrinol., 138 (1997) 3613.
133. A.C. Trakatellis, K. Tada and K. Yamaji, Int. Congress. Biochem. 9. Stockholm, (1973) 452.
134. P. Miahle, Hebd. Seances Acad. Sci., 235 (1952) 94.
135. P.K. Lund, R.H. Goodman, M.R. Montminy, P.C. Dee and J. F. Habener, J. Biol. Chem., 258 (1983) 3280.
136. E.M. Plisetskaya and T.P. Mommsen, Int. Rev. Cyt., 168 (1996) 187.

137. J. Gutierrez, J. Fernandez, J. Blasco, J.M. Gesse and J. Planas, Gen. Comp. Endocrinol., 63 (1986) 328.
138. P.C. Andrews and P. Ronner, J. Biol. Chem., 260 (1985) 3910.
139. J.M. Conlon, N. Hazon and L. Thim, Peptides, 15 (1994) 163.
140. C. Ottolenghi, E. Fabbri, A.C. Puviani, M.E. Gavioli and L. Brighenti, Mol. Cell. Endocrinol., 60 (1990) 163.
141. B.L. Umminger and D. Benziger, Gen. Comp. Endocrinol., 25 (1975) 96.
142. L. Brighenti. A.C. Puviani, M.E. Gavioli, E. Fabbri and C. Ottolenghi, Gen. Comp. Endocrinol, 82 (1991) 131.
143. D.K. Chan and N.Y.S. Wo, Gen. Comp. Endocrinol., 35 (1978) 216.
144. A.Gerhard, P. Gohlke and W. Hanke, Acta. Endocrinol., 117 (1988) 222.
145. T.P. Mommsen, E. Danulat and P.J. Walsh, Gen. Comp. Endocrinol., 85 (1992) 316.
146. T.D.O. Petersen, P.W. Hochachka and R.K. Suarez, J. Exp. Zool., 243 (1987) 173.
147. G.D. Foster , K.B. Storey and T.W. Moon, Gen. Comp. Endocrinol., 73 (1989) 382.
148. J.C. Murat and E.M. Plisetskaya, Seances Soc. Biol. Ses Fil., 171 (1977) 1302.
149. T.P Mommsen. and T.W. Moon, Fish Physiol. Biochem., 7 (1989) 279.
150. A. Mallat, C. Pavoine, M. Dufor, S. Lotersztajn, D. Bataille and F. Pecker, Nature, Lond., 325 (1987) 620.
151. I. Navarro and T. W. Moon, J. Endocrinol., 140 (1994) 217.
152. B. Ørskov, Diabetologia, 35 (1992) 701.
153. T.P. Mommsen and E.M. Plisetskaya, Fish Physiol. Biochem., 11 (1993) 429.
154. T.P. Mommsen, P.C. Adrews and E.M. Plisetskaya, FEBS Lett., 219 (1987) 227.
155. M.A. Sheridan and E.M. Plisetskaya, Amer. Zool., 28 (1988) 56.
156. T.W. Moon, G.D. Foster and E.M. Plisetskaya, Can. J. Zool., 67 (1989) 2189.
157. J.G. Eals, Amer. Zool., 28 (1988) 351.
158. K.A. Sevarino, P. Stork, R.Ventimiglia, G. Mandel and R.H. Goodman, Cell., 57 (1989) 11.
159. M.A. Sheridan, C.D. Eilertson and E.M. Plisetskaya, Gen. Comp. Endocrinol., 81 (1991) 365.
160. S.L. Migram, J.K. McDonald and B.D. Noe, Amer. J. Physiol., 261 (1991) 444.
161. P. Ronner and A. Scarpa, Amer. J. Physiol., 243 (1982) E352.
162. P. Ronner and A. Scarpa, Amer. J. Physiol., 246 (1984) E506.
163. N.M. Carneiro, C.D. Eilertson and M.A. Sheridan, Fish Physiol. Biochem., 15 (1996) 447.
164. M.A. Sheridan and T.P. Mommsen, Gen. Comp. Endocrinol., 81 (1991) 473.
165. M. J. Pesek and M.A. Sheridan, J. Endocrinol., 150 (1996) 179.
166. C.D. Eilertson, J. Kittilson and M. Sheridan, Gen. Comp. Endocrinol., 99 (1995) 211.
167. M.A. Sheridan, Comp. Biochem. Physiol., 107B (1994) 495.
168. C.D. Eilertson and M. Sheridan, J. Comp. Physiol. B-Biochem. Systemic and Environmental, 164 (1994) 256.
169. E.M. Plisetskaya and S.J. Duguay, in: The Endocrinology of Growth, Development, and Metabolism in Vertebrates. M.P. Schreibman, C.G. Scanes, and P.K.T. Pang (eds.), Academic Press, New York, 1993.
170. J.S. Harmon, C.D. Eilertson, M.A. Sheridan and E.M. Plisetskaya, Amer. J. Physiol., 261 (1991) 609.
171. P. Ronner and A. Scarpa, Gen. Comp. Endocrinol., 65 (1987) 354.

458

172. P. Brazeau, W. Vale, R. Burgus, N. Ling, M. Butcher, J. Rivier and R. Guillemin, Science, 29 (1973) 77.
173. T.A. Marchant, R.A. Fraser, P.C. Andrews and R.E. Peter, Reg. Pept., 17 (1987) 41.
174. T.A. Marchant and R.E. Peter, Fish Physiol. Biochem., 7 (1989) 133.
175. C.D. Eilertson, J. Kittilson and M. Sheridan, Gen. Comp. Endocrinol., 92 (1993) 62.
176. J.M. Conlon, C. Bjenning, T.W. Moon, J.H. and L.Thim, Peptides, 12 (1991) 221.
177. J.M. Conlon, A. Balsubramaniam and N. Hazon, Endocrinology, 128 (1991) 2273.
178. A. Balsubramaniam, D.F. Riegel, W.T. Chance, M. Stein, J. E. Fisher, D. King and E.M. Plisetskaya, Peptides, 11 (1990) 673.
179. J.T. Silverstein, J. Breininger, D.G. Baskin and E.M. Plisetskaya, Gen. Comp. Endocrinol., 110 (1998) 157.

PostScript

Dear Reader,

Animal performance has never been as important as now. Society expects animal breeding to be as ethical and humane as possible, while new and higher standards are constantly being set for product quality. Antibiotics are no longer accepted as a growth promoters in European husbandry, while nitrogen and phosphorus emission are now in focus.

With this in mind we need to put the animal on a pedestal. Without doubt we are at the beginning of a new era, where we should be able to find new ways of raising the quality of life for animals. For each of us who are experts in any area of animal production or welfare, it is an exciting situation!

Hopefully this book will be a help in setting up a new research frontiers, enabling us to continue with the development of high-quality animal production.

Hans G Jungvid
GRAMINEER INTERNATIONAL AB